The Organization of the Cerebral C

The Organization of the Cerebral Cortex

Proceedings of a Neurosciences Research
Program Colloquium

Editors
Francis O. Schmitt
Frederic G. Worden
George Adelman
Stephen G. Dennis

Contributing Editors
Floyd E. Bloom
W. Maxwell Cowan
Gerald M. Edelman
Ann M. Graybiel
Herbert H. Jasper
Brenda A. Milner
Pasko Rakic

The MIT Press
Cambridge, Massachusetts, and
London, England

MIT Press

026219189X

ADELMAN
ORG CEREBRAL CORTEX

Acknowledgment of Sponsorship and Support

The Neurosciences Research Program, a research center of the Massachusetts Institute of Technology, is an interdisciplinary, interuniversity organization with the primary goal of facilitating the investigation of how the nervous system mediates behavior including the mental processes of man. To this end, the NRP, as one of its activities, conducts scientific meetings to explore crucial problems in the neurosciences. The NRP is supported in part through Massachusetts Institute of Technology by National Institute of Mental Health Grant No-MH23132, National Institute of Neurological and Communicative Disorders and Stroke Grant NS15690, The National Science Foundation, and Max-Planck-Gesellschaft, and through the Neurosciences Research Foundation by The Arthur Vining Davis Foundations, The Camille and Henry Dreyfus Foundation, Inc., The Beverly and Harvey Karp Foundation, van Ameringen Foundation, Inc., The G. Unger Vetlesen Foundation, and Vollmer Foundation, Inc.

This book was set in VIP Palatino by Achorn Graphic Services, Inc.

Library of Congress Cataloging in Publication Data
Main entry under title:

The organization of the cerebral cortex.

Includes bibliographies and indexes.
1. Cerebral cortex—Congresses. I. Schmitt, Francis Otto, 1903-   II. Neurosciences Research Program. [DNLM: 1. Cerebral cortex—Physiology—Congresses. WL307 069 1979]
QP383.073   599.01'88   80-22427
ISBN 0-262-19189-X

Contents

Preface
ix

Keynote   W. Maxwell Cowan
xi

**Development, Plasticity, and
Evolution of Neocortex**

Introduction   Pasko Rakic
3

1. Developmental Events Leading   Pasko Rakic
to Laminar and Areal
Organization of the Neocortex
7

2. The Postnatal Development   Simon LeVay, Torsten N. Wiesel,
and Plasticity of   and David H. Hubel
Ocular-Dominance Columns in
the Monkey
29

3. Induced Ocular-Dominance   Martha Constantine-Paton
Zones in Tectal Cortex
47

4. Development and Plasticity of   Patricia S. Goldman-Rakic
Primate Frontal Association
Cortex
69

**Functional Microorganization in
the Cerebral Cortex**

Introduction   W. Maxwell Cowan
101

5. Intrinsic Organization of the Primate Visual Cortex, Area 17, As Seen in Golgi Preparations
105

J. S. Lund

6. The Electron-Microscopic Analysis of the Neuronal Organization of the Cerebral Cortex
125

M. Colonnier

7. Thalamocortical Synaptic Relations
153

Edward L. White

8. Laminar Specialization and Intracortical Connections in Cat Primary Visual Cortex
163

Charles D. Gilbert and Torsten N. Wiesel

Organization and Connections of the Neocortex

Introduction
195

Ann M. Graybiel

9. Anatomy of Cerebral Cortex: Columnar Input–Output Organization
199

E. G. Jones

10. Organization of Somatosensory Cortex in Primates
237

J. H. Kaas, R. J. Nelson, M. Sur, and M. M. Merzenich

11. Functional Studies of the Motor Cortex
263

Edward V. Evarts

12. On the Relation between Transthalamic and Transcortical Pathways in the Visual System
285

Ann M. Graybiel and David M. Berson

Chemical Signaling and Circuitry in Cerenral Cortex and its Interconnections

Introduction
323

Floyd E. Bloom

13. Anatomical Chemistry of the
Cerebral Cortex
325

P. C. Emson and S. P. Hunt

14. Neurotransmodulatory
Control of Cerebral Cortical
Neuron Acitivity
347

D. A. Taylor and T. W. Stone

15. Chemical Signaling and
Cortical Circuitry: Integrative
Aspects
359

Floyd E. Bloom

**The Role of Cerebral Cortex in
Higher Brain Function**

Introduction
373

Herbert H. Jasper

16. Problems of Relating Cellular
or Modular Specificity to
Cognitive Functions: Importance
of State-Dependent Reactions
375

Herbert H. Jasper

17. Why Are There So Many
Visual Areas?
395

A. Cowey

18. The Cerebral Cortex in Visual
Learning and Memory, and in
Interhemispheric Transfer in the
Cat
415

Giovanni Berlucchi and
James M. Sprague

19. Scalp-Recorded Cerebral
Event-Related Potentials in Man
as Point of Entry into the
Analysis of Cognitive Processing
441

John E. Desmedt

**Impact of Theoretical Constructs
and Modeling of Cortical
Function**

Introduction
477

Gerald M. Edelman

20. Distributed Memory in the
Central Nervous System: Possible
Test of Assumptions in Visual
Cortex
479

Leon N Cooper

21. An Information-Processing
Approach to Understanding the
Visual Cortex
505

Francis H. C. Crick,
David C. Marr,
and Tomaso Poggio

22. Group Selection as the Basis
for Higher Brain Function
535

Gerald M. Edelman

List of Authors
565

Participants, Proceedings of a
Neurosciences Research Program
for Cerebral Cortex Colloquium,
1979
567

Name Index
569

Subject Index
581

Preface

This volume and the week-long conference at the Marine Biological Laboratory, Woods Hole, Massachusetts, on which it is based grew out of the fourth in a series of Neurosciences Intensive Study Programs (ISP) planned and held under the auspices of the Neurosciences Research Program (NRP). The ten-day program in Boulder, Colorado, in the summer of 1977 dealt with circuitry at the structural, bioelectrical, and biochemical levels. Considerable emphasis was placed on the processing of information in local domains involving the structural and electrical properties of neuronal local circuits.

In his keynote lecture at the outset of the ISP, V. B. Mountcastle suggested that requisite for any fruitful theory of higher brain function is an understanding of the unique structure and function of the cerebral cortex, and that central to its functions are the ensemble actions of very large numbers of neurons organized in multiply replicated local neuronal circuits comprising functional units (columns, modules).

Not inappropriately, the ISP concluded on a challenging note with the presentation by G. M. Edelman of a novel theory for certain "higher brain functions" based on selection (rather than instruction) and on phasic reentry into neuronal ensembles located primarily in the cerebral cortex. The closely related papers of Edelman and Mountcastle were published shortly afterward in a single volume (Edelman and Mountcastle, 1978).

This work had great impact on the subsequent interests and activities of NRP. Almost immediately after the close of the 1977 ISP, there was organized an ongoing colloquy, appropriately dubbed the "Cortex Colloquium," that was participated in primarily by NRP Associates and Staff especially knowledgeable about, and interested in, the cerebral cortex.

Four tangible activities were nucleated by the Cortex Colloquium. First, a substantial portion of the program of each of the next three stated meetings of the NRP Associates was focused on one or another aspect of cortical morphology, development, or function. Second, a comprehensive inquiry was made of individuals whose publications dealt in one way or another with the cerebral cortex. This resulted in the receipt of letters and reprints from more than a hundred individuals worldwide. Third, a series of lectures at the NRP Center by eight authorities on aspects of cortical science was arranged; the lecturers were Drs. A. M. Graybiel, E. G. Jones, W. J. H. Nauta, S. L. Palay, D. N.

Pandya, A. Peters, T. P. S. Powell, and P. Rakic. Fourth, the foregoing activities led to the conclusion that the time might be ripe to call the attention of the neuroscience community to the recent research advances that might set the stage for establishing new concepts about the role of the cerebral cortex in "higher functions" of the brain. To this end a planning session was held on January 25, 1979; included among the conferees were Drs. W. M. Cowan, G. M. Edelman, A. M. Graybiel, H. H. Jasper, P. Rakic, and the NRP Center Staff. It was decided that the conference and its published proceedings should not aim to deal exhaustively with particular cortical issues. Rather, it should convey the highlights of the topic, beginning with a series of presentations on the ontogenetic and morphogenetic development of the cerebral cortex and followed by a systematic review of the remarkable explosion during the last decade of our knowledge of the cellular organization and connectivity of the cortex. Also significant have been recent advances in the chemical organization of the cortex as well as new directions in the study of perception, learning, and memory; these were made the subject of conference sessions. The conference was concluded by a short series of theoretical contributions.

As it happened, the sequence of presentations had to be modified to accommodate changes in schedules of some of the participants; but for the publication it seemed appropriate to present the various papers not in the sequence in which they were given but in the more logical progression originally planned.

When this conference was being planned, the question was raised whether the time was opportune for such a meeting. During the 1977 ISP, and especially during the followup Cortex Colloquium, ample evidence emerged to support a consensus that indeed it would be timely for NRP to organize a meeting to examine the current status of research on cortex and the possibilities for developing new understanding and new directions for experimental programs. In retrospect, this was perhaps an overly ambitious undertaking; indeed areas of active scientific endeavor had of necessity to be either omitted or covered in only the most cursory manner. Yet the conference proved to be extremely valuable to the participants, and we present these proceedings to the neuroscience community at large with the hope that they will stimulate and call forth creative new approaches to the study of the neural substrates of behavior including "higher brain function."

Reference

Edelman, G. M., and V. B. Mountcastle, eds., 1978. *The Mindful Brain: Cortical Organization and the Group-Selective Theory of Higher Brain Function.* Cambridge, MA: MIT Press.

Boston, Massachusetts

Francis O. Schmitt
Frederic G. Worden and
Stephen G. Dennis

Keynote

W. Maxwell Cowan

The history of cortical studies spans a period of almost a century. For convenience we may think of it as comprising three principal epochs: (i) from about the middle of the nineteenth century to the end of World War I—this era includes the now classical clinical studies of Broca, Wernicke, and Charcot on the European continent and of Gowers, Horsley, Hughlings Jackson, Henry Head, and Gordon Holmes in Great Britain, as well as the earliest anatomical and physiological studies; (ii) from the 1920s until the late 1950s, during which so many of the great experimental neuroanatomical and neurophysiological studies were carried out; and (iii) from the physiological identification of the columnar organization of the cortex to the present.

Since experimental studies have so dominated the recent history of the study of the cerebral cortex, it is worth reminding ourselves that much of what we know about the human cerebral cortex has its origin in the careful clinical observation of patients with strokes, tumors, or seizures. These studies not only established the principle of localization of function in the cortex but also served to identify the anatomical locus of most of the major functional areas in the human brain. And while the first fruits of this rich harvest had clearly been garnered by the 1920s, we should not forget that the tradition established by the founding fathers of clinical neurology has continued more or less uninterruptedly to the present, and it is not invidious to mention in this context the names of Wilder Penfield and Roger Sperry, who have brought many of the analytic tools of modern neuroscience to bear upon some of the problems that are uniquely posed by the human brain.

While focusing upon these important clinical contributions, it would be a mistake not to mention that this same epoch saw the beginning of cortical cytoarchitectonics with the monumental studies of Baillarger, Campbell, Flechsig, Brodmann, and Maximilian Rose, the first detailed analyses of the neuronal organization of the cortex by Golgi, Ramón y Cajal, and Kölliker (to name only the most prominent workers), and the beginnings of cortical physiology in the electrical stimulation studies of Fritsch and Hitzig, of Ferrier and Horsley, and Sherrington and Leyton.

It is difficult to place a precise date on the beginning of the second epoch. If one has to be selected it might be the beginning of Polyak's important series of publications on what he termed "the main afferent fiber system of the cerebral cortex in primates," which culminated in his seminal monograph of the same title in 1932. These experimental studies, which were based on the Marchi method, certainly provided the stimulus for the long and important series of papers by Earl Walker in this country and by Le Gros Clark in England, which together laid the foundation for much of what we know about the organization of thalamocortical connections. These studies, in turn, paved the way for Rose and Woolsey's (1948, 1949) tripartite definition of a cortical field, as an area that (a) has a distinctive cytoarchitecture, (b) bears a unique relationship to a specific thalamic nucleus, and (c) in some cases, at least, can be shown to be coextensive with a physiologically definable area. Rose and Woolsey's studies may be said also finally to have answered the skepticism expressed by Lashley and Clark (1946) about the validity of cortical cytoarchitectonics—a skepticism engendered in part by the excesses of the more exuberant cytoarchitectonicists and in part by behavioral experiments of rather dubious significance.

The period between the two world wars also gave birth to the "evoked-potential method" for mapping cortical areas, a development that will always be associated with the names of Marshall, Woolsey, and Bard in this country and of Adrian and Bremer in Great Britain and Belgium, respectively. We have become so familiar with the maps of the various sensory areas of the cerebral cortex (in almost every class of mammal, from pigs and ponies to macaques and chimps) that it is difficult to believe that this major accomplishment occurred over a period of less than twenty years. And almost forty years later, we are still trying to make sense of one of the most unexpected discoveries of that period, namely, the multiple cortical representations of each of the major sensory modalities. What are we to make of the thirteen auditory areas that have been identified in the cat, or the half-dozen visual areas found in the monkey?

The apotheosis of this period coincided with the introduction of microelectrode recording into cortical studies and the beginning of what we may legitimately call the modern era. We can date this, I believe, quite precisely. It coincides with two fundamental discoveries. The first was Mountcastle's (1957) observation that the neurons in the somatosensory cortex are arranged in modality-specific, vertical columns; and the second was Hubel and Wiesel's (1959) finding that the functional properties of neurons in the visual cortex are quite different from those in either the retina or the lateral geniculate nucleus. It is probably true to say that much of the work of the past two decades has been built upon this foundation and has been directed toward the elucidation of the dual issues of the columnar organization of the cortex and the sequential processing of information within the cortex that determines the functional properties of its intrinsic neurons.

W. Maxwell Cowan

To an unusual extent this modern era has been shaped by a succession of technical developments. I have alluded already to the critical role played by microelectrode recording in its inception, and to a large extent this approach remains central to neurophysiological studies of the cortex. At the same time there have been a number of neuroanatomical developments that have had far-reaching consequences. Interestingly, the first of these has been the revival of interest in the Golgi method. As Mountcastle has repeatedly pointed out, the essentially columnar organization of the cortex was first demonstrated in Lorente de Nó's Golgi studies, which were so succintly summarized and brought together in the chapter he wrote for Fulton's monograph, *Physiology of the Nervous System* (Lorente de Nó, 1938). But in addition to focusing attention on the vertical organization of the cortex (as opposed to the horizontal, laminar organization that had preoccupied cytoarchitectonicists for so long), Lorente de Nó drew attention to the bewildering variety of cell types present, to the existence of two quite different types of subcortical input to the cortex (his so-called specific and nonspecific afferents), and to the importance of what we would now term serial processing in the cortex. But for sheer prescience, no comment was more perceptive than this bold statement: "From the functional point of view [the cortex] is a unitary system composed of vertical chains of neurons, among which anatomically the most important are those starting at the articulation of the specific afferents and the cells of the external [i.e., IVth] lamina." It is closely rivaled, however, by his summary statement on architectonics:

The cortex is composed of an enormous number of elementary units, not simply juxtaposed but overlapping. Each elementary unit has a series of axonal and dendritic processes, where the synapses between intracortical elements and afferent fibers with cortical cells are established. The bodies of the cells which form similar links in the intracortical chains are grouped in horizontal layers. Therefore any change in the constitution of the intracortical chains must produce a variation also in the . . . Nissl pattern.

Since much of the recent Golgi work is reviewed by Jennifer Lund elsewhere in this volume, I need only add that this, the oldest of the analytic tools of neuroanatomy, continues (in the right hands) to yield valuable new data, especially since the sterile, statistical approach to cortical connectivity that at one time threatened to dominate the field has been abandoned.

For all its virtues the Golgi method has one serious drawback: the impregnation of neurons is random and unpredictable. Hence the recent development of techniques for selectively labeling identified neurons must be seen as a major achievement. The first successful study of this kind, by Kelly and van Essen (1974), involved the intracellular injection of the fluorescent dye Procion yellow. Among other things this work established that although most *complex* and *hypercomplex* cells (to use Hubel and Wiesel's classificatory terms for cells in the visual cortex) are pyramidal in form, not all *simple* cells are stellate neurons, as had been suggested at one time. More recently this approach has been improved by the use of the enzyme marker HRP (horseradish peroxidase), which has two significant advantages: it does not fade rapidly with repeated examination; and it often fills the entire neuron, including its axon and axon collaterals. The power of this new approach to the intrinsic structure of the cortex is strikingly illustrated by Gilbert and Wiesel's chapter in this volume. Its further application, including its extension to the electron-microscopic level (for the elucidation of synaptic organization of the identified cells, and the three-dimensional analysis of the cells), should permit us, for the first time, to fully reconstruct the morphology of a small segment of the cortex.

Such a reconstruction has been one of the unspoken goals of many neuroanatomists, ever since the introduction of the electron microscope to the study of central nervous tissue in the early 1950s. Until recently the complexity of the problem and the enormous number of micrographs that such reconstructions require have been powerful deterrents to this type of undertaking. There can be no doubt, however, that they would be eminently worthwhile, as can be judged from the insights gleaned from Ed White's reconstruction of the dendritic processes of a single stellate neuron in the mouse cerebral cortex, in this volume. In the meantime much is to be learned (and, indeed, has been learned) from the careful study of single thin sections. Colonnier, who first introduced the useful and now widely adopted classification of synaptic types according to the symmetry or asymmetry of their membrane specializations in one of his earlier studies of the fine structure of the cortex (Colonnier, 1966), has provided us in his chapter to the volume with an excellent review of the extensive body of work that has accumulated on this subject in the past two decades. I think we can be fairly confident that some combination of intracellular marking with HRP (or the Golgi precipitate) combined with the selective labeling of certain afferent fibers—thalamic or corticocortical—will shortly help to crack the problem of cortical circuitry and, in doing so, pave the way for a functional analysis as complete as that that we now have for the cerebellar cortex. In mentioning the cerebellar cortex, however, one should sound a note of caution against the naive and overly optimistic view that "if we only knew the detailed anatomy of the cortex we could easily deduce its function." The morphology of the cerebellar cortex has been known in principle since the time of Ramón y Cajal (1889, 1890) and its synaptic organization has been known in considerable detail for at least a decade (see Palay and Chan-Palay, 1974), but we are still hard pressed to say what the cerebellum "does." Is it too pessimistic to guess that it may take even longer to be able to understand what the cerebral cortex "does" and "how it does it"?

One of the most striking uses of HRP histochemistry has been the demonstration that the pyramidal cells in the various layers of the cortex have distinctive efferent projections. This finding (which had been anticipated by earlier electrophysiological studies involving the antidromic firing from various subcortical regions of neurons at different levels within the visual cortex; Toyama et al., 1974; Palmer and Rosenquist, 1974) was first demonstrated for the visual cortex by Gilbert and Kelly (1975) who succeeded in retrogradely labeling different populations of cortical neurons by injections of HRP into the lateral geniculate nucleus and the superior colliculus. The findings in this seminal study have been confirmed and also extended to other cortical areas and to other efferent projections. As a result it is now clear that one of the principles underlying the horizontal stratification of cortical neurons is that each layer of pyramidal cells (or in some cases, each sublayer) consists of a population of neurons that share a common efferent projection. Thus, the pyramidal and fusiform cells in layer VI invariably send their axons to the thalamus (those in the more superficial part of the layer projecting to the corresponding principal thalamic nucleus and those in the deeper part of the layer to one of the adjoining nonspecific or intralaminar thalamic nuclei; Catsman-Berrevoets and Kuypers, 1978). Similarly, the pyramidal cells in layer V project to various subcortical regions (other than the thalamus) and, again, the neurons in the various sublaminae within this layer appear to have different subcortical projections to the striatum, brain stem, or spinal cord (Jones et al., 1977). And at least in monkeys, most corticocortical projections arise from the supragranular layers of the cortex: those that project to the opposite hemisphere arise from the deeper part of layer III; while those that project to other cortical fields on the same side arise either from pyramidal cells in the more superficial part of layer III or in layer II (Jones and Wise, 1977; and see Jones, this volume). The implications of the laminar segregation of neurons in the various layers remain to be determined, but for the moment it is perhaps worth recalling that the cells in the various laminae are generated at different times during gestation, and that they migrate outward to the cortical plate in well-defined sequences; those that come to occupy the deepest cortical layer are formed first, while those that finally reside in the most superficial layers invariably are generated at a much later period in development (Rakic, 1974; and see Rakic, this volume).

The introduction in the early 1970s of the autoradiographic method for tracing connections also has added significantly to our knowledge of cortical connectivity. In particular it has thrown light not only on the laminar distribution of the various classes of cortical afferents but also on the columnar organization of the cortex. Since Jones, who has been at the forefront of this work, has reviewed the evidence for the localized termination of the specific and nonspecific thalamic and corticocortical (including callosal) afferents elsewhere in this volume, I need not comment further upon it except to say that it poses, in an especially acute form, the problem as to how, during development, the various classes of ingrowing fibers selectively determine the appropriate levels at which they should terminate. The fact that in the reeler mouse the afferents still reach their appropriate levels (even if they have to follow extremely devious routes) when the cortical lamination is grossly disrupted (in fact, the laminar pattern is almost the reverse of that seen in normal animals) argues rather strongly for a high degree of prespecification of both the incoming fibers and their cortical targets (Caviness and Rakic, 1978).

One of the most striking applications of the autoradiographic technique has come from experiments that take advantage of the transsynaptic transport of label introduced into the eye. In such experiments the IVth layer of the monkey visual cortex appears as an alternating series of labeled and unlabeled bands, each about 0.5 mm in width. The arrangement, ontogenetic appearance, and modifiability of these "eye dominance columns" have been studied extensively by Hubel and Wiesel and their colleagues (Hubel, Wiesel, and LeVay, 1977; LeVay, Hubel, and Wiesel, 1975), and more recently by Rakic (1977). Again, since much of this work is reviewed elsewhere in this volume by LeVay and Rakic, only two remarks need be made. The first is that the arrangement of these eye dominance columns could not have been predicted from the earlier physiological studies that had indicated that the cells in layer IV are driven by one or the other eye; it required the imaginative combination of electrophysiology and a new neuroanatomical technique to reveal the organization of the eye dominance bands across the extent of the visual cortex. The second remark is that, a priori, there was no reason to guess that the definitive form of the eye dominance bands would be the end product of a progressive refining and sharpening process. Nor would one have predicted that visual deprivation (produced by monocular eyelid suture) would produce a dramatic reduction in the width of the "deprived" columns, or that after a period of deprivation, reverse suturing of the eyelids would cause a reexpansion of the formerly reduced columns. Some of the implications of this remarkable degree of plasticity are evident; their full import remains to be uncovered.

One of the most intriguing observations reported in the past year may prove to be of considerable importance for our understanding of how the eye dominance patterns are generated, even though the experiments were carried out with a quite different goal in mind and on a totally different system. This is the finding that if a supernumerary eye is implanted close to one of the normal eyes of a developing frog, the retinal fibers from the two adjoining eyes to the contralateral optic tectum seem to compete with each other for the available space and finally become arranged in a series of alternating bands, the dimensions of which are rather similar to those of the eye dominance columns in the primate visual cortex. Again, as Martha Constantine-Paton, who first made this remarkable observation, has pointed out in her chapter, it could only have been made by the application of the newer neuroanatomical technology.

Another recent technique that promises to be of considerable use in cortical studies is that involving the labeled glucose analogue, 2-deoxyglucose. Shortly after this methodology had been perfected by Lou Sokoloff and his colleagues (1977), it was applied by Hubel, Wiesel, and Stryker (1978) in an attempt to directly visualize the so-called orientation columns in the cortex. While the results obtained so far in animals subjected to prolonged exposure to oriented visual stimuli are extremely suggestive, the method clearly requires further refinement before the morphology of the orientation columns can be said to have been established. One obvious difficulty in the use of this approach is the absence of a built-in control that would effectively monitor whether the selective distribution of the labeled material is directly related to the presented visual stimulus or reflects some other feature in the organization of the cortex.

For some years one facet of cortical studies seemed to lag appreciably behind the others: this includes the related fields of neurochemistry and neuropharmacology. Of course there had been many studies dealing with what one might call the general biochemistry of the cortex, but comparatively few studies focused on those aspects of the cortex that make it distinctive. This hiatus is being filled rapidly. Beginning with the discovery of the extensive aminergic input to the cortex, there has been a veritable explosion of new knowledge about synaptic transmitters (both well established and putative) in the cortex. Again this development has been due in no small part to the emergence of new techniques as well as to the refinement of older methods. The outstanding example of this development is the methods that permit the identification of neurons or fibers that contain specific transmitters. This identification is commonly made by taking advantage of the capacity of certain neurons to take up, with high affinity, exogenous transmitters, or by immunohistochemical procedures that utilize antibodies of high specificity directed against the transmitter itself or certain enzymes involved in its synthesis. Different aspects of this exciting body of work are reviewed at length in this volume by Bloom, Taylor and Stone, and Emson and Hunt, so I shall not deal with them here. I cannot resist one comment, however: Who would have guessed even three years ago that the vasoactive intestinal peptide (VIP) would turn out to be one of the major transmitter candidates in the cerebral cortex? It will hardly be surprising if a number of equally unexpected developments occur in the next decade. This is clearly one of the most rapidly burgeoning areas in the whole of neuroscience, and from the dual points of view of cortical physiology and clinical therapy, clearly one of the most important.

The development of adequate techniques for recording from cells of the cortex in conscious, behaving animals had been a major goal of neurophysiologists for some time. Many of the technological problems were resolved by Edward Evarts a few years ago, and since that time his method has yielded a substantial body of data both from his own laboratory and that of several others. I think it would be fair to say that Evarts's own work completely revolutionized our thinking about the role of the motor cortex in skilled movements. At the same time the technique has opened up an entirely new approach to the study of the association areas of the cortex (see, for example, Mountcastle, 1976).

It is worth dwelling on this point for a moment, if only because we know so little about the functional significance of the association areas. Historically it is not difficult to see why their study has lagged so far behind that of the various sensory areas or the motor cortex. It is not only that we lack a straightforward means of activating most of the associational areas; for many of these areas we hardly know what types of questions to pose. Yet as Le Gros Clark pointed out almost 50 years ago, the growth in size and the progressive elaboration in the complexity of the cortical association fields (and their related thalamic nuclei) are two of the most striking features in the evolution of the mammalian brain (Le Gros Clark, 1932).

Much of what we know about these "silent areas" (to use a term that was popular in the 1940s and regrettably is still appropriate) has come from clinical and diagnostic studies of human neurological patients, or from studies on nonhuman subjects in which analogous syndromes have been produced. Although such studies are usually difficult to interpret, they have often provided useful insights, especially when the patients and experimental animals were examined by skilled behavioral scientists. An example is outlined in the chapter by Berlucchi and Sprague. In a somewhat different way, the increasingly sophisticated method of evoked-potential analysis has been used to monitor simultaneously certain properties of the nervous system and the overt behavior of the experimental subject; see the discussion by Desmedt. The general problems of linking cortical physiology and anatomy with function are discussed by Jasper and Cowey, with the latter specifically addressing the question I raised previously: Why are there so many distinct anatomical areas for each sensory modality? It is evident that new methodological approaches are needed if we are to understand the role of the cortex in complex behavior (and especially human behavior). This problem remains one of the greatest challenges to neuroscience; but if the past is any guide to the future, progress in this direction is likely to be painfully slow.

Apart from the technical and methodological difficulties, perhaps the most serious obstacle in the way of real advance in the study of those aspects of cortical activity that are commonly (if obscurely) referred to as "higher brain functions," is the absence, in most of neuroscience, of a sure theoretical framework. Indeed hardly any area of biology has been so singularly lacking in theory as neurobiology; it is almost as if neurobiologists as a group not only have eschewed theory, but even despise it. This is unfortunate. It takes no great insight to see that if substantial progress is to be made in the understanding of such phenomena as perception, learning, memory, and emotion, we shall have to have theories that are cogent and testable. It was for this reason that the closing session of the program at Woods Hole was devoted to certain theoretical issues; and it is perhaps not without significance that those who were invited to lead these discussions were drawn from other disciplines and were certainly not identified as "card-carrying" neuroscientists.

It would be inappropriate to attempt to summarize the theoretical contributions that comprise the final section of this book. But it is worth remarking, if only for the benefit of those who view all theorizing with skepticism (healthy or otherwise), that the theories discussed are of several types. Some, like that presented by Francis Crick, Tomaso Poggio, and David Marr, are highly focused and address a very specific issue in visual physiology (albeit one that has broader implications for visual perception). At the other end of the spectrum is Gerald Edelman's contribution, which is a bold attempt to provide a very general theory of cortical function that is obviously colored by his background in immunology, but is also informed by his remarkably broad reading in neuroscience. Between these two extremes, there is Leon Cooper's intermediate-level theory of memory—intermediate in that while it addresses a specific issue, and draws heavily on certain types of experimental evidence, it goes well beyond the evidence in suggesting a rather general mode of cerebral action. Clearly we can expect a great many more theoretical contributions of this kind in the next decade; and certainly we may hope that neuroscientists will become increasingly open to the contributions of theoreticians, and even that a new "breed" of theoretical neurobiologists will emerge.

References

Catsman-Berrevoets, C. E., and H. G. J. M. Kuypers, 1978. Differential laminar distribution of cortico-thalamic neurons projecting to the VL and the center median. An HRP study in the cynomolgus monkey. *Brain Res.* 154:359–365.

Caviness, V. S., and P. Rakic, 1978. Mechanisms of cortical development: A view from mutations in mice. *Ann. Rev. Neurosci.* 1:297–326.

Colonnier, M., 1966. The structural design of the neocortex. In *Brain and Conscious Experience.* J. C. Eccles, ed. New York: Springer-Verlag, pp. 1–23.

Evarts, E. V., 1964. Temporal patterns of discharge of pyramidal tract neurons during sleep and waking in the monkey. *J. Neurophysiol.* 27:152–171.

Gilbert, C. D., and J. P. Kelly, 1975. The projections of cells in different layers of the cat's visual cortex. *J. Comp. Neurol.* 163:81–106.

Hubel, D. H., and T. N. Wiesel, 1959. Receptive fields of single neurones in the cat's striate cortex. *J. Physiol. (London)* 148:574–591.

Hubel, D. H., T. N. Wiesel, and S. LeVay, 1977. Plasticity of ocular dominance columns in monkey striate cortex. *Phil. Trans. Roy. Soc. B* 278:377–409.

Hubel, D. H., T. N. Wiesel, and M. P. Stryker, 1978. Anatomical demonstration of orientation columns in macaque monkey. *J. Comp. Neurol.* 177:361–380.

Jones, E. G., and S. P. Wise, 1977. Size, laminar and columnar distribution of efferent cells in the sensory-motor cortex of monkeys. *J. Comp. Neurol.* 175:391–438.

Jones, E. G., H. Burton, and R. Porter, 1975. Commissural and cortico-cortical "columns" in the somatic sensory cortex of primates. *Science* 190:572–574.

Jones, E. G., J. D. Coulter, H. Burton, and R. Porter, 1977. Cells of origin and terminal distribution of corticostriatal fibers arising in the sensory-motor cortex of monkeys. *J. Comp. Neurol.* 173:53–80.

Kelly, J. P., and D. C. van Essen, 1974. Cell structure and function in the visual cortex of the cat. *J. Physiol. (London)* 238:515–547.

Lashley, K. S., and G. Clark, 1946. The cytoarchitecture of the cerebral cortex of Ateles: A critical examination of cytoarchitectonic studies. *J. Comp. Neurol.* 85:223–305.

Le Gros Clark, W. E., 1932. The structure and connections of the thalamus. *Brain* 55:406–470.

LeVay, S., D. H. Hubel, and T. N. Wiesel, 1975. The pattern of ocular dominance columns in macaque visual cortex revealed by a reduced silver stain. *J. Comp. Neurol.* 159:559–576.

Lorente de Nó, R., 1938. Cerebral cortex: Architecture, intracortical connections, motor projections. In *Physiology of the Nervous System*. J. F. Fulton, ed. New York: Oxford University Press, pp. 291–339.

Mountcastle, V. B., 1957. Modality and topographic properties of single neurons of cat's somatic sensory cortex. *J. Neurophysiol.* 20:408–434.

Mountcastle, V. B., 1976. The world around us: Neural command functions for selective attention. F. O. Schmitt Lecture. *Neurosci. Res. Prog. Bull.* 14 (Suppl. 1).

Palay, S. L., and V. Chan-Palay, 1974. *Cerebellar Cortex: Cytology and Organization*. New York: Springer-Verlag.

Palmer, L. A., and A. C. Rosenquist, 1974. Visual receptive fields of single striate cortical units projecting to the superior colliculus in the cat. *Brain Res.* 67:27–42.

Rakic, P., 1974. Neurons in rhesus monkey visual cortex: Systematic relation between time of origin and eventual disposition. *Science* 183:425–427.

Rakic, P., 1977. Prenatal development of the visual system in the rhesus monkey. *Phil. Trans. Roy. Soc. B* 278:245–260.

Ramón y Cajal, S., 1889. Sur l'origine et la direction des prolongations nerveuses de la couche moléculaire du cervelet. *Int. Mschr. Anat. Physiol.* 6:158–174.

Ramón y Cajal, S., 1890. Sur les fibres nerveuses de la couche granuleuse du cervelet et sur l'évolution des éléments cérébelleria. *Int. Mschr. Anat. Physiol.* 7:12–30.

Rose, J. E., and C. N. Woolsey, 1948. Structure and relations of the limbic cortex and anterior thalamic nuclei in rabbit and cat. *J. Comp. Neurol.* 89:279–348.

Rose, J. E., and C. N. Woolsey, 1949. The relations of thalamic connections, cellular structure and evocable electrical activity in the auditory region of the cat. *J. Comp. Neurol.* 91:441–466.

Sokoloff, L., M. Reivich, C. Kennedy, M. H. Des Rosiers, C. S. Patlak, K. D. Pettigrew, O. Sakurada, and M. Shinohara, 1977. The [^{14}C]-deoxyglucose method for the measurement of local cerebral glucose utilization: Theory, procedure, and normal values in the conscious and anesthetized albino rat. *J. Neurochem.* 28:897–916.

Toyama, K., K. Matsunami, T. Ohno, and S. Takashiki, 1974. An intracellular study of neuronal organization in the visual cortex. *Exp. Brain Res.* 21:45–66.

Development, Plasticity, and
Evolution of Neocortex

Introduction

Pasko Rakic

The human neocortex consists of billions of neurons that are interconnected with each other and with subcortical structures by afferent and efferent processes of various length. If the cortex were flattened, it would be an average 3 mm thick and occupy an area of about 80,000 mm². Traditionally the neocortex has been divided into six to ten layers and into numerous cytoarchitectonic areas. The significance of this radial and tangential parcellation is only now beginning to be fully appreciated. For example, the newest addition to our understanding of cortical organization is the discovery that various axonal inputs to, and outputs from, the neocortex form distinct, discontinuous terminal fields referred to as columns, stripes, bands, or patches. It is also becoming evident that the columns or stripes are present not only in the sensory systems where they were initially discovered but also in the highly developed association cortex in nonhuman primates. Importantly, the application of reduced-silver methods to human brain tissue reveals that a similar parcellation of afferents may also exist in the human neocortex.

In spite of conflicting morphological details, confusing terminology, and even formal disagreement among neuroscientists in conceptual views and interpretations, it is generally accepted that neurons, which are defined by specific afferents and interconnected by local circuits along the radial dimension of the cortex, operate as structural and also functional units. The main subject of the chapters in this part is to review and to discuss how this complex neuronal assembly may be put together during ontogenetic development.

The chapter by Pasko Rakic provides an account of experimental studies in nonhuman primates on the critical cellular events that lead to the laminar and areal organization of the neocortex. As a first step, an appropriate number of cortical neurons are generated exclusively in the proliferative centers situated outside of the developing cortex—allowing an orderly production of various cell classes according to specific spatial and temporal parameters. As a next step, postmitotic cells migrate from the proliferative centers to the developing cortical plate along elongated, radially arranged glial fibers. The consequence of this mode of migration is that several generations of neurons which originate at a common restricted location on the ventricular surface eventually accumulate in the same radially oriented column in the cortex. This column can be referred to as an ontogenetic column because somata of neurons generated later take up positions external to the somata of their predecessors. The existence of glial guides also assures reproduction of the mosaicism of the proliferative zones on the expanding and curving cortical mantle of the gyrencephalic primate cerebrum.

Recent studies on the genesis of efferent and afferent cortical connections have considerably changed our views of the mechanisms involved in cortical ontogeny. Thus, in the short time since fetal neurosurgery in primates became practical we have learned that the development of thalamocortical afferents proceeds in three distinct phases that are separated in time and apparently governed by different mechanisms. In the first phase fibers enter the appropriate cerebral lobe and accumulate in the intermediate zone below the cortical plate. In the second phase axons enter the cortex but are distributed in a diffuse manner. The third phase is one in which terminal fields of initially intermixed fibers sort out. In rhesus monkey this phase continues after birth—thus providing an opportunity for the external environment to play a role in the establishment of synaptic circuits.

This important third stage of corticogenesis, which in monkey occurs mainly in the postnatal period, is discussed in the chapter by Simon LeVay. He gives an account of recent advances that he and his colleagues David Hubel and Torsten Wiesel have made in delineating the critical periods of structural and functional maturation and in exposing the capacity and mechanism of modifiability of afferent connections in the visual cortex of rhesus monkeys. Their recent analysis of the effect of reverse lid suture shows that the sorting out of geniculocortical input may be caused both by curtailment of development as well as by reexpansion of terminal fields. The series of studies performed by this group on the interplay between genetic endowment and sensory environment in determining structural and functional properties of the neocortex provides compelling evidence of neural plasticity in primates.

The experiments by Martha Constantine-Paton give an instructive example of how studies done in amphibia can be used to advantage in analyzing the basic neural mechanisms involved in the development of the mammalian neocortex. Her discovery that retinal fibers of an experimentally implanted extra eye form alternating bands of terminal fields in the frog optic tectum which are strikingly similar to the ocular-dominance stripes in monkey cortex provides a useful model for analysis of cellular interactions involved in segregation of input fibers in target structures. Another finding that is of particular interest to the topic of the present work is that bands of terminal fibers develop from an overlapping phase to a segregated phase just as ocular-dominance stripes do in the primate visual cortex.

The analysis of development and plasticity in prefrontal association cortex of the rhesus monkey by Patricia Goldman-Rakic provides evidence that many of the basic findings on cortical development in sensory and motor systems also apply to the more complex primate association cortex. Her studies demonstrate that advanced neurobiological techniques can be applied with success and often with advantage to this until recently neglected neocortical area. Her discovery that the corticocortical and corticosubcortical connections in the primate brain can be rearranged after perinatal removal of one frontal lobe has important implications for clinical neurology as well as for theories of neuroplasticity. Finally, she reminds us that if we are to understand higher cortical functions, eventually we will have to study association cortex.

The chapters in this part indicate that, at present, we know more about various morphological phenomena involved in the process of cortical development than about the underlying mechanisms. However, the data accumulated so far provide an excellent empirical base from which to build a coherent model of cortical development in which cell movement and establishment of neuronal connections are viewed dynamically in space and time. The present studies probably expose only a small fraction of the various cellular processes that lead to cortical organization in the adult, but they demonstrate that the development of the mammalian neocortex can be analyzed by technology currently available and that significant advances may be expected in the near future.

1

Developmental Events Leading to Laminar and Areal Organization of the Neocortex

Pasko Rakic

ABSTRACT Evidence from a series of studies on the development of the primate neocortex indicates that the tangential (horizontal) coordinates of each cortical neuron are determined by the relative position of its precursor cell in the proliferative zones lining the cerebral ventricle, while the radial (vertical) position is determined by the time of its genesis and rate of migration. Thus, the development of topography and/or modality are determined by spatial parameters, while the hierarchical organization of neurons within each radial columnar unit is determined by temporal factors.

Radial glial fibers connect proliferative zones and the developing cortical plate and serve as guides which specify the positions of cortical neurons and assure that the mosaicism of the ventricular surface will be faithfully represented on the expanding cortical mantle. The existence of glial guides minimizes the amount of information needed by each neuron to reach the correct locus and to establish correct synaptic relations within the cortex.

The development of thalamocortical connections can be divided into three phases. In the first phase, thalamic fibers grow into the intermediate zone of the cerebral wall and accumulate below the developing cortical plate; in the second phase, fibers enter the appropriate cortical region but distribute in a relatively diffuse manner; finally, in the third phase, fibers sort out into specific terminal fields. The three phases are separated in time and are probably regulated by different mechanisms.

The tangential parcellation of the neocortical mantle into cytoarchitectonic areas and "modular" structural–functional units along with the radial stratification of its neurons into layers and sublayers is determined by a complex series of developmental processes. The end result of this complex chain of events is that each neuron attains a unique position within the cortex, and based on this position a unique set of afferent, local, and efferent connections. It is obvious, then, that factors which enable a neuron to attain the correct map locus during ontogeny may be of paramount importance for the normal development of this structure. Since, as described below, all cortical neurons are generated outside of the cortex itself, how then do they reach their proper coordinates? For example, are tangential coordinates, which denote cell position along the cortical surface, and radial coordinates,[1] which de-

PASKO RAKIC Yale University, School of Medicine, New Haven, Connecticut 06510

1 In describing the coordinates of the position of neurons within the cortex we have adopted the terms "radial" and "tangential" rather than "vertical" and "horizontal." The latter terms refer to the orientation of cells in diagrams of the cortex in which the pial surface faces the top of the page. However, due to the curved and convoluted shape of the

note cell depth within the cortex, specified in the same way or at the same time? Is the position of each cortical neuron determined before or after it leaves the proliferative zone? How and when does it become incorporated into synaptic circuitry?

In this chapter, I shall review published and unpublished data related to the following factors and cellular events which may play a role in the coding of position-dependent differentiation of cortical neurons: (1) acquisition of radial or layer-specific positions of cortical neurons; (2) acquisition of tangential or area-specific positions of cortical neurons; and (3) formation of synaptic connections. The evidence to be presented is based primarily on work done on rhesus monkeys in my laboratory. In this species, as in man, the major events that are critical for formation of the neocortex occur mainly before birth.

Acquisition of Laminar Positions

Time and Place of Origin

The entire population of cortical neurons present in adult human neocortex is generated over about a 100-day period during midgestation (e.g., see Poliakov, 1965; Rakic, 1978). In the rhesus monkey the corresponding span of genesis for all neocortical neurons is 60 days (Rakic, 1974). It is important to emphasize that not a single one of the enormous number of neurons that constitute primate neocortex is actually produced within the cortical plate itself. Rather, as shown by analysis of monkey fetuses sacrificed 1 hr after [³H]-thymidine ([³H]-TdR) injections, all prospective neocortical neurons are generated in the proliferative zones which are situated around the cavities of the cerebral ventricles (Rakic, 1975). In the monkey, young neurons are initially produced almost exclusively in the ventricular zone;[2] during middle stages of cortical development they seem to be generated in both ventricular and subventricular zones; and by the end of the proliferative period, the subventricular zone appears to become the predominant and, finally, the only source of new cells. In man, prospective neocortical neurons are also generated exclusively in the ventricular and subventricular zones (Rakic and Sidman, 1968). It is therefore safe to conclude that in both primate species all neocortical neurons are produced outside of the cortical plate and must migrate a considerable distance in order to reach their final positions. The redistribution of such a vast number of cells during development undoubtedly provides opportunities for establishment of essential relationships and key contacts that eventually determine the radial and tangential coordinates of each neuron in the

---

mammalian neocortex in general, and in the gyrencephalic primate brain in particular, the terms radial (for Z) and tangential (for X and Y) reflect more accurately the relationships which exist in vivo.

2 Nomenclature recommendation of the Boulder Committee (1970), *Anat. Rec.* 166:257–262, has been adopted.

3-dimensional map of the neocortex. Thus, the separation of proliferative centers from the final residence of neurons is of great biological
significance.

To analyze in more detail the manner in which neurons attain their
radial positions within the cortex, we have conducted a series of studies
on the genesis of the primary and secondary visual cortices in rhesus
monkeys that were exposed to [^{3}H]-TdR at selected embryonic (E) and
postnatal (P) days and sacrificed at various intervals (Rakic, 1974, 1975,
1976b). As a first step, we explored the question whether the time at
which a neuron is generated correlates with its final position.

Radioactive cells in the cortical laminae of areas 17 and 18 were plotted in five consecutive autoradiograms (Figure 1) and the positions of
simultaneously generated cells compared in the two cytoarchitectonic
fields (Figure 2). The results show that all visual cortical neurons are
generated between E40 and E100 of the 165-day gestational period in
this primate species. In both visual areas, the final position of neurons
in the cortex is systematically related to the time of cell origin; neurons
destined for positions in deeper cortical layers are generated earlier,
and those situated more superficially progressively later (Rakic, 1974).
Thus, the spatiotemporal gradient is inside-to-outside, as described in
rodents (Angevine and Sidman, 1961; Berry and Rogers, 1965). In pri-

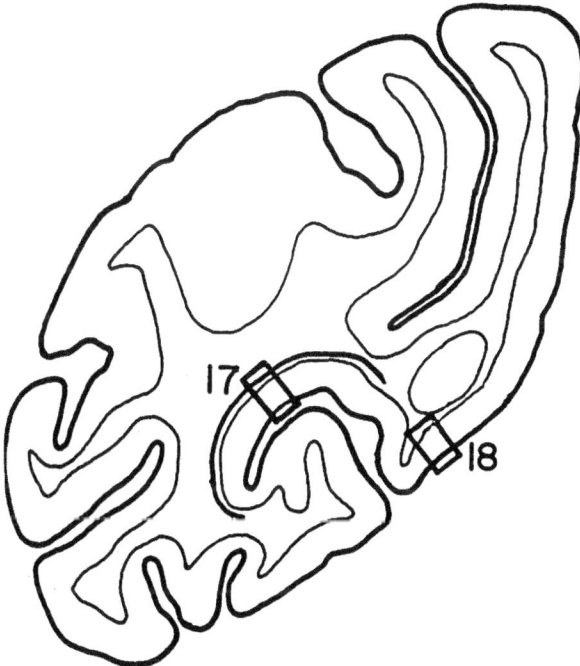

Figure 1 An outline of a coronal section through the occipital lobe of a 3-month-old
rhesus monkey. The two frames indicate selected strips of cortex in areas 17 and 18 of
Brodmann (1905) in which the positions of the [^{3}H]-TdR-labeled neurons were plotted in
Figure 2. (From Rakic, 1976a.)

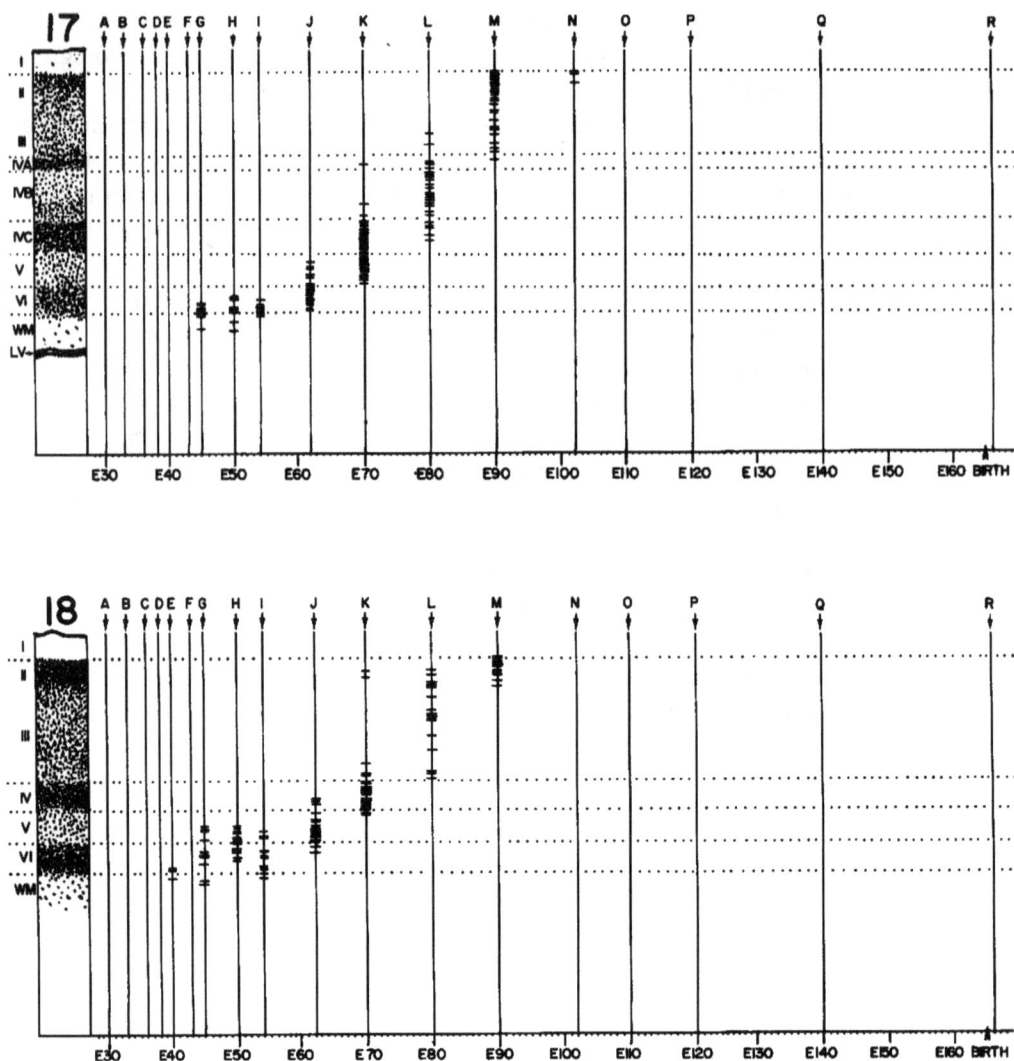

Figure 2 Diagrammatic representation of the positions of heavily labeled neurons in the visual cortex of juvenile monkeys, each of which had been injected with [³H]-TdR at selected embryonic days: top, area 17; bottom, area 18 of Brodmann (1905). On the left side of each diagram is a drawing of the cortex from cresyl-violet-stained sections, in which subdivisions into cortical layers are indicated by Roman numerals according to the classification of Brodmann (1905). Embryonic days (E) are represented on the horizontal line, starting on the left with the end of the first fetal month (E27) and ending on the right at term (E165). Positions of vertical lines (A to R) indicate the embryonic day on which one animal received a pulse of [³H]-TdR. On each vertical line short horizontal markers indicate positions of all heavily labeled neurons encountered in one 2.5-mm-long strip of the cortex. Abbreviations: LV, obliterated posterior horn of the lateral ventricle; WM, white matter. (Based on Rakic, 1974, 1976a.)

mates, however, the relationship between the time of origin and position of cells within the cortex is more accurate and more rigid (Rakic, 1974).

A corollary issue is whether neurons that eventually form a given cortical layer are generated simultaneously across the different cytoarchitectonic areas. A new and to some extent surprising finding was obtained when the positions of labeled neurons in areas 17 and 18 were compared to each other (Rakic, 1976b). From inspection of the cell plots in Figure 2, it is evident that, although the production of neurons destined for two selected cortical areas overlap considerably in time, both the beginning and end of neurogenesis occur at slightly earlier ages for neurons that are destined for area 18 than for those that will form area 17. Preliminary examination of neurogenesis in area 19 indicates that neurons destined to reside in corresponding laminae in this cytoarchitectonic area are generated during even slightly earlier periods than in area 18. Since the positions of labeled neurons in Figure 2 are compared within the same animal and on the very same tissue sections (see Figure 1), the recorded differences in cell positions, even when relatively small, are significant (Rakic, 1976b).

The differences in the time of origin of neurons in corresponding cortical layers among cytoarchitectonic subdivisions indicate that neurons which are generated simultaneously in neighboring regions of the ventricular zone may end up in different layers in adjacent cortical areas, and thus will eventually assume different morphological and functional characteristics. The fact that each cortical layer in areas 18 and 19 acquires its neurons somewhat earlier than the corresponding layer in area 17 would not be expected from what is known about the sequence of morphological and functional differentiation in these regions. For example, area 17 myelinates (Flechsig, 1920) and differentiates (Poliakov, 1965; Preobrazhenskaya, 1965) earlier in ontogeny than adjacent secondary visual areas. Comparison of the timing of cell origin with the schedule of cellular differentiation indicates that the time of neuron origin and onset of differentiation may be independent developmental processes probably regulated by different genetic mechanisms. A similar hypothesis has been postulated for the explanation of position-dependent differentiation of stellate cells in the molecular layer of the cerebellar cortex (Rakic, 1973).

Rate of Neuronal Migration
The final position of a cortical neuron along the radial axis depends not only on the time of its origin but also on the time it requires to attain its final destination. For example, assuming that the rate[3] of cell migration

---

3 It is important to distinguish between the term "speed" of cell migration, which designates the actual change in position of cells along the migratory pathway per unit time, and the "rate" of cell arrival at the cortical plate, which designates the fraction of cells which

is uniform and constant in all telencephalic regions and at all stages, all simultaneously generated neurons would arrive at the outermost edge of the developing cortical plate at the same time. In this case, regional differences in positions of simultaneously generated cells would depend entirely on the variability in the length of migrating trajectories. Alternatively, if the rate of neuronal migration is nonuniform, then many simultaneously generated cells would arrive at different cortical depths; those arriving first would end up deeper in the cortex while those arriving last would settle at more superficial positions.

Our autoradiographic analysis of a series of monkey fetuses sacrificed at various times following exposure to [^{3}H]-TdR indicates that at early stages of cerebral development (between E40 and E50), young neurons arrive at the cortical plate synchronously and quite rapidly—in less than 3 days after the last cell division (Rakic, 1975). At later stages, however, the interval between the last cell division and the time when a given cell reaches its final destination is generally much longer than would be predicted from the extension of the cell's migratory pathway. Thus, the majority of cells generated around E80 or E85 require more than a week to arrive at their destination, and some need more than two weeks. Furthermore, we found that there is considerable variability in the time of arrival of simultaneously generated cells at these later stages. As a consequence, neurons generated early in development come to occupy a relatively narrow zone of the cortex, while those generated later come to be distributed over a somewhat wider span along the radial axes (Rakic, 1974). Also, neurons generated more than one week apart may have the same position within one layer (Rakic, 1975).

In spite of the significance of cell position along the radial axis for future synaptic connectivity within the cortex, the mechanism that determines the rate of cell migration is not understood. So far, we know that the rate of neuronal migration may vary from approximately 10 μm to over 100 μm per day in two adjacent telencephalic regions. For example, neurons of the hippocampal formation reach the superficial part of the developing cortical plate ten times more rapidly than neurons in the adjacent subiculum (Nowakowski and Rakic, 1980). Such an abrupt and marked difference in the rate of migration for cells generated in neighboring areas of the proliferative zone supports the hypothesis that cell position may already be determined in these zones (Rakic, 1977a).

---

have reached their destination at any moment in time. These definitions are necessary since the "rate" of cell arrival may depend on many factors, such as the length of the generation cycle, lag in the initiation of cell movement, intermittent migration (i.e., with stops), the duration of the stops, the total length of the pathways, as well as the "speed" of cell migration. Since the "speed" of cell migration cannot be determined by our experimental design, all the data used in this chapter refer to the rate of migration as defined above.

Mode of Neuronal Migration

The final position of each neuron class, and perhaps of each individual neuron, seems to be determined by a mechanism of cell migration which delivers the neuron to appropriate laminae within the cortex. In all mammalian species studied so far, young postmitotic neurons migrate radially to the developing cortical plate (see references quoted in Rakic, 1975). In primates, as the intermediate zone expands, these neurons traverse increasingly longer distances and more complex trajectories to reach the superficial strata of the developing cortical plate (Rakic, 1971, 1972). The length of the migratory pathway in the large primate cerebrum is not matched by a corresponding elongation of the migrating cells themselves. The fact that the length of migrating cells at later stages of corticogenesis is only a fraction of their total pathway has to be taken into consideration in any explanation of cell movement in densely packed neural tissue.

Our electron-microscopic analysis in the rhesus monkey demonstrates that migrating cells are continuously apposed to elongated radial glial fibers which span the fetal cerebral wall at early ages. This class of glial cells, which is illustrated in Figure 3, may assume somewhat different forms in other brain regions (see review in Varon and Somjen, 1979). In the mammalian telencephalon, they exist only during ontogenetic development (Schmechel and Rakic, 1979b). Recent autoradiographic studies using [³H]-TdR-labeled DNA demonstrate that during midgestation many radial glial cells stop dividing for about two months (Schmechel and Rakic, 1979a), although their fibers increase in length and curve with the expansion of the convoluted cerebral wall (Figures 3 and 4). Toward the end of gestation, however, radial glial cells reenter the mitotic cycle and ultimately disappear, many becoming transformed into protoplasmic or fibrillary astrocytes (Ramón y Cajal, 1911; Schmechel and Rakic, 1979b).

Until recently it was not possible to identify with complete security the glial nature of radial cells at very early stages. The evidence for their glial identity was based on the Golgi-impregnated material both in monkey (Rakic, 1975; Schmechel and Rakic, 1979b) and in man (Kostovic, Krmpotic-Nemanic, and Kelovic, 1975). Recent use of immunoperoxidase staining of the antibody to glial acidic fibrillary protein in the fetal monkey telencephalon has allowed us to positively identify radial glial fibers by E47 in this species (Levitt and Rakic, 1980). Since in man some radial fibers are positively stained by immunofluorescence as early as the tenth fetal week (Antanitus, Choi, and Lapham, 1976), it appears that in both primate species radial glial cells are present during the period of intensive cell migration to the cortex.

At all embryonic stages, neuronal growth and development are predominantly along the radial path that extends from the ventricular cavity toward the periphery. Orientation and guidance is at first provided

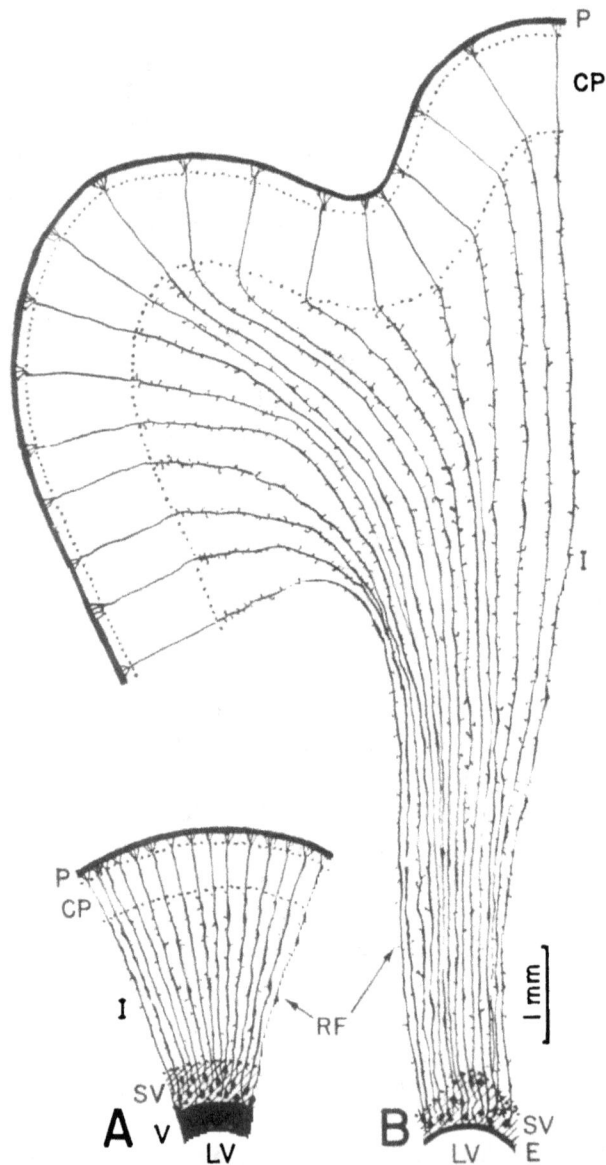

Figure 3 Semischematic drawing of the distribution of radial glial cells in the tel-encephalon of two monkey fetuses stained with the Golgi-impregnation method. (A) Dorsal portion of the occipital lobe of an 81-day-old fetus (E81). (B) Section from the corresponding region of the cerebrum in an E138 fetus. Due to the increased thickness of the cerebral wall and expansion of the cortical plate during the intervening period, radial glial fibers that traverse the cerebral wall from the subventricular zone near the lateral ventricle to the pial surface become several times longer and considerably curved. Abbreviations: CP, cortical plate; E, ependyma; I, intermediate zone; LV, lateral ventricle; P, pial membrane; RF, radial fiber; SV, subventricular zone; V, ventricular zone. (From Schmechel and Rakic, 1979a.)

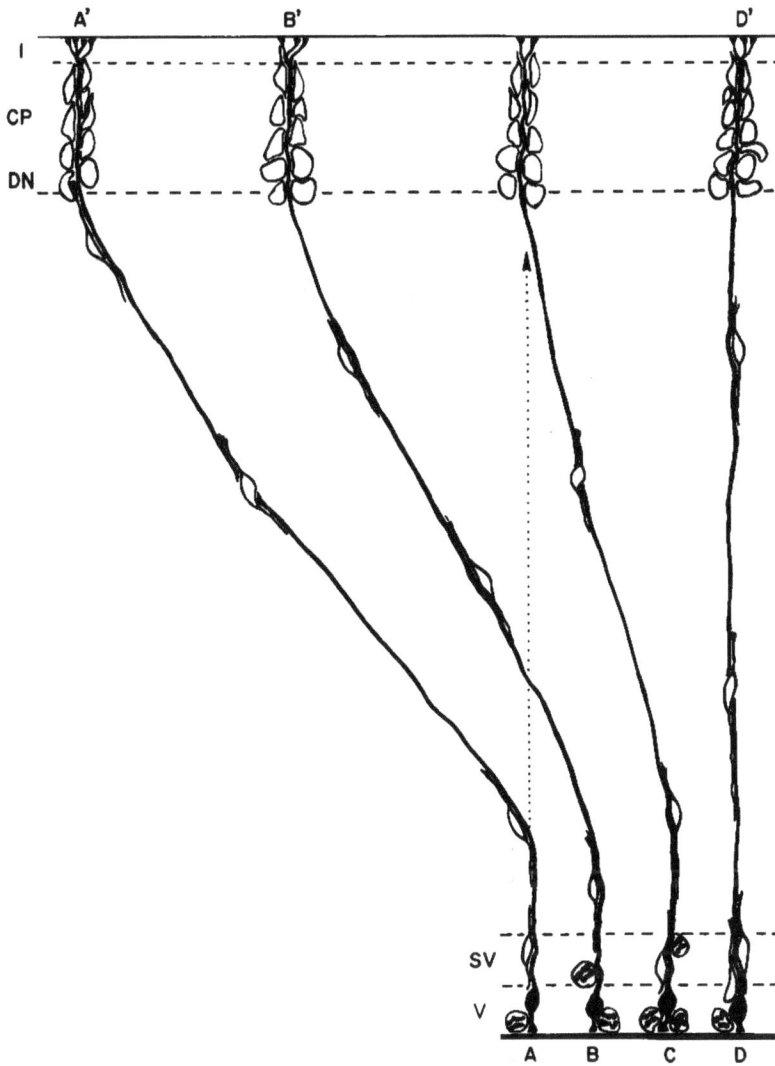

Figure 4 Diagrammatic illustration of the pattern of neuronal migration along radial glial fibers. Only four radial glial cells and cohorts of associated migrating neurons are drawn at approximately equal distances from each other to render the diagram legible. All neurons in the ventricular (V) and subventricular (SV) zones produced around a given glial fascicle (proliferative units A–D) migrate in succession along the same fiber fascicle to the cortical plate (CP), where they establish ontogenetic radial columns A'–D'. Within each radial column the newly arrived cells assume the most superficial position at the border-line between the developing cortical plate and the first cortical layer (I). On their way, they bypass deep neurons (DN) that were generated earlier. In spite of a considerable shift in the position of this growing cerebral surface (see also Figures 3 and 7), the topographic relationships between generations of neurons produced in proliferative units and their final position in the cortex are preserved by glial guides. This mechanical aid prevents the possibility of mismatching, for example, between A' and C', illustrated by a dotted line and arrow. Further explanation in text.

by undifferentiated columnar epithelial ventricular cells. Later, however, this role is served by immature glial cells and/or the processes of previously generated neurons, and even later by more clearly differentiated and dramatically elongated radial glial cells (Rakic, 1972, 1978). Thus electron-microscopic studies indicate that the elongated processes of radial glial cells guide young neurons across the complex assembly of closely spaced cells and processes that make up the developing primate telencephalon (Figures 5, 6; Rakic, 1971, 1972). As shown in relatively low-magnification electron micrographs (Figure 6), migrating neurons are in intimate contact with numerous cell processes, but they follow faithfully only radial glial guides.

Acquisition of Areal Positions

While the time of origin and rate of cell migration may be essential for the position of neurons along the radial axis within the cortex, the site of last cell division in the proliferative zones seems to determine the tangential coordinates of cells along the cortical surface. We have suggested that fascicles of radial glial cells provide lateral constraints for the migratory neurons (Rakic, 1978). This may be of crucial importance for preserving initial cell relationships. The concept of lateral constraints is illustrated schematically in Figure 7, which displays a 3-dimensional reconstruction of the medial cerebral wall of the occipital lobe at the level of the calcarine fissure. According to this concept, communities of neurons generated at adjacent proliferative units (illustrated in Figure 8A) migrate along adjacent radial glial fascicles (Figure 5), and thus these neurons retain a strict and constant relationship to one another. As a consequence, they finally form neighboring radially oriented columns in the cortical plate (Figure 8B).

The aggregates of cells aligned along one radial fascicle in the developing cortical plate has been referred to as a "minicolumn" by Mountcastle (1979) and an "ontogenetic column" by Edelman (1979). Our best approximation is that in fetal monkey telencephalon the number of proliferative units in the ventricular zone about equals the number of ontogenetic columns in the cortical plate. Thus, each proliferative unit may have a corresponding ontogenetic column. Obviously, ontogenetic columns widen considerably in the course of subsequent development as individual neurons grow, differentiate, and acquire synaptic connections from local and extrinsic sources (compare Figures 8A and 8B). However, we do not know at present whether any relationship exists between these transient ontogenetic columns and the disjunctive terminal fields of afferent fibers systems (e.g., ocular-dominance stripes) of the adult cortex. We can only say that the ontogenetic column represents a consequence of the sequential migration of many generations of neurons all of which have arrived along the same radial glial fascicle from a single proliferative unit. Further, since

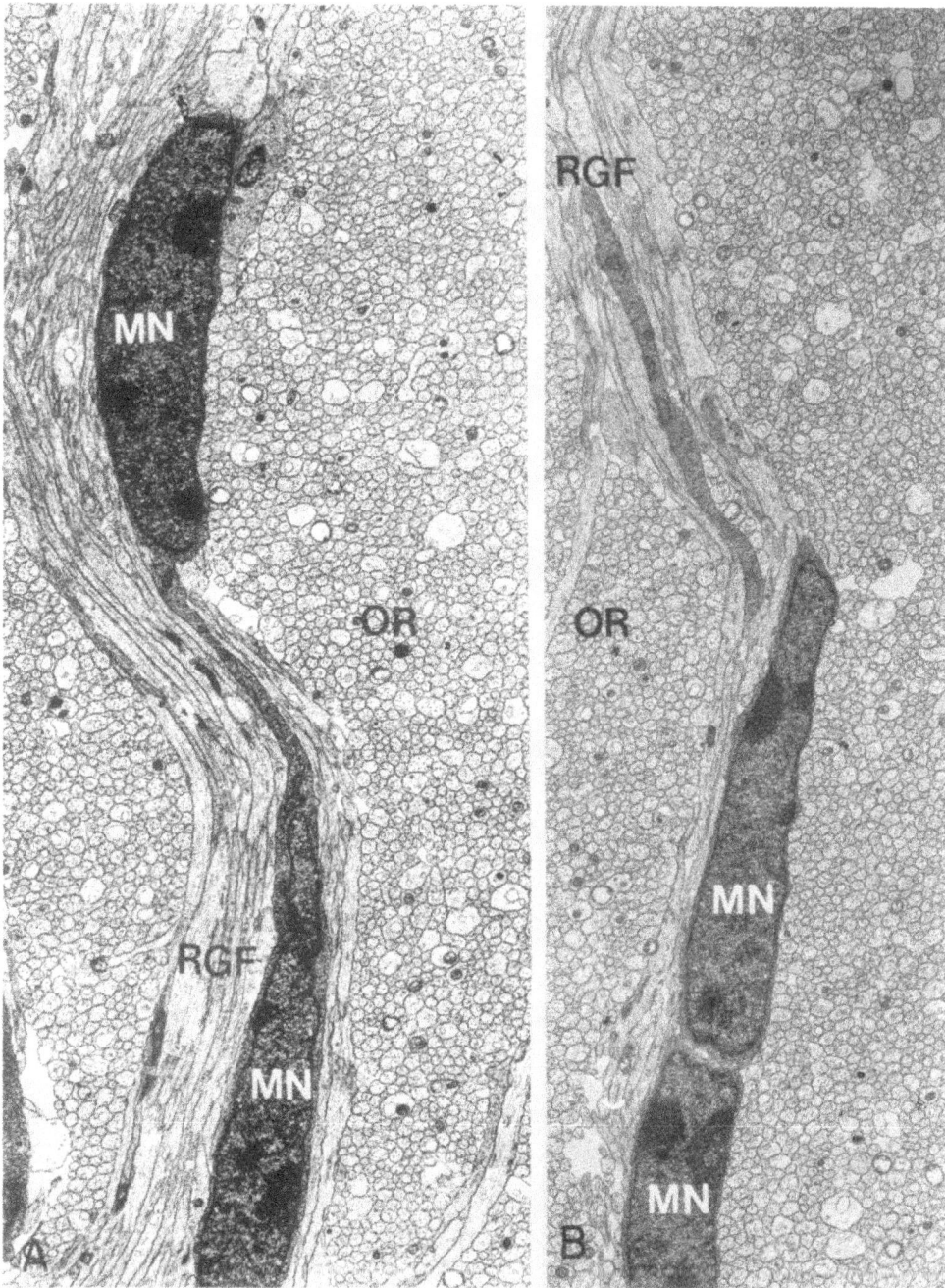

Figure 5 Two electron micrographs prepared from the cerebral wall of a 97-day-old monkey fetus. The sections are cut parallel to the cell movement, which proceeds from the bottom to the top of each photograph. The migrating neurons (MN) are aligned closely with fascicles of radial glial fibers (RGF) in the intermediate zone of the occipital lobe which is filled with transversely cut fibers of the optic radiation (OR).

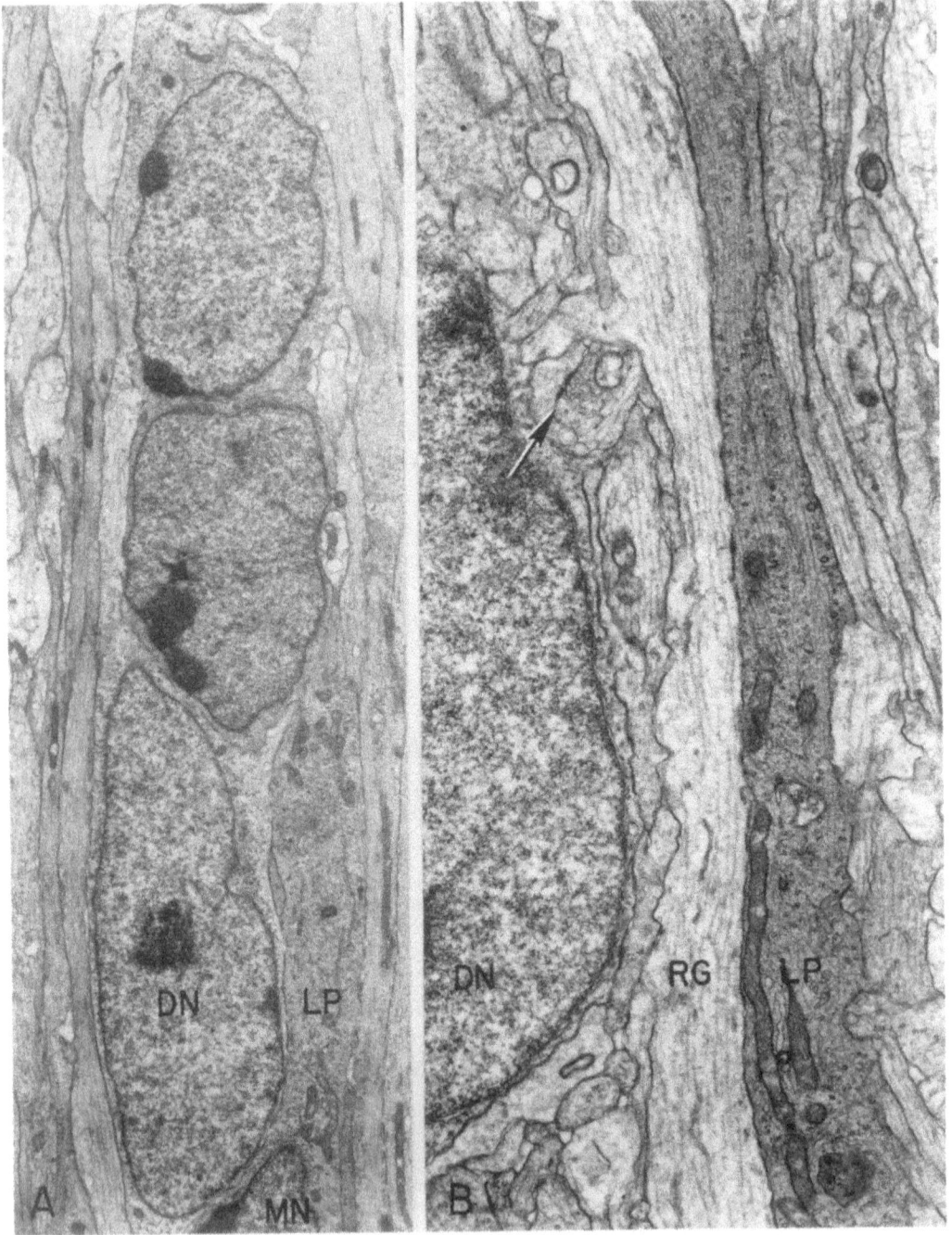

Figure 6 Electron micrographs of a portion of a radial ontogenetic column similar to those illustrated at the light-microscopic level in Figure 8B. A migrating neuron (MN) and its leading process (LP) are aligned with more mature, earlier-generated deep neurons (DN) and with the pale profile of radial glial fibers (RG). The presence of an occasional synapse illustrates the presence of highly interconnected cells and processes that have to be penetrated by a migrating neuron on its way to the superficial border of the developing cortical plate.

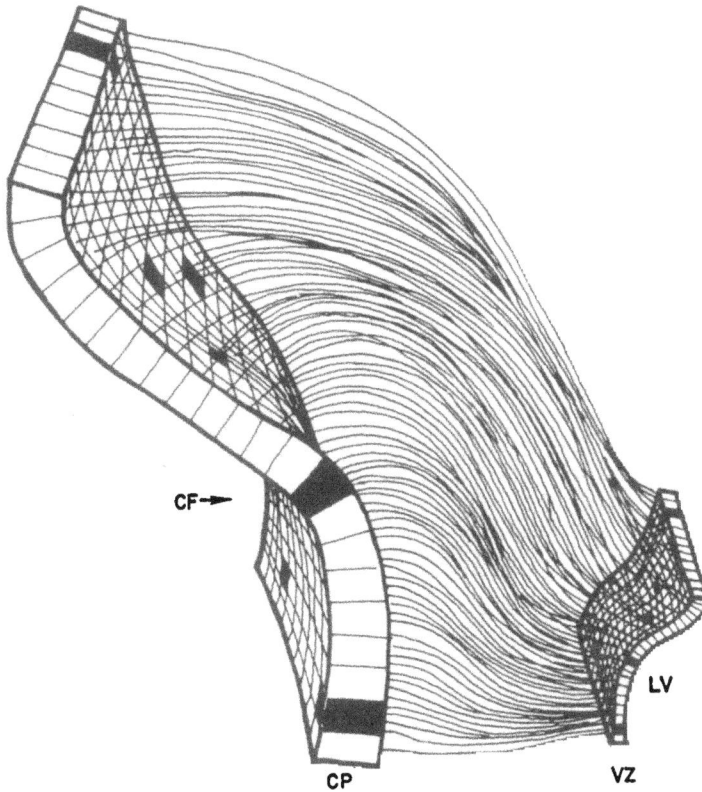

Figure 7 Schematic 3-dimensional reconstruction of a portion of the occipitoparietal junction on the medial cerebral wall of an 80-day-old monkey fetus. The reconstruction is confined to the level of the incipient calcarine fissure (CF) to display the relationship between the parcellation of the ventricular zone (VZ) and that of the cortical plate (CP). Although, during midgestation, the calcarine fissure deepens and the adjacent cortical regions rapidly grow, radial fibers stretch and curve, but their contact with both the ventricular and pial surface remains preserved (see also Figure 3 for illustration of this point). As a result, the corresponding regions of the proliferative zone and cortical plate are connected by radial glial fibers which span the full thickness of the cerebral wall from the lateral ventricle (LV) to the pial surface. It is postulated that these elongated cords provide lateral constraints during cell migration and enable precise reproduction of the mosaic of the ventricular zone on the enlarged and distorted cerebral surface. (From Rakic, 1978.)

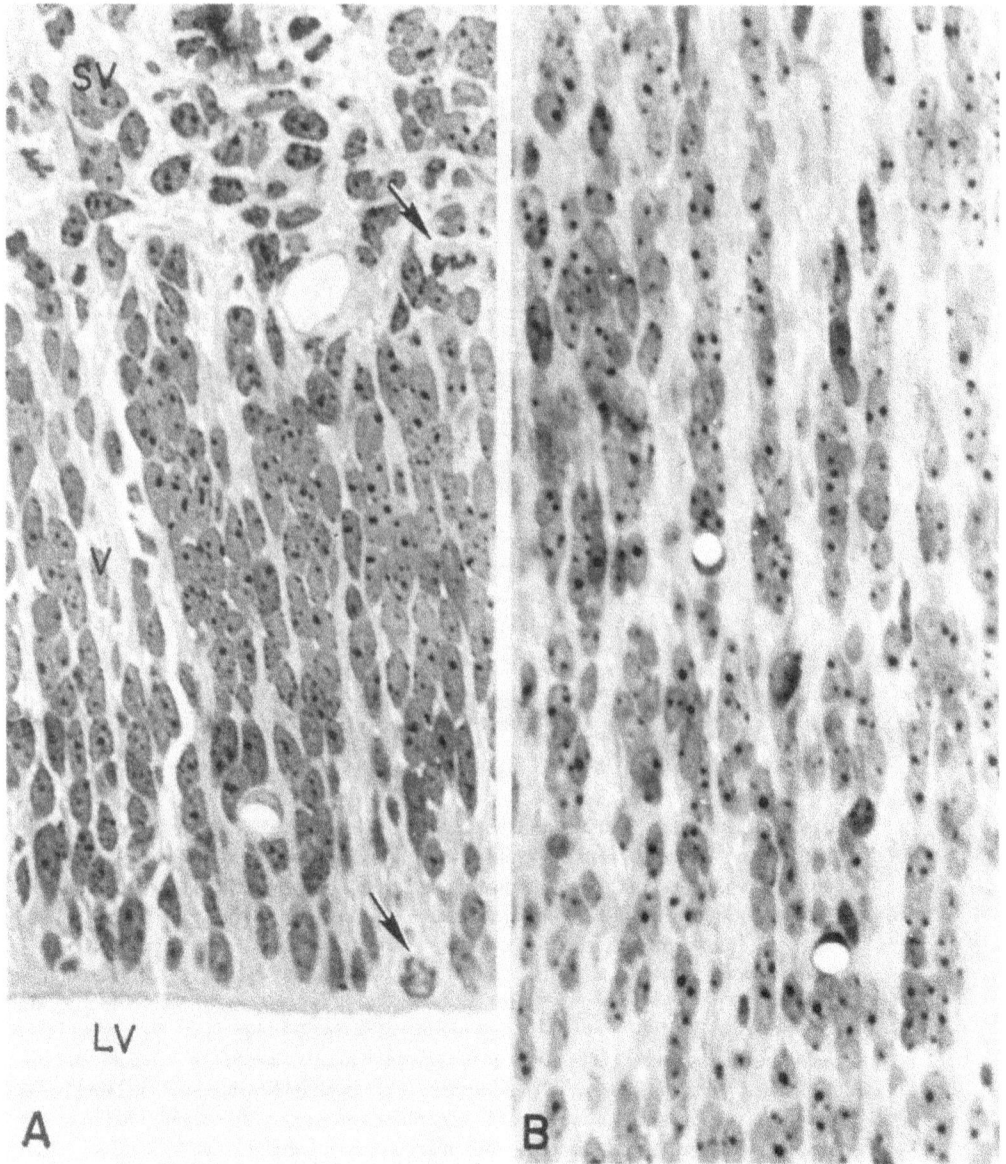

Figure 8 (A) Ventricular (V) and subventricular (VZ) zones in the monkey fetus which contain dividing cells, some of which are in the mitotic phase (arrows). Note that most cells are aligned in the vertical direction along radial glial cells. Their fibers, which are in this section, can be recognized as unstained tracts. All cells within one vertical column form a proliferative unit. (B) A portion of the fetal cortical plate which illustrates the ontogenetic radial columnar arrangement of the fetal cortex prominent at this developmental stage.

each proliferative unit (Figure 8A) may possibly have a matching ontogenetic radial column in the cortical plate (Figure 8B), and since the two are connected with elongated glial cords (Figure 7), the relationship between the ventricular zone and expanding cortex remains preserved in spite of considerable morphogenetic changes in the cerebral surface. Thus, glial guides not only minimize the amount of information needed for neurons to reach the correct map locus, but may also prevent the disaster that could conceivably occur if neurons produced in the ventricular zone at point A in Figure 4, which are destined to arrive at the cortex at point A', end up instead at a completely different cortical area, point C'.

The role of radial guides in establishing orderly areal cortical organization is based mainly on evidence from combined Golgi, electron-microscopic, immunoperoxidase, and [³H]-TdR autoradiographic analysis. At present, no other cellular constituents of the developing brain are viable candidates for this role. At one time the distribution of thalamic afferents was considered a possible determinant of cortical-cell position (Hicks and D'Amato, 1968; Sidman and Rakic, 1973). However, recent experimental evidence shows that specific thalamocortical and corticocortical fibers follow rather than precede cell migration to the cortex (Rakic, 1976a, 1977b; Lund, 1976; Wise and Jones, 1976). Also, the displaced neurons in both cerebral and cerebellar cortex of the reeler mutant mouse appear to attract appropriate afferents in spite of aberrant locations along the radial axes (Caviness and Rakic, 1978). Thus, it is unlikely that thalamocortical axons play a significant part in positioning of migrating neurons at early stages of cortical development.

The acquisition of laminar and areal positions of neurons is to be considered as separate cellular events. Although radial glial fibers may play a role in determining both the radial and tangential coordinates of a neuron, these coordinates are nevertheless probably achieved by different cellular mechanisms. While the delivery of neurons to an appropriate cytoarchitectonic area depends exclusively on the spatial position of its precursors in the proliferative zones, attainment of laminar position depends, in addition, on timing. For example, in the reeler mutant mouse, cortical cells apparently arrive at appropriate cytoarchitectonic areas but do not stop in the appropriate layers (Caviness and Rakic, 1978). Thus, acquisition of laminar and areal position of cortical neurons may be regulated by different genes.

Formation of Synaptic Connections

After the young neurons reach their proper vertical and horizontal coordinates, they then establish afferent, local, and efferent synaptic connectivity. Since long tract connections of the primate telencephalon are laid down before birth, until recently very little was known about the timing and mode of development of synaptic connectivity of the neocortex. However, the prospect for analysis of prenatal genesis of cortical connections in primates has changed considerably in the last few years with the refinement of techniques for performing fetal neuro-surgery (Rakic, 1976a, 1977b, 1980; Goldman and Galkin, 1978; Goldman-Rakic, 1980, and this volume) and by the advent of methods utilizing axonal (Cowan et al., 1972) and transneuronal (Grafstein, 1971; Wiesel, Hubel, and Lam, 1974) transport of radioactive macromolecules for tracing neuronal pathways. Although at present we cannot say much about prenatal development of local synaptic circuits of the cortex, a recent study of the genesis of geniculocortical projections in the rhesus monkey gives some insight into the formation of extrinsic connections (Rakic, 1976a, 1977b, 1979, 1980). The mechanism of establishment of visual connections may serve as a useful paradigm for understanding the development of other neocortical areas. Indeed, it appears that the basic principles which have evolved from the study of the visual system may also apply to the development of frontal association cortex (Goldman-Rakic, this volume).

The advantage of studying thalamocortical afferents of the visual system is that geniculocortical connections can be labeled transneuronally following unilateral eye injection of a mixture of [^{3}H]-proline and [^{3}H]-fucose into one eye of monkey fetuses. Each fetus is first exteriorized by histerotomy (Rakic, 1976a, 1977b, 1980) and, after intraocular injection of isotopes, returned to the uterus. Fourteen days later, when sufficient radioactivity has been transferred from retinal axons to dorsal lateral geniculate nucleus (LGd) neurons, the fetus is removed by a second cesarean section, fixed, and its brain processed for autoradiography.

So far, we have successfully processed five fetuses injected at different ages. This series of experiments has already provided basic information on the mode of development of thalamocortical visual connections (Figure 9). In the youngest fetus of our series, injected at E64 and sacrificed at E78, geniculate neurons form a sizable axonal pathway which enters the occipital lobe and forms a typical optic radiation (OR in Figure 9A). However, at this fetal age, geniculate axons do not enter the developing cortical plate (Rakic, 1976a). Instead, LGd axons accumulate in the intermediate zone below the cortical plate (Figure 9A). We have referred to these transient axonal plexuses as a "waiting compartment" (Rakic, 1979). It should be emphasized that at this fetal age only cells of prospective layers V and VI and a small fraction of layer IVC cells are present in the visual cortex (Rakic, 1974, and Figure 9A).[4] Thus, most of the neurons destined for layer IV migrate

4 Our recent study on the development of efferents from the visual cortex in rhesus monkey (Shatz and Rakic, 1978) shows that even at this early fetal age, neurons of layers V and VI project to their subcortical targets even though formation of the afferent geniculocortical system has not been completed and most neurons that receive the bulk of afferent terminals have not been generated.

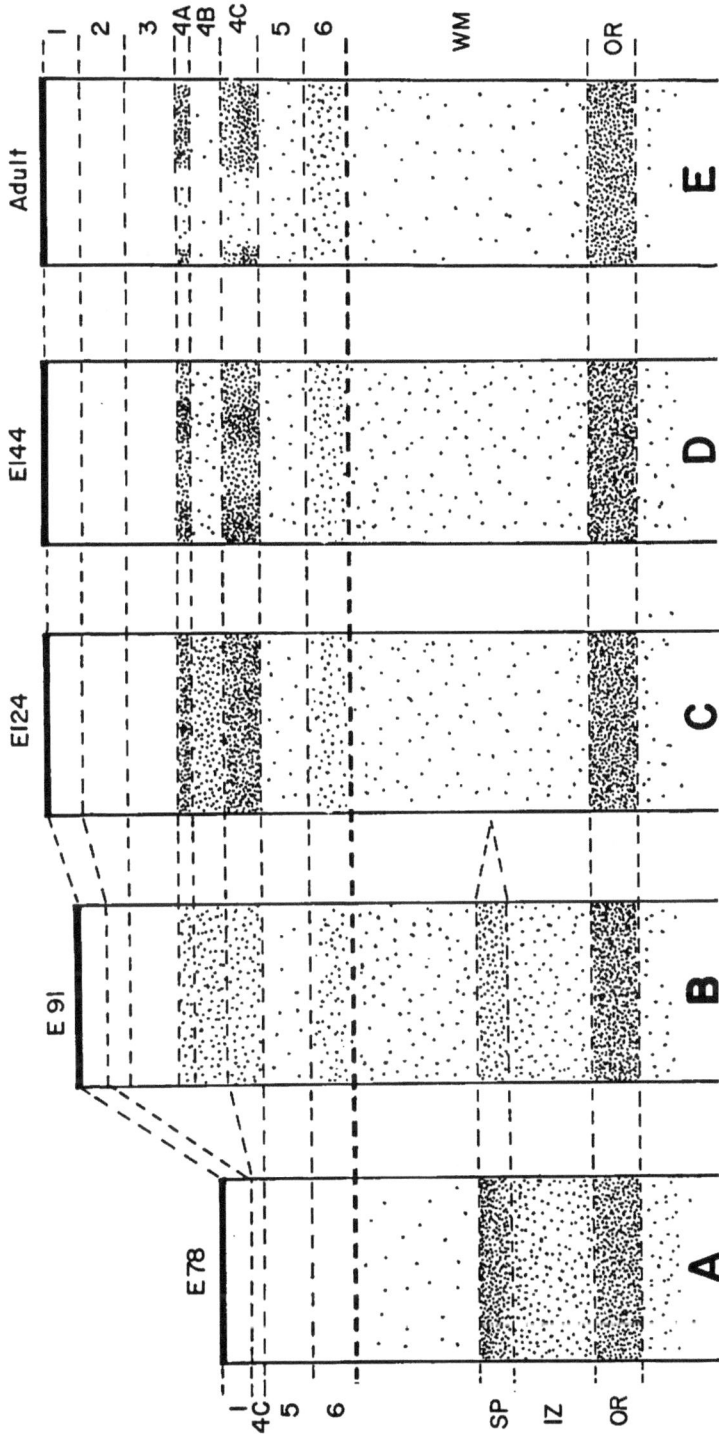

Figure 9 Semidiagrammatic summary of the development of geniculocortical connections and ocular-dominance columns in the occipital lobe of the rhesus monkey from the end of the first half of pregnancy to adulthood. Each drawing [(A) to (E)] illustrates a portion of the lateral cerebral wall in the region of area 17 as seen in autoradiograms of animals that had received unilateral eye injections of a mixture of [³H]-proline and [³H]-fucose 14 days earlier. The age of animals at the time of sacrifice is provided at the top of each drawing in embryonic (E) and postnatal (P) days. Cortical layers I–VI are delineated according to Brodmann's (1905) classification. Note that at E78 the cortical plate consists of only layers VI, V, and a portion of IVC. Abbreviations: OR, optical radiation; SP, deep portion of subplate layer; WM, white matter. (From Rakic, 1980.)

through the transient axonal compartment, which consists of thalamic fibers, and have àn opportunity to make contact with their prospective synaptic partners. The significance of this temporary interaction in the intermediate zone for the establishment of eventual permanent synaptic connectivity in the cortex is unknown.

In a slightly older specimen (E91) some geniculocortical axons have invaded the territory of the primary visual cortex. They are uniformly distributed within layer IV, and do not display evidence of preferential horizontal segregation into ocular-dominance stripes or vertical segregation into layers IVA and IVC (Figure 9B). After all cortical neurons destined for the primary visual cortex have been generated (Rakic, 1974) and have attained their final positions (Rakic, 1975), the number of LGd axons entering the cortex increases, so that somewhere between E110 and E124 vertical segregation into sublayers IVA and IVC becomes apparent (Figure 9C). However, alternating territories corresponding to ocular-dominance stripes are not yet discernible at this age (Figure 9C).

The vertical segregation of input into sublayers IVA and IVC becomes even more visible in a fetus injected about three weeks later, at E130, and sacrificed at E144 (Figure 9D). Most important, however, the horizontal segregation of axons carrying input from the two eyes into incipient ocular-dominance stripes begins to emerge. Although a subtle fluctuation in density of grains is difficult to discern upon simple inspection of the slides, grain counts per unit area expose alternating 250–300-μm-wide territories containing higher and lower grain densities (Rakic, 1976a). The process of segregation of geniculocortical afferents into ocular-dominance stripes continues during the immediate postnatal period and is completed by about three weeks of age (Hubel, Wiesel, and LeVay, 1977), when the final pattern, present in the adult, is attained (Figure 9E). It has subsequently been shown that the process of segregation of the geniculocortical projection obeys a similar progression in the visual cortex of the cat, except that corresponding stages occur later with respect to birth (LeVay, Stryker, and Shatz, 1978).

Based on our study of monkey fetuses, the development of specific thalamic afferent connections can be divided into three phases. In the first phase, axons enter the occipital lobe and become distributed in the "waiting" compartment. In the second phase, thalamic axons enter the cortex but their endings are distributed in layer IV in a diffuse manner; in the third phase, the axon terminals become segregated into patterned territories (e.g., IVA and IVC and ocular-dominance stripes). Each phase is not only separated in time, but apparently governed by different genetic mechanisms since one can be eliminated by experimental manipulation without disturbing the other (Rakic, 1979).

The existence of the "waiting" compartments and the process of segregation from a diffuse to a patterned termination of neuronal connections is apparently not confined to the visual system. Thus, the cells of origin of the corpus callosum seem to be initially widespread (Innocenti, Fiore, and Caminiti, 1977), and callosal columns of the frontal association cortex are initially continuously distributed before becoming segregated in the second half of gestation (Goldman-Rakic, this volume). Likewise, in the pyriform cortex, olfactory and association input initially overlap before becoming separated into different strata of the molecular layer (Price, Moxley, and Schwob, 1976). Intricate corticocaudate projections in forms of patches and rings described in the neostriatum of postnatal monkeys (Goldman and Nauta, 1977) are also initially diffuse during fetal stages (Goldman-Rakic, 1980, and this volume). Therefore, the phenomenon of transformation from diffuse to patterned organization of neuronal connections may be a general principle of synaptic development (Goldman-Rakic, 1980).

The mechanism for segregation of terminals is not known. Selective cell death and rearrangement of synaptic contacts are among the mechanisms that have been most often considered. At present, it is likely that segregation may develop by way of transient synaptic arrangements. Temporary synapses have been described during development of connections in the visual system (LeVay and Stryker, 1979), spinal cord (Knyihar, Csillik, and Rakic, 1978), and other systems (e.g., Ramón y Cajal, 1911; Giordano and Cunningham, 1978; Changeux and Danchin, 1976; Rakic, 1979), and this mechanism most likely is also involved during development of cortical connections. However, the sheer size and complexity of connections within the neocortex have so far precluded more detailed studies of synaptogenesis in this important structure. The application of new techniques, approaches, and models for study, as well as a renewed interest in the mammalian neocortex, promises a new and exciting future in this field.

Acknowledgments

This study was supported by National Institutes of Health Grants NS 14841 and EY 02593. Pregnant monkeys were obtained from New England Regional Primate Research Center, Southborough, Massachusetts. I am thankful to Dr. P. K. Seghal for his generous help in surgery and care of animals.

References

Angevine, J. B., Jr., and R. L. Sidman, 1961. Autoradiographic study of cell migration during histogenesis of cerebral cortex in the mouse. *Nature* 192:766–768.

Antanitus, D. B., B. H. Choi, and L. W. Lapham, 1976. The demonstration of glial fibrillary acidic protein in the cerebrum of the human fetus by indirect immunofluorescence. *Brain Res.* 103:613–616.

Berry, M. and A. W. Rogers, 1965. The migration of neuroblasts in the developing cortex. *J. Anat.* 99:691–709.

Brodmann, K., 1905. Beitrage zur histologischen Lokalization der Grosshirnride. Dritte Mitteilung: Die Rinderfelder niederen Affen. *J. Psychol. Neurol. Leipzig* 9:177–226.

Caviness, V. S., Jr., and P. Rakic, 1978. Mechanisms of cortical development: a view from mutations in mice. *Ann. Rev. Neurosci.* 1:279–326.

Changeux, J.-P., and A. Danchin, 1976. Selective stabilization of developing synapses as mechanism for the specification of neuronal networks. *Nature* 264:705–712.

Cowan, W. M., D. I. Gottlieb, A. Hendrickson, J. L. Price, and T. A. Woolsey, 1972. The autoradiographic demonstration of axonal connections in the CNS. *Brain Res.* 37:21–51.

Edelman, G. M., 1979. Group selection and phasic reentrant signaling: A theory of higher brain function. In *The Neurosciences: Fourth Study Program.* F. O. Schmitt and F. G. Worden, eds. Cambridge, MA: MIT Press, pp. 1115–1144.

Flechsig, P., 1920. *Anatomie des menschichen Gehirns und Ruckenmarks auf myelogenetischer Grundlage.* Leipzig: George Thieme.

Giordano, D. L., and T. J. Cunningham, 1978. Naturally occurring neuron death in the superior colliculus of the postnatal rat. *Anat. Rec.* 190:402.

Goldman, P. S., and T. W. Galkin, 1978. Prenatal removal of frontal association cortex in the rhesus monkey: Anatomical and functional consequences in postnatal life. *Brain Res.* 52:451–485.

Goldman, P. S., and W. J. H. Nauta, 1977. An intricately patterned prefrontocaudate projection in the rhesus monkey. *J. Comp. Neurol.* 171:369–386.

Goldman-Rakic, P., 1980. Prenatal development of cortico-striatal connections in the rhesus monkeys: Transformation from diffuse to patterned projections. (Submitted for publication.)

Grafstein, B., 1971. Transneuronal transfer of radioactivity in the central nervous system. *Science* 172:177–179.

Hicks, S. P., and C. J. D'Amato, 1968. Cell migrations to the isocortex in the rat. *Anat. Rec.* 160:619–634.

Hubel, D. H., T. N. Wiesel, and S. LaVay, 1977. Plasticity of ocular dominance columns in monkey striate cortex. *Phil. Trans. Roy. Soc. B* 278:377.

Innocenti, G. M., L. Fiore, and R. Caminiti, 1977. Exuberant projection into corpus callosum from the visual cortex of newborn cats. *Neurosci. Lett.* 4:237–242.

Knyihar, E., B. Csillik, and P. Rakic, 1978. Transient synapses in the embryonic primate spinal cord. *Science* 202:1206–1209.

Kostovic, I., J. Krmpotic-Nemanic, and Z. Kelovic, 1975. The early development of glia in human neocortex. *Rad. Jug. Akad. Znan. Umijet. Natural Science Series* 17:155–159.

LeVay, S., and M. P. Stryker, 1979. The development of ocular dominance columns in the cat. In *Aspects of Developmental Neurobiology.* J. A. Fernandelli, ed. Bethesda: Society of Neuroscience Symposia 4, pp. 83–97.

LeVay, S., M. P. Stryker, and C. J. Shatz, 1978. Ocular dominance columns and their development in layer IV of the cat's visual cortex: A quantitative study. *J. Comp. Neurol.* 179:223–244.

Levitt, P. R., and P. Rakic, 1980. Immunoperoxidase localization of glial fibrillary acid protein in radial glial cells and astrocytes of the developing rhesus monkey brain. *J. Comp. Neurol.* (in press).

Lund, R. D., 1976. The development of laminar connections in the mammalian visual cortex. *Exp. Brain Res. Suppl.* 1:255–258.

Mountcastle, V. B., 1979. An organizing principle for cerebral function: The unit module and the distributed system. In *The Neurosciences: Fourth Study Program.* F. O. Schmitt and F. G. Worden, eds. Cambridge, MA: MIT Press, pp. 21–42.

Nowakowski, R. S., and P. Rakic, 1980. Site of origin and route and rate of migration of neurons to the hippocampal region of the rhesus monkey. *J. Comp. Neurol.* (submitted for publication).

Poliakov, G. I., 1965. Development of the cerebral neocortex during first half of intrauterine life. In *Development of the Child's Brain.* S. A. Sarkisov, ed. Leningrad: Medicina, pp. 22–52. [In Russian.]

Preobrazhenskaya, N. S., 1965. Occipital area, lateral geniculate body, pulvinar, and other subcortical structures of the visual analyser. In *Development of the Child's Brain.* S. A. Sarkisov, ed. Leningrad: Medicina, pp. 87–127. [In Russian.]

Price, J. L., G. F. Moxley, and J. E. Schwob, 1976. Development and plasticity of complementary afferent fiber systems to the olfactory cortex. *Exp. Brain Res. Suppl.* 1:148–154.

Rakic, P., 1974. Neurons in rhesus monkey visual cortex: Systematic relation between 33:471–476.

Rakic, P., 1972. Mode of cell migration to the superficial layers of fetal monkey neocortex. *J. Comp. Neurol.* 145:61–84.

Rakic, P., 1973. Kinetics of proliferation and latency between final division and onset of differentiation of the cerebellar stellate and basket neurons. *J. Comp. Neurol.* 147:523–546.

Rakic, P., 1974. Neurons in rhesus monkey visual cortex: systematic relation between time of origin and eventual disposition. *Science* 183:425–427.

Rakic, P., 1975. Timing of major ontogenetic events in the visual cortex of the rhesus monkey. In *Brain Mechanisms in Mental Retardation.* N. A. Buchwald, and M. Brazier, eds. New York: Academic Press, pp. 3–40.

Rakic, P., 1976a. Prenatal genesis of connections subserving ocular dominance in the rhesus monkey. *Nature* 261:467–471.

Rakic, P., 1976b. Differences in the time of origin and in eventual distribution of neurons in areas 17 and 18 of visual cortex in rhesus monkey. *Exp. Brain Res. Suppl.* 1:244–248.

Rakic, P., 1977a. Genesis of the dorsal lateral geniculate nucleus in the rhesus monkey: Site and time of origin, kinetics of proliferation, routes of migration and pattern of distribution of neurons. *J. Comp. Neurol.* 176:23–52.

Rakic, P., 1977b. Prenatal development of the visual system in the rhesus monkey. *Phil. Trans. Roy. Soc. B* 278:245–260.

Rakic, P., 1977c. Effects of prenatal unilateral eye enucleation on the formation of layers and retinal connections in the dorsal lateral geniculate nucleus (LGd) of the rhesus monkey. *Neuroscience Abst.* 3:573.

Rakic, P., 1978. Neuronal migration and contact guidance in primate telencephalon. *Postgrad. Med. J.* 54:25–40.

Rakic, P., 1979. Genetic and epigenetic determinants of local neuronal circuits in the mammalian central nervous system. In *The Neurosciences: Fourth Study Program*. F. O. Schmitt, and F. G. Worden, eds. Cambridge, MA: MIT Press, pp. 109–127.

Rakic, P., 1980. Mode of genesis of central visual connections revealed by orthograde axonal flow and transneuronal transport of radioactive tracers following unilateral eye injection in temporarily exteriorized monkey fetuses. (In preparation.)

Rakic, P., and R. L. Sidman, 1968. Supravital DNA synthesis in the developing human and mouse brain. *J. Neuropath. Exp. Neurol.* 27:246–276.

Ramón y Cajal, S., 1911. *Histologie du système nerveux de l'homme et des vertébrés.* Paris: Maloine. [Reprinted by Consejo Superior de Investigaciones Científicas, Madrid, 1955, Vols. I and II.]

Schmechel, D. E., and P. Rakic, 1979a. Arrested proliferation of radial glial cells during midgestation in rhesus monkey. *Nature* 277:303–305.

Schmechel, D. E., and P. Rakic, 1979b. A Golgi study of radial glial cells in developing monkey telencephalon: Morphogenesis and transformation into astrocytes. *Anat. Embryol.* 156:115–152.

Shatz, C., and P. Rakic, 1978. Prenatal development of efferent projections from the visual cortex in the rhesus monkey. *Neurosci. Abst.* 4:654.

Sidman, R. L., and P. Rakic, 1973. Neuronal migration, with special reference to developing human brains: A review. *Brain Res.* 62:1–35.

Varon, S. S., and G. G. Somjen, 1979. Neuron-glia interaction. *Neurosci. Res. Prog. Bull.* 17:1–239.

Wiesel, T. N., D. H. Hubel, and D. M. K. Lam, 1974. Autoradiographic demonstration of ocular dominance columns in the monkey striate cortex by means of transneuronal transport. *Brain Res.* 79:273–279.

Wise, S. P., and E. G. Jones, 1976. The organization and postnatal development of the commissural projection of the rat somatic sensory cortex. *J. Comp. Neurol.* 168:313–344.

2

The Postnatal Development and Plasticity of Ocular-Dominance Columns in the Monkey

Simon LeVay, Torsten N. Wiesel, and David H. Hubel

ABSTRACT In the striate cortex of the newborn macaque monkey, ocular-dominance columns are only partially formed. Their further development, which involves the sorting out of the terminals of the left- and right-eye geniculocortical afferents into alternating, parallel bands in layer IVC, is complete by 3 to 6 weeks of postnatal age. Monocular lid suture at birth causes the afferents to sort out into bands of unequal width, those for the open eye being about three times wider than the bands for the closed eye. Besides distorting the normal sorting process, monocular deprivation can also cause a reexpansion of afferents that have already segregated out into columns. This latter kind of plasticity may be demonstrated both in normal animals, by later eye closures, and in animals deprived monocularly from birth, by reverse suture.

Introduction

In view of the prolonged gestation period in monkeys, and the elaborate, orderly sequence of developmental events that take place in utero (see the chapter by Rakic, in this volume), it is not surprising that at the time of birth the visual cortex displays a considerable functional maturity. Recordings from very young, visually inexperienced monkeys (Wiesel and Hubel, 1974) have demonstrated the same map of the visual field, the same receptive field types, the same selectivity for stimulus orientation, and the same orderly arrangement of orientation columns as are found in adult animals.

In one important aspect of their physiology, however, cortical neurons in newborn macaque monkeys are not fully mature. This is their eye preference or ocular dominance. The visual cortex of adult monkeys is parcellated into vertical columns, within which cells respond better to stimulation of one eye or the other. This pattern of organization is most well defined in layer IVC, the layer which receives most of the specific visual afferents from the lateral geniculate nucleus. If an electrode is passed horizontally along layer IVC, in an adult monkey, one records responses to one eye only, for a few hundred micrometers; then there is an abrupt shift to the other eye, which dominates completely for about

SIMON LEVAY, TORSTEN N. WIESEL, and DAVID H. HUBEL Department of Neurobiology, Harvard Medical School, Boston, Massachusetts 02115

the same distance, and so on for as long as the electrode remains within the layer. In the layers above and below layer IVC, the basic columnar pattern of organization is similar, but there is more mixing of the influence of the two eyes, as if the second-order projections from layer IVC to the other layers are predominantly vertical (intracolumnar) but also include some oblique (intercolumnar) axons. In newborn monkeys (Hubel, Wiesel, and LeVay, 1977) similar tangential penetrations in layer IVC revealed the same basic columnar organization, but there was considerable mixing of left- and right-eye activity, such as is never seen in adults, and column boundaries were poorly defined. The probable anatomical basis for this difference between newborn and adult monkeys has been demonstrated by autoradiography, after injection of one eye with [^{3}H]-fucose or [^{3}H]-proline. Such injections label by transneuronal transport the complete set of geniculocortical afferents serving the injected eye (Specht and Grafstein, 1973; Wiesel, Hubel, and Lam, 1974), and in adult monkeys they give, in tangential sections of layer IVC, a pattern of sharply defined, more or less parallel bands, each about 400 μm wide and separated by unlabeled bands of the same width. These labeled and unlabeled bands have been shown by combined physiology and autoradiography to correspond precisely to the ocular-dominance columns for the injected and the noninjected eyes. In newborn monkeys similar injections produced a cortical labeling pattern that is continuous throughout the extent of layer IVC, although a periodic waxing and waning in grain density was seen, as if the two sets of afferents were in the process of sorting themselves out. Rakic (1976) has been able to study earlier stages of this sequence by injecting the eyes of fetal monkeys. Initially, the left- and right-eye afferents are completely intermingled, and traces of a columnar pattern appear by about 3 weeks before birth.

It is tempting to try to relate the lateness of development of ocular-dominance columns to their remarkable plasticity shown in response to monocular visual deprivation in infancy (Wiesel and Hubel, 1963; Hubel and Wiesel, 1970; Hubel, Wiesel, and LeVay, 1977; Shatz and Stryker, 1978). Such deprivation leads to a loss of responsiveness of most cortical neurons to stimulation of the deprived eye, and a corresponding increase in the influence of the seeing eye. Anatomically, the afferents for the seeing eye occupy abnormally wide bands in layer IVC (about 650 μm instead of 400 μm) and the afferents for the closed eye occupy narrow, fragmented bands (about 150 μm). The unequal visual input via the deprived and seeing eyes apparently allows the geniculocortical afferents for the seeing eye to gain control of a disproportionate share of their target neurons in the cortex.

It has been thought that the effects of monocular deprivation depend on some kind of competitive interaction between the left- and right-eye afferents that is operative during normal postnatal life. Such an interaction would explain why monocular deprivation leads, not merely to a reduction in the effectiveness of the closed eye, but also to an increase in the influence of the open eye and an expansion of its afferents in layer IVC. It would also account for the observation that *binocular* deprivation, though certainly detrimental to cortical function, has far less effect than might be predicted by summing the effects of separate left- and right-eye closures (Wiesel and Hubel, 1965). A competitive interaction may most easily be imagined to take place when the left- and right-eye afferents are in close proximity, particularly if they converge on the same target cells. As described above, this is the situation in the fourth layer of newborn monkeys, but not in adults. Thus one is presented with a potential explanation for the greater susceptibility of very young animals to the effects of monocular deprivation: it might be that such deprivation allows the seeing eye to gain sole possession of regions of binocular overlap in layer IVC, but does not allow its afferents to reinvade territory which has already become the possession of the other eye.

We have tested this idea by examining the time course of normal columnar development in the rhesus monkey, and by determining the effects of lid suture instituted at various postnatal ages. One would predict that the anatomical effect of lid suture would vary according to the state of columnar development at the time of suture, and the age of completion of the normal segregation process would also be the age at which anatomical effects could no longer be produced by monocular deprivation. In addition, we have asked whether the effects of monocular deprivation, once established, can be reversed by reopening the deprived eye and closing the experienced eye. A physiological recovery can be induced by reverse suture, if performed early enough (Blakemore and Van Sluyters, 1974; Blakemore, Garey, and Vital-Durand, 1978). We would predict, however, by the model described above, that recovery would not be possible once the initial period of deprivation had induced the segregation of the two sets of afferents into their abnormal pattern of wide and narrow bands. The present chapter summarizes the results of these experiments; a fuller account is presented elsewhere (LeVay, Wiesel, and Hubel, 1980).

Normal Development

The process of segregation of the left- and right-eye afferents into ocular-dominance columns is illustrated in Figure 1, which shows autoradiographs of tangential sections of the visual cortex of three monkeys, aged 1, 3, and 6 weeks. Each of them had received an injection of [³H]-proline or [³H]-fucose into the ipsilateral eye about 1 week previously. The autoradiographs show a progressive sharpening of the columnar pattern. At 1 week of age, the label is distributed continuously, but the periodic waxing and waning in grain density is an indication that the process of segregation is already under way. By 3 weeks the

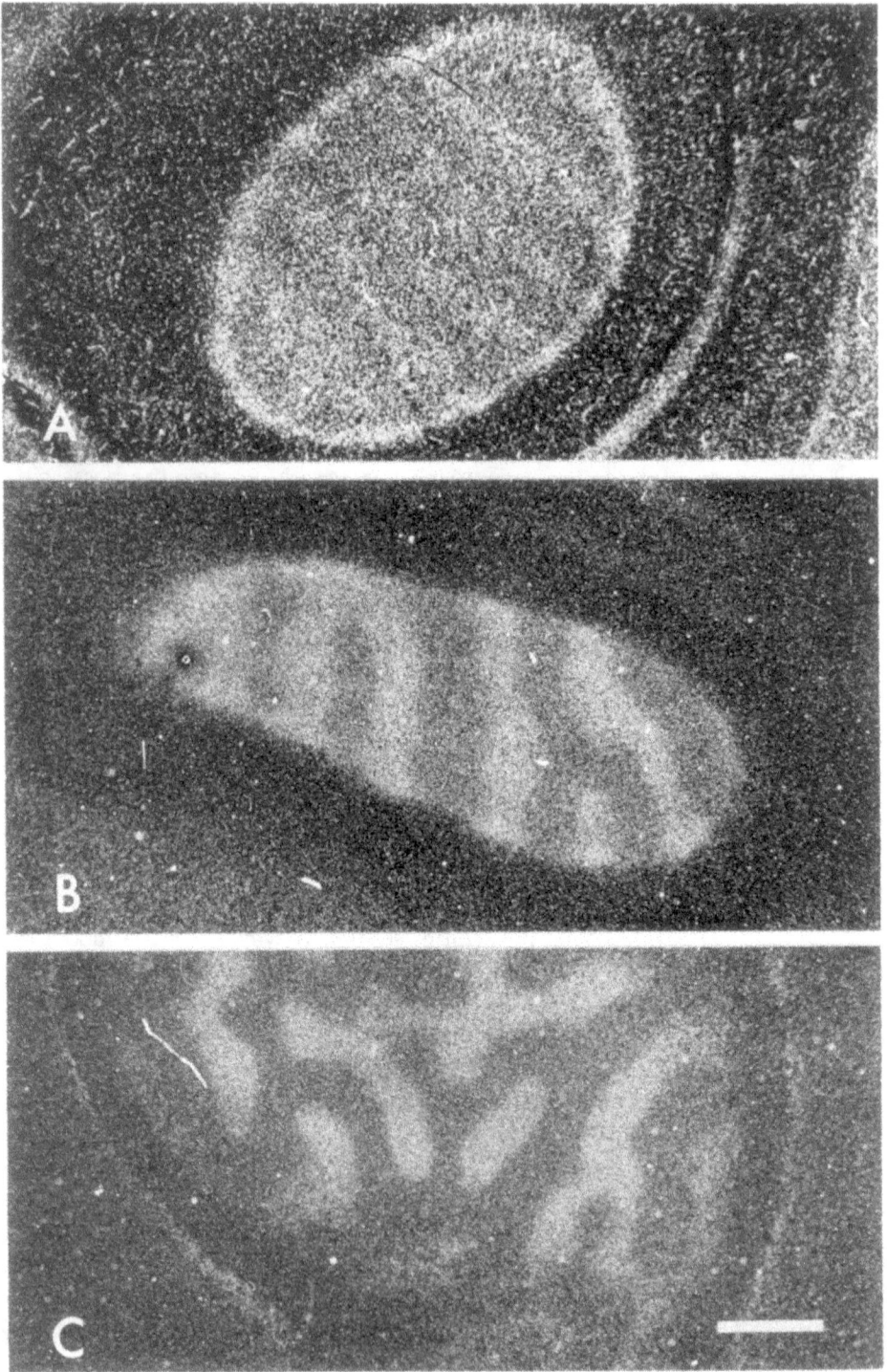

Figure 1 The normal postnatal development of ocular-dominance columns studied autoradiographically. These are single tangential sections, grazing layer IVC, from the striate cortex ipsilateral to the injected eye in rhesus monkeys aged 1 week (A), 3 weeks (B), and 6 weeks (C). In the 1-week-old monkey the emerging columns are visible only as

columnar pattern is much sharper; in fact the only difference from the adult pattern is a slight lack of definition of the borders of columns. By 6 weeks the labeling pattern is as sharp as in adults. On the contralateral side the process seems to lag slightly, and even at 6 weeks there is a little more label in the gaps between labeled bands than there was on the ipsilateral side.

In a previous study of the same developmental process in the cat (LeVay, Stryker, and Shatz, 1978), evidence was produced that in young animals the transneuronal labeling pattern is degraded to some extent by leakage of labeled compounds between laminae of the lateral geniculate nucleus. This leakage (spillover) was considerably more severe on the contralateral than on the ipsilateral side. Although we have not measured spillover in monkeys, we suspect that it accounts for the difference in the cortical labeling pattern on the two sides, and that the labeling pattern on the ipsilateral side is the more faithful image of the distribution of the geniculocortical afferents. Thus we believe that the left- and right-eye afferents are partially overlapping at 1 week, are nearly completely segregated by 3 weeks, and are completely so by 6 weeks of age.

This conclusion is supported by the results of physiological experiments in which tangential electrode penetrations were made in layer IVC and the ocular dominance of single units or (more commonly) multiunit activity was determined. At 1 week of age a columnar organization in layer IVC was already detectable, and in fact some small regions already responded only to stimulation of one or the other eye. Mixed left- and right-eye activity was recorded, however, at the majority of sites. At 3 weeks, the physiology was only slightly different from that of an adult. A reconstruction of an electrode penetration is shown in Figure 2. As the electrode traversed successive columns, ocular dominance swung from complete left-eye to complete right-eye dominance and back. The transition, however, was rather less sharp than is seen in adults, and at one recording site a binocularly activated single unit was recorded. (In adults, all single units that can be isolated in layer IVC are monocular.) Recordings from a 6-week-old monkey gave results that were indistinguishable from those obtained in adults.

Effects of Lid Suture at Different Ages

We examined the effects of monocular deprivation begun at various ages in ten monkeys. The right eye was closed at ages ranging from 2 days to adult, and the animals were allowed to survive for at least several months after the operation.

---

a gentle fluctuation in labeling density, even though the micrograph was printed at relatively high contrast. At 3 weeks the columnar pattern is much clearer, but the borders of the labeled bands are slightly less sharply defined than in adults. At 6 weeks the picture is indistinguishable from that seen in adults. Bar = 1 mm.

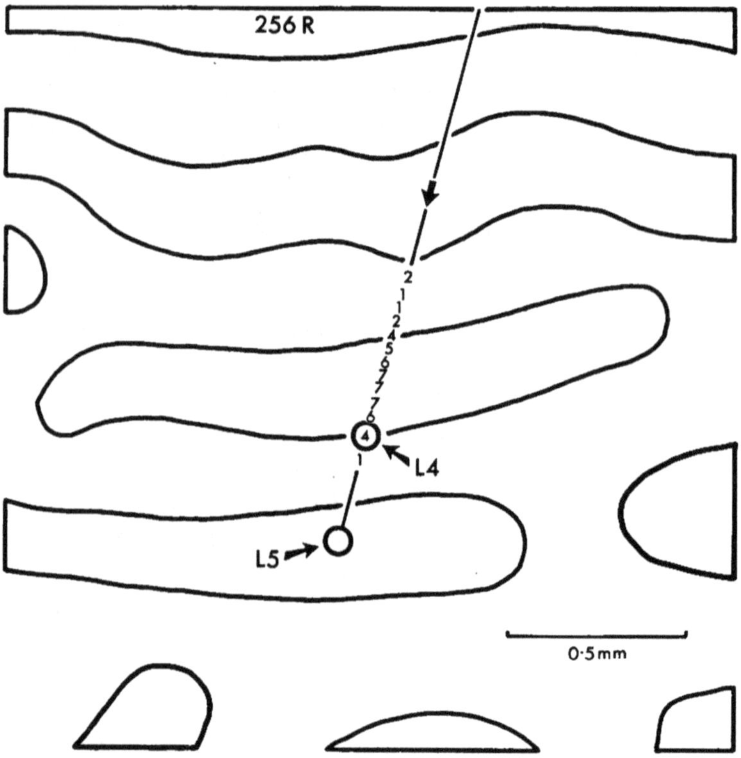

Figure 2 The state of columnar development in layer IVC, studied physiologically, at 3 weeks postnatal age. This is a reconstruction in surface view of part of an electrode penetration that traveled tangentially in layer IVC. The string of numbers gives the ocular dominance of the neural activity (mostly multiunit) recorded at various positions along the track (within layer IVC only). The circles marked L1 and L2 are the positions of electrolytic lesions; only L1 marks a transition in ocular dominance; L2 marks the end of the penetration. Also reconstructed is the autoradiographic labeling pattern in the area. The labeled bands (columns for the ipsilateral eye) are shown closed off at the borders of the figure; the unlabeled bands for the contralateral eye are left open. Eye preference swung from one extreme of ocular dominance to the other, as the electrode traversed successive columns, but, compared with the adult, the zones of overlap of left- and right-eye activity at column borders were rather wide. For a more detailed description of the physiological results in this and the other animals, see LeVay, Wiesel, and Hubel (1980).

Anatomically, closures performed at any age up to and including $5\frac{1}{2}$ weeks had approximately the same effect; the layer-IVC bands for the nondeprived eye were enlarged, and those for the deprived eye were shrunken (Figure 3A,B). The ratio of the cortical areas occupied by the experienced and deprived eyes, measured from the autoradiographs, was about $3:1$, a marked difference from the normal value of $1:1$.

The physiological picture in layer IVC closely matched the autoradiography. On tangential penetrations, relatively long stretches in which activity was completely dominated by the experienced eye alternated with short regions in which responses to the deprived eye were obtained. During the penetrations, marking lesions were made at points of transition in eye preference. These lesions were used to reconstruct the tracks histologically and to match them to the autoradiographic labeling pattern in the area. An example of such a track re-

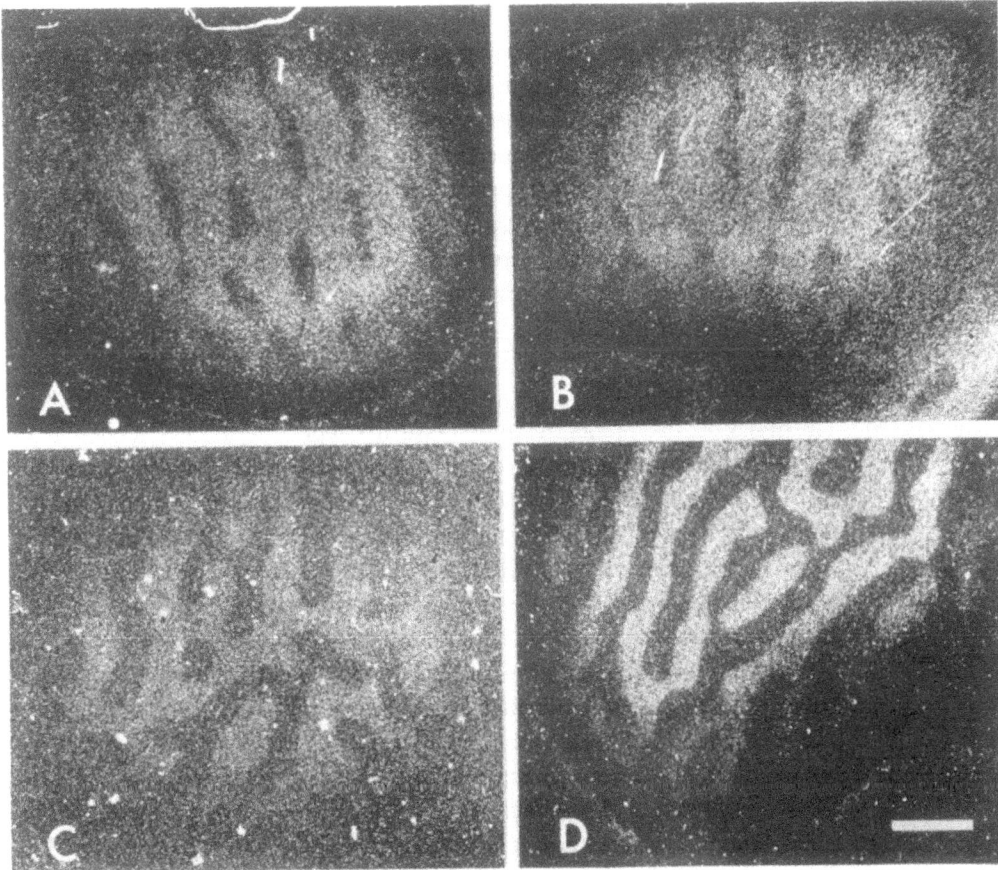

Figure 3 The anatomical effects of long-term monocular deprivation begun at 2 weeks (A), $5\frac{1}{2}$ weeks (B), 10 weeks (C), and adult (D). In each case the nondeprived eye was injected. The main decline in susceptibility to the anatomical effects of deprivation occurs between $5\frac{1}{2}$ and 10 weeks, although even at the latter age there was a small expansion of the open-eye's afferents in the hemisphere ipsilateral to the lid suture. The picture in (D) is indistinguishable from normal. Bar = 1 mm.

construction, from the monkey deprived at 5½ weeks, is shown in Figure 4. It seems then that, as in normal animals, the eye preference of layer-IVC cells is dictated by the distribution of left- and right-eye geniculate afferents, and is not greatly influenced by intracortical connections. There were no obvious differences in the effects of deprivation on the α and β sublaminae of layer IVC, the divisions that receive the afferents from the magno- and parvocellular laminae of the lateral geniculate nucleus.

In the layers above and below layer IVC, the influence of the deprived eye was very weak indeed: the vast majority of cells responded exclusively to the open eye. It seems as if there had been a further weakening of the projections from layer IVC to the other layers, within the deprived eye's columns.

Closures at later ages had progressively less effect. Thus a closure at 10 weeks led to only a modest expansion of the columns for the nondeprived eye (Figure 3C), and this expansion was limited to the right hemisphere (ipsilateral to the deprived eye). As before, the layers above and below layer IVC were dominated almost entirely by the left eye. Closure at a year of age did not induce any changes in column width in layer IVC, although there was still a moderate swing in eye preference toward the nondeprived eye in the upper cortical layers. Monocular suture in an adult monkey led to no detectable anatomical or physiological changes (Figure 3D). Even monocular eye enucleation, in an adult, did not induce sprouting of the geniculocortical afferents for the other eye.

Reverse Suture

To interpret the results of reverse-suture experiments it is necessary to know the state of the ocular-dominance columns after the initial period of deprivation, that is, at the time of the reversal. We therefore first studied monkeys whose right eyes were closed from shortly after birth until 3 or 6 weeks of age. The three monkeys deprived from birth to 3 weeks of age showed a physiological picture very similar to that seen after long-term deprivation: that is, the great majority of cells outside of layer IVC were driven only by the nondeprived left eye, and within layer IVC tangential penetrations encountered alternating stretches of left-eye and right-eye activity, with the left-eye regions being 2–3 times longer than the right-eye regions. Injection of the left eye produced a labeling pattern of expanded columns in layer IVC, and injection of the right eye (in another animal) labeled shrunken columns (Figure 5A). The picture differed from that seen in long-term deprived animals in that the labeled bands were not as sharply defined and there were more silver grains in the gaps between them. As in the case of the normal 3-week-old monkey, we attribute most of this blurring of the pattern to technical factors, especially to the leakage of radioactivity between

S. LeVay, T. N. Wiesel, and D. H. Hubel

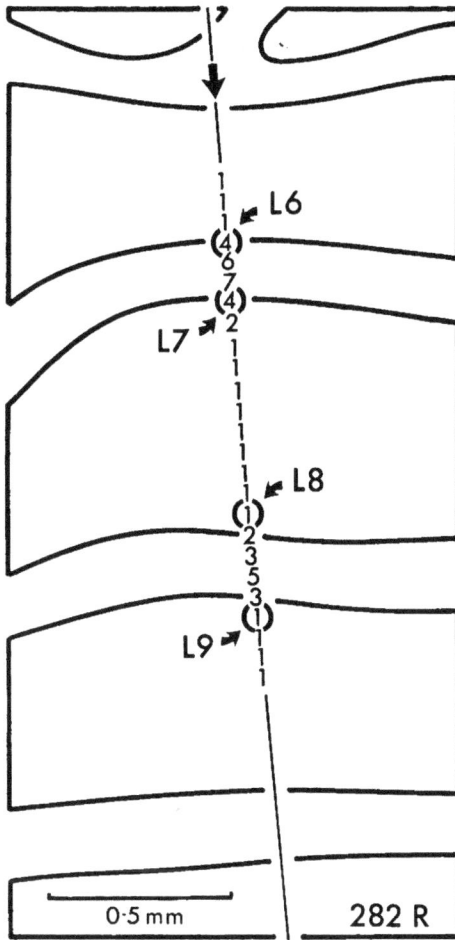

Figure 4 Reconstruction of an electrode track in a monkey whose right eye was closed at 5½ weeks of age. This is the same monkey of which an autoradiograph is shown in Figure 3B. Conventions in the reconstruction are the same as in Figure 2. The contralateral eye dominated completely (ocular dominance group 1) for most of the pass through layer IVC, but there were two short stretches, matching with gaps in the autoradiographic labeling, in which the deprived eye dominated. Only at one point, however, was the influence of the nondeprived eye entirely absent (group 7).

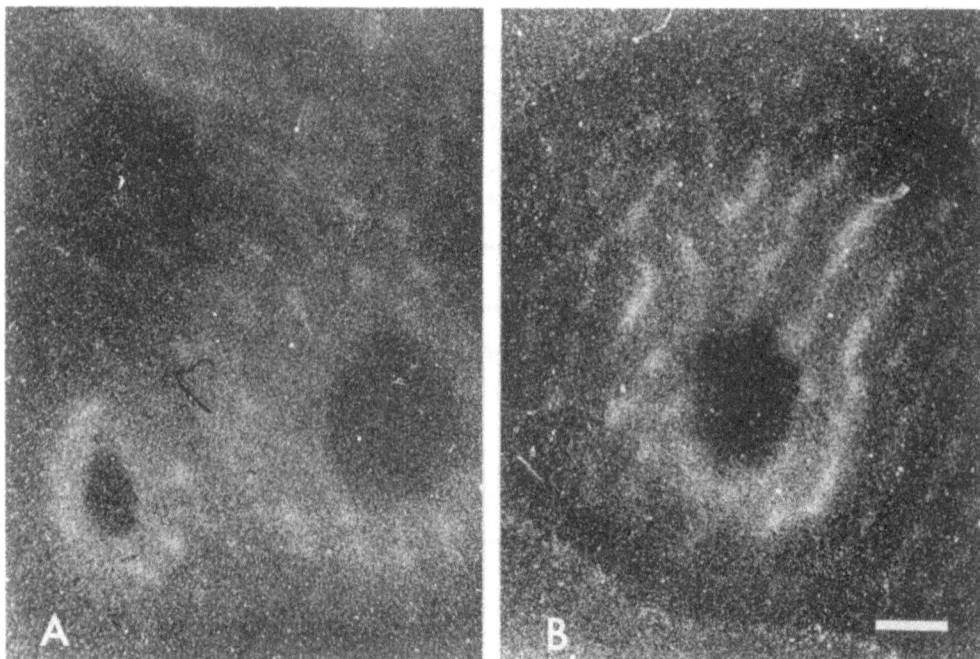

Figure 5 Autoradiographs of the labeling pattern in layer IVC of two monkeys deprived monocularly from the first week of life until 3 weeks (A) and 6 weeks (B) of age. In both cases the deprived eye was injected. Both autoradiographs show a narrowing and fragmentation of the columns for the deprived eye. In (A), the picture is somewhat blurred by the presence of a fairly high grain density in the gaps between the heavily labeled bands; this may be an artifact due to leakage of radioactivity in the lateral geniculate nucleus (see text). In (B), the picture is similar to that seen after long-term deprivation. Scale = 1 mm.

laminae of the lateral geniculate nucleus, but we cannot exclude the possibility that the afferents have not fully settled out into separate columns. After 6 weeks of closure (Figure 5B) the labeling pattern closely resembled that seen after much longer periods of deprivation. Thus columnar development seems to go forward at about the same rate in normal and monocularly deprived animals, being very nearly completed at 3 weeks of age and fully complete by 6 weeks. The difference lies of course in the relative size of the two sets of columns.

Three monkeys were subjected to reverse suture, the reversals being performed at 3 weeks, 6 weeks, and 1 year of age. In each case the right eye was the initially deprived eye, and several months were allowed after the reversal for possible recovery.

In the animal reverse sutured at 3 weeks, the autoradiographic findings were remarkable in that quite different labeling patterns were obtained in the two subdivisions of layer IVC (Figure 6A). The initially deprived right eye had been injected. In layer IVCα, the sublamina that receives the afferents from the magnocellular laminae of the lateral geniculate nucleus (LGN), the injection had led to labeling of ab-

S. LeVay, T. N. Wiesel, and D. H. Hubel

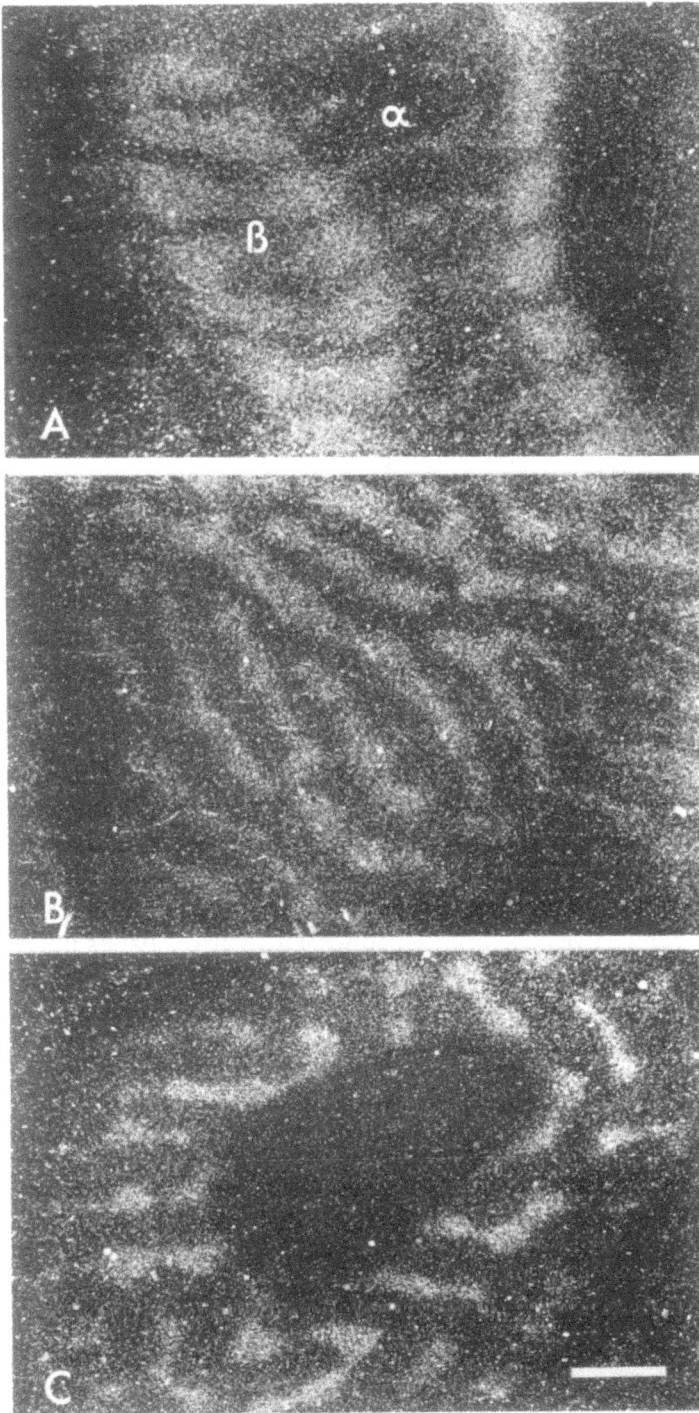

Figure 6 Autoradiographs from three reverse-sutured animals, in each case after injection of the initially deprived eye. In (A), reverse suture was performed at 3 weeks of age. There has been a reexpansion of the columns for the initially deprived eye, but only in the β subdivision of layer IVC. In IVCα the labeled bands are shrunken, indicating a failure of recovery. In (B), reverse suture was performed at 6 weeks of age. There was a recovery, in

normally narrow bands. In layer IVCβ, on the other hand, the sub-lamina that receives the parvocellular afferents, the labeled bands were much wider than normal. The two sets of labeled bands lay in register with each other just as they do in normal animals. It seems therefore that the reverse suture at 3 weeks had induced a reexpansion of the par-vocellular afferents for the deprived eye, so that they actually occupied a greater-than-normal share of the cortical territory, but the operation did not induce any recovery of the magnocellular afferents at all. Physio-logically, most cells in the layers outside of layer IVC were driven only by the right eye, indicating a complete reversal in ocular dominance from the situation at the time of reverse suture. Within layer IVC, both left-eye-and right-eye-dominated regions were encountered, but, on ac-count of unsatisfactory histology, these regions could not be identified with particular columns or sublaminae.

Reverse suture at 6 weeks also led to anatomical and physiological re-covery of the columns for the initially deprived eye. Again, recovery was limited to the parvocellular geniculate afferents. In contrast to the previous monkey, however, the right-eye parvocellular afferents only reexpanded to a normal column width, and did not go beyond that to take over the territory of the later-deprived left eye (Figure 6B). Physio-logically, the picture in layer IVC was in good agreement with the au-toradiography (Figure 7): there were approximately equal-sized regions of left- and right-eye dominance. In the other layers, the initially de-prived eye was strongly dominant, again indicating an almost complete reversal of eye preference with reverse suture at 6 weeks.

Reverse suture at 1 year of age did not seem to produce any signifi-cant recovery. The labeled geniculocortical afferents for the initially de-prived eye still occupied abnormally narrow bands in layer IVC (Figure 6C), and this pattern was confirmed by physiological recording in this layer. In the other layers the left eye, which had been open during the first year of life, dominated very strongly.

Discussion

The results of this study establish an approximate time course both for the sequence of normal development of ocular-dominance columns in the monkey and for the effects of monocular deprivation. The rela-tionship between the two appears to be less simple than we initially had hoped.

The normal process of columnar development, which begins prena-tally (Rakic, 1976), goes to completion quite soon after birth. By 3 weeks

---

IVCβ, of the columns for the initially deprived eye back to an approximately normal size, but not an expansion beyond that as in (A). In (C), reverse suture was performed at 1 year of age. There is little evidence of any anatomical recovery. Bar = 1 mm.

S. LeVay, T. N. Wiesel, and D. H. Hubel

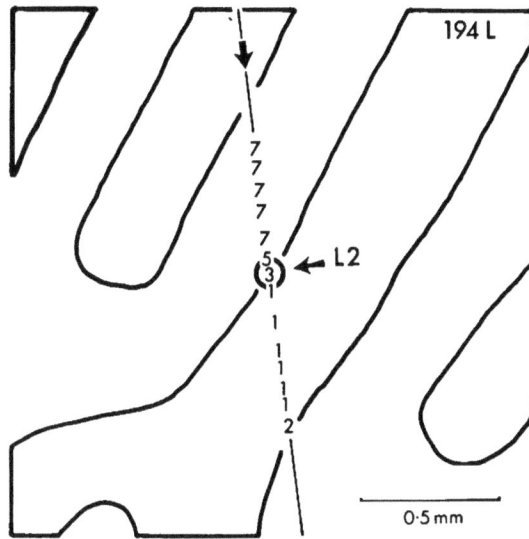

Figure 7 Reconstruction of an electrode pass through layer IVC in the monkey that was reverse sutured at 6 weeks of age. In agreement with the autoradiography, there was a restoration of an approximately even balance between the eyes. Except for the first two recording sites, the pass was entirely within the sublamina IVCβ.

of age the columns in layer IVC differ from those in adult monkeys only in a slight blurring of their borders—a blurring that is seen both in the autoradiographs and in the physiology. By 6 weeks the columns appear fully mature. Columnar development therefore takes place at an earlier age in macaque monkeys than it does in cats: in the latter species segregation does not begin until about 3 weeks of postnatal age, and is completed by about 7 weeks (LeVay, Stryker, and Shatz, 1978). This difference is, of course, consistent with the overall maturity of the monkey's visual system at birth. There may, in fact, be species in which columnar development is completed in utero; the sheep, for example, whose visual system is particularly well developed at birth (Rama-chandran, Clarke, and Whitteridge, 1977) is a likely candidate.

This sequence of normal development appears not to be dependent on visual experience, in the monkey at least, since there is both physiological (Wiesel and Hubel, 1974) and autoradiographic (LeVay, Wiesel, and Hubel, 1980) evidence for the presence of columns in layer IVC in dark-reared or binocularly lid-sutured monkeys. The effects of monocular deprivation should therefore be viewed as a distortion of normal growth processes, and not as evidence for an instructional role of visual experience in cortical development.

When one eye is closed at birth, segregation proceeds at about its normal pace, but most of the retraction is done by the afferents for the deprived eye. The seeing-eye's afferents are thus left in possession of abnormally wide fourth-layer bands, and presumably strengthen their connections within these bands. Of course, the autoradiographic and physiological methods tell us little about the exact nature of the sorting process, either in normal or deprived animals. There is some indication from work on the cat (LeVay and Stryker, 1979) that it may involve a redistribution of terminal branches rather than bulk movements of entire axons.

While the effects of monocular suture at birth can be interpreted in terms of a misrouting of normal development, the set of experiments in which one eye was closed at successively later ages provides evidence for a different kind of plasticity, more akin to axon sprouting. The critical experiments here are the closures at 3, 5½, and 10 weeks. If all that monocular deprivation could do was to allow the open-eye's afferents to obtain sole possession of cortical territory which they still shared with the other eye, then by comparison with the normal series of animals one would expect closure at 3 weeks to have quite a small effect on column size, compared with that of closure at birth, and one would expect closures at 5½ or 10 weeks to have no effect. In fact, closure at 3 and 5½ weeks both had an effect as great as closure at birth, and even the closure at 10 weeks had a small effect on column size, although apparently it was restricted to the hemisphere ipsilateral to the deprived eye. In other words, the period of anatomical plasticity extends beyond the period of overlap of left- and right-eye afferents in layer IVC, even if only by a few weeks. These later closures seem to evoke a reexpansion of the open-eye's afferents into territory which they previously had relinquished. Again, we must emphasize our ignorance of the details of this process—in particular, whether it was an actual reinvasion of entire axons or simply a redistribution of terminals.

The results of the reverse-suture experiments reinforce the conclusion that a reexpansion can occur. The physiological effects of reverse suture have been described previously both for the cat (Blakemore and Van Sluyters, 1974) and for the monkey (Blakemore, Garey, and Vital-Durand, 1978). Our results confirm these studies in showing that the operation, if performed early enough, permits the initially deprived eye to regain its influence and in fact to become the physiologically dominant eye. The autoradiographic results suggest that this recovery involves an actual reexpansion of the shrunken bands in layer IVC. Thus it is not necessary, on the present evidence, to invoke the concept of suppression and derepression of intact synapses in order to explain the effects of reverse suture (Blakemore, Garey, and Vital-Durand, 1978). A more detailed anatomical study is obviously needed, however, to clarify the events occurring in the cortex of reverse-sutured animals.

An interesting aspect of the reverse-suture experiments is the observation that only the parvocellular geniculate afferents, and not the magnocellular afferents, were induced to reexpand. This could mean either that the magnocellular afferents had suffered more severely in the initial period of deprivation, impeding their ability to recover, or that the period of anatomical plasticity simply ends earlier for the magnocellular than for the parvocellular afferents. Whatever the mechanism, a cortex in which the magno- and parvocellular receiving layers are dominated by different eyes offers an unusual opportunity to study the relative contributions of these two sets of afferents to cortical function.

Whether or not the sensitive period ends at different ages in the two sublaminae of layer IVC, a very noticeable difference does exist between layer IVC as a whole and the other cortical layers. In the layers outside of IVC (most of our recordings were from the upper layers) ocular dominance can be influenced by eye closure at 1 year of age and perhaps later, although not in the fully mature animal. We have not studied plasticity in these layers with anatomical techniques, but we would not be surprised if here too the physiological changes were accompanied by changes in the distribution of left- and right-eye afferents, in this case the intracortical projections from layer IVC to the upper layers.

The present study has not pinned down the events responsible for ending the period of anatomical plasticity in the visual cortex. They seem, however, to operate shortly after the segregation of the left- and right-eye geniculocortical afferents is complete, as if the main function of the plastic period were to permit the normal segregation process. Among the morphological events that come into question here are the myelination of the geniculocortical arborizations (LeVay and Stryker, 1979) and the completion of synaptogenesis and spine formation (Cragg, 1972; Boothe et al., 1979). Biochemically, attention has been drawn by the experiments of Kasamatsu and Pettigrew (1979) and Kasamatsu, Pettigrew, and Ary (1979) to a possible role for norepinephrine in cortical plasticity. This concept would be greatly strengthened if changes in endogenous norepinephrine levels, or changes in the distribution of noradrenergic afferents, could be demonstrated to accompany the decline in susceptibility to visual deprivation.

Acknowledgments

This study was supported by National Institutes of Health Grants EY00605, EY00606, and EY01960. S. L. is the recipient of a National Institutes of Health Research Career Development Award.

References

Blakemore, C., and R. C. Van Sluyters, 1974. Reversal of the physiological effects of monocular deprivation in kittens: Further evidence for a sensitive period. *J. Physiol. (London)* 237:195–216.

Blakemore, C., L. J. Garey, and F. Vital-Durand, 1978. The physiological effects of monocular deprivation and their reversal in the monkey's cortex. *J. Physiol. (London)* 261:423–444.

Boothe, R. G., W. T. Greenough, J. S. Lund, and K. Wrege, 1979. A quantitative investigation of spine and dendrite development of neurons in visual cortex (area 17) of *Macaca nemestrina* monkeys. *J. Comp. Neurol.* 186:473–489.

Cragg, B. G., 1972. The development of synapses in cat visual cortex. *Invest. Ophthal.* 11:377–384.

Hubel, D. H., and T. N. Wiesel, 1970. The period of susceptibility to the physiological effects of unilateral eye closure in kittens. *J. Physiol. (London)* 206:419–436.

Hubel, D. H., T. N. Wiesel, and S. LeVay, 1977. Plasticity of ocular dominance columns in monkey striate cortex. *Phil. Trans. Roy. Soc. B* 278:377–409.

Kasamatsu, T., and J. D. Pettigrew, 1979. Preservation of binocularity after monocular deprivation in the striate cortex of kittens treated with 6-hydroxydopamine. *J. Comp. Neurol.* 185:139–162.

Kasamatsu, T., J. D. Pettigrew, and M. Ary, 1979. Restoration of visual cortical plasticity by local microperfusion of norepinephrine. *J. Comp. Neurol.* 185:163–182.

LeVay, S., and M. P. Stryker, 1979. The development of ocular dominance columns in the cat. *Soc. Neurosci. Symp.* 4:83–98.

LeVay, S., M. P. Stryker, and C. J. Shatz, 1978. Ocular dominance columns and their development in layer IV of the cat's visual cortex: A quantitative study. *J. Comp. Neurol.* 179:223–244.

LeVay, S., T. N. Wiesel, and D. H. Hubel, 1980. The development of ocular dominance columns in normal and visually deprived monkeys. *J. Comp. Neurol.* (in press).

Rakic, P., 1976. Prenatal genesis of connections subserving ocular dominance in the rhesus monkey. *Nature* 261:467–471.

Ramachandran, V. S., P. G. H. Clarke, and D. Whitteridge, 1977. Cells selective to binocular disparity in the cortex of newborn lambs. *Nature* 268:333–335.

Shatz, C. J., and M. P. Stryker, 1978. Ocular dominance in layer IV of the cat's visual cortex and the effects of monocular deprivation. *J. Physiol. (London)* 281:267–283.

Specht, S. C., and B. Grafstein, 1973. Accumulation of radioactive protein in mouse cerebral cortex after injection of ^{3}H-fucose into the eye. *Exp. Neurol.* 41:705–722.

Wiesel, T. N., and D. H. Hubel, 1963. Single-cell responses in striate cortex of kittens deprived of vision in one eye. *J. Neurophysiol.* 26:1003–1017.

Wiesel, T. N., and D. H. Hubel, 1965. Comparison of the effects of unilateral and bilateral eye closure on cortical unit responses in kittens. *J. Neurophysiol.* 28:1029–1040.

Wiesel, T. N., and D. H. Hubel, 1974. Ordered arrangement of orientation columns in monkeys lacking visual experience. *J. Comp. Neurol.* 158:307–318.

Wiesel, T. N., D. H. Hubel, and D. M.-K. Lam, 1974. Autoradiographic demonstration of ocular-dominance columns in the monkey striate cortex by means of transneuronal transport. *Brain Res.* 79:273–279.

3

Induced Ocular-Dominance Zones in Tectal Cortex

Martha Constantine-Paton

ABSTRACT   Work on the tectal cortex of the frog is presented as an experimental system in which to study the periodic segregation of afferent projections. Retinal ganglion-cell terminals will segregate as interdigitating eye-specific bands within the optic fiber layers of the frog optic tectum whenever two eyes are forced to innervate a single tectal lobe. This segregation develops from an initial state of overlap, and electrophysiological studies indicate that both retinas maintain a roughly normal topographical projection onto the banded tecta.

Banded frog tecta are strikingly similar to the ocular-dominance columns of cat and monkey visual cortex. However, two retinas never project throughout one tectal lobe in normal *Rana*; thus this frog never shows, nor has it any need for, tectal ocular-dominance zones. Our results suggest that the cellular interactions which produce periodic input segregation may be common to most instances of synaptogenesis, and some possible mechanisms are discussed.

The subdivision of afferent projections into periodic bands of terminal neuropil is emerging as a basic component of organization in diverse regions of the mammalian brain. This segregation has been documented in a variety of commissural and corticocortical projections (Grant, Landgren, and Silfvenius, 1975; Jones, Burton, and Porter, 1975; Shanks, Rockel, and Powell, 1975; Goldman and Nauta, 1977; Imig and Brugge, 1976; Wise and Jones, 1976; Gould, 1978), in projections to the superior colliculus (Goldman and Nauta, 1976; Graybiel, 1975, 1978; Rakic, 1977; Hubel, LeVay, and Wiesel, 1975; Wise and Jones, 1977; Pollack and Hickey, 1979), and in the cerebellum (Voogd, 1969; Oscarsson, 1973; Groenewegen and Voogd, 1977; Groenewegen, Voogd, and Freedman, 1979). However, the ocular-dominance columns of cat and primate visual cortex remain the best known and the most dramatic examples of the striped pattern (Hubel and Wiesel, 1969, 1972, 1978; Wiesel, Hubel, and Lam, 1974; LeVay, Hubel, and Wiesel, 1975; Shatz, Lindström, and Wiesel, 1977; Tigges, Tigges, and Perachio, 1977; Hendrickson, Wilson, and Ogren, 1978; Tigges and Tigges, 1979).

The reports by Drs. Rakic and LeVay in this volume illustrate the considerable information available on the function, the normal develop-

MARTHA CONSTANTINE-PATON   Biology Department, Princeton University, Princeton, New Jersey 08544

ment, and the plasticity of mammalian ocular-dominance columns (Rakic, 1976, 1977; Hubel, Wiesel, and LeVay, 1977; LeVay, Stryker, and Shatz, 1978; Shatz and Stryker, 1978). In the present chapter, I describe an experimentally induced example of banding that is strikingly similar to the neocortical ocular-dominance system, and I discuss the types of cellular interactions that may be involved in establishing this form of terminal organization.

Banding in Three-Eyed Frogs

We work on the retinal afferents to the optic tectum of the anuran amphibian *Rana pipiens*. This pathway has received considerable attention from neuroanatomists and it is consequently well described on both the light- and electron-microscope level (Knapp, Scalia, and Riss, 1965; Lázár and Székely, 1967; Scalia et al., 1968; Potter, 1969, 1972; Lázár, 1971; Székely, Sétáló, and Lázár, 1973; Scalia and Colman, 1974; Scalia and Fite, 1974). Figure 1A is a coronal section through a normal frog's midbrain, and it illustrates the retinotectal synaptic zone with light-microscope autoradiography. Three days prior to sacrifice, this animal's left eye was injected with 10uCi of [^{3}H]-proline. Retinal ganglion-cell terminals appear as a dense black region of developed silver grains that fill the superficial neuropil of the right tectal lobe. The retinotectal projection of normal *Rana pipiens* is crossed except for a few ipsilateral fibers that terminate in the deep laminae of the anterior tectum (Levine, 1980). Consequently there is no label in the left optic tectum of Figure 1A.

In our experiments, the normal anatomy of this system is altered by adding a third eye primordium to a young frog embryo soon after closure of the neural folds (Shumway developmental stage 16–18; Shumway, 1940). At the time of the operation, the prospective eye is only a flattened evagination from the prosencephalic vesicle, but differentiation of optic and retinal elements will generally continue undisturbed in anomalous locations (Constantine-Paton and Law, 1978). As these animals mature, most supernumerary eyes develop optic nerves that penetrate the anterior diencephalon and send fibers to innervate either the ipsilateral or contralateral tectal lobe along with one of the host's normal eyes. The result is that a single, previously uninnervated optic lobe receives a projection from two complete retinas.

We have studied the retinal inputs to the tecta in 27 of these three-eyed animals using light-microscope autoradiography and the anterograde transport of the enzyme horseradish peroxidase (HRP) (Scalia and Colman, 1974; Adams, 1977).

In every animal, regardless whether the normal or third eye had been labeled, the deposition of retinotectal synapses was dramatically altered within the doubly innervated tectum. All cases exhibited the pattern illustrated in Figure 1B. Instead of the normal continuous labeled zone, ≈200-μm-wide regions of dense autoradiographic grains alter-

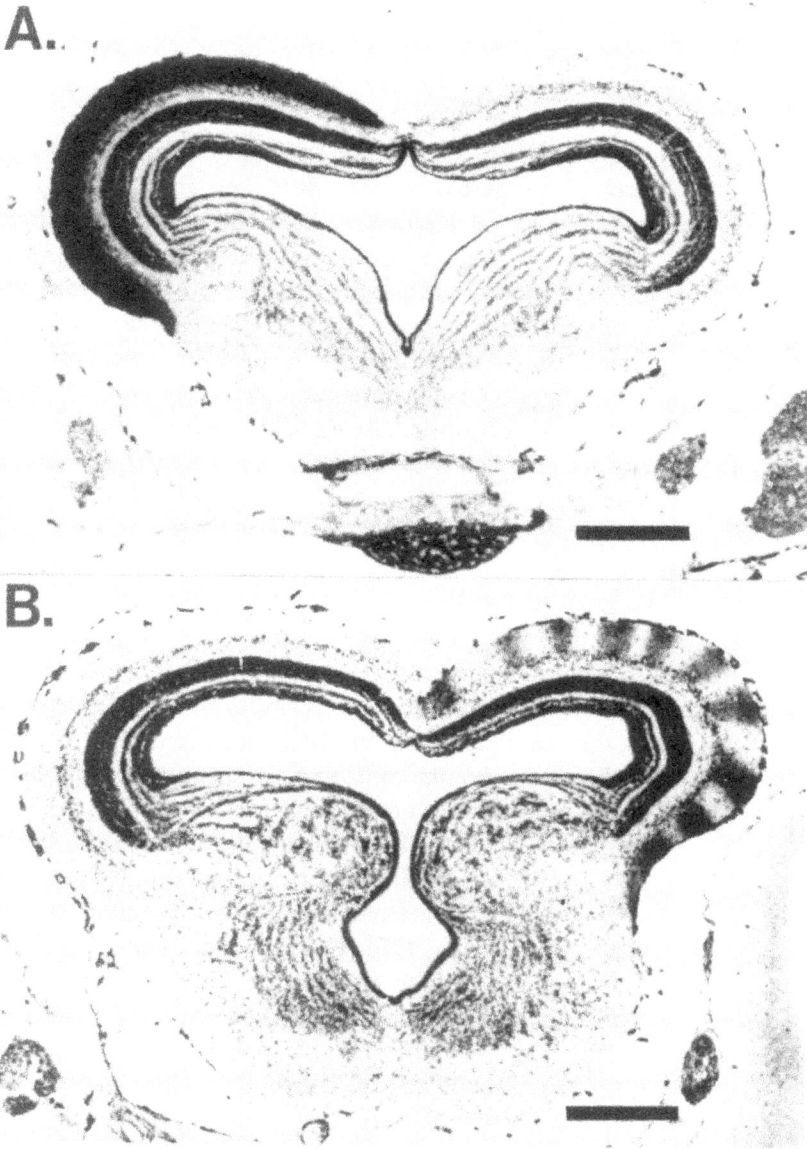

Figure 1 (A) Autoradiograph of a coronal section through the midbrain of a normal frog. This animal's left eye was injected with 10uCi of [³H]-proline 3 days before it was killed. The entire superficial neuropil of the right optic lobe (left side of the picture) is filled with developed silver grains indicating the region occupied by synaptic terminals from the labeled (contralateral) eye. (B) Autoradiograph of a coronal section through the midbrain of a three-eyed frog following intraocular injection of 10uCi of [³H]-proline into its normal right eye. The left optic lobe of this animal was innervated by the labeled eye plus the supernumerary eye. The normally continuous retinotectal synaptic zone of the contralateral eye has consequently been divided into regularly spaced bands of terminal neuropil. Bar = 400 μm. Tissue shrinkage during histological processing is ≈45%.

nated periodically with areas of low grain density, and serial reconstructions showed these regions to be cross sections of rostrocaudally oriented bands (Constantine-Paton and Law, 1978; Law and Constantine-Paton, 1978, 1981).

Eye-specific segregation of retinal ganglion-cell terminals was strongly suggested by our initial data; first, because the discontinuous pattern was established by both the normal and supernumerary eye; and second, because grain densities in the interband region fell to tissue background, indicating little or no input from the labeled retina (Constantine-Paton and Law, 1978). We have now been able to demonstrate directly interdigitation of the two projections in three-eyed animals where the supernumerary eye is labeled with [^{3}H]-proline and the normal projection is labeled with HRP. Spaces between the bands of one eye are filled with terminals from the second retina. There is minimal overlap ($\simeq$30 μm) between the two sets of inputs (Law and Constantine-Paton, 1981).

Genesis of Bands

Considerable information is available on the normal development of the retinotectal system in anuran amphibians. Tritiated thymidine studies on these animals have amply demonstrated that retinal- and tectal-cell proliferation occurs continuously throughout tadpole life. The retina grows as a series of nearly concentric rings (Straznicky and Gaze, 1971; Hollyfield, 1968, 1971) or ellipses (Jacobson, 1976; Beach and Jacobson, 1979), while tectal-cell proliferation and differentiation progresses in an anterolateral-to-posteromedial sequence (Straznicky and Gaze, 1972; Currie and Cowan, 1974, 1975).

Retinal axons span the distance between the developing eye and midbrain in the hatchling larvae (Currie and Cowan, 1974, 1975) and during the 2–6-month tadpole period the enlarging visual projection spreads within the tectal neuropil in close register with the wave of neuronal differentiation (Currie and Cowan, 1974, 1975; Lázár, 1973; Scott, 1974; Jacobson, 1977). Moreover, several lines of evidence now indicate that functional synaptic contacts are present in rostral tectum while caudomedial segments are still being generated (Gaze, Chung, and Keating, 1972; Chung, Bliss, and Keating, 1974; Scott, 1974).

Projections from supernumerary eyes develop at nearly the same time as the axons from the host's retinas. It is consequently possible to study the development of bands by labeling either one of the eyes projecting to the dually innervated tectum and examining the distribution of fibers at different tadpole ages and at different tectal levels.

Two distinct conclusions arise from this work. First, band width, as measured across the medial lateral axis of the tectum, is a constant. Young and old tadpoles and postmetamorphic frogs all have bands of approximately 200 μm. The system accommodates to the increasing numbers of retinal and tectal cells by simply adding more bands, so that a young Taylor and Kollros (T&K) stage IV tadpole (Taylor and Kollros, 1946) will generally have 4 bands, whereas 12–13 bands are typically present in postmetamorphic frogs (Constantine-Paton and Law, 1978, 1981; Law and Constantine-Paton, 1981). Second, banding develops from an initial state of relatively uniform distribution with extensive overlap. Subsequently, the axons sort out according to their retina of origin (Constantine-Paton and Law, 1978, 1981).

Figure 2 illustrates these points in two autoradiographs from a young (T&K stage IV) tadpole. The section in Figure 2A was taken from a rostral region of this animal's midbrain and four distinctly labeled bands are evident in the superficial neuropil of the left tectal lobe. Figure 2B is a section through the caudal tectum of the same animal. Tectal lamination is poorly established in this region, and uniformly distributed grains can be seen as a thin dark strip in the superficial neuropil. In this particular case, the third eye had been labeled with [^{3}H]-proline. We have seen the same rostral-to-caudal difference in a doubly innervated tectum when the projection from the host's eye was labeled with HRP (Constantine-Paton and Law, 1981).

Striped tecta can also be produced during axonal regeneration. When one tectal lobe is surgically removed in late tadpoles and young frogs, the severed retinal afferents to that lobe will frequently grow across the dorsal midline of the mesencephalon and send axons ipsilaterally at the optic chiasm in order to innervate the remaining optic tectum. Two out of the sixteen single-tectum animals that we have analyzed by labeling either one or both optic tracts showed striped tecta that were essentially indistinguishable from those seen in three-eyed frogs. Three other animals with postoperative survivals of less than 4 months showed no evidence of terminal segregation in the remaining tectum, and the other frogs were only partially banded because some axons from the ipsilateral eye failed to reach the remaining lobe. Nevertheless, whenever they occurred, eye-specific termination bands were $\simeq$ 150–200 μm in width and ran in the same rostrocaudal direction (Law and Constantine-Paton, 1980).

Figure 3 shows several ipsilateral-eye termination bands in a single-tectum frog after the optic nerve was labeled with HRP (Law and Constantine-Paton, 1980). Retinal ganglion-cell axon terminals appear as dense powder in this photomicrograph, and the axons of passage can be seen to run between the bands. In this animal, the contralateral eye was labeled with [^{3}H]-proline. Autoradiographs demonstrated that the normal contralateral projection was localized to the regions between the HRP-labeled terminals of the ipsilateral eye. During tectal-lobe ablation, considerable care is taken to leave the projection to the remaining lobe undisturbed. It, therefore, seems that the forces involved in

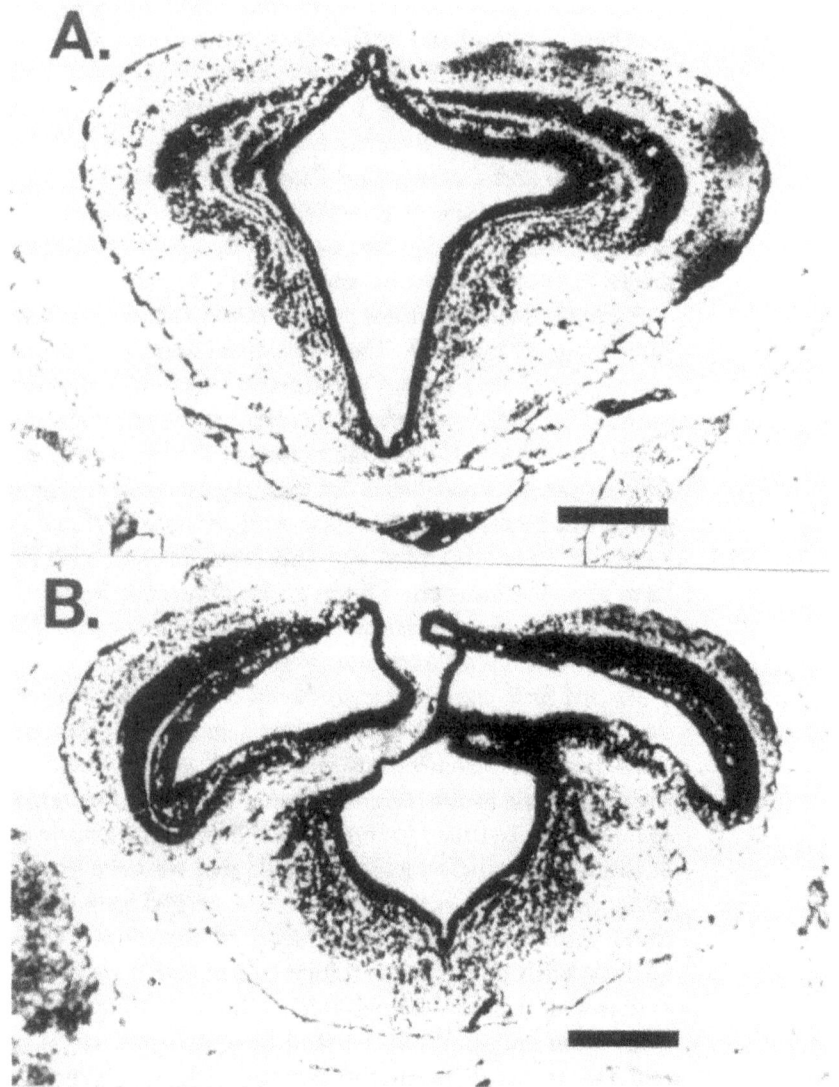

Figure 2 (A) Autoradiograph of a coronal section through the rostral midbrain of a young (T&K stage-IV) three-eyed tadpole following injection of 5uCi of [³H]-proline into the supernumerary eye. (B) Autoradiograph of a coronal section through the caudal midbrain of the same animal. Bar = 200 μm.

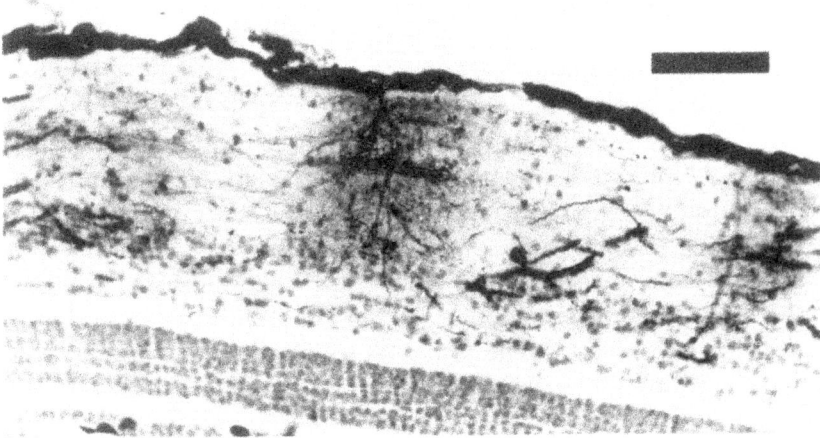

Figure 3 Retinotectal termination bands from the recrossed ipsilateral projection in a single tectum frog 4½ months after removal of the contralateral tectal lobe. Retinal ganglion-cell axons and axon terminals have been labeled with HRP by placing a pledget saturated with the enzyme on the cut stump of the optic nerve 3 days before killing the animal. Bar = 100 μm.

banding are quite strong. They enable regenerating terminals from the ipsilateral eye to displace the established synaptic contacts from the contralateral retina (Law and Constantine-Paton, 1980).

Our frog studies suggest that banding will result whenever two sets of retinal afferents attempt to share the same tectal area. A somewhat similar distribution of retinal terminals has been observed following tectal ablations and axonal regeneration in goldfish (Levine and Jacobson, 1975; Schmidt, Cicerone, and Easter, 1978; Meyer, 1979). However, neither the goldfish regeneration studies nor the majority of our frog regeneration preparations consistently shows the periodic pattern observed in three-eyed frogs and tadpoles. In the frogs, this seems due to failure of some regenerating axons to reach the remaining optic tectum (Law and Constantine-Paton, 1980). The variability of segregated patterns in single-tectum goldfish may result from the same factor (Meyer, 1979).

Banding is not seen following neonatal single-tectum ablations in mammals (Schneider, 1973; Miller and Lund, 1975; So and Schneider, 1978; So, 1979). Instead, the retinal axons to the missing lobe establish an exclusive projection zone in the most medial region of the other tectum (Miller and Lund, 1975; So and Schneider, 1978; So, 1979). However, Miller and Lund (1975) report a "patchy" distribution of anomalous (recrossed) ipsilateral terminals in the superior colliculus of rats when one tectum was ablated on fetal day 17 before the arrival of any retinal fibers. It may consequently be that the absence of induced banding in mammals is related to age-dependent decreases in axonal regeneration and synaptic flexibility within their central nervous systems (CNS; Miller and Lund, 1975; So and Schneider, 1978; So, 1979).

Competition for Tectal Space

In both three-eyed and single-tectum frogs, axons from two retinas project to a target region that normally receives input from only one eye. Electrophysiology indicates that some fibers from both of these eyes establish functional synaptic contacts with tectal cells (unpublished observation), and volume estimates suggest that the amount of post-synaptic membrane has not doubled in the superinnervated tecta. Apparently three-eyed and single-tectum frogs represent competitive situations in which two sets of retinal axons are attempting to innervate limited postsynaptic space. Two lines of evidence suggest that these are local interactions in which particular ganglion-cell terminals compete for postsynaptic space in particular regions of the tectal lobe.

Anatomical support for such localization is illustrated in the camera lucida tracings of Figure 4. These sections were taken through the midbrain of an animal in which only the caudal half of the left tectum was removed. After 4 months' survival, the projection from the right eye was labeled with [³H]-proline, and stippling indicates the position and relative density of the retinal input. Label is heavy in the rostral region where the remnant of the left tectal lobe remained. There is some light label, but no evidence of banding within the rostral right tectal lobe. In more caudal sections, the left tectum is completely absent and bands become obvious in the bilaterally equivalent parts of the right lobe (Law and Constantine-Paton, 1980).

It is significant that label in the caudal region of the right lobe is not only discontinuous but also more plentiful, suggesting a high density of ipsilateral axons. If these axons were not competing for specific tectal regions, the ipsilateral fibers should distribute themselves throughout the rostrocaudal length of the right lobe. They do not do this.

Additional evidence supporting spatially specific interactions comes from electrophysiological experiments that demonstrate an organized projection of the visual field through both eyes within the banded optic tecta. These investigations are conducted on curarized animals positioned in an ophthalmic projection perimeter so that the position of a 3° light spot can be systematically varied. We use gold-and-platinum-plated tungsten microelectrodes (≈5–7 MΩ impedance) to record single or multiunit activity from retinal ganglion-cell terminals in the superficial tectal layers, and our penetrations are made at fixed (200-μm) intervals to assure an unbiased survey of the dorsal tectal surface.

In dually innervated tecta, the characteristic radial distribution of ganglion cell-response types (Lettvin et al., 1959, 1961; Maturana et al., 1960) remains relatively normal, and at most recording positions some

Martha Constantine-Paton

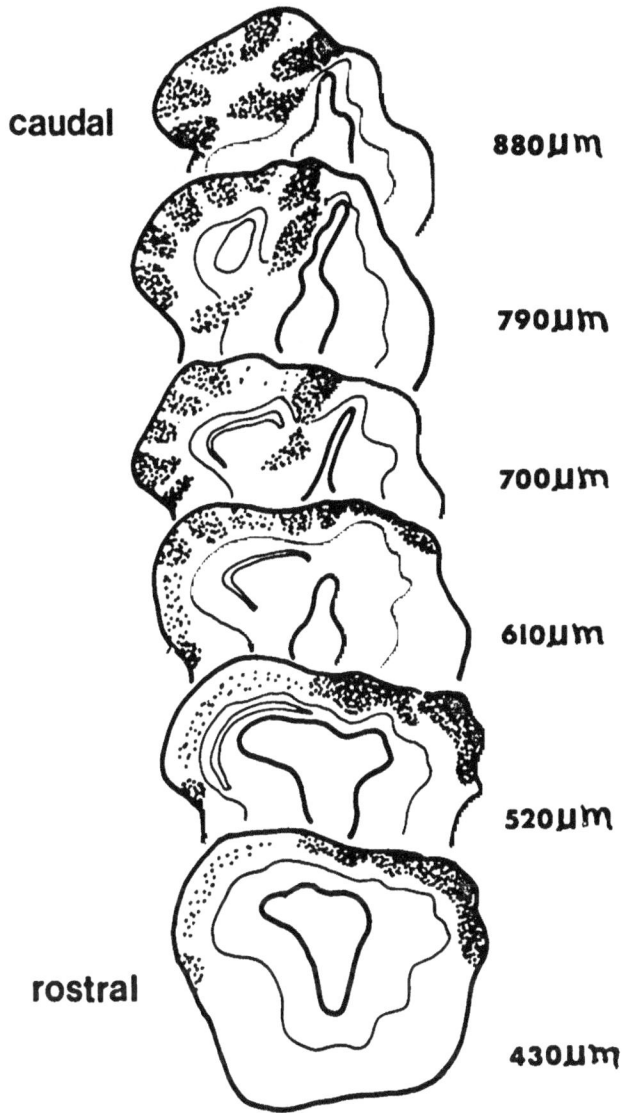

caudal

880μm

790μm

700μm

610μm

520μm

rostral

430μm

Figure 4 Camera lucida tracing of coronal sections through the last 450 μm of the mid-brain in a frog that had the caudal region of its left tectal lobe (right side of the figure) removed 4 months earlier. The eye contralateral to the partially ablated tectum had been labeled with [³H]-proline, and stippling indicates the position and relative density of the label.

activity can be driven through either retina. In general, however, the activity elicited through one of the eyes is more pronounced and remains that way throughout any penetration that is perpendicular to the tectal surface (Law and Constantine-Paton, 1981). We map the visuotectal projections in these preparations by occluding all but one eye and advancing the electrode until one or at most three units stand out from the background activity. After the receptive field of this activity is plotted using the perimeter light spot, we switch the occluder to the other eye and repeat the procedure to determine the receptive field for that recording site as seen through the second retina.

Figure 5 shows the results of one such experiment in a striped unitectal animal. In this case, the animal's nose was centered on the vertical meridian of the perimeter arc and pointed 15° below the perimeter's fixation point. This allows for more complete mapping of the superior visual field. Both the left and right eyes can be seen to project to the remaining right tectal lobe, and, at most tectal sites, activity could be driven through each of the eyes from nearly mirror-symmetrical positions around the vertical meridian. This result has been reported previously in unitectal adult frogs and goldfish (Sharma, 1973; Ingle, 1973; Easter and Schmidt, 1977; Meyer, 1979). The mirror-symmetrical pattern is expected if both eyes map to the single tectum normally; that is, nasal retina to caudal tectum, temporal retina to rostral tectum, inferior retina to medial tectum, and superior retina to lateral tectum.

The situation becomes complicated in three-eyed frogs because the eyes have abnormal alignments and also because the visuotectal maps frequently show a number of local distortions that we have not seen in either unitectal or normal animals.

Figure 6 presents results from one three-eyed frog chosen for ease of illustration because the dorsoventral alignment of the supernumerary eye was normal, and it was located on the midline between the two lateral eyes. This animal was positioned in the same orientation as the unitectal animal shown above, except that its nose was pointed directly at the perimeter's fixation point.

Visual-field positions that elicited activity through the two lateral eyes are shown in the left-hand side of the figure. The right-hand side of the figure shows visual-field positions projected through the supernumerary eye onto the left tectal lobe. The arrows are convenient references. They take into account the inversion produced by the eyes' lenses and mark sequences of points in visual space and along the rostrocaudal axes of the tecta that are relayed by progressively more nasal regions of all three retinas. The transplanted eye shows a visuotectal map that is roughly comparable to that of a normal right eye. Images falling on successively more nasal regions of this retina are projected to progressively more caudal tectal sites. (The arrows for both the normal right eye's visual-field map and the supernumerary-eye map are pointed from left to right.) Generally normal organization is also

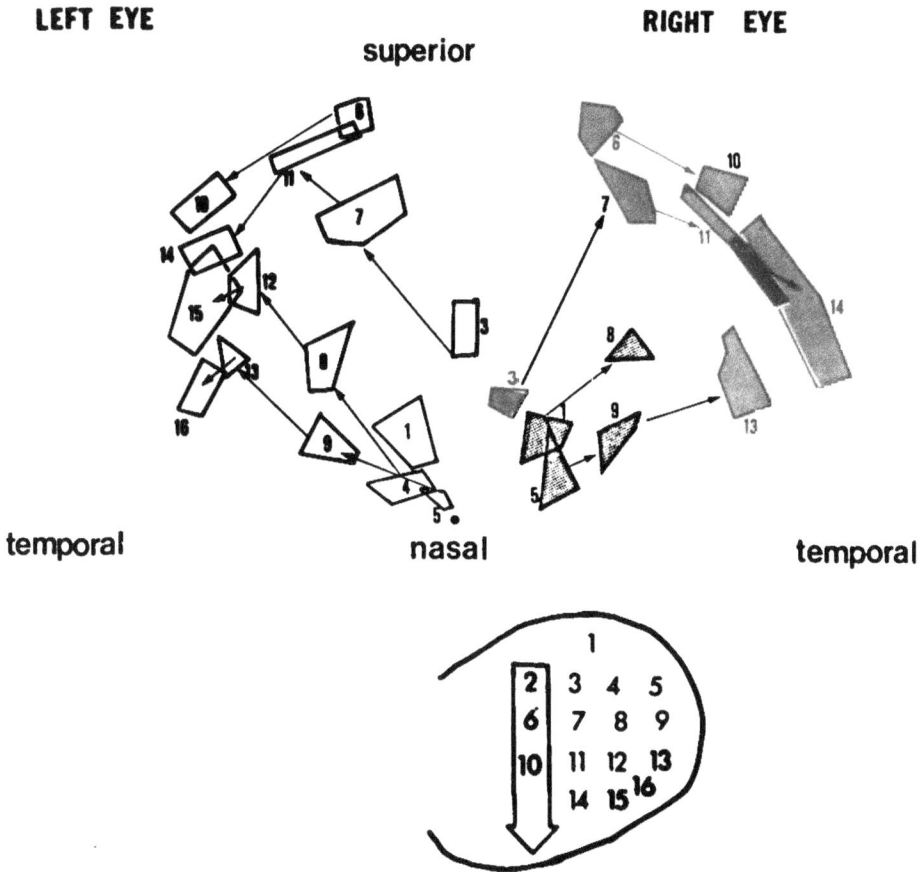

Figure 5 The visuotectal map obtained from the remaining right tectal lobe of a frog 8 months after metamorphosis. The left tectal lobe of this animal had been removed 6 months earlier. Tectal recording positions are 200 μm apart. Each eye was mapped independently at each electrode position. The limits of the visual field areas in which a 3° light spot could drive activity at the numbered recording sites are shown in the perimeter plot. The arrow indicates the progression of visual fields at successively more caudal tectal recording positions.

TRANSPLANT EYE

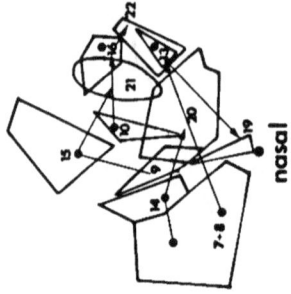

NORMAL EYES

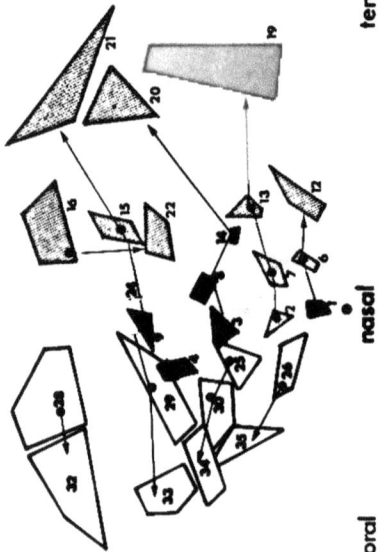

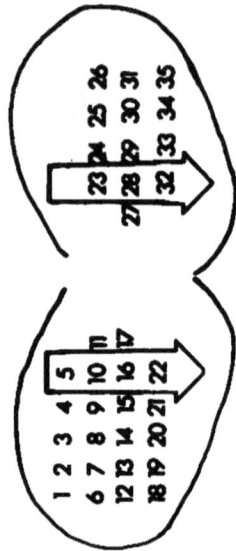

Figure 6 The visuotectal maps obtained from the right and doubly innervated (left) tectal lobes of a three-eyed frog. Conventions are the same as in Figure 5. This animal's supernumerary eye was centered on the tip of its nose. All visual-field positions are represented on the same perimeter coordinates. Visual-field areas for the host's eyes are shown on the left-hand side. Visual-field areas for the supernumerary eye are shown on the right. In this particular animal supernumerary visual-field areas were large because of an unusual texturing on the corneal surface. However, despite several local discontinuities, the sequence of visual-field areas projected through this transplant is from left to right, similar to that seen in the host's right eye.

present in the third eye's map relative to the mediolateral axis of the tectum, with superior visual-field positions shifting to more inferior positions in increasingly lateral tectal penetrations.

The presence of organized maps in striped tecta indicates that ganglion-cell terminals retain the retinal position-dependent identity of the ganglion-cell body (Sperry, 1948; Székeley, 1954; Stone, 1960; Jacobson, 1968; Hunt and Jacobson, 1974; Sharma and Hollyfield, 1974). Competitive exclusion of terminals apparently occurs among positionally similar ganglion cells which have a predetermined affinity for a particular subset of tectal cells.

Determinants of Banding

Figure 7 is a photographic reconstruction of bands made from ventrolateral horizontal sections of a dually innervated tectum. It graphically emphasizes the parallels between the geniculocortical projection in cat and monkey and eye-specific banding in frog. In both cases, the segregated pattern develops from an initial state of overlap (Rakic, 1976; Hubel, Wiesel, and LeVay, 1977; LeVay, Stryker, and Shatz, 1978) and, in both systems, the interdigitating slabs of neuropil

ROSTRAL

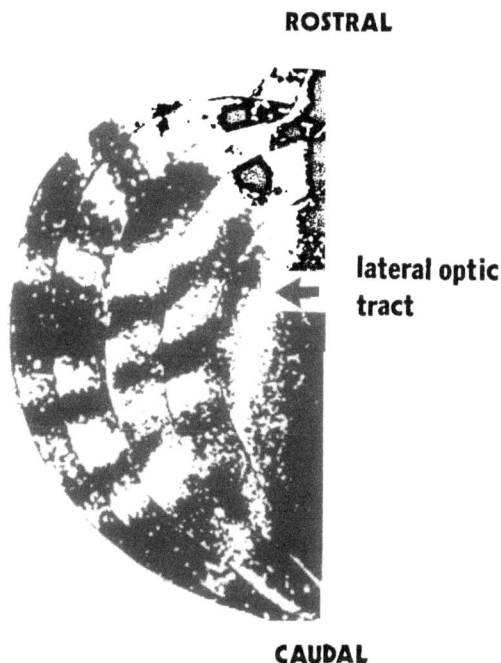

lateral optic tract

CAUDAL

Figure 7 Photographic reconstruction of bands in a dark field autoradiograph from a single-tectum frog after the ipsilateral eye was labeled with 10uCi of [³H]-proline. The brain was horizontally sectioned and the ventrolateral side of the doubly innervated tectal lobe is shown. The lateral optic tract runs along the edge of the tectal plate, and bands of retinal ganglion-cell terminals diverge from the tract to run in a generally rostrocaudal direction.

are superimposed on a retinotopic representation of the visual world (Hubel and Wiesel, 1962, 1972). These similarities suggest that a single mechanism is responsible for both the normal and induced patterns. Thus, the determinants of striped tecta in frogs may, at least tentatively, be applied to the mammal.

Banding in frogs seems to represent a competitive balance between two opposing sets of interactions. One of these is a relative, but not absolute, tendency for ganglion cells within a particular region of the retina to terminate within a particular region of the tectum (Sperry, 1963). A second mechanism causes ganglion cells from the same retina to stay together in their target areas.

Figure 8 schematically illustrates how these two mechanisms interact to produce bands. Figure 8A depicts the situation of complete overlap that would be expected if ganglion cell axons from both retinas simply grew to their predetermined address on the tectal lobe. Figure 8B shows one of several patterns of binary tectal partitioning that could result if all the axons from the same retina stayed together and simply reestablished the relative order of the ganglion-cell bodies in the presynaptic sheet. The final pattern (Figure 8C) represents the banded compromise that is expected if ganglion cell axons from two retinas sort so as to (1) maximize contact between particular regions of each retina and particular regions of the tectal lobe, and (2) maximize the spatial contiguity between terminals from neighboring retinal ganglion-cell bodies.

This explanation arises directly from work on amphibian and goldfish retinotectal specificity. In these species there is experimental

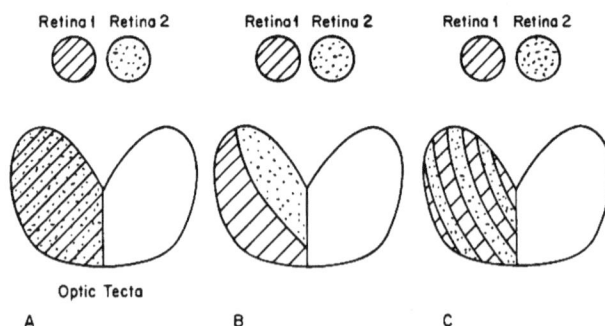

Figure 8 Schematic explanation of banding when retinal ganglion cells from two eyes (retina 1 and retina 2) innervate one tectal lobe. (A) Complete overlap of the terminals from the two eyes. Expected if only retinal ganglion cell-to-tectal cell affinities are involved in generating the retinotectal map. (B) One of several ways the two retinal projections could divide the tectal plate. Expected if ganglion-cell axons merely obtained some aligning cue from the tectal plate and sorted so as to reestablish the nearest-neighbor relationships of the retinal ganglion-cell bodies. (C) Interdigitating termination bands. Expected if ganglion cell terminals from each retina sorted so as to maximize contact with particular regions of the tectum *and* maintain the nearest-neighbor relationships of their retinal-cell bodies.

Martha Constantine-Paton

support for regionally graded affinities between the retina and the tectum (Yoon, 1972a; Levine and Jacobson, 1974; Jacobson and Levine, 1975a,b; Gaze and Hope, 1976; Meyer, 1978) and evidence for relatively strong interactions among ganglion cells from the same retina (for example, see Sharma, 1972; Yoon, 1972b; Jacobson and Levine, 1975a; Udin, 1977; Meyer, 1978, 1979; Schmidt and Easter, 1978; Schmidt, Cicerone, and Easter, 1978). However, virtually the same ideas were advanced independently by LeVay, Hubel, and Wiesel (1975) to explain ocular-dominance columns in monkey striate cortex.

Conclusion

We do not know the basis of neurospecificity in the frog, in the mammal, or in any animal for that matter. We also do not know how afferents from different sources distinguish each other, but given our ability to induce banding in the frog, we can begin to rule out the following possibilities:

(1) This interdigitating pattern of eye-specific terminals is not based on some genetically dictated prepattern in the postsynaptic sheet. The frog never shows, and it does not need, tectal ocular-dominance zones, so it seems more likely that this segregation develops from interactions that are normally involved in synaptogenesis.

(2) Two left eyes, two right eyes, or two eyes on the same side of the head will band equally well, suggesting that optic terminals do not make distinctions on the basis of the laterality of the eye.

(3) Banding does not seem to be based on the segregation of axons during growth or the temporal sequence with which axons enter the tectal plate. We see no evidence of two distinct optic tracts in the diencephalon, and the same termination pattern can result during regeneration in unitectal frogs.

(4) Banding is in some way dependent on the target cell population because diencephalic visual nuclei are not striped (Law and Constantine-Paton, 1980, 1981), though they are confronted with a double complement of afferents, and they normally contain maps of visual space.

In short, our observations indicate that highly elaborate patterns of interdigitating bands are not under direct genetic control. They probably reflect interactions that are fundamental to most instances of synaptogenesis. I suggest that banding results from these interactions when two sets of identically "specified" presynaptic terminals are forced to compete for space on the same postsynaptic sheet. It is likely that these interactions are mediated through the postsynaptic neuron, and that terminal segregation is related to the proximity of the presynaptic cell bodies.

Acknowledgments

I wish to thank Margaret I. Law and John A. Paton for their useful criticisms of this manuscript. Much of the research discussed in this chapter has been performed in my laboratory by Margaret I. Law as part of her doctoral dissertation. The work has been supported by National Institutes of Health Grant EYO 1872 and by a Whitehall Foundation Grant to the Princeton University Biology Department. Several of the experiments were performed during the 1978 CNS Workshop at Cold Spring Harbor, Long Island.

References

Adams, J. C., 1977. Technical considerations in the use of horseradish peroxidase as a neuronal marker. *Neuroscience* 2:141–145.

Beach, D. H., and M. Jacobson, 1979. Patterns of cell proliferation in the retina of the clawed frog during development. *J. Comp. Neurol.* 183:603–614.

Chung, S. H., T. V. P. Bliss, and M. J. Keating, 1974. The synaptic organization of optic afferents in the amphibian tectum. *Proc. Roy. Soc. B* 187:421–447.

Constantine-Paton, M., and M. I. Law, 1978. Eye-specific termination bands in tecta of three-eyed frogs. *Science* 202:639–641.

Constantine-Paton, M., and M. I. Law, 1981. Genesis of eye-specific bands in three-eyed tadpoles. (In preparation.)

Currie, J., and W. M. Cowan, 1974. Some observations on the early development of the optic tectum in the frog *Rana pipiens* with special reference to the effects of early eye removal on mitotic activity in the larval tectum. *J. Comp. Neurol.* 156:123–142.

Currie, J., and W. M. Cowan, 1975. The development of the retino-tectal projections in *Rana pipiens*. *Develop. Biol.* 46:103–119.

Easter, S. S., and J. T. Schmidt, 1977. Reversed visuomotor behavior mediated by induced ipsilateral projections in goldfish. *J. Neurophysiol.* 40:1245–1254.

Gaze, R. M., and R. A. Hope, 1976. The formation of continuously ordered mappings. *Prog. Brain Res.* 45:327–455.

Gaze, R. M., S. H. Chung, and M. J. Keating, 1972. The development of the retinotectal projection in *Xenopus*. *Nature* 236:133–135.

Goldman, P. S., and W. J. H. Nauta, 1976. Autoradiographic demonstration of a projection from prefrontal association cortex to the superior colliculus in the rhesus monkey. *Brain Res.* 116:145–149.

Goldman, P. S., and W. J. H. Nauta, 1977. Columnar distribution of cortico-cortical fibers in the frontal association, limbic, and motor cortex of the developing rhesus monkey. *Brain Res.* 122:393–413.

Gould, H. J., 1978. Periodicity in the visual commissural projections of the grey squirrel. *Neurosci. Abst.* 4:630.

Grant, G., S. Landgren, and H. Silfvenius, 1975. Columnar distribution of U-fibres from the post cruciate cerebral projection area of the cats' group I muscle afferents. *Exp. Brain Res.* 24:57–74.

Graybiel, A. M., 1975. Anatomical organization of retinotectal afferents in the cat. An autoradiographic study. *Brain Res.* 96:1–23.

Graybiel, A. M., 1978. A stereometric pattern of distribution of acetylthiocholinesterase in the deep layers of the superior colliculus. *Nature* 272:539–541.

Groenewegen, H. J., and J. Voogd, 1977. The parasagittal zonation within the olivo-cerebellar projection. I. Climbing fiber distribution in the vermis of cat cerebellum. *J. Comp. Neurol.* 174:417–488.

Groenewegen, H. J., J. Voogd, and S. L. Freedman, 1979. The parasagittal zonation within the olivo-cerebellar projection. II. Climbing fiber distribution in the intermediate and hemispheric parts of the cat cerebellum. *J. Comp. Neurol.* 183:551–602.

Hendrickson, A. E., J. R. Wilson, and M. P. Ogren, 1978. The neuroanatomical organization of pathways between the dorsal lateral geniculate nucleus and visual cortex in Old and New World primates. *J. Comp. Neurol.* 182:123–136.

Hollyfield, J. G., 1968. Differential addition of cells to the retina in *Rana pipiens* tadpoles. *Develop. Biol.* 18:163–179.

Hollyfield, J. G., 1971. Differential growth of the neural retina in *Xenopus laevis*. *Develop. Biol.* 24:264–286.

Hubel, D. H., and T. N. Wiesel, 1962. Receptive fields, binocular interaction and functional architecture in the cats' visual cortex. *J. Physiol.* 160:106–154.

Hubel, D. H., and T. N. Wiesel, 1969. Anatomical demonstration of columns in the monkey striate cortex. *Nature* 221:747–750.

Hubel, D. H., and T. N. Wiesel, 1972. Laminar and columnar distribution of geniculo-cortical fibers in the macaque monkey. *J. Comp. Neurol.* 146:421–450.

Hubel, D. H., and T. N. Wiesel, 1978. Distribution of inputs from the two eyes to striate cortex of squirrel monkeys. *Neurosci. Abst.* 4:632.

Hubel, D. H., S. LeVay, and T. N. Wiesel, 1975. Mode of termination of retinotectal fibers in macaque monkey: An autoradiographic study. *Brain Res.* 96:25–40.

Hubel, D. H., T. N. Wiesel, and S. LeVay, 1977. Plasticity of ocular dominance columns in monkey striate cortex. *Phil. Trans. Roy. Soc. B* 278:377–409.

Hunt, R. K., and M. Jacobson, 1974. Specification of positional information in retinal ganglion cells of *Xenopus laevis*. Intraocular control of the time of specification. *Proc. Nat. Acad. Sci. USA* 71:3616–3620.

Imig, T. J., and J. F. Brugge, 1976. Relationship between binaural interaction columns and commissural connections of the primary auditory field (A1) in the cat. *Neurosci. Abst.* 2:19.

Ingle, D., 1973. Two visual systems. *Science* 181:1053–1055.

Jacobson, M., 1968. Development of neuronal specificity in retinal ganglion cells of *Xenopus. Develop. Biol.* 17:202–218.

Jacobson, M., 1976. Histogenesis of retina in the clawed frog with implications for the pattern of development of retinotectal connections. *Brain Res.* 103:541–545.

Jacobson, M., 1977. Mapping the developing retinotectal projection in frog tadpoles by a double label autoradiographic technique. *Brain Res.* 127:55–67.

Jacobson, M., and R. L. Levine, 1975a. Plasticity in the adult frog brain: Filling the visual scotoma after excision or translocation of parts of the optic tectum. *Brain Res.* 88:339–345.

Jacobson, M., and R. L. Levine, 1975b. Stability of implanted duplicate tectal positional markers serving as targets for optic axons in adult frogs. *Brain Res.* 92:468–471.

Jones, E. G., H. Burton, and R. Porter, 1975. Commissural and cortico-cortical "columns" in the somatic sensory cortex of primates. *Science* 190:572–574.

Knapp, H., F. Scalia, and W. Riss, 1965. The optic tracts of *Rana pipiens. Acta Neurol. Scand.* 41:325–355.

Law, M. I., and M. Constantine-Paton, 1978. Alternating retinal ganglion cell termination bands in doubly innervated frog optic tecta. *Neurosci. Abst.* 4:118.

Law, M. I., and M. Constantine-Paton, 1980. Right and left eye bands in frogs with unilateral tectal ablations. *Proc. Nat. Acad. Sci. USA* 77:2314–2318.

Law, M. I., and M. Constantine-Paton, 1981. Anatomy and physiology of experimentally produced striped tecta. (In preparation.)

Lázár, G., 1971. The projection of retinal quadrants on the optic centres in the frog: A terminal degeneration study. *Acta Morphol. Acad. Sci. Hung.* 19:325–334.

Lázár, G., 1973. The development of the optic tectum in *Xenopus laevis*: A Golgi study. *J. Anat.* 116:347–355.

Lázár, G., and G. Székely, 1967. Golgi studies on the optic center of the frog. *J. Hirnforsch.* 9:329–344.

Lettvin, J. Y., H. R. Maturana, W. S. McCulloch, and W. H. Pitts, 1959. What the frog's eye tells the frog's brain. *Proc. IRE* 47:1940–1951.

Lettvin, J. Y., H. R. Maturana, W. H. Pitts, and W. S. McCulloch, 1961. Two remarks on the visual system of the frog. In *Sensory Communication.* W. A. Rosenblith, ed. Cambridge, MA: MIT Press, pp. 757–776.

LeVay, S., D. H. Hubel, and T. N. Wiesel, 1975. The pattern of ocular dominance columns in macaque visual cortex revealed by a reduced silver stain. *J. Comp. Neurol.* 159:559–576.

LeVay, S., M. P. Stryker, and C. J. Shatz, 1978. Ocular dominance columns and their development in layer IV of the cat's visual cortex: A quantitative study. *J. Comp. Neurol.* 179:223–244.

Levine, R. L., 1980. An autoradiographic study of the retinal projection in *Xenopis laevis* with comparisons to *Rana. J. Comp. Neurol.* 189:1–30.

Levine, R. L., and M. Jacobson, 1974. Deployment of optic nerve fibers is determined by positional markers in the frog's tectum. *Exp. Neurol.* 43:527–538.

Levine, R., and M. Jacobson, 1975. Discontinuous mapping of retina onto tectum innervated by both eyes. *Brain Res.* 98:172–176.

Maturana, H. R., J. Y. Lettvin, W. S. McCulloch, and W. H. Pitts, 1960. Anatomy and physiology of vision in the frog (*Rana pipiens*). *J. Gen. Physiol.* Suppl. 43:129–175.

Meyer, R., 1978. Deflection of selected optic fibers into a denervated tectum in goldfish. *Brain Res.* 155:213–227.

Meyer, R., 1979. Extra optic fibers exclude normal fibers from tectal regions in goldfish. *J. Comp. Neurol.* 183:883–902.

Miller, B. F., and R. D. Lund, 1975. The pattern of retinotectal connections in albino rats can be modified by fetal surgery. *Brain Res.* 91:119–125.

Oscarsson, O., 1973. Functional organization of spinocerebellar paths. In *Handbook of Sensory Physiology, Vol. 2: Somatosensory System.* A. Iggo, ed. Berlin: Springer Verlag, pp. 339–380.

Pollack, J. G., and J. C. Hickey, 1979. The distribution of retino-collicular terminals in Rhesus monkey. *J. Comp. Neurol.* 185:587–602.

Potter, H. D., 1969. Structural characteristics of cell and fiber populations in the optic tectum of the frog (*Rana catesbiana*). *J. Comp. Neurol.* 136:203–232.

Potter, H. D., 1972. Terminal arborizations of retinotectal axons in the bullfrog. *J. Comp. Neurol.* 144:269–283.

Rakic, P., 1976. Prenatal genesis of connections subserving ocular dominance in the rhesus monkey. *Nature* 261:467–471.

Rakic, P., 1977. Prenatal development of the visual system in rhesus monkey. *Phil. Trans. Roy. Soc. B* 278:245–260.

Scalia, F., and D. K. Colman, 1974. Aspects of the central projection of the optic nerve in the frog as revealed by the anterograde migration of horseradish peroxidase. *Brain Res.* 79:496–504.

Scalia, F., and K. Fite, 1974. A retinotopic analysis of the central connections of the optic nerve in the frog. *J. Comp. Neurol.* 158:455–477.

Scalia, F., H. Knapp, M. Halpern, and W. Riss, 1968. New observations on the retinal projection in the frog. *Brain Behav. Evol.* 1:324–353.

Schmidt, J. T., and S. S. Easter, Jr., 1978. Independent biaxial reorganization of the retinotectal projection: A reassessment. *Exp. Brain Res.* 31:155–169.

Schmidt, J. T., C. M. Cicerone, and S. S. Easter, Jr., 1978. Expansion on the half retinal projection to the tectum in goldfish: An electrophysiological and anatomical study. *J. Comp. Neurol.* 177:257–278.

Schneider, G. E., 1973. Early lesions of superior colliculus: factors affecting the formation of abnormal retinal projections. *Brain Behav. Evol.* 8:73–109.

Scott, T. M., 1974. The development of the retino-tectal projection in *Xenopus laevis:* An autoradiographic and degeneration study. *J. Embryol. Exp. Morphol.* 31:409–414.

Shanks, M. F., A. J. Rockel, and T. P. S. Powell, 1975. The commissural fibre connections of the primary somatic sensory cortex. *Brain Res.* 98:166–171.

Sharma, S. C., 1972. Reformation of retinotectal projections after various tectal ablations in adult goldfish. *Exp. Neurol.* 34:171–182.

Sharma, S. C., 1973. Anomalous retinal projections after removal of the contralateral optic tectum in adult goldfish. *Exp. Neurol.* 41:661–669.

Sharma, S. C., and J. G. Hollyfield, 1974. Specification of retinal central connections in *Rana pipiens* before the appearance of the first post-mitotic ganglion cell. *J. Comp. Neurol.* 155:395–408.

Shatz, C. J., and M. P. Stryker, 1978. Ocular dominance in layer IV of the cat's visual cortex and the effects of monocular deprivation. *J. Physiol. (London)* 281:267–283.

Shatz, C. J., S. H. Lindström, and T. N. Wiesel, 1977. The distribution of afferents representing the right and left eyes in the cat's visual cortex. *Brain Res.* 131:103–116.

Shumway, W., 1940. Stages in the normal development of *Rana pipiens*. I. External forms. *Anat. Rec.* 83:309–315.

So, K. F., 1979. Development of abnormal recrossing retinotectal projections after superior colliculus lesions in newborn syrian hamsters. *J. Comp. Neurol.* 186:241–258.

So, K. F., and G. E. Schneider, 1978. Abnormal recrossing retinotectal projections after early lesions in syrian hamsters: Age-related effects. *Brain Res.* 147:277–295.

Sperry, R. W., 1948. Orderly patterning of synaptic associations in regeneration of intracentral fiber tracts mediating visuomotor coordination. *Anat. Rec.* 102:63–75.

Sperry, R. W., 1963. Chemoaffinity in the orderly growth of nerve fiber patterns and connections. *Proc. Nat. Acad. Sci. USA* 50:703–710.

Stone, L. S., 1960. Polarization of the retina and development of vision. *J. Exp. Zool.* 145:85–93.

Straznicky, K., and R. M. Gaze, 1971. The growth of the retina in *Xenopus laevis:* An autoradiographic study. *J. Embryol. Exp. Morphol.* 26:67–79.

Straznicky, K., and R. M. Gaze, 1972. The development of the tectum in *Xenopus laevis:* An autoradiographic study. *J. Embryol. Exp. Morphol.* 28:87–115.

Székely, G., 1954. Zur Ausbildung der lokalen funktionellen Spezifitat der Retina. *Acta Biol. Acad. Sci. Hung.* 5:157–167.

Székely, G., G. Sétálo, and G. Lázár, 1973. Fine structure of the frog's optic tectum: Optic fiber termination layers. *J. Hirnforsch.* 14:189–225.

Taylor, A. C., and J. J. Kollros, 1946. Stages in the normal development of *Rana pipiens* larvae. *Anat. Rec.* 94:7–28.

Tigges, J., and M. Tigges, 1979. Ocular dominance columns in the striate cortex of chimpanzee (*Pan troglodytes*). *Brain Res.* 166:386–390.

Tigges, J., M. Tigges, and A. Perachio, 1977. Complementary laminar terminations of afferents to area 17 originating in area 18 and in lateral geniculate nucleus in squirrel monkey. *J. Comp. Neurol.* 176:87–100.

Udin, S., 1977. Rearrangements of the retinotectal projection in *Rana pipiens* after unilateral caudal half-tectum ablation. *J. Comp. Neurol.* 173:561–582.

Voogd, J., 1969. The importance of fiber connections in the comparative anatomy of the mammalian cerebellum. In *Neurobiology of Cerebellar Evolution and Development.* R. Llinás, ed. Chicago: American Medical Association, pp. 493–514.

Wiesel, T. N., D. H. Hubel, and D. M. K. Lam, 1974. Autoradiographic demonstration of ocular-dominance columns in the monkey striate cortex by means of transneuronal transport. *Brain Res.* 79:273–279.

Wise, S. P., and E. G. Jones, 1976. The organization and postnatal development of the commissural system of the somatic sensory cortex in the rat. *J. Comp. Neurol.* 168:313–343.

Wise, S. P., and E. G. Jones, 1977. Cells of origin and terminal distribution of descending projections of the rat somatic sensory cortex. *J. Comp. Neurol.* 175:129–158.

Yoon, M. G., 1972a. Transposition of the visual projection from the nasal hemiretina onto the foreign rostral zone of the optic tectum in goldfish. *Exp. Neurol.* 37:451–462.

Yoon, M. G., 1972b. Reversibility of the reorganization of retinotectal projection in goldfish. *Exp. Neurol.* 35:565–577.

4

Development and Plasticity of Primate Frontal Association Cortex

Patricia S. Goldman-Rakic

ABSTRACT   The neuronal organization and connections of the prefrontal association cortex in primates are beginning to be understood as these features are brought increasingly to light by the use of advanced morphological techniques. In the present report, the corticocortical and corticostriatal fiber systems of the prefrontal cortex have been selected to illustrate the timing, sequence, mode, and mechanisms of development and plasticity of the prefrontal cortex. At early fetal ages, axons of prefrontal corticocortical and corticostriatal systems are distributed in a diffuse manner in their target structures. This initial stage is followed by a progressive sorting out of terminal fields into specific territories which take the form of alternating "stripes" in prefrontal cortex and cylinders with elliptical cores in the neostriatum. In the rhesus monkey, the segregation of projections into the adult-typical "modular" type of organization in these two systems is attained at least 2 weeks before birth. Both corticocortical and corticostriatal fiber systems display a considerable capacity for rearrangement in response to surgical resection of their target structures at critical periods of development. Thus, callosal fibers connect heterotopic cortical areas in the absence of a homotopic target, and strong contralateral corticostriatal projections develop when the ipsilateral corticostriatal projections are removed by unilateral resection of prefrontal cortex. The remarkable neuronal plasticity exhibited by the output neurons of the developing primate neocortex may be an important biological mechanism for recovery of function following injury to the telencephalon at various stages of prenatal and early postnatal development.

Introduction

The frontal association cortex reaches its peak phylogenetic development in the human brain, in which it comprises almost a fourth of the entire surface area of the cerebral cortex (Filimonov, 1949). This large and functionally important region of primate neocortex commanded the attention of the nineteenth-century scholars and clinicians (e.g., Harlow, 1868; Ferrier, 1886; Fritsch and Hitzig, 1870) and was a subject of intense scientific inquiry in the early part of the twentieth century (e.g., Franz, 1907; Bianchi, 1922; Jacobsen, 1936; Denny-Brown, 1951; Fulton, 1951). After midcentury, however, scholarly interest and experimental research on the association areas of the frontal lobe declined, and just a

P. S. GOLDMAN-RAKIC Yale University, School of Medicine, New Haven, Connecticut 06510

few years ago the frontal granular cortex was among the least-studied, and as Nauta (1971) has pointed out, among the least-understood structures in the central nervous system. Relatively slow progress in understanding prefrontal association cortex is unquestionably related to its intrinsic complexity as well as to limitations in methods that have been applied to the subject in the past. It may also be due in part to the cautionary view prevalent in the 1960s that the structural and functional complexity of this region virtually prohibits scientific analysis.

The prospects for scientific inquiry of functionally and anatomically complicated structures like the frontal association cortex have changed considerably over the last decade. In recent years, it has become possible to begin to build a coherent picture of the intrinsic and extrinsic organization of frontal-lobe connections and to relate this knowledge to relevant biochemical, electrophysiological, and behavioral data. These gains have been possible because of the advent of new methods, for example, axonal transport of macromolecules for tracing pathways in the central nervous system, 2-deoxyglucose metabolic mapping, monoamine biochemistry and histofluorescence, electrophysiological recording in chronic behaving animals and, finally, the refinement of techniques for performing neurosurgery in the primate fetus. As this volume of papers on the cerebral cortex attests, the application of these powerful neurobiological techniques has led to major advances in unraveling structure–function issues in the primary sensory and motor cortical areas. Most of these same experimental techniques can and have now been used to study the prefrontal association cortex of primates. In the following pages, I will describe some recent findings from my laboratory on the development and plasticity of selected prefrontal cortical connections in fetal and neonatal rhesus monkeys. By way of introduction, I will review certain morphological characteristics of the prefrontal association cortex and selected aspects of its organization and topography in the adult brain. This background may be particularly appropriate for a discussion of the prefrontal cortex, the boundaries of which are much less widely known than are areas like the visual cortex.

Morphology and Thalamic Connections of Prefrontal Cortex

In primates, the cortical mantle anterior to the central sulcus is considered frontal neocortex. This large cortical expanse can be divided into two major territories: a posterior "motor" area and an anterior "prefrontal" area separated by an intermediate transition zone, the premotor cortex including the frontal eye fields (Figure 1). The prefrontal cortex is the projection field of thalamocortical fibers originating in the mediodorsal (MD) nucleus of the dorsal thalamus (e.g., Walker, 1940; Mettler, 1947; Pribram, Chow, and Semmes, 1953; Akert, 1964). These

Patricia S. Goldman-Rakic

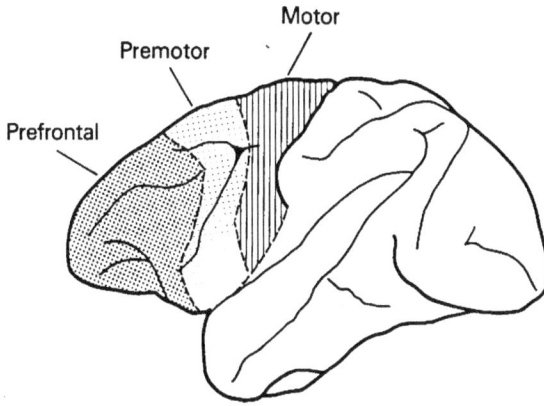

Figure 1 Diagram illustrating the three major subdivisions of neocortex in the frontal lobe of rhesus monkey based on cytoarchitectonic and hodological criteria. The prefrontal cortex (dense dots), which is highly developed in primates, extends onto the ventral surface of the frontal lobe, and a large proportion of it is buried within the banks and depths of sulci.

afferent projections are topographically organized. According to our recent horseradish peroxidase (HRP) study, thalamic neurons display a concentric organization in which dorsolateral cortical areas receive input from cells in the lateral subdivision of the nucleus and ventromedially situated cortex is innervated by cells situated in the medial subdivision of MD (see Figure 2 for details).

In addition to its reciprocal connections with the dorsal thalamus, the prefrontal cortex is interconnected with many other areas of cortex and with numerous subcortical structures located at all levels of the neuroaxis. Many of these pathways have been reviewed elsewhere (Nauta, 1971) or described in recent reports (e.g., Pandya, Dye, and Butters, 1971; Van Hoesen, Pandya, and Butters, 1975; Goldman and Nauta, 1976; Tanaka and Goldman, 1976; Kievit and Kuypers, 1977; Goldman and Nauta, 1977a,b; Jacobson and Trojanowski, 1975; 1977a,b; Jacobson, Butters, and Tovsky, 1978; Künzle, 1978; Goldman, 1979). Two classes of prefrontal connections are of particular relevance to the subject of this report: (i) the corticocortical fibers linking the dorsolateral prefrontal cortex of each hemisphere with synaptic targets situated in the same hemisphere (associational) as well as with targets situated in the opposite hemisphere (callosal); and (ii) the corticostriatal fibers, particularly the major descending projection from the dorsolateral prefrontal cortex to the head of the caudate nucleus. These connections have a specific pattern of organization (Goldman and Nauta, 1977 a,b) and exhibit a remarkable degree of structural plasticity in response to brain injury (Goldman, 1978). These two classes of prefrontal projections and experimental manipulation of their development will be described and discussed in greater detail below.

PREFRONTAL CORTEX

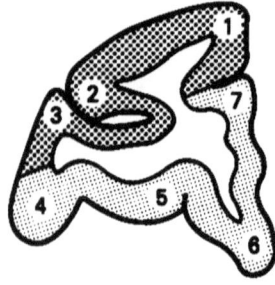

MEDIODORSAL NUCLEUS

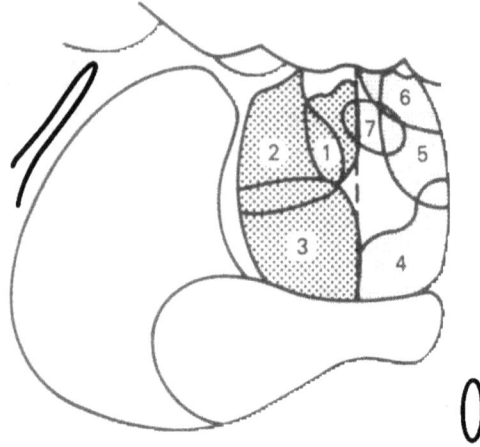

Figure 2 Summary diagram of the topography of thalamocortical connections in the pre-frontal cortex of the rhesus monkey. The parcellation of the thalamic mediodorsal (MD) nucleus into medial (magnocellular) and lateral (parvocellular) subdivisions has long been appreciated (e.g., Walker, 1940; Mettler, 1947; Pribram, Chow, and Semmes, 1953; Akert, 1964). However, the detailed arrangement of thalamocortical cell groups is revealed most distinctly by recent studies employing retrograde cell labeling with horseradish peroxidase (HRP) in seven cases arbitrarily numbered 1 to 7. With the arbitrary number-ing system used, the MD neurons and their synaptic targets in the prefrontal cortex are in register and exhibit a counterclockwise organization. (From Goldman-Rakic and Porrino, unpublished observations.)

Corticocortical Connections

Adult Organization

A recent finding of great significance for understanding the functions of the frontal association cortex is the recent discovery that its corticocortical projections are organized in "columns," "stripes," or "bands" (Goldman and Nauta, 1977a). A disjunctive pattern in the terminal fields of axons originating in prefrontal cortex is especially explicit in its ipsilateral projections to the retrosplenial cortex (Figure 3) and in its callosal projections to homotopic prefrontal cortex in the contralateral cerebral hemisphere (Figure 5). Although the concept that the neocortex has vertical structural units dates back to Lorente de Nó (1938), modern anatomical methods have only recently shown that specific thalamic afferents terminate in vertically oriented alternating territories of primary visual cortex (LeVay, Hubel, and Wiesel, 1975; Hubel and Wiesel, 1977).

The anatomical demonstration of terminal fiber bands in association and limbic cortex serves to emphasize that vertical segregation of afferent input is not unique to specific sensory cortex and therefore is not just a mechanism for "point-to-point" mapping of the peripheral receptor surface onto cerebral cortex. This not withstanding, the pattern of distribution of corticocortical connections within the dorsolateral prefrontal cortex and in anatomically related cortical regions outside the frontal lobe differs in several respects from the vertical organization of the thalamic input to the somatosensory and visual regions of the cortical mantle (e.g., Mountcastle, 1957, 1978; Hubel and Wiesel, 1977). For example, ocular-dominance stripes in the primate visual cortex represent a single sensory modality, and alternating bands are equivalent fiber systems subserving the two eyes. In prefrontal cortex, the source of fiber input interpolated between corticocortical territories is not yet known, but certainly will not be reducible to a single sense modality. Another difference between the "columnar organization" of sensory and association cortex is that the distribution of thalamocortical terminals in primary sensory regions is usually confined to subdivisions of layer IV whereas the callosal input to the frontal granular or retrosplenial limbic cortex is distributed throughout the full thickness of the cortex (Figures 3 and 4). In this respect, the distribution of callosal fibers in the prefrontal areas differs from that of callosal fibers interconnecting the somatosensory regions of the two hemispheres. The latter terminate principally in layers II–IV (Jones, Coulter, and Hendry, 1978).

An important question that has arisen in studying the development of the prefrontal cortex is whether in adult monkeys the disjunctive callosal and associational fiber systems of cortex terminate in a pattern of segregated cylinders as originally indicated by Mountcastle's physiological studies of somatosensory cortex (Mountcastle, 1957), or whether they are arranged as bands or stripes similar to the distribution

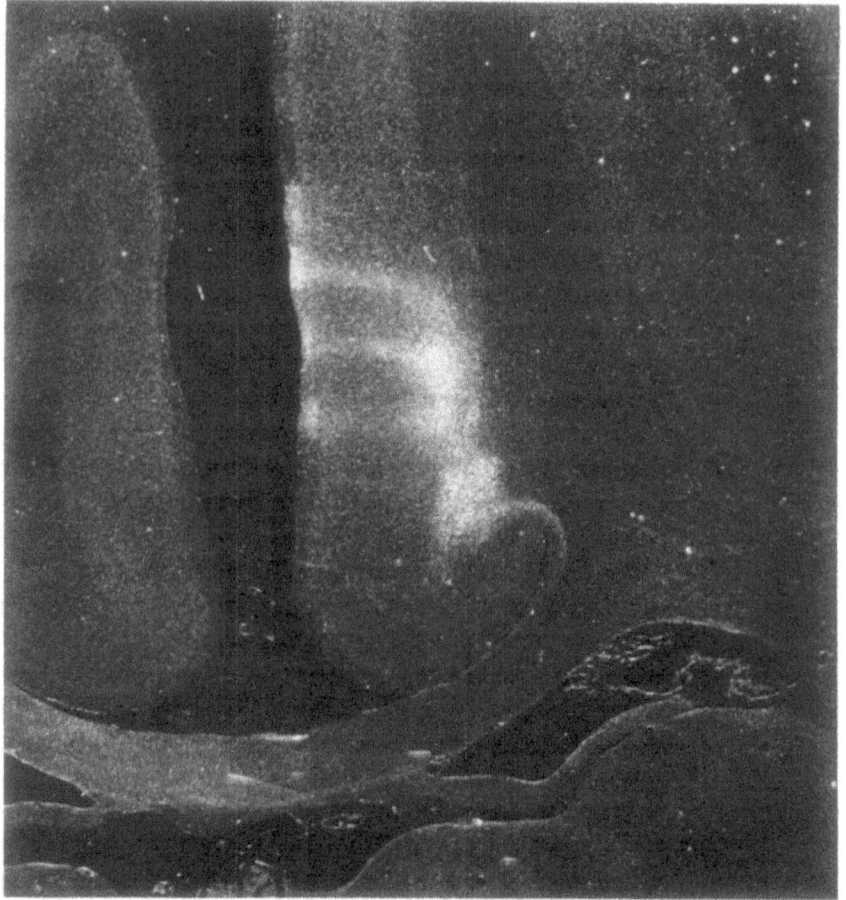

Figure 3 Dark-field autoradiogram of the retrosplenial cortex in a young rhesus monkey whose ipsilateral principal sulcus was injected with [³H]-leucine and [³H]-proline at 4 days of age. The photograph illustrates the distribution and spatial periodicity of the terminal fields of the prefrontoretrosplenial projection. Although this associational fiber system spreads over all six layers of the cortex, it is not yet known whether these fibers make synaptic connections in all layers.

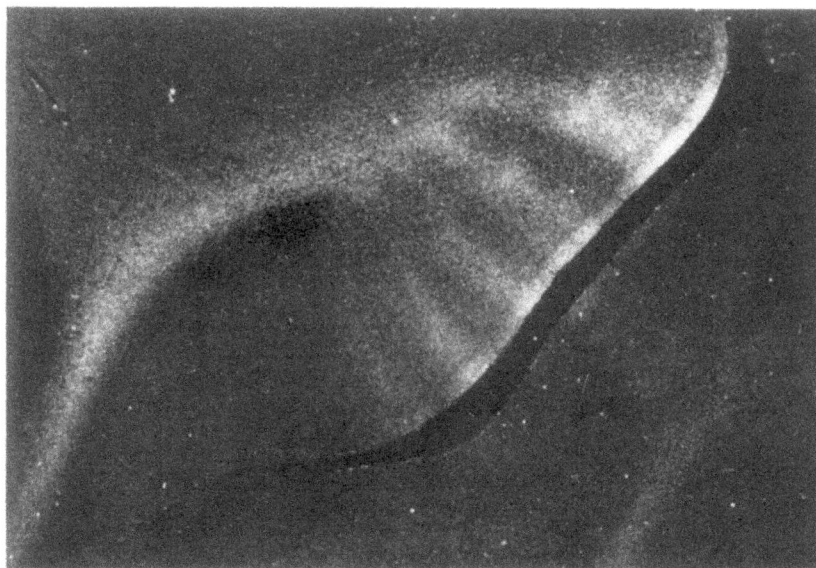

Figure 4 Photograph under dark-field illumination of the principal sulcus in the hemisphere opposite to that in which a mixture of [³H]-leucine and [³H]-proline was deposited in the corresponding homotopic cortex. The photograph displays the pattern of alternating "stripes" which characterizes the terminal fields of prefrontal callosal efferent fibers. Again, callosal fibers are found in all six layers of the cortex, with prominence in layers I and IV.

of the ocular-dominance system in primary visual cortex (Hubel and Wiesel, 1977). To answer this question we prepared autoradiograms from a gapless series of sections through one frontal lobe of a rhesus monkey that had received an injection of [³H]-leucine and [³H]-proline in the principal sulcus of the opposite hemisphere. Each autoradiogram was photographed in dark-field illumination, and the prints were used to reconstruct the homotopic area contralateral to the injected hemisphere. Figure 4 is an example of one of the more than 400 autoradiograms on which this reconstruction was based, which illustrates explicitly the spatial periodicity in the distribution of callosal fibers within the cortex. Because the principal sulcus is deeply invaginated, morphometric techniques were used to flatten out the sulcus and project the reconstruction upon a flat surface. As shown in Figure 5, a partial "face-on" surface reconstruction of a roughly 8-mm² area revealed that the callosal afferents to prefrontal cortex are distributed in the form of stripes. Although only a portion of the prefrontal cortex has so far been reconstructed, our present data display a pattern of callosal terminal fields viewed at the surface that are remarkably similar to that of the ocular-dominance stripes in visual cortex (Hubel and Freeman, 1977). In both cytoarchitectonic areas, the dominant pattern is one of alternating stripes across the cortical surface. In the principal sulcus, the stripes are oriented diagonally with respect to the fundus of the sulcus. As is the case with ocular-dominance stripes, prefrontal stripes exhibit x- and

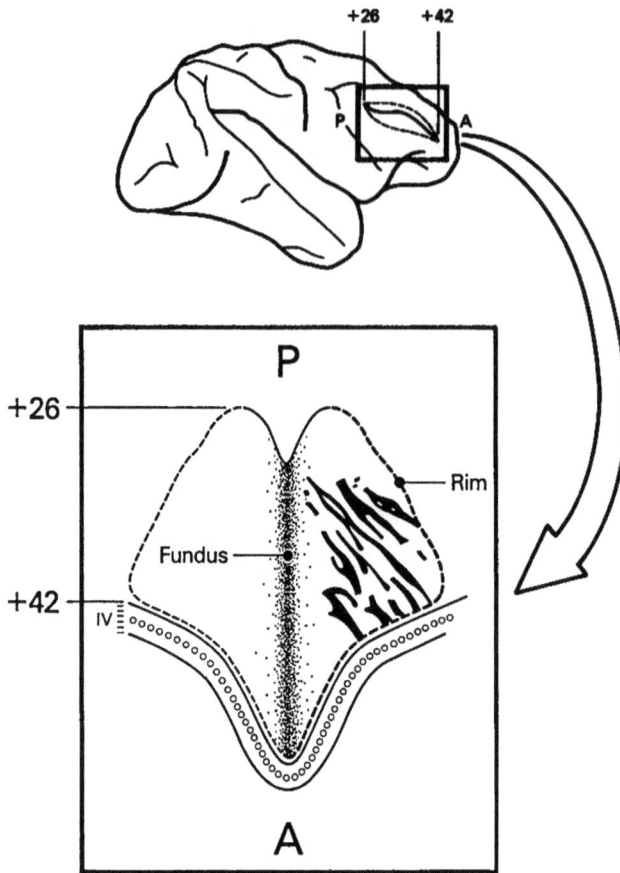

Figure 5 Semidiagrammatic illustration of a partial surface reconstruction of the pattern of innervation of the dorsal bank of the principal sulcus by callosal fiber efferents from the homotopic area in the opposite hemisphere. The findings were obtained in a rhesus monkey given a single 3-μl injection of 100 μC/μl in the middle of the dorsal bank of the principal sulcus and allowed to survive 1 week. The reconstruction was based on over 400 serial sections cut through the relevant prefrontal region located between stereotaxic coordinates +26 at the posterior (P) ends of the sulcus and +42 anteriorly (A). Within the frame shown in the lower half of the figure is an enlarged "bird's-eye" view of the cortex lining the dorsal bank of the principal sulcus. The fundus of the sulcus is running vertically and the superior rim of the sulcus is to the right. The distribution of label in layer IV was recorded in this reconstruction. (From Goldman-Rakic and Galkin, unpublished observations.)

Patricia S. Goldman-Rakic

y-shaped bifurcations, cross linkages, and blind endings as well as territories of more regular periodicity (Figure 5).

The functional significance of the disjunctive arrangement of corticocortical terminal fields in the frontal association and limbic cortex is unknown. One approach we are taking to this problem makes use of the recently developed and potentially powerful 2-deoxyglucose method for observing regional differences in functional activity based on glucose consumption (Sokoloff et al., 1977; Kennedy et al., 1976). This method has been used to expose certain features of the functional organization of cortical columns in the visual cortex: [^{14}C]-autoradiographs of the striate cortex of monkeys that viewed vertical stripes with both eyes open showed vertical bands of label extending through the full thickness of the cortex (Hubel, Wiesel, and Stryker, 1978). The same method has been used to demonstrate a one-to-one relationship of a single mystical vibrissa to a single cortical column in the rat somatosensory cortex (Hand, Miselis, and Reivich, 1977; Hand et al., 1978). Preliminary studies in my laboratory reveal that frontal association cortex also has metabolic "columns" (Bugbee and Goldman-Rakic, unpublished observations). As illustrated in Figure 6, metabolically active bands display an alternating pattern resembling the afferent-fiber distribution demonstrated by axonal transport (Goldman and Nauta, 1977a). However, only further studies combining the 2-deoxyglucose metabolic labeling method with anatomical and behavioral techniques will determine whether and how the two banding patterns are related to each other as well as to behavior.

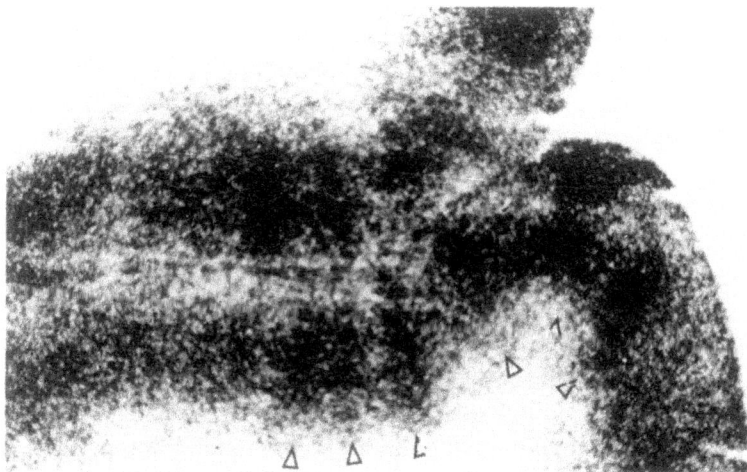

Figure 6 Photograph of an X-ray film of a section through the principal sulcus in a rhesus monkey given a pulse label of [^{14}C]-2-deoxyglucose 45 minutes before sacrifice. The photograph displays stripe-like areas of higher and lower glucose utilization within the cortex resembling the "columnar" pattern in the terminal distribution of the callosal pathways. "Stripes" in the ventral bank of the principal sulcus are marked by arrowheads.

Development and Plasticity of Primate Frontal Association Cortex

Mode of Development

All neurons of the frontal association cortex in primates are generated well before birth (Rakic and Wikmark, personal communication). Since the basic connections of the primate brain are also formed to a large extent well before birth, it is not surprising that until recently we had little idea of the mode of their development. Actually, only a few experimental anatomical studies exist on the development of connections in the nonhuman primate brain, and these studies have been limited to a very few brain regions: the spinal cord (Bodian, 1966; 1970), motor cortex (Kuypers, 1962; Kemper, Caviness, and Yakovlev, 1973), cerebellum (Rakic, 1971, 1972, 1973), and visual system (Rakic, 1975, 1976, 1977a,b; Hubel, Wiesel, and LeVay, 1977; LeVay, Wiesel, and Hubel, this volume). These investigations have not only established the feasibility of applying advanced morphological methods to various developmental issues in primates, they have also revealed the advantages of studying their large and slowly developing brains.

In order to study the development of prefrontal connections, I injected a mixture of $[^3H]$-proline and $[^3H]$-leucine into the prospective dorsolateral prefrontal cortex of rhesus monkey fetuses varying in age between 69 and 152 embryonic days (E69 and E152). After the intracortical injections were completed, the fetuses were returned to the uterus. Twenty-four to 72 hours later a second Caesarean section was performed, the fetus was removed and perfused intracardially with buffered formalin, and its brain processed for autoradiography by standard procedures.

The youngest fetus studied was injected at E69. At this stage of primate-brain development, the cortex is little more than a thick shell covering the balloon-shaped cerebral vesicles. Only a small fraction of the neurons that compose the cerebral cortex have been generated, and many of these have not yet completed their migrations to the cortex (Rakic, 1975). The cortical plate at E69 is densely packed with darkly stained neurons and does not yet exhibit any laminar differentiation. Although the corpus callosum is recognizable as such, it is thin and many fibers have not yet reached the midline. Ipsilateral corticocortical fiber tracts such as the cingulum bundle are even less well defined. However, the internal capsule, though small in size in comparison to later stages, is well demarcated by the cell masses of the anlage of the basal ganglia which abut it.

In the fetus injected at E69 and sacrificed at E70, labeled fibers descend from the injection site to the subjacent intermediate zone (prospective white matter) and into the developing corpus callosum. However, few if any callosal fibers enter or even approach the boundaries of the prospective homotopic prefrontal cortex (Figure 7, E69–70). Likewise, within the injected hemisphere, labeled fibers could not be visualized in the prospective white matter along the medial wall of the hemisphere to form a fascicle resembling the cingulum bundle, which

Patricia S. Goldman-Rakic

is the prominent intrahemispheric pathway of prefrontal fibers to the adult retrosplenial cortex. Hence the ipsilateral association-fiber connections are also not evident at this embryonic age. On the other hand, fibers in the anterior limb of the internal capsule are heavily labeled at E60, indicating that the survival time of 24 hours alloted in our experiments was more than sufficient for labeled tracers to reach distant structures by axonal transport.

The prospective dorsolateral prefrontal cortex was also injected with radioactive amino acids in fetuses at midgestation (E85, E95, and E104). The cortical mantle of the fetal brain at these ages is still essentially lissencephalic. Although all neurons that will compose the dorsolateral convexity cortex have been generated before E100 (Rakic and Wikmark, personal communication), they have not completed their migratory journeys to this region of the telencephalon from their "birthplace" in the germinal ventricular and subventricular zones lining the lateral cerebral ventricles. At midgestation, numerous bipolar cells, presumably migrating neurons, are distributed throughout the intermediate zone between the ventricular surface and the developing cortical plate (Goldman and Galkin, 1978). In areas subjacent to the immature neopallium, some larger and paler cells form the so-called cortical subplate of Kostovic and Molliver (1974). At E105 in the monkey, these cells lie considerably below the densely packed cortical plate (Goldman and Galkin, 1978). Histological examination of the cortex in fetal brains at midgestation reveals the emergence of laminar segregation, but the cellular organization is far from mature.

Examination of specimens injected between E85 and E104 reveals a progressive increase in the density of radioactive label over associational and callosal fibers as well as an extension of the distance over which they have grown from their site of origin in the prospective dorsolateral prefrontal cortex over this period. Even at these embryonic ages, however, the callosal and associational fibers display an immature pattern of distribution which is different from the adult (Figure 7, E95–96). Within the injected hemisphere of an E104 fetus, the oldest in this series, it was possible to identify the anlage of the cingulum bundle, but the labeled fibers in this bundle were confined to the frontal lobe and did not extend very far caudally into the parietal and temporal lobes. Thus, they did not reach the retrosplenial cortex, which is their main target. In the hemisphere contralateral to the injection site, labeled fibers were dispersed in the prospective white matter but, like the associational system on the ipsilateral side, gave no evidence of attaining their specific cortical targets. In the same fetus, fibers of the internal capsule and other classes of descending axons (corticothalamic, corticobulbar) were relatively heavily labeled.

Between E104 and E123, when the next injection was made, the gross morphology of the developing telencephalon changes considerably. Fissuration is well advanced as primary and secondary sulci become

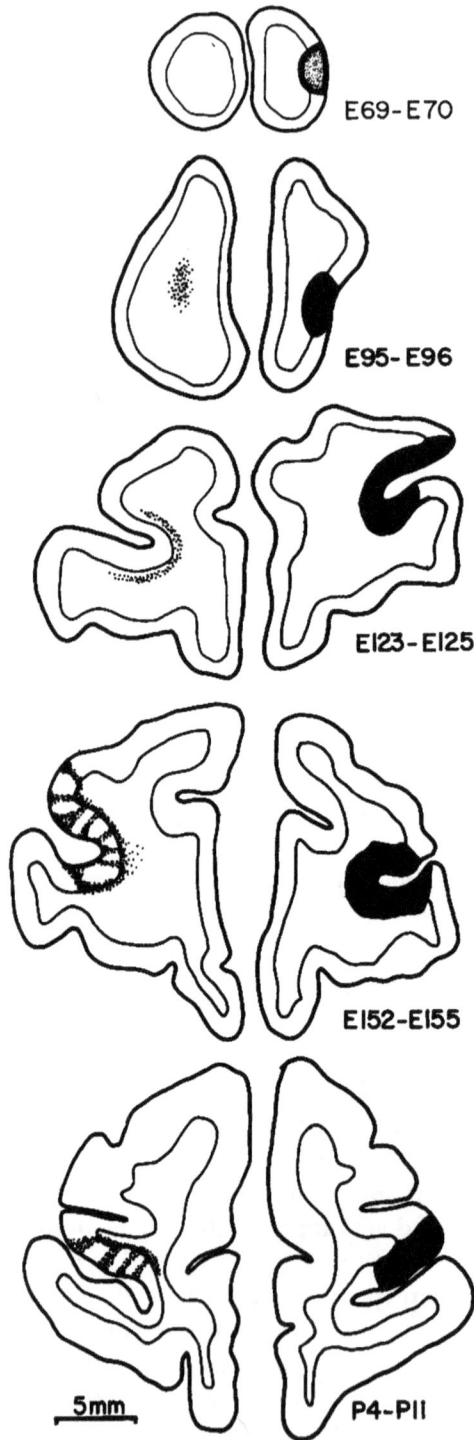

Figure 7 Diagrammatic illustration of the development of callosal fibers at different embryonic (E) and postnatal (P) ages. The first number in the label below each outline drawing indicates the age in days when the animal was injected and the second number refers to the age in days at which it was sacrificed. Callosal fibers do not reach the con-

clearly identifiable. The six-layered pattern of cortical lamination is distinct though neurons still stain darkly in Nissl preparations and are relatively densely packed in comparison with mature brain. The subplate layer lies closer to the cortical plate and forms a narrow band below it. In the fetus injected at E123 and sacrificed at E125, labeled fibers are not only more numerous as judged by the density of radioactivity in autoradiograms, but many of them now reach the border of their cortical targets. In the prefrontal cortex, callosal fibers are lined up in the outer part of the intermediate zone beneath the cortical plate subjacent to layer VI of the developing cortex. Silver grains form a continuous line beneath the cortex lining the principal sulcus, which becomes prominent at this age, but do not enter the cortical plate (Figure 7, E123–125). Further, terminal fields show no indication of segregating into bands or columns. In the same specimen, the ipsilateral associational fibers to the retrosplenial cortex show a somewhat more advanced level of development. Alternating areas of higher and lower grain density are observable over the region of the subplate layer, and some fibers penetrate the overlying cortex at these points of concentration. In these cortical regions, radioactivity extends only as far as layer III and at this stage does not enter layer I.

In a fetus injected at E152 and sacrificed at E155, both the associational and callosal fibers have entered their respective cortical targets and their terminals are distributed in the mature pattern (Figure 7, E152–155). The retrosplenial cortex in the ipsilateral hemisphere and the homotopic prefrontal cortex in the contralateral hemisphere display a clear pattern of alternating bands that extend through all layers of the cortex in a manner nearly identical to that in postnatal animals. The differentiation of these pathways therefore takes place prenatally about 2 months earlier than that described for thalamocortical fibers of the primary visual system of the same species (Rakic, 1976; Hubel, Wiesel, and LeVay, 1977).

Plasticity of Callosal Connections

Over the past decade, numerous studies have established that connections of the developing mammalian central nervous system are considerably more modifiable than previously thought. Our recent experiments in monkeys provide new evidence for plasticity of neuronal connections that can occur in the frontal association cortex in developing primates. We removed the dorsolateral prefrontal cortex in one hemisphere in fetuses and in neonates 1–8 weeks after birth. Following the unilateral resections, the monkeys survived at least two

---

tralateral hemisphere until after E70 and do not even enter the cortical plate before E123. Rather, at this embryonic age, callosal fibers accumulate in the "waiting" compartment in the intermediate zone below the developing cortical plate. Callosal axons invade the cortex between E125 and E152, and by the end of this period they are already segregated into the "modular" pattern characteristic of the neocortex in postnatal monkeys (e.g., P4–11).

months. After this period we injected microquantities of [³H]-leucine and [³H]-proline into the dorsal bank of the principal sulcus in the unoperated hemisphere corresponding to the area resected in the opposite brain half. One or three weeks later, the animals were sacrificed and their brains processed for autoradiography.

The main purpose of this experiment was to examine the mode of development of the dorsolateral prefrontal callosal projections in the absence of their normal synaptic target in the contralateral hemisphere. Our preliminary analyses show that the callosal fibers that would normally innervate the homotopic cortex in the principal sulcus can be displaced to the dorsomedial frontal cortex dorsal to the callosal marginal sulcus (Goldman-Rakic, 1980b, and Figure 8). This frontal region normally receives projections from the prefrontal cortex in the ipsilateral principal sulcus. Thus, it is an area that was partially deafferented by the prefrontal resection within the same hemisphere. Although at present we do not know whether the same cortical area normally receives callosal fibers, it is interesting that the displaced fibers are distributed in a discontinuous pattern, as they would be in their normal field of termination. A "columnar" mode of organization is thus preserved in the anomalous afferent fibers innervating a foreign territory.

The mechanisms underlying this extraordinary rearrangement of callosal connections remain to be determined. The simplest and perhaps most parsimonious explanation is that in the absence of their targets, callosal fibers which normally project to the resected frontal cortex enter a nearby cortical region. The locus and degree of this rerouting may be determined by the absence of association-fiber input from the resected cortex. However, it is also possible that the aberrant distribution of callosal fibers is influenced indirectly by rearrangements of thalamocortical fibers which may occur more immediately following resection. During normal development, callosal fibers enter the cortex only after the thalamocortical system is established. Thus, if thalamocortical fibers are displaced as a result of our resection, the callosal fibers may follow them into their aberrant positions. There is some indication from studies of the visual system that the distribution of geniculocortical afferents may alter the distribution of callosal fibers (Shatz, 1979; Lund and Mitchell, 1979). Thus, the rearrangement of callosal terminals in our material could conceivably occur secondarily to thalamocortical rearrangements.

Corticostriatal Connections

Adult Organization
It is widely accepted that the dorsolateral prefrontal cortex influences behavior through its principal output pathway—the corticostriatal projection. Paradoxically, in spite of its considerable size, the existence of a corticostriatal fiber system was denied for most of this century.

Patricia S. Goldman-Rakic

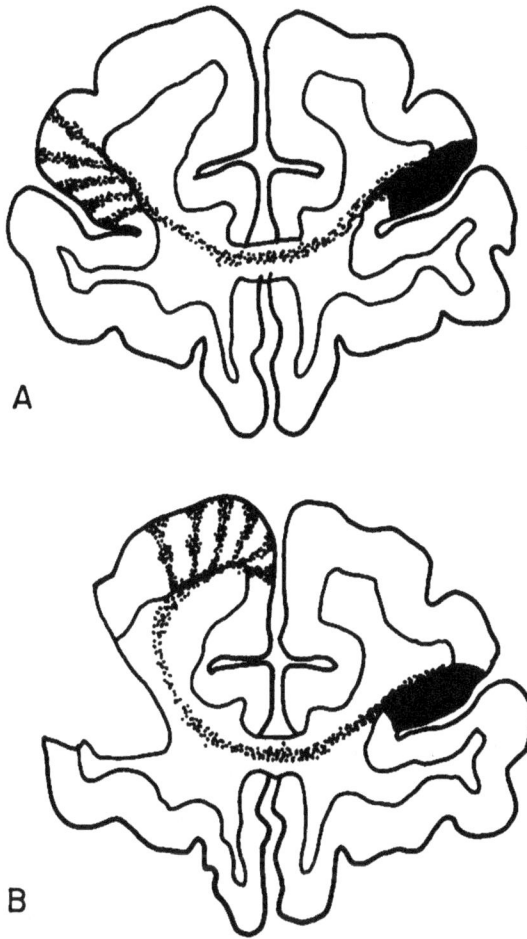

Figure 8 Drawing of prefrontal cortex in the left and right hemispheres. (A) Normal rhesus monkey whose principal sulcal cortex in the right hemisphere was injected with a mixture of [³H]-leucine and [³H]-proline 3 weeks before being sacrificed. The drawing illustrates the pattern of alternating callosal fiber bundles in the homotopic cortex of the left hemisphere. (B) Monkey in which the dorsolateral prefrontal cortex was resected in the left hemisphere at 8 weeks of age. Two months later intracortical injections were placed in the principal sulcus of the right hemisphere and the monkey survived 3 weeks before being sacrificed. Callosal fibers deprived of their normal target in the contralateral hemisphere pass by the resected area and become redistributed in the cortex dorsal and medial to the resected area. The anomalous pathway retains its pattern of spatial periodicity.

Only in the last two decades has this massive cortical efferent system become firmly established by studies in rats and cats (Webster, 1961, 1965), rabbit (Carman, Cowan, and Powell, 1963), and monkey (DeVito and Smith, 1964; Johnson, Rosvold, and Mishkin, 1968; Kemp and Powell, 1970). More recently, autoradiographic studies (Künzle, 1975; Goldman and Nauta, 1977b; Yeterian and Van Hoesen, 1978) have exposed the full extent of these connections as well as the nature of their terminal distribution within the neostriatum.

The higher resolution of the autoradiographic method for tracing central neuronal connections has revealed some important new information that has revised our view about the size and topographic relations of corticostriatal projections as well as introduced new concepts that are essential for understanding the development and plasticity of this system. For example, early investigations employing silver degeneration methods indicated that the corticostriatal projection in primates is organized according to an anterior-posterior plan such that the frontal cortical regions projected to the head of the nucleus while more posterior cortical zones terminated in the body and tail of the caudate (Kemp and Powell, 1970). Autoradiography after injection of [^{3}H]-leucine into prefrontal cortex of one hemisphere shows that even a small zone of cortex in the middle third of the dorsal bank of the principal sulcus projects not only to the head of the caudate nucleus, as previously shown, but also throughout the entire rostrocaudal extent of the nucleus to its tail in the temporal lobe (Goldman and Nauta, 1977b). These prefrontal-striatal projections overlap with those originating in other cortical areas (Yeterian and Van Hoesen, 1978) as well as with those from the substantia nigra (Carpenter, 1976) and thalamus (Kalil, 1978; Royce, 1978). The sizeable projection of prefrontal cortex upon the caudate nucleus stands in contrast to the sparse innervation of this structure by motor cortex (Goldman and Nauta, 1977b; Künzle, 1975) and provides a neural basis for the cognitive deficits that have long been known to result from lesions of the caudate nucleus (Battig, Rosvold, and Mishkin, 1960; Divac, 1968; Goldman and Rosvold, 1972).

Another new observation that is particularly relevant to the issue of neuronal plasticity in the mode of organization of corticostriatal projections is the configurational pattern of its terminal field (Goldman and Nauta, 1977b). Our autoradiographic study revealed that the corticocaudate projections terminate in the form of clusters of fields surrounding round or elliptically shaped territories which are devoid of prefrontal afferents (Figure 9). Presumably, these label-free territories are innervated by other sources of input, the identity of which has not been determined. The clustering of corticostriatal terminals is interesting in light of evidence for clustering of dopamine-containing fibers from the substantia nigra (Olson, Seiger, and Fuxe, 1972; Tennyson et al., 1972) as well as more recent data indicating dense and light zones of acetylcholinesterase staining within the fetal and mature striatum of the

Patricia S. Goldman-Rakic

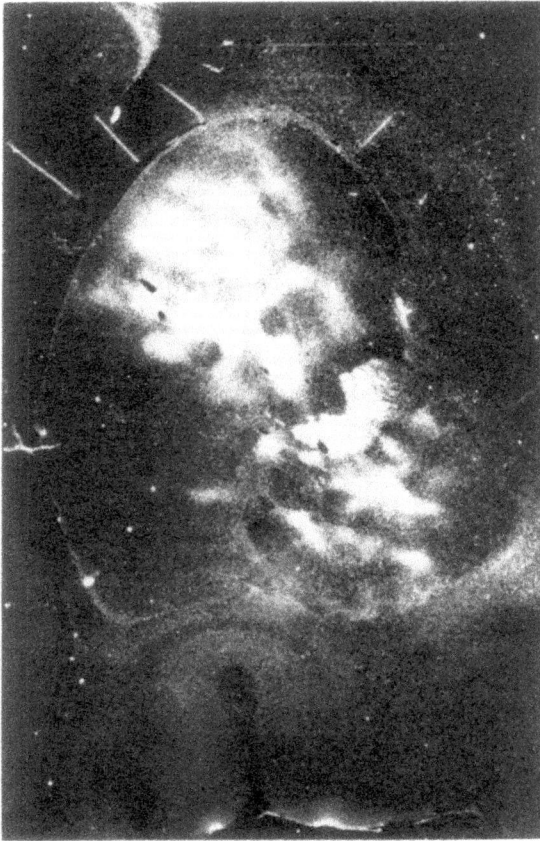

Figure 9 Photograph under dark-field illumination of the caudate nucleus in a normal rhesus monkey whose homolateral principal sulcus was injected with tritiated amino acids. The dark-field autoradiogram displays the intricate pattern of fiber clusters originating in prefrontal cortex. These fiber clusters often surround elliptically shaped territories devoid of prefrontal input.

rat (Butcher and Hodge, 1976), cat (Graybiel and Ragsdale, 1979), and monkey (Goldman-Rakic, unpublished). Another part of the primate neostriatum, the putamen, also receives its cortical (Künzle, 1975) and thalamic (Kalil, 1978) input in discontinuous patterns. Detailed knowledge of how the various intrinsic and extrinsic fiber systems are intercalated within the neostriatum is still lacking. However, the structural information presently available can be used to advantage in studying the development and modifiability of this system in primates.

Development of Corticostriatal Connections
The development of corticostriatal fibers was studied autoradiographically in fetuses ranging in age from E69 to E155 and in monkeys of selected postnatal ages. In contrast to the slow and protracted outgrowth of the corticocortical fiber systems of the prefrontal cortex,

prefrontostriatal axons reach their target structure very early during prenatal development (Goldman-Rakic, 1980a). Thus, in a fetus injected at E69, many radioactively labeled fibers can be detected in the homolateral caudate nucleus, even though at this age this nucleus is still acquiring additional neurons and glial cells from the proliferative zone of the ganglionic eminence (Brand and Rakic, 1979). The most notable finding is that the cortical projections are distributed *uniformly* throughout the prospective caudate nucleus rather than as segregated patches characteristic of the prefrontal corticostriatal terminals in neonatal and adult monkeys (Figure 10).

By E85, all neurons destined to become caudate neurons have been generated (Brand and Rakic, 1979). In fetuses injected at this and slightly older fetal ages (E85, E95, and E104) the caudate nucleus is replete with silver grains (Goldman-Rakic, 1980a). However, fiber clusters or "patches" are still not present at any of these ages. Rather, prefrontal terminals seem to be distributed in a uniform fashion throughout the head of the caudate (Figure 10A,B).

As in the case of the corticocortical fibers, the first evidence of segregation of fibers was found in the fetus injected at E123 and sacrificed at E125. In the caudate nucleus of this fetus, areas of higher and lower grain density begin to emerge (this specimen is not illustrated in Figure 10). However, the boundaries between these areas are less distinct than in postnatal monkeys processed in an identical manner.

In synchrony with the maturation of disjunctive arrangements of corticocortical fibers, the corticocaudate projection appears to attain a virtually adult configuration at least 2 weeks before birth at E152–155 (Figure 10C,D). The labyrinthine network of fiber clusters surrounding elliptical or irregularly shaped cores that are free of prefrontal input is fully evident in the monkey injected at E152 and sacrificed at E155 (Figure 10C). Thus, the development of corticostriatal terminals goes through a phase of relatively diffuse terminal distribution before entering a phase of terminal fiber segregation. Although at present we do not know precisely the source of the interlocking input in the areas that become "vacated," the mode of segregation is reminiscent of the biphasic development of lamination in the lateral geniculate body of the thalamus (Rakic, 1976). It thus appears that the same basic mechanisms are at play in the formation of two very different neural systems.

Plasticity of Prefrontocaudate Projection
We have recently described the existence of anomalous crossed prefrontocaudate projections in monkeys in which the prospective dorsolateral prefrontal cortex was removed 6 weeks before birth (Goldman, 1978). These results have now been confirmed in, and extended to, monkeys in which the dorsolateral cortex was resected as late as 2 months after birth (Goldman-Rakic, 1980b).

Patricia S. Goldman-Rakic

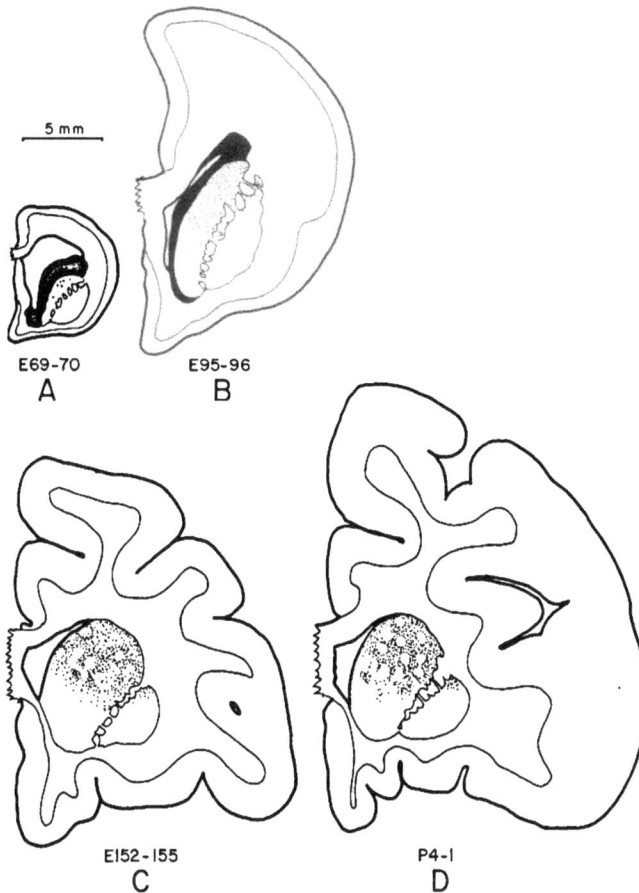

Figure 10 Illustration of the time and mode of establishment of prefrontocaudate connections in the rhesus monkey. Prefrontal fibers enter the caudate nucleus as early as E69 but they are distributed uniformly at this and subsequent embryonic ages. Segregation of cortical terminals begins at or around E123 (not shown), and is well developed, if not virtually completed, by E152.

In both prenatally and postnatally operated monkeys the projection to the ipsilateral caudate nucleus is, as might be expected, similar in topography and configuration to that observed in normal monkeys of the same age. The projection to the contralateral caudate nucleus, however, differs markedly from that of controls (Figure 11). Whereas in normal animals the contralateral caudate nucleus contains silver grains that only barely exceed background, in the previously operated monkeys dense concentrations of label can be traced in consecutive serial sections throughout the entire extent of the contralateral nucleus, that is, over a distance of several centimeters (Goldman, 1978). Significantly, the crossed projection is expanded predominantly in those areas that were deafferented by the unilateral dorsolateral lesions. Furthermore,

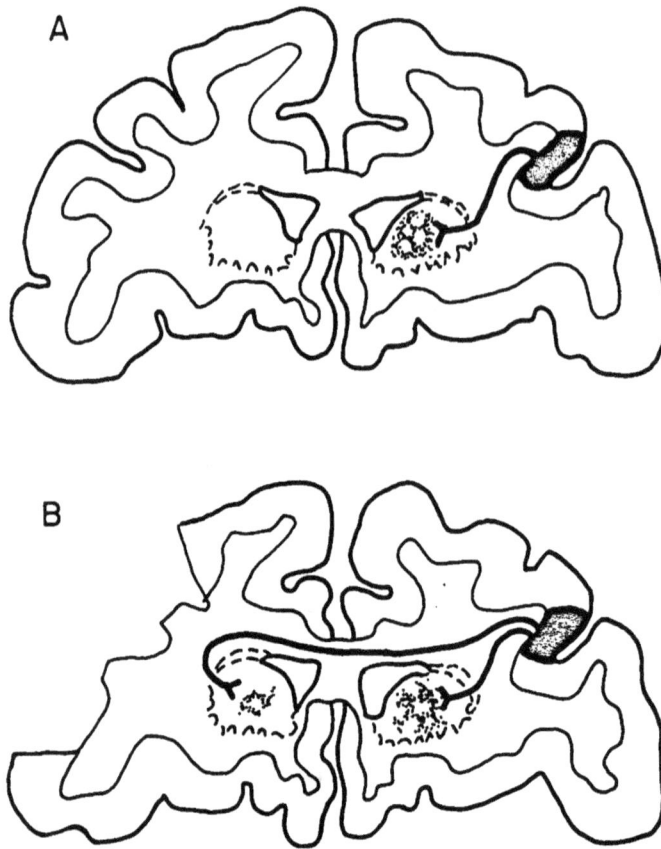

Figure 11 Diagrammatic illustration of the head of the caudate nuclei in the left and right hemispheres. (A) Normal monkey that received an injection of mixed [³H]-proline and [³H]-leucine in the right hemisphere at 5 days of age. The monkey was sacrificed one week later and its brain processed for autoradiography. The drawing shows the intricate and dense pattern of labeling in the right (ipsilateral) caudate nucleus. (B) Monkey whose prospective dorsolateral prefrontal cortex in the left hemisphere was resected at E119, 6 weeks before birth. The fetus was returned to the uterus and subsequently delivered near term. On the fifth postnatal day, the right prefrontal cortex was injected with tritiated amino acids and sacrificed 1 week later. Note intricate pattern of grains in the right (ipsilateral) caudate nucleus, but also a distinct projection to the left (contralateral) caudate. (Based on Goldman, 1978.)

Patricia S. Goldman-Rakic

the anomalous contralateral projections exhibit the same "annular" pattern of termination that characterize the normal projections (Figure 11).

Several mechanisms may be involved in the reorganization of corticocaudate projections consequent to unilateral prefrontal resection, and some of them have already been discussed (Goldman, 1978). One possibility is that the abnormally large contralateral projections result from arresting development at an embryonic stage when corticostriatal projections might normally be bilateral. It now appears that this mechanism is unlikely to be involved because of our recent autoradiographic data on prenatal development of connections (see previous section and Goldman-Rakic, 1980a), which provides no evidence of strong bilateral prefrontocaudate projections at any stage of development between E69 and E155. Therefore, the phenomenon of neuronal rearrangement cannot simply be explained as a failure of selective elimination of contralateral projections. However, a considerable number of fibers enters the contralateral hemisphere and collects along the dorsal margin of the internal capsule at these same fetal ages (Goldman, 1979). It is thus possible that some axons that would normally descend into the internal capsule of the contralateral hemisphere invade the deafferented caudate nucleus, which lacks its normal input from the resected cortex.

A related but more likely possibility is that axons forming anomalous connections belong to the class of efferent neurons that normally issue a *minor* projection to the contralateral caudate nucleus. These corticostriatal neurons, which are not easy to detect by the autoradiographic method in developing animals, may expand their terminal fields and occupy a number of synaptic spaces on caudate neurons vacated by degeneration of their ipsilateral prefrontal input. Such a mechanism has been postulated for neuronal plasticity in a variety of other systems (e.g., Hicks and D'Amato, 1970; Schneider, 1973; Lund, Cunningham, and Lund, 1973; Lynch, Stanfield, and Cotman, 1973).

Finally, we have not ruled out the possibility that the anomalous crossed corticostriatal fibers originate from callosal neurons which, in the absence of their homotopic target cells in the operated hemisphere, invade the caudate nucleus subjacent to the lesion to join with the normally meager complement of crossed corticostriatal fibers. Thus, callosal fibers, in the absence of their normal terminal field, may split into two groups: one that is rerouted to heterotopic cortex (described in the previous section), and another that enters the completely foreign territory of the neostriatum. This hypothesis is testable, and if rewiring of callosal fibers to subcortical targets should prove to be the case, it would represent a type of rewiring that is unprecedented in the mammalian nervous sytem. However, in order to choose between the various mechanisms that have been proposed and perhaps to reveal new possibilities that have not been considered, further experimental anatomical studies are essential.

Concluding Remarks

The cellular organization and neuronal connections of the prefrontal association cortex in primates are beginning to be understood at a level of analysis that was not possible before introduction of new neuroanatomical methods. The corticocortical connections of prefrontal cortex have discontinuous terminal fields that form a "modular" type of organization that in several respects is both similar to, and different from, the spatially periodic afferent-fiber input described previously for the various sensory specific cortices (e.g., Hubel and Wiesel, 1977; Jones, Coulter, and Hendry, 1978; Imig and Brugge, 1978). Further, this mode of cellular organization is also reflected in the disjunctive distribution of its subcortical efferents, for example, to the superior colliculus (Goldman and Nauta, 1976), to the thalamus (Goldman, 1979) and most notably, to the caudate nucleus as described above (Goldman and Nauta, 1977b). Analyses of the sequence of outgrowth and plasticity of these connections have yielded new insights into brain development and modifiability.

The results of experiments performed on monkey fetuses indicate that the two classes of efferent prefrontal connections develop unexpectedly early both in comparison with other species and in relation to other systems of the primate brain. Thus, callosal stripes in the prefrontal cortex are well delineated at least 2 weeks before birth whereas oculardominance stripes in the primary visual cortex do not become fully segregated until approximately 6 weeks after birth (Hubel, Wiesel, and LeVay, 1977). The biological significance of the sequences and disparities in timetables of development of fiber terminal fields is not known.

Regardless of differences in the onset of outgrowth and differentiation of the corticocortical and corticostriatal fiber systems, these two classes of connections follow a common program of development that can be divided into at least three stages. The first stage is the stage of outgrowth of axons before they reach their target structures. The present material does not provide the precise time when this stage begins for any of the fiber classes studied but indicates that it ends earlier for the corticostriatal (around or before E69) than for the corticocortical (around or before E123) connections of prefrontal cortex.

In the second stage, which spans the middle third of gestation, the two classes of fibers reach and/or enter their target structures. The corticostriatal fibers initially innervate the neostriatum in a diffuse and uniform manner. The segregation of terminals into fiber clusters surrounding fiber-free cores that characterizes the mature pathway is not evident before E123. A similar lack of spatial segregation is displayed by the corticocortical fibers; but unlike the corticostriatal fibers which enter their target, the uniformly distributed cortical terminals remain just below the cortical plate in the "waiting compartment." Further-

Patricia S. Goldman-Rakic

more, when they do enter, they do so in a segregated fashion from the very beginning. We have not observed a periodic distribution of their terminals within the cortex itself in any of our material studied to date. To the contrary, the available evidence shows that the corticocortical fibers enter the cortex only at nodal points, rather than in a uniform "front." Thus, it appears that the mode of development of corticocortical fibers differs from that of thalamocortical (Rakic, 1976) and corticostriatal fibers (Goldman-Rakic, 1980a), both of which are initially distributed in a diffuse manner within their target structures. A plausible reason for this difference may be that the late-forming corticocortical fibers follow the earlier-developing thalamic fibers, which "stake out" their synaptic territories first and "force" the corticocortical fibers to enter the cortex only through narrow and "vacant" channels.

The third stage of development of connectivity of prefrontal cortex begins during the last third of gestation. During this period, fibers become fully segregated into bands in all cortical layers and clusters in the caudate nucleus. The development of connections from diffuse to patterned termination has previously been reported for thalamocortical pathways of the primary visual system in the same species (Rakic, 1976). In this system, axons derived from the two eyes invade the tectum, the lateral geniculate body, and visual cortex in an overlapping manner before becoming segregated from one another into patches, laminae, and stripes, respectively. Thus a transformation from overlapping-and-diffuse to segregated-and-patterned innervation appears to reflect a general rule governing the formation of central connections—one that applies not only to ascending fiber systems but to corticocortical, both associational and callosal, connections—and to the great descending corticostriatal pathway as well.

One of the salient attributes of the developing brain is its modifiability. Our studies on the plasticity of prefrontal connections have revealed their capacity for reorganization, which is comparable to, and in certain respects greater than, that described for other systems in both primate and nonprimate mammals. A high degree of plasticity should perhaps be expected from the prefrontal cortex, which also displays a high order of functional resilience in response to changes in the internal and external environment. However, it should be emphasized that the anomalous prefrontal connections demonstrated in our studies retain to a remarkable degree the orderliness and spatial regularity that characterize their normal distributions. This finding suggests that the same rule which governs the local distribution of pathways during initial development may also govern their redevelopment.

The capacity of the central nervous system to reorganize its synaptic connectivity in response to deprivation or lesions is of interest not only because of its theoretical significance but also because new connections are potentially the most important biological mechanism underlying resilience of function. It is generally accepted that the severity of behavioral deficits caused by focal injury to the mammalian nervous system is strongly influenced by the age at which the lesion is sustained. Although the critical period for lesion-induced alterations in the callosal and corticostriatal connections of the primate brain is still unknown, evidence of rewiring of these cortical efferents following perinatal brain injury leads naturally to the hypothesis that anomalous connections may play an important role in restitution of function in primates. It is noteworthy that the dorsolateral prefrontal cortex, the connections of which exhibit considerable anatomical plasticity, is part of the same neural system that has been shown to exhibit modifiability in response to early experience (Goldman, 1976; Goldman and Mendelson, 1977) and hormones (Goldman and Brown, 1975), as well as a marked capacity for functional reorganization following both prenatal (Goldman and Galkin, 1978) and postnatal (Goldman, 1971) cortical injury. Although at the present state of technology, we have had to use a reasonably large surgical ablation to reveal the structural plasticity of frontal-lobe connections, there is every reason to believe that these connections can also be modified in more subtle ways by relevant extrinsic stimulation and experience. Such changes in the connections of prefrontal association cortex can be expected to be of profound significance for the behavior and personality of the individual.

References

Akert, K., 1964. Comparative anatomy of the frontal cortex and thalamocortical connections. In *The Frontal Granular Cortex and Behavior*. J. M. Warren and K. Akert, eds. New York: McGraw-Hill, pp. 372–396.

Battig, K., H. E. Rosvold, and M. Mishkin, 1960. Comparison of the effects of frontal and caudate lesions on delayed response and alternation in monkeys. *J. Comp. Physiol. Psychol.* 53:400–404.

Bianchi, L., 1922. *The Mechanism of the Brain and the Function of the Frontal Lobes*. J. H. MacDonald, transl. New York: W. Wood & Co.

Bodian, D., 1966. Development of fine structure of spinal cord in monkey fetuses. I. The motoneuron neuropil at the time of onset of reflex activity. *Bull. Johns Hopkins Hosp.* 119:129–149.

Bodian, D., 1970. A model of synaptic and behavioral ontogeny. In *The Neurosciences: Second Study Program*. F. O. Schmitt, ed. New York: Rockefeller University Press, pp. 129–140.

Brand, S., and P. Rakic, 1979. Genesis of the primate neostriatum: ^{3}H-thymidine autoradiographic analysis of the time of neuron origin in the rhesus monkey. *Neuroscience* 4:767–778.

Butcher, L. L., and C. G. Hodge, 1976. Postnatal development of acetylcholinesterase in the caudate-putamen nucleus and substantia nigra of rats. *Brain Res.* 106:223–240.

Patricia S. Goldman-Rakic

Carman, J. B., W. M. Cowan, and T. P. S. Powell, 1963. The organization of corticostriate connections in the rabbit. *Brain* 86:525–560.

Carpenter, M. B., 1976. Anatomical organization of the corpus striatum and related nuclei. In *The Basal Ganglia.* M. D. Yahr, ed. New York: Raven Press, pp. 1–35.

Denny-Brown, D., 1951. The frontal lobes and their function. In *Modern Trends in Neurology.* A. Feiling, ed. New York: Hoeber, Inc., pp. 13–89.

DeVito, J. L., and O. A. S. Smith, Jr., 1964. Subcortical projections of the prefrontal lobe of the monkey. *J. Comp. Neurol.* 123:413–424.

Divac, I., 1968. Functions of the caudate nucleus. *Acta Biol. Exp. (Warsaw)* 28:107–120.

Ferrier, D., 1886. *The Functions of the Brain,* 2nd ed. New York: G. P. Putnam's Sons.

Filimonov, I. N., 1949. Cortical cytoarchitecture—general concepts. Classification of the architectonic formations. In *Cytoarchitecture of the Cerebral Cortex in Man.* S. A. Sarkisov, I. N. Filimonov, and N. S. Preobrazenskaya, eds. Moscow: Medgiz, pp. 11–32. (In Russian.)

Franz, S. I., 1907. On the functions of the cerebrum: The frontal lobes. *Arch. Psychol.* 2:1–64.

Fritsch, G., and E. Hitzig, 1870. Über die elektrische Erregbarkeit des Grosshirns. *Arch. Anat. Physiol. Wiss. Med.* 37:300–332. [Transl. in Bonin (1960): *Some Papers on the Cerebral Cortex.* Springfield, Illinois: Charles C. Thomas.]

Fulton, J. F., 1951. *Frontal Lobotomy and Affective Behavior.* New York: W. W. Norton & Co.

Goldman, P. S., 1971. Functional development of the prefrontal cortex in early life and the problem of neuronal plasticity. *Exp. Neurol.* 32:366–387.

Goldman, P. S., 1976. The role of experience in recovery of function following prefrontal lesions in infant monkeys. *Neuropsychologia* 14:401–412.

Goldman, P. S., 1978. Neuronal plasticity in primate telencephalon: anomalous crossed cortico-caudate projections induced by prenatal removal of frontal association cortex. *Science* 202:768–770.

Goldman, P. S., 1979. Contralateral projections to the dorsal thalamus from frontal association cortex in the rhesus monkey. *Brain Res.* 166:166–171.

Goldman, P. S., and R. M. Brown, 1975. The influence of neonatal androgen on the development of cortical function in the rhesus monkey. *Neurosci. Abst.* 1:494.

Goldman, P. S., and T. W. Galkin, 1978. Prenatal removal of frontal association cortex in the rhesus monkey: Anatomical and functional consequences in postnatal life. *Brain Res.* 52:451–485.

Goldman, P. S., and M. J. Mendelson, 1977. Salutary effects of early experience on deficits caused by lesions of frontal association cortex in developing rhesus monkeys. *Exp. Neurol.* 57:588–602.

Goldman, P. S., and W. J. H. Nauta, 1976. Autoradiographic demonstration of a projection from prefrontal association cortex to the superior colliculus in the rhesus monkey. *Brain Res.* 116:145–149.

Goldman, P. S., and W. J. H. Nauta, 1977a. Columnar distribution of corticocortical fibers in the frontal association, limbic, and motor cortex of the developing rhesus monkey. *Brain Res.* 122:393–413.

Goldman, P. S., and W. J. H. Nauta, 1977b. An intricately patterned prefrontocaudate projection in the rhesus monkey. *J. Comp. Neurol.* 171:369–386.

Goldman, P. S., and H. E. Rosvold, 1972. The effects of selective caudate lesions in infant and juvenile rhesus monkeys. *Brain Res.* 43:53–66.

Goldman-Rakic, P. S., 1980a. Prenatal development of corticostriatal projections in the rhesus monkey. *Neurosci. Abst.* (in press).

Goldman-Rakic, P. S., 1980b. Rearrangement of callosal terminal fields following ablation of developing neocortex in primates. (In preparation.)

Graybiel, A. M., and C. W. Ragsdale, 1979. Histochemically distinct compartments in the striatum of human being, monkey and cat demonstrated by the acetylthiocholinesterase staining method. *Proc. Nat. Acad. Sci. USA* 75:5723–5726.

Hand, P. J., R. R. Miselis, and M. Reivich, 1977. A (^{14}C)-2-deoxyglucose metabolic mapping study of the rat posteromedial barrel subfield. *Neurosci. Abst.* 3:483.

Hand, P. J., J. H. Greenberg, R. R. Miselis, W. L. Weller, and M. Reivich, 1978. A normal and altered cortical column: A quantitative and qualitative (^{14}C)-2-deoxyglucose (2DG) mapping study. *Neurosci. Abst.* 4:553.

Harlow, J. M., 1868. Recovery after severe injury to the head. *Pub. Mass. Med. Soc.* 2:329.

Hicks, S. P., and C. J. D'Amato, 1970. Motor-sensory and visual behavior after hemispherectomy in newborn and mature rats. *Exp. Neurol.* 29:416–438.

Hubel, D. H., and D. C. Freeman, 1977. Projection into the visual field of ocular dominance columns in macaque monkey. *Brain Res.* 122:336–343.

Hubel, D. H., and T. N. Wiesel, 1977. Functional architecture of macaque monkey visual cortex. *Proc. Roy. Soc. B* 193:1–59.

Hubel, D. H., T. N. Wiesel, and S. LeVay, 1977. Plasticity of ocular dominance columns in monkey striate cortex. *Phil. Trans. Roy. Soc. B* 278:377–409.

Hubel, D. H., T. N. Wiesel, and M. P. Stryker, 1978. Orientation columns in macaque monkey visual cortex demonstrated by the 2-deoxyglucose autoradiographic technique. *Nature* 269:328–330.

Imig, T. J., and J. F. Brugge, 1978. Sources and terminations of callosal axons related to binaural and frequency maps in primary auditory cortex of the cat. *J. Comp. Neurol.* 182:637–660.

Jacobsen, C. F. 1936. Studies of cerebral function in primates. *Comp. Psychol. Monogr.* 13:1–68.

Jacobson, S., and J. Q. Trojanowski, 1975. Amygdaloid projections to prefrontal granular cortex in rhesus monkey demonstrated with horseradish peroxidase. *Brain Res.* 100:132–139.

Jacobson, S., and J. Q. Trojanowski, 1977a. Prefrontal granular cortex of the rhesus monkey. I. Intrahemispheric cortical afferents. *Brain Res.* 132:209–233.

Jacobson, S., and J. Q. Trojanowski, 1977b. Prefrontal granular cortex of the rhesus monkey. II. Interhemispheric cortical afferents. *Brain Res.* 132:235–246.

Jacobson, S., N. Butters, and N. J. Tovsky, 1978. Afferent and efferent subcortical projections of behaviorally defined sectors of prefrontal granular cortex. *Brain Res.* 159:279–296.

Johnson, T. N., H. E. Rosvold, and M. Mishkin, 1968. Projections from behaviorally-defined sectors of the prefrontal cortex to the basal ganglia, septum, and diencephalon of the monkey. *Exp. Neurol.* 21:20–34.

Jones, E. G., J. D. Coulter, and S. H. C. Hendry, 1978. Intracortical connectivity of architectonic fields in the somatic sensory, motor and parietal cortex of monkeys. *J. Comp. Neurol.* 181:291–348.

Kalil, K., 1978. Patch-like termination of thalamic fibers in the putamen of the rhesus monkey: An autoradiographic study. *Brain Res.* 140:333–339.

Kemp, J. M., and T. P. S. Powell, 1970. The cortico-striate projection in the monkey. *Brain* 93:525–546.

Kemper, T. L., W. F. Caviness, and P. I. Yakovlev, 1973. The neuronographic and metric study of the dendritic arbours of neurons in the motor cortex of macaca mulatta at birth and at 24 months of age. *Brain* 96:765–782.

Kennedy, C., M. des Rosiers, O. Sakurada, M. Shinohara, M. Reivich, J. Jehle, and L. Sokoloff, 1976. Metabolic mapping of the primary visual system of the monkey by means of the autoradiographic (^{14}C)-deoxyglucose technique. *Proc. Nat. Acad. Sci. USA* 73:4230–4234.

Kievit, J., and H. G. J. M. Kuypers, 1977. Organization of the thalamocortical connexions to the frontal lobe in the rhesus monkey. *Exp. Brain Res.* 29:299–322.

Kostovic, I., and M. Molliver, 1974. A new interpretation of the laminar development of cerebral cortex: synaptogenesis in different layers of neopallium in the human fetus. *Anat. Rec.* 178:395.

Künzle, H., 1975. Bilateral projections from precentral motor cortex to the putamen and other parts of the basal ganglia. *Brain Res.* 88:195–210.

Künzle, H., 1978. An autoradiographic analysis of the efferent connections from premotor and adjacent prefrontal regions (areas 6 and 9) in *Macacca fascicularis*. *Brain Behav. Evol.* 15:185–234.

Kuypers, H. G. J. M., 1962. Corticospinal connections: Postnatal development in rhesus monkey. *Science* 138:678–680.

LeVay, S., D. H. Hubel, and T. N. Wiesel, 1975. The pattern of ocular dominance columns in macaque visual cortex revealed by a reduced silver stain. *J. Comp. Neurol.* 159:559–576.

Lorente de Nó, R., 1938. The cerebral cortex: Architecture, intracortical connections and motor projections. In *Physiology of the Nervous System*. J. F. Fulton, ed. Oxford: Oxford University Press, pp. 291–339.

Lund, R. D., and E. D. Mitchell, 1979. Plasticity of visual callosal projections. *Soc. Neurosci. Symp.* 4:142–152.

Lund, R. D., T. J. Cunningham, and J. S. Lund, 1973. Modified optic projections after unilateral eye removal in young rats. *Brain Behav. Evol.* 8:51–72.

Lynch, G., B. Stanfield, and C. W. Cotman, 1973. Developmental differences in post-lesion axonal growth in the hippocampus. *Brain Res.* 59:155–168.

Mettler, F. A., 1947. Extracortical connections of the primate frontal cerebral cortex. II. Cortico-fugal connections. *J. Comp. Neurol.* 86:119–166.

Mountcastle, V. B., 1957. Modality and topographic properties of single neurons of cat's somatic sensory cortex. *J. Neurophysiol.* 20:408–434.

Mountcastle, V. B., 1978. An organizing principle for cerebral function: The unit module and the distributed system. In *The Mindful Brain*. G. M. Edelman and V. B. Mountcastle, eds. Cambridge, MA: MIT Press, pp. 7–50.

Nauta, W. J. H., 1971. The problem of the frontal lobe: A reinterpretation. *J. Psychiat. Res.* 8:167–187.

Olson, L., A. Seiger, and K. Fuxe, 1972. Heterogeneity of striatal and limbic dopamine innervation: Highly fluorescent islands in developing and adult rats. *Brain Res.* 44:283–288.

Pandya, D., P. Dye, and N. Butters, 1971. Efferent cortico-cortical projections of the prefrontal cortex in the rhesus monkey. *Brain Res.* 31:35–46.

Porrino, L. J., and P. S. Goldman, 1979. Selective distribution of amygdala projections to the prefrontal cortex of the rhesus monkey. *Neurosci. Abst.* 5:280.

Pribram, K. H., K. L. Chow, and J. Semmes, 1953. Limit and organization of the cortical projection from the medial thalamic nucleus in monkey. *J. Comp. Neurol.* 98:433–448.

Rakic, P., 1971. Neuron-glia relationship during granule cell migration in developing cerebellar cortex. A Golgi and electronmicroscopic study in macacus rhesus. *J. Comp. Neurol.* 141:283–312.

Rakic, P., 1972. Mode of cell migration to the superficial layers of fetal monkey neocortex. *J. Comp. Neurol.* 145:61–84.

Rakic, P., 1973. Kinetics of proliferation and latency between final cell division and onset of differentiation of cerebellar stellate and basket neurons. *J. Comp. Neurol.* 147:523–546.

Rakic, P., 1975. Timing of major ontogenetic events in the visual cortex of the rhesus monkey. In *Brain Mechanisms and Mental Retardation*. N. A. Buchwald and M. A. B. Brazier, eds. New York: Academic Press, pp. 3–40.

Rakic, P., 1976. Prenatal genesis of connections subserving ocular dominance in the rhesus monkey. *Nature* 261:467–471.

Rakic, P., 1977a. Prenatal development of the visual system in rhesus monkey. *Phil. Trans. Roy. Soc. B* 278:245–260.

Rakic, P., 1977b. Effects of prenatal unilateral eye enucleation on the formation of layers and retinal connections in the dorsal lateral geniculate nucleus (LGd) of the rhesus monkey. *Neurosci. Abst.* 3:573.

Royce, J. G., 1978. Cells of origin of subcortical afferents to the caudate nucleus: a horseradish peroxidase study in the cat. *Brain Res.* 153:465–475.

Schneider, G. E., 1973. Early lesions of superior colliculus: Factors affecting the formation of abnormal retinal projections. *Brain Behav. Evol.* 8:73–109.

Shatz, C.   1979. Abnormal connections in the visual system of siamese cats. *Soc. Neurosci Symp.* 4:121–141.

Sokoloff, L., M. Reivich, C. Kennedy, M. des Rosiers, C. Patlak, K. Pettigrew, O. Sakurada, and M. Shinohara, 1977. The (^{14}C)-deoxyglucose method for the measurement of local cerebral glucose utilization. Theory, procedure, and normal values in the albino rat. *J. Neurochem.* 28:897–916.

Tanaka, D., and P. S. Goldman, 1976. Silver degeneration and autoradiographic evidence of a projection from the mid-region of the principal sulcus to the septum in the rhesus monkey. *Brain Res.* 103:535–540.

Tennyson, V. M., R. E. Barrett, G. Cohen, L. Cote, R. Heikkila, and C. Mytilineou, 1972. The developing neostriatum of the rabbit: Correlation of fluorescence histochemistry, electron microscopy, endogenous dopamine levels and (^{3}H)-dopamine uptake. *Brain Res.* 46:251–285.

Van Hoesen, G. W., D. N. Pandya, and N. Butters, 1975. Some connections of the entorhinal (area 28) and perirhinal (area 35) cortices of the rhesus monkey. II. Frontal lobe afferents. *Brain Res.* 95:25–38.

Walker, A. E., 1940. The medial thalamic nucleus: A comparative anatomical, physiological and clinical study of the nucleus medialis dorsalis thalami. *J. Comp. Neurol.* 73:87–115.

Webster, K. E., 1961. Cortico-striate interrelations in the albino rat. *J. Anat.* 95:532–545.

Webster, K. E., 1965. The cortico-striatal projection in the cat. *J. Anat.* 99:329–337.

Yeterian, E. H., and G. W. Van Hoesen, 1978. Cortico-striate projections in the rhesus monkey: The organization of certain cortico-caudate connections. *Brain Res.* 139:43–63.

Functional Microorganization in the
Cerebral Cortex

Introduction

W. Maxwell Cowan

No aspect of cortical studies has made more progress in the past twenty-five years than the analysis of the intrinsic organization of the neocortex. As I have pointed out in the introduction to this volume, the initial impetus for this rapid advance was Mountcastle's seminal observation that the cells in the somatosensory cortex are organized functionally into modality-specific columns orthogonal to the cortical surface. In view of the impact that this discovery has had on all later work on the cortex, it was appropriate that the session of the Neurosciences Research Program colloquium at Woods Hole, Massachusetts, on the microorganization of the cortex should begin with a general overview of the functional organization of the cortex by Vernon Mountcastle. In reviewing much of the evidence on which our current understanding of cortical organization is based, Mountcastle took the opportunity to further develop his concept of the cortical module and to clarify some of the confusion that has arisen over the use of the term "column." As he first used the term in 1957, its meaning was quite explicit. It was operationally defined in terms of vertical electrode penetrations into the cortex; each cell encountered in a given penetration was found to be responsive to the same sensory modality and had its receptive field in more or less the same part of the sensory periphery. Later usage, by others, has been less explicit; it is not uncommon to hear reference to "ontogenetic," or "developmental" columns, to "commissural" columns and "eye-dominance columns" (even though those are hardly columnar in any topographic sense). The field is obviously in a state of some turmoil; every few months sees the publication of interesting new data, and it is difficult at this time to attempt any general synthesis. But clearly, when such a synthesis becomes possible, the fundamental notion that the cortex is in some important sense modular in its structural and functional organization will remain as the keystone of our understanding.

The last decade has witnessed a remarkable revival of interest in the use of the Golgi method. And although so much had been harvested in this field before World War II, the systematic analysis of neuronal types in specific cortical areas continues to throw new light on the cellular organization of the cortex. In this area few people have been more productive, in recent years, than Dr. Jennifer Lund, whose careful analyses of the striate cortex in a variety of forms, but especially in the macaque monkey, are generally recognized as definitive. At the Woods Hole meeting, Dr. Lund presented a synopsis of her recent studies, and her chapter in this section provides a convenient summary, not only of her own work, but also of much of the relevant literature. To "isolate and partially characterize" a number of generally identifiable cell types, from the almost staggering array one encounters when first exposed to a well-impregnated Golgi preparation, is no easy task; by producing a degree of order out of this potential chaos, Dr. Lund has performed a valuable service.

If a cursory glance at a Golgi preparation is bewildering, to look at an ultrathin section of the cerebral cortex in the electron microscope is to risk forever being lost in an impenetrable undergrowth. And to the non-electron microscopist, even the literature on the fine structure of the cerebral cortex has become almost as impenetrable. We were fortunate therefore in being able to persuade Dr. Marc Colonnier, whose own contributions in this area have provided the basis for much of the recent work on cortical synaptology, to review this field. In fact the scholarly chapter he has written for this monograph is more than just an overview of the field: in reviewing the literature, he has culled from it a coherent and useful body of information which should provide an effective starting point for anyone approaching this field for the first time, and a satisfying overview of the literature for those reasonably familiar with it.

A natural extension of these pioneering electron-microscopic studies of the cortex, which were based largely on isolated thin sections, is the reconstruction, from serial thin sections, of a small segment of the cortex, or of individual cortical neurons. Dr. Ed White's account of his own painstaking work on the analysis of the synaptic connections of single cortical cells, and especially of their thalamic input, clearly points the way for future electron-microscopic studies. The task confronting a neuroanatomist who wishes to wholly reconstruct a small segment of the cortex is a formidable one; it will require not only great technical skill and patience, but also great courage. Fortunately, as we have learned from comparable analyses of other systems (especially the retina and cerebellar cortex), the rewards are likely to be commensurately great. We can hardly expect to make much progress toward understanding how information is processed within the cortex if we do not know upon which cells the various classes of incoming afferents (thalamic, associational, and callosal) synapse, to say nothing of the varieties of intracortical connections that remain to be elucidated.

The combination of electron microscopy and Golgi impregnation shows promise of facilitating this endeavor. However, at present it seems likely that this approach will always be limited by the vagaries of the Golgi method. For this reason the development of intracellular labeling procedures that permit one to selectively mark functionally identified cell types must be seen as a major advance. We are therefore fortunate in being able to include in this section a report by Gilbert and Wiesel of their ongoing analysis of horseradish peroxidase- (HRP-) filled neurons in the striate cortex of the cat. To many people this work stands as one of the most significant recent contributions to cortical morphology. Its importance lies not only in the fact that the labeled cells have been functionally identified as to type, but also because in many cases the injected marker has labeled the entire cell, and it has been possible to trace out the course of individual axons, with all their collateral ramifications. The logical extension of this work to the analysis of the synaptic organization of such identified cells may yet be a distant prospect, but it is already evident that this approach probably holds the key to the whole problem of the "wiring" of the cortex. As an important first step toward this goal, the chapter by Gilbert and Wiesel at once provides a striking demonstration of the current state of the art, and is a clear harbinger of things to come.

5 Intrinsic Organization of the Primate Visual Cortex, Area 17, As Seen in Golgi Preparations

J.S. Lund

ABSTRACT The macaque monkey visual cortex (area 17) is anatomically divided between white matter and pia into a series of well-defined laminae. The identity of each lamina is established by a unique afferent and efferent relationship to regions outside area 17, as has been demonstrated by a variety of anatomical tracing techniques. However, the axons and dendrites of neurons within a particular lamina may reach beyond its boundaries to establish specific links with one or more of the other laminae. These interlaminar links must underlie the physiologically identified systems of ocular dominance and orientation-specific responsiveness that stretch in columnar fashion between pia and white matter. The Golgi technique has been used to trace these interlaminar links in an effort to determine the course traveled by visual information entering the cortex from different divisions of the dorsal lateral geniculate nucleus, and other afferent sources, to its eventual departure from area 17 via one or other population of efferent projection neurons. The roles of neurons with spiny dendrites and those with smooth dendrites in excitatory and inhibitory functions is debated.

The structure of the primary visual cortex of the monkey has probably received the most attention of all areas of neocortex studied. The striking laminar groupings of the neuron-cell bodies (shown in Figure 1) and distinct fiber architecture makes it an intriguing region for anatomists concerned with neocortical structure, and its primary association with sensory relays from the eyes has encouraged physiological analysis of its function. Currently almost every technique available to the neurobiologist is being used to enlarge our knowledge of the region from the older Golgi methods to the newest [^{14}C]-deoxyglucose and immunocytochemical procedures. This chapter points out the correlations that can be made between the Golgi architecture of the region and information obtained by other techniques and suggests some ways of looking at cortical organization which may be useful in future investigations.

Neuron Morphology within Area 17

A simplistic view of the neurons within the striate cortex would divide them into two main groups differing in morphology and synaptology.

J.S. LUND Department of Ophthalmology, Storm Eye Institute, Medical University of South Carolina, Charleston, South Carolina 29403

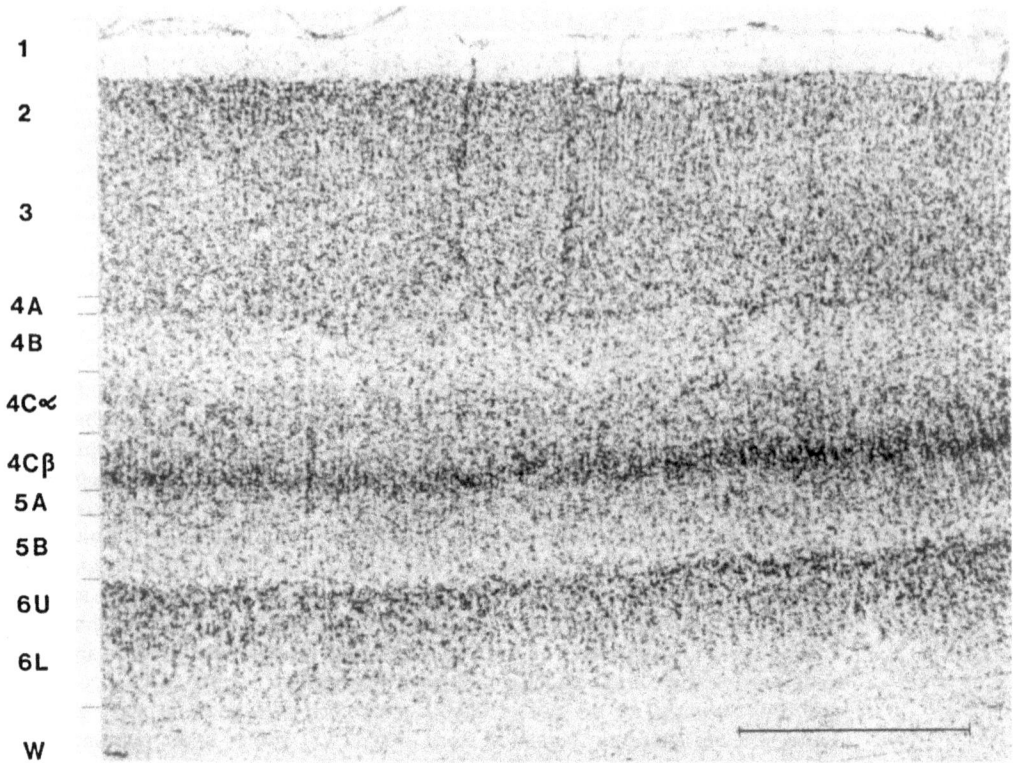

Figure 1 Nissl-stained section of macaque monkey visual cortex, area 17. Scale bar = 500 μm.

In Golgi preparations of adult monkey cortex (Valverde, 1971; Lund, 1973) one group is characterized by their dendrites bearing a marked population of spines (with narrow stalk and dilated tip). These spiny neurons include both the classical cortical pyramidal neuron, where one dendrite on the pial side—the "apical" dendrite—is greatly elongated relative to the rest of the dendrites (see Figure 2) and also stellate forms with dendrites all roughly the same length (see Figure 4A). It has been found in electron-microscopic studies of both normal cortex and of Golgi-impregnated neurons identified first by light microscopy (see chapters by Colonnier and White, this volume) that all spine-bearing neurons examined have a common pattern of synapses (Gray, 1959; Colonnier, 1968; Lund and Lund, 1970; LeVay, 1973; Somogyi, 1978). The soma and the main dendrite shafts (particularly the initial portions) are contacted only by axon terminals making symmetric (type II) specializations and containing flattened vesicles (in tissue fixed with aldelyde with appropriate buffer and osmolarity). In contrast the dendrite spine tips are contacted by axons making asymmetric (type I) specializations and containing round vesicles. The axons of these spiny neurons make only type I contacts with other neurons. The other major group of neurons within the cortex has a general stellate morphology

J. S. Lund

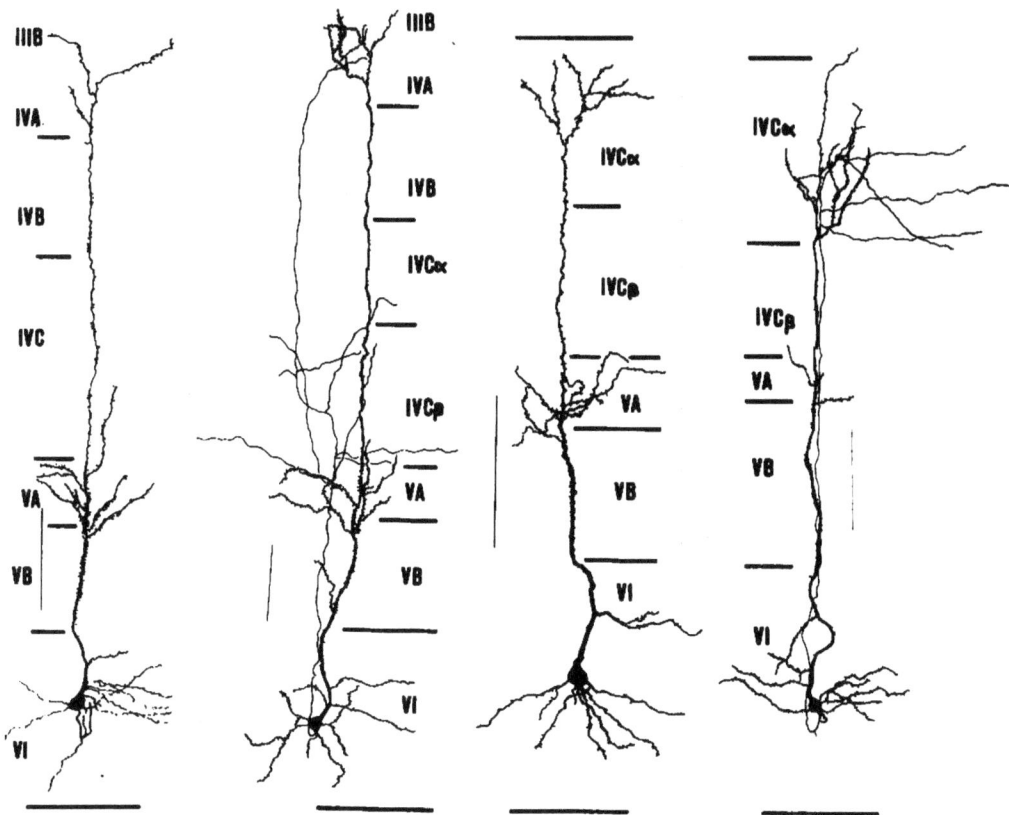

Figure 2 Drawings of Golgi-impregnated pyramidal neurons typical of the upper half of lamina 6 in *Macaca nemestrina*, area 17. (A), (B) Pyramidal neurons with principal arborization of the apical dendrite in laminae 5A and 4A-3B; the recurrent axon collaterals of such neurons arborize in lamina 4Cβ and 4A-3B. (C), (D) Pyramidal neurons typical of the lower half of lamina 6 with principal arborization of the apical dendrite in laminae 5A and 4Cα; the recurrent axon collaterals of such neurons arborize in lamina 4Cα. Scale bar on all drawings = 100 μm.

with either smooth dendrites or with only very occasional spines or thorn-like projections. These cells, where examined by electron microscopy (Colonnier, 1968; Lund and Lund, 1970; LeVay, 1973; Somogyi, 1977; Peters and Fairén, 1978), have both type I and type II contacts intermixed on soma and dendrites. The axons of such cells make type II contacts. Where type I or type II axon contacts have been correlated in the nervous system with excitation or inhibition, the type II contact has been in an inhibitory relationship (some identified as GABAergic) and the type I excitatory (Uchizono, 1965; McLaughlin et al., 1974; Peters, Palay, and Webster, 1976; Ribak, 1977; Ribak, Vaughn, and Saito, 1978). This would suggest that in the visual cortex the smooth dendritic neurons exert an inhibitory effect, whereas the spiny neurons should be excitatory.

While acknowledging that inhibition and excitation within area 17 must be vastly more complex in terms of transmitter substances and neuron–neuron interrelations than simply the two groups of neurons outlined above, it is of interest to consider the relative numbers of neurons in each of these two groups. In lamina 6 and divisions α and β of 4C, where we (Mates and Lund, 1979, and work in progress) have conducted counts by electron microscopy of cell bodies having only type I contacts versus those that have both type I and type II, only 3–4% of the neuron-cell bodies have both types of contact. This indicates that there are many more spiny neurons (pyramids in lamina 6, stellate in lamina 4C) than smooth dendritic neurons. This is probably true of all laminae, but the proportion of smooth dendritic neurons may be slightly higher in laminae 2 and 3. The implication of this finding is that one inhibitory neuron (or perhaps a small cluster) controls a much larger pool of excitatory spiny neurons. The spatial distribution of these relatively few smooth or sparsely spined cells may be crucial in determining the patterns of activity emerging from the excitatory substrate of spiny neurons, and information concerning their distribution is sorely needed. Their relative discontinuity in the cortical matrix may give rise to the functional discontinuities observed in physiological recording experiments examining horizontal segregation of neuron properties.

Physiologically, the visual cortex generally shows low spontaneous activity with the exception of certain complex cells characteristic of lamina 5 (Finlay, Schiller, and Volman, 1976). It may be that the *release* of inhibition, allowing excitation to follow particular routes within the cortex, is a predominant feature of cortical organization. The placement of excitatory input upon dendritic spines, segregated from inhibitory input on main dendritic trunks, soma and axon initial segment, in the one neuron class—as opposed to the lining of the surface of dendrites and soma with both types of input in the other class—may have important functional consequences. Since it would be of great interest to be able to identify the smooth dendritic neurons during physiological recording experiments, it is worth considering what these functional consequences might be. One suggestion could be that the smooth dendritic neurons may show gradual increase and decrease in firing rate, always pooling the results of the activity of neighboring synapses. In contrast, for the spiny neurons the inhibitory contacts could hold the neuron in a state of inactivity despite excitatory input on the spines, the inhibition preventing invasion of the spine activity into the main body of the cell. Only when the balance of inhibition falls below a crucial level can the activity of the spine synapses invade the dendrites and generate an action potential. This synaptology could explain low spontaneous activity and powerful, stimulus-related responsiveness. More information is needed about the firing patterns of neurons identified by intracellular injection techniques as either spine bearing or smooth or sparsely spined cells (see chapter by Gilbert and Wiesel, this volume).

Neurons with Smooth or Sparsely Spined Dendrites

Only in the adult brain can this group of neurons be characterized by their smooth or sparsely spined dendrites. In the immature brain the dendrites and cell bodies of these neurons are covered in projections, some having dilated tips but the majority being thorn-like without end dilations. As the cortex matures, these projections (which may bear synaptic contacts in the young animal; LeVay, 1973) are retracted or lost and the adult neuron is largely spine free. These neurons are distinguished from the true spine-bearing neurons in the young animal by the prevalence of thorn-like projections rather than spines, by the axon origin being often on the pial side of the cell, and by their particular dendritic and axonal branching patterns (Lund, Boothe, and Lund, 1977).

The morphology of the adult smooth or sparsely spined neurons is very diverse, with greatest variety probably occurring in laminae 2 and 3. Examples are shown in Figure 3. It is not certain whether any particular forms are unique to the visual cortex, and certainly many resemble those described for other cortical areas (see Jones, 1975, for details of such cells in somatosensory cortex) and in the visual cortex of other species (Ramón y Cajal, 1911; O'Leary, 1941; Lorento de Nó, 1949; Szentágothai and Arbib, 1974; Colonnier, 1966; Lund et al., 1979). The clearest distinguishing feature between varieties in Golgi material is the morphology of the axon arborizations, particularly the arrangement of the terminal dilations which occur in very distinctive patterns. For instance, the "chandelier" cell of Szentágothai (Szentágothai and Arbib, 1974; see also Jones, 1975, type 4) has vertically arranged "cylinders" of terminal dilations (Figure 4B) that have been shown by Somogyi (1977) to surround the initial axon segments of pyramidal neurons in the rat cortex. These cells are impregnated in Golgi material in laminae 2 and 3 in the primate visual cortex and probably synapse in the same relationship to pyramidal neurons as in the rat—their synaptic relationship to the initial axon segment being a particularly powerful one for inhibiting

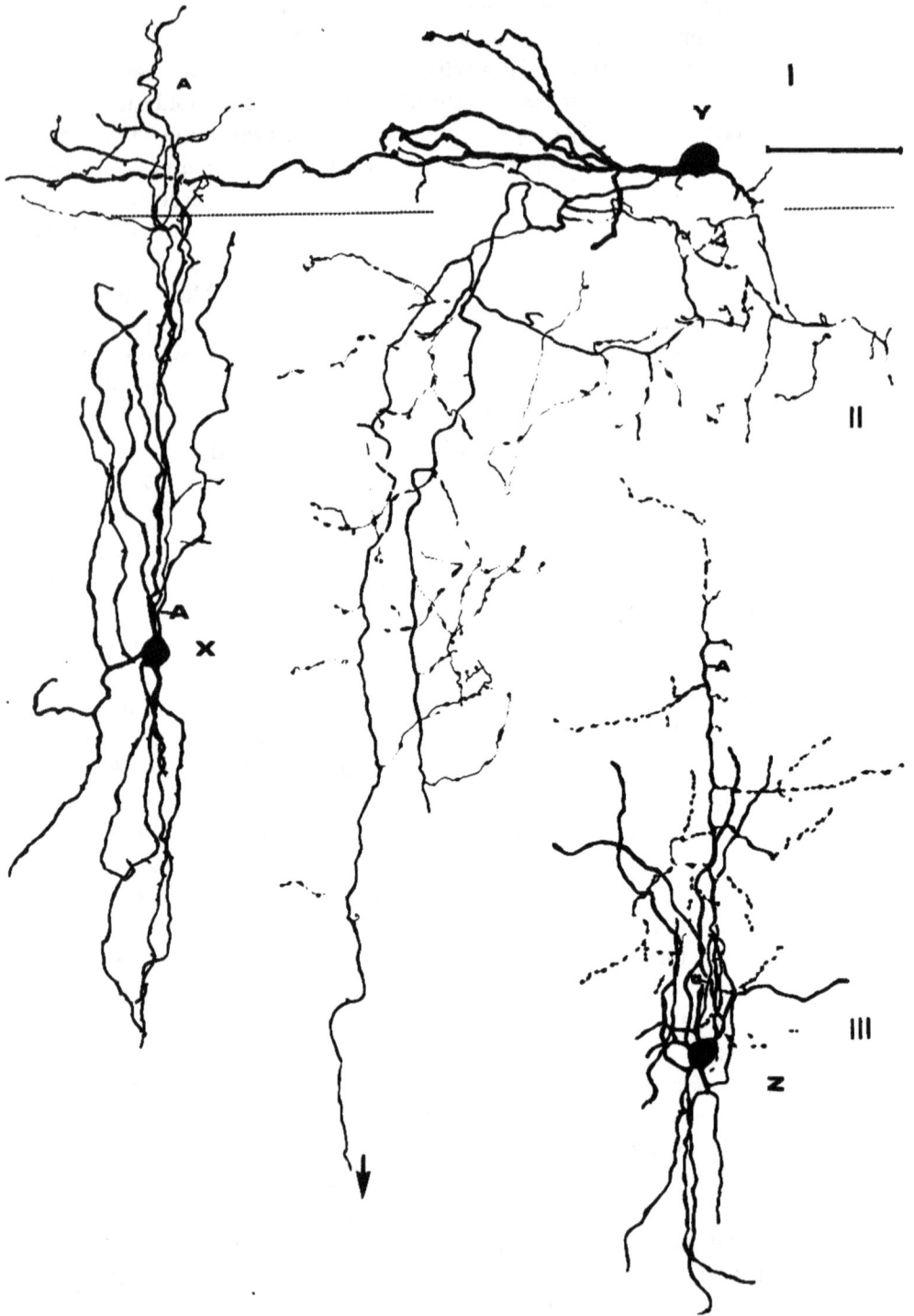

Figure 3 Three examples of stellate neurons with smooth or sparsely spined dendrites found in the upper laminae of the macaque monkey visual cortex, area 17. Drawings from Golgi rapid preparations. Scale bar = 50 μm.

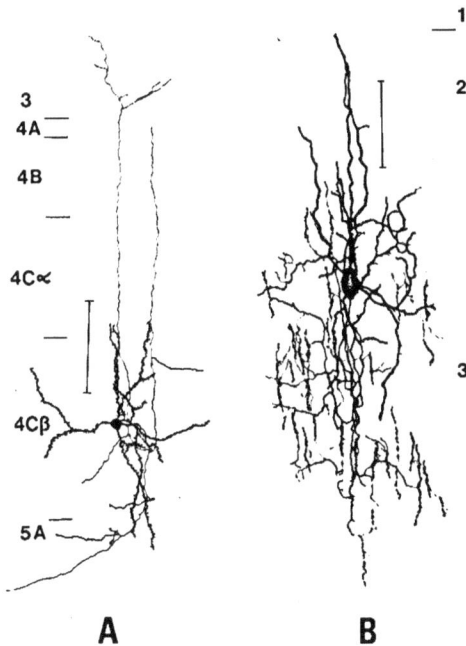

Figure 4 (A) A spiny stellate neuron of lamina 4Cβ. The rising axon collaterals with arborization in lamina 3B is typical of such cells of 4Cβ. Scale bar = 100 μm. (B) Immature "chandelier" neuron from 3-month-old macaque monkey visual cortex, area 17. Note the vertically oriented arrays of axon terminals believed to surround pyramidal-neuron initial axon segments (Somogyi, 1977). Scale bar = 50 μm.

the pyramidal neuron's firing. The axon initial segment of spiny stellate neurons in area 17 does not seem to bear a marked population of type II contacts, in contrast to many of the pyramidal-neuron populations (Lund and Mates, work in progress), and the smooth dendritic neurons also seem to have few contacts on the axon initial segment (Peters and Fairén, 1978). It is noticeable that "chandelier" cells are found in the granule cell zone of layer 4 of area 18 in the monkey. This mass of small cells, however, is largely of pyramidal neurons, and does not include spiny stellate cells.

Axons of other varieties of smooth dendritic neurons of area 17 may have swirling configurations surrounding cell bodies, vertical arrays, and other configurations whose contact relationships have not been clearly defined. In most cases the axon terminal fields of these neurons are confined to a region not much greater in lateral extent than the dendrites of the same neuron. This field may be around the dendrites themselves or vertically above or below the cell in another lamina, the axon forming long trunks traveling from the soma to their distant arborization. Sometimes the axon can have two separate fields of arborization vertically separated. This has been described for the cat (Lund et al., 1979) but is also true for the primate. The implication of these variously placed axon arborizations is that such neurons may form interlaminar modulatory links that complement the more obvious interlaminar axonal relays shown by the spiny neurons. There are a few varieties of the smooth dendritic neurons in the visual cortex whose axons spread horizontally within a lamina, but even these exhibit relatively restricted horizontal spread compared to the collaterals of pyramidal-neuron axons, which often spread several millimeters, particularly axons of the pyramids in the upper cortical layers. One question of great importance for understanding these smooth dendritic neurons is whether, despite their heterogenous morphology, they represent a homogeneous functional class. How many properties do they have in common with one another in terms of the transmitter substances they use and their inhibitory or modulatory effect on the cells postsynaptic to them? As discussed by Emson and Hunt (this volume), some smooth dendritic neurons may use peptides as transmitter substances, and these peptides appear to have a powerful *excitatory* effect. Will such neurons have flattened vesicles in their axon terminals and make type II contacts? If they do, such a finding will alter the prevailing concept of such contacts as being inhibitory. Conversely, if these peptide-containing neurons have axons making type I contacts, it will alter the prevailing view that such smooth dendritic neurons make only type II axon contacts.

Neurons with Spiny Dendrites

The precise number of dendritic spines (and therefore presumably also the number of type I synapses) borne by the spiny neuron in the adult animal seems to be determined during a period of postnatal maturation, and the number is influenced by the afferent activity the cortex receives during this period (Ruiz-Marcos and Valverde, 1969). During the first few postnatal weeks a superabundance of spines forms upon these neurons with a subsequent loss of up to two thirds their numbers as the animal matures further. The spiny neurons of each lamina and even different parts of the apical dendrite of pyramidal neurons show an individual sequence of spine accumulation and loss during maturation (Boothe et al., 1979). A similar maturational sequence of superabundance and subsequent loss occurs in the type II synaptic contacts on the cell bodies of spiny neurons (Mates and Lund, 1979).

In the primate visual cortex, area 17, the two forms of spiny neurons, stellate and pyramidal, differ in their lamina distribution. The stellate forms are confined to a band of cortex in middle depth called lamina 4. The various subdivisions of lamina 4 are associated with thalamic input from the dorsal lateral geniculate nucleus—dLGN (lamina 4A and 4C)—or with input from a cortical visual-association region in the superior temporal sulcus (lamina 4B) called STS (Zeki, 1974) or MT by homology with the apparently equivalent area in the New World primates (see review by Van Essen, 1979). The dendrites of the spiny stellate neurons within each subdivision of lamina 4 are largely restricted to that single division, although there is some interweaving of dendrites at lamina borders. These neurons have axons which usually arise from the white-matter side of the cell and which form trunks projecting to other laminae. The axons of the cells of each subdivision of lamina 4 have specific and differing interlaminar projections (Lund and Boothe, 1975). Only the spiny stellate neurons of lamina 4B give rise to efferent projections leaving the striate cortex (Lund et al., 1975).

The pyramidal neurons also restrict their basal dendrites largely to single laminae. Their cell bodies occur in all laminae except 4C. Their apical dendrites cross laminar boundaries and allow the pyramidal neuron to "listen in" to ongoing activity in laminae superficial to that sampled by their basal dendritic field. The apical dendrite greatly increases its input in a specifiic and restricted fashion to only certain laminae by emitting a number of side branches in only these laminae. We shall see later that these patterns of apical dendrite arborization are not random, but are very much related to the way in which information is relayed through the cortical laminae (Lund and Boothe, 1975). The relative importance of input to the apical dendrite as compared to the basal dendrites of pyramidal neurons is open to conjecture. It is conceivable that the apical-dendrite input may provide a kind of modulatory influence which acts to enhance the neuron's responsiveness to particular basal dendritic inputs, perhaps by the relative timing of events impinging on apical and basal dendrites. The average lateral spread of the basal dendrites of pyramidal neurons (and of apical dendrites in lamina 1) is shown in Figure 5. Also shown for comparison is the spread of spiny-stellate-neuron dendrites. The width of dendritic fields is shown relative to the approximate width of ocular-dominance and orientation columns as defined physiologically (Hubel and Wiesel, 1974). So far, no marked asymmetry has been detected in dendritic fields that might relate to physiological properties such as orientation-specific responsiveness. It is clear that single orientation columns (25–50 μm) are narrower than the average dendritic extent of the spiny neurons, and that certain classes of pyramidal neurons should bridge almost an entire ocular-dominance hypercolumn. Observations on thalamic-axon distribution within lamina 4 in both Golgi impregnations and horseradish peroxidase-filled axons indicate that the lateral spread of individual axons is much greater than the dendritic spread of individual neurons (Ferster and LeVay, 1978, for the cat; Humphrey, Mates, and Lund, work in progress).

The pyramidal neurons of all laminae, except lamina 5A, have axons that form efferent trunks leaving the cortex (Lund et al., 1975). In addition, each pyramidal-neuron axon emits collaterals, both rising on the pial side of the neuron and off the descending efferent trunk in laminae deeper in the cortex. The intracortical collaterals innervate in a specific fashion one or more of the cortical laminae. This is particularly evident

Ocular-dominance hypercolumn 770 μ

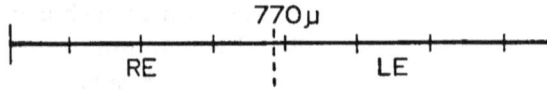

770 μ

RE   LE

Orientation hypercolumn 570 μ

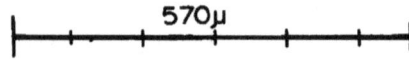

570μ

Change in orientation every 25-50μ

Lateral spread of spiny dendrites:—

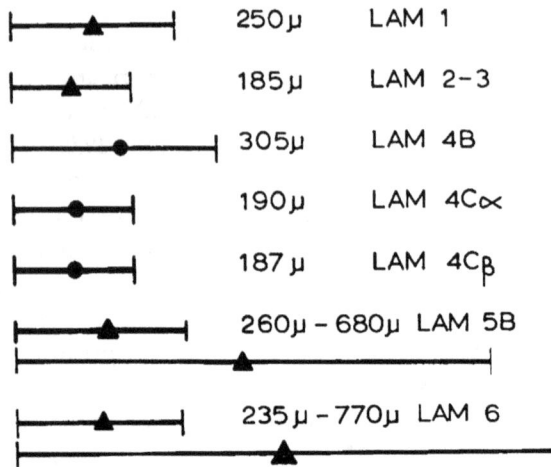

250 μ   LAM 1

185 μ   LAM 2-3

305μ   LAM 4B

190 μ   LAM 4Cα

187 μ   LAM 4Cβ

260μ – 680μ LAM 5B

235 μ – 770μ LAM 6

Figure 5 Average lateral spread of the dendrites of spiny neurons within area 17 of the macaque monkey compared to the width of ocular-dominance and orientation columns (Hubel and Wiesel, 1974). The lateral spread in lamina 1 refers to pyramidal-neuron apical dendrite aborizations, while the spread in laminae 2, 3, 5B, and 6 refers to pyramidal-neuron basal dendrites. The lateral spread of dendrites of spiny stellate neurons is shown for lamina 4. In laminae 5B and 6 the dendritic spread of the largest classes of pyramidal neurons is indicated separately from the rest of the pyramid population. Allowance has been made for shrinkage during fixation and Golgi impregnation so as to make comparison with physiological data more accurate.

for the pyramidal neurons of lamina 6 (Figure 2). These specific axon and apical dendritic arborizations are determined in the early growth of the neuron and are not the result of later pruning of a wider distribution (Lund, Boothe, and Lund, 1977). Intracortical pyramidal-neuron axon collaterals can spread considerable distances laterally, particularly the axons of pyramidal neurons in laminae 2 and 3, and may have very geometrically arranged branching patterns. The collaterals rising from the parent axon trunk of a pyramidal neuron in lamina 3 mimic the angles of dendritic branching patterns of the surrounding population of pyramidal neurons. These axons travel in very straight trajectories, and it could be hypothesized that they form a system of axons that establish *en passant* synapses with the dendrites of similar neurons at predictable distances and cortical depths relative to the cell of origin (see also Szentágothai, 1975). If such an *en passant* type of synaptic relationship is established, it would imply that each pyramidal neuron receives a maximum number of synapses from each of rather a limited number of axons. This would be in contrast to the type of synaptology seen between the cerebellar Purkinje cell and parallel-fiber system, where the Purkinje cell receives a minimal number of synapses from each of a great number of parallel fibers.

The apical dendrite of the pyramidal neuron, in having a morphology and distribution that differs from the rest of the cell's dendrites, is a defining characteristic of this class of neurons. There are, however, some groups of pyramidal neurons for which the apical dendrite is modified from the usual pattern. One group of pyramids—those of lamina 5A—have a fine, unbranched, spine-free apical dendrite that appears vestigial. Another group, the giant pyramids of lamina 6, have a rather reduced apical dendrite that branches chiefly in lamina 5, then peters out in the more superficial laminae; the basal dendrites of the same cells spread nearly a millimeter in lamina 6, thus exceeding the apical dendrite in total length. As well as increasing their synaptic surface by increased branching in particular laminae, the apical dendrites may also reduce their synaptic surface as they traverse a lamina, not only by not giving off branches, but also by reducing the number of spines on the shaft of the apical dendrite. This is seen on the apical dendrites of the pyramidal neurons below lamina 4 as they traverse lamina 4C; here they show a marked reduction in the numbers of spines on their surface, suggesting an avoidance of this type of synaptic input in this lamina (Lund, 1973).

The efferent-cell groups of the visual cortex are grouped in laminar fashion and have been shown to occupy the positions illustrated in Figure 6 in studies using the retrograde transport of horseradish peroxidase (Lund et al., 1975). It will be evident from Figure 6 that the physiological entity described as a cortical column or slab (Hubel and Wiesel, 1968, 1974) in which both ocular dominance and orientation-specific responsiveness are similar from pia to white matter, contains

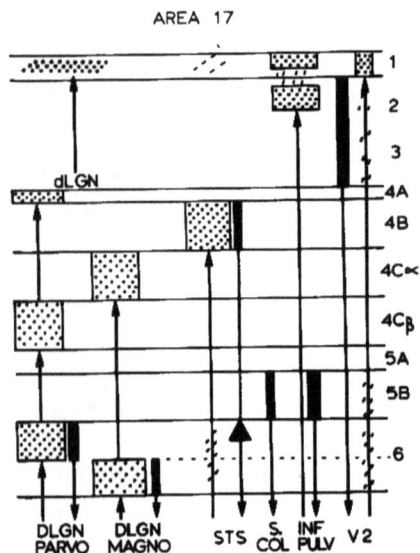

AREA 17

Figure 6 Diagram of relative laminar positions of afferent-fiber terminal fields and efferent neuron-cell bodies in area 17 of the macaque monkey.

within its pia-to-white matter dimension considerable diversity and laminar segregation of afferent-axon terminations and efferent-cell groups. The physiological nature of this diversity in depth has scarcely been explored despite considerable investigation (Hubel and Wiesel, 1968; Dow, 1974; Schiller, Finlay, and Volman, 1976a,b; Poggio and Fischer, 1977; Poggio, Doty, and Talbot, 1977; Michael, 1978a,b,c), perhaps because recording from apical-dendrite extensions of pyramidal neurons, as well as from their cell bodies, obscures laminar segregation of neuron properties.

Interlaminar Axonal Relays of Spiny Neurons

It has proved more feasible to trace the axon relays of the spine-bearing neurons (Lund and Boothe, 1975) than the smooth dendritic neurons since the spiny cells are much more frequently impregnated in Golgi material. As mentioned earlier, their real frequency can only be assessed by electron microscopy and it indeed seems that at least 90% of the cortical neurons are of the spine-bearing type. Assuming that the spiny neurons are the main excitatory elements in the cortex, it is of interest to trace via their axon relays the possible chains of neurons through which incoming information can be channelled. It is also of interest to consider whether different types of afferent information can retain a separate identity even to particular efferent-cell groups, and how different types of input can be combined on a single neuron.

The main intrinsic spiny-cell-axon relays and their relationship to afferents and efferent-cell grouping are shown in Figure 7. The laminar

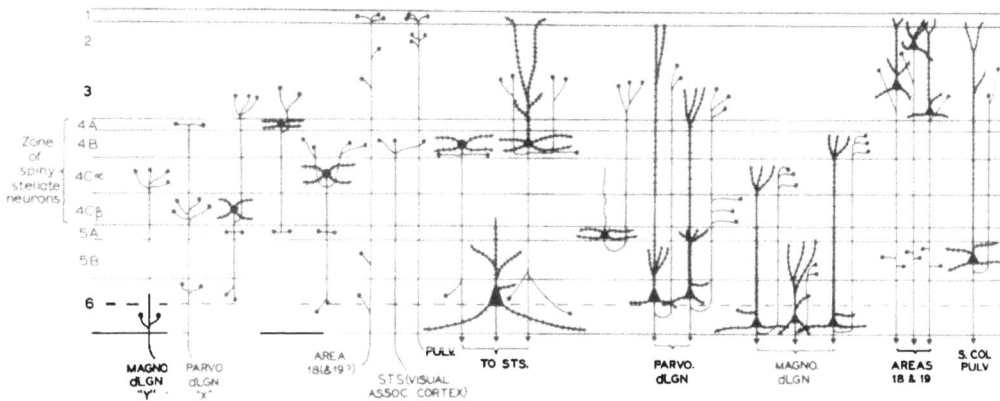

Figure 7 Diagram summarizing the interlaminar intrinsic axon relays of spiny neurons in relation to afferent terminations and efferent-cell groups in area 17 of the macaque.

distribution of the parvocellular and magnocellular dLGN inputs have been shown by degeneration techniques and by autoradiography (Hubel and Wiesel, 1972; Wiesel, Hubel, and Lam, 1974). These inputs are segregated into separate zones of termination for the two eyes in an alternating band-like fashion, but each eye distributes fibers in a similar laminar fashion in the pattern shown in Figure 7. The input from the parvocellular laminae distributes in two main tiers in laminae 4Cβ and 4A and also makes a sparse contribution to upper lamina 6 (Hendrickson, Wilson, and Ogren, 1978). Spiny stellate neurons in laminae 4A and 4Cβ both send their principal axon projections to lamina 3 (see Figure 4A), with sparser collaterals to laminae 5A and 6. Pyramidal neurons of lamina 5A have totally recurrent axon projections to laminae 2 and 3. The axons of pyramidal neurons of laminae 2 and 3 are efferents to the visual association areas ringing area 17, and on their way out of area 17 they contribute a heavy projection to lamina 5B. Pyramidal neurons of lamina 5B project to the superior colliculus and inferior pulvinar nucleus (Lund et al., 1975), the pulvinar sending back a projection to laminae 1 and 2 organized in a periodic fashion (Ogren and Hendrickson, 1977). Pyramidal neurons of the upper half of lamina 6 project back to the parvocellular laminae of the dLGN. The apical dendrites of many of these neurons arborize specifically in both laminae 5A and lower 3, the relay zones of spiny stellate neurons of 4Cβ. The recurrent axon trunks of these pyramids arborize within 4Cβ itself and again in lower lamina 3 (Lund and Boothe, 1975)—see Figures 2A,B and 7.

The axons of the cells of the magnocellular dLGN laminae distribute chiefly within lamina 4Cα with a sparse projection to lower lamina 6 (Hubel and Wiesel, 1972; Hendrickson, Wilson, and Ogren, 1978). Spiny stellate neurons of lamina 4Cα project chiefly upon lamina 4B immediately superficial to them and also have a fine descending axon arborizing in lamina 5A and lamina 6. Lamina 4B receives a heavy projection from cortical area STS, and the spiny stellate neurons as well as the pyramids in 4B can project to STS. The descending axon trunks of these 4B neurons do not contribute collaterals to lamina 5, although they probably do contribute a projection to lamina 6. It is noticeable that the axons of pyramidal neurons of laminae 2 and 3 do not project upon any division of lamina 4, so that the only input from laminae 2 and 3 to 4B (and presumably the only means of parvocellular relays influencing 4B neurons) is via the apical dendrites of pyramids in 4B. These same 4B pyramids send ascending axon collaterals into laminae 2 and 3. Neurons efferent to the magnocellular division of the lateral geniculate nucleus lie in the deep half of lamina 6. Many of these pyramids of deeper lamina 6 have apical dendrites and rising axon collaterals that arborize specifically either in 4Cα (with dendritic branches also in 5A—Figure 2C,D) or in 4B, but not in both. One particular population of pyramidal neurons in lamina 6—the largest pyramids in the striate cortex in somal size and spread of basal dendrites—does not project back to the dLGN. Instead these large neurons project to the same STS region of cortex as the spiny neurons of 4B (Lund et al., 1975; Spatz, 1975, 1977). Developmentally it is indeed difficult to understand how this dichotomy of efferent projections to STS and dLGN is generated from lamina 6. There is evidence in at least the marmoset (Spatz, 1977) that MT (the STS homolog) contributes a light projection to laminae 6 and 1 of area 17 as well as to 4B. Lamina 4B and its reciprocal relationship to a distant visual association area is apparently a special feature of the primate cortex and this lamina has no direct homolog in the cat (Lund et al., 1979). It is interesting that the STS cortical input is placed in close proximity to input from the dLGN, that both STS and dLGN inputs are associated with spiny stellate neurons, and that both STS and the dLGN receive feedback from lamina 6. These similarities suggest a special, almost thalamic-like, relationship of area STS input to the function of area 17.

It is clear from a study of these spiny-cell relays (see Figure 7) that there is not necessarily continued segregation of parvocellular and magnocellular inputs within the cortex, in the sense that the sequence of relays from neurons upon which the two impinge does not retain absolute dendritic and axonal separation. Rather, it appears that the two streams may eventually reach all efferent neurons, but they do so by different routes, often involving one stream in more synaptic delay than the other. The two streams may also eventually engage different parts of the same efferent neuron (e.g., apical versus basal dendrites), which presumably will affect the way in which the two inputs interact to fire the neuron. The interlaminar relays suggest that magnocellular input will be relayed from 4Cα to 4B and may therefore be particularly important in determining the physiological nature of the relationship between area 17 and STS. However, it is apparent that the pyramids of 4B will receive input on their apical dendrites from laminae 2 and 3, which is the principal relay zone of parvocellular information from 4Cβ.

In the same fashion, while the neurons of laminae 2 and 3 will receive parvocellular relays from $4C\beta$, they will also be influenced by ascending axon collaterals of the pyramidal neurons of lamina 4B. Lamina 5B presents a particular puzzle since the physiology of the cells (large fields, responsiveness to fast movement, poor orientation tuning; Finlay, Schiller, and Volman, 1976) suggests derivation from magnocellular relays. However, anatomically these neurons of 5B receive the bulk of their input from neurons of laminae 2 and 3, on both basal and apical dendrites, and, apart from a small segment of the apical dendrite shaft as it passes through $4C\alpha$ and 4B, there is not much opportunity for direct magnocellular dLGN input. Physiologically the neurons of laminae 2–3 have small fields, are often hypercomplex and tightly tuned for orientation, and prefer slow movements, that is, contrasting in their properties with the cells of lamina 5B. The projection from laminae 2 and 3 to lamina 5B is more or less vertically organized with little lateral spread within lamina 5 (Nauta, Butler, and Jane, 1973). However, neurons within lamina 5B send axon collaterals horizontally for long distances within the lamina, and one population of large pyramids in lamina 5B has basal dendrites spreading up to 700 μm. This suggests that the physiological properties identified for neurons of lamina 5B could be generated within the lamina itself, rather than being evoked by direct magnocellular input to these neurons, and perhaps could be the properties of only the largest cells in the lamina. Considerably more information is needed in physiological analysis of the monkey visual cortex in order to determine how the anatomical linkages observed subserve the function of the neurons.

While it is highly likely in the visual cortex that the different efferent groups of neurons in cortical depth differ in their physiological properties (Palmer and Rosenquist, 1974; Finlay, Schiller, and Volman, 1976; Gilbert, 1977; Henry, Harvey, and Lund, 1979), it is also clear from the studies of Hubel and Wiesel (1968, 1974) that eye dominance and preferred orientation of line stimulus are properties that are reflected in common in columnar fashion between pia and white matter. [^{14}C]-deoxyglucose experiments have confirmed this physiological columnar organization for both ocularity and orientation (Kennedy et al., 1976; Hubel, Wiesel, and Stryker, 1978). Such experiments have also indicated that an interesting periodicity of high-activity levels can occur beyond that so far predicted by physiological experiments (Hendrickson and Wilson, 1979). A regular punctate pattern of high-activity zones, particularly evident in the upper cortical laminae can be found with either monocular or binocular stimulation with all orientations of stimulus presented (see Figure 8). These experiments indicate the need for further anatomical studies to try to uncover the axonal and dendritic linkages that underly these geometric arrays. It would be predicted that all neuron types will play a part in generating these activity patterns by interaction of excitation and inhibition. Also the interplay and geomet-

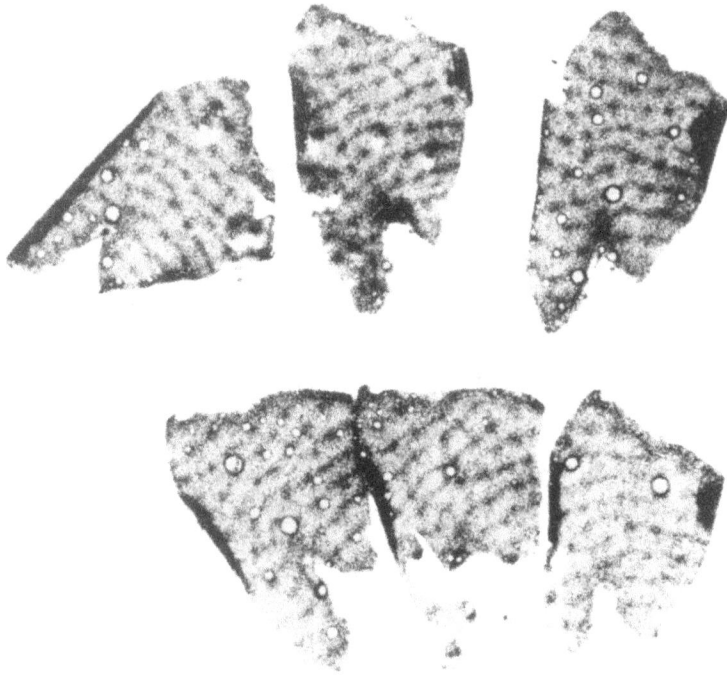

Figure 8 Autoradiograph of tangential sections of macaque visual cortex (laminae 2 and 3) showing [^{14}C]-deoxyglucose incorporation during monocular exposure in the alert animal to lines of all orientations. Note a punctate pattern of heaviest incorporation superimposed upon bands of label overlying the input relayed to layer IV from the exposed eye (Hendrickson and Wilson, 1979).

ric distribution of afferent-fiber groups may be crucial in determining which particular patterns of activity emerge. It needs to be determined, however, whether there is a rigid anatomical framework within the cortex beyond that governed by geometry of afferents, or whether the cortical neurons can provide a substrate for a variety of fluid patterns of spatial activation.

References

Boothe, R. G., W. T. Greenough, J. S. Lund, and K. Wrege, 1979. A quantitative investigation of spine and dendrite development of neurons in visual cortex (area 17) of *Macaca nemestrina* monkeys. *J. Comp. Neurol.* 186:473–490.

Colonnier, M., 1966. The structural design of the neocortex. In *Brain and Conscious Experience*. J. E. Eccles, ed. Berlin, Heidelberg, New York: Springer, pp. 1–23.

Colonnier, M., 1968. Synaptic patterns on different cell types in the different laminae of the cat visual cortex. An electron microscope study. *Brain Res.* 9:268–287.

Dow, B. M., 1974. Functional classes of cells, and their laminar distribution in monkey visual cortex *J. Neurophysiol.* 37:927–946.

Ferster, D., and S. LeVay, 1978. The axonal arborization of lateral geniculate neurons in the striate cortex of the cat. *J. Comp. Neurol.* 182:923–944.

Finlay, B. L., P. H. Schiller, and S. F. Volman, 1976. Quantitative studies of single cell properties in monkey striate cortex. IV. Corticotectal cells. *J. Neurophysiol.* 39:1352–1361.

Gilbert, C. D., 1977. Laminar differences in receptive field properties of cells in cat primary visual cortex. *J. Physiol.* 268:391–421.

Gray, E. G., 1959. Axosomatic and axodendritic synapses of the cerebral cortex. *J. Anat.* 93:420–433.

Hendrickson, A. E., and J. R. Wilson, 1979. A difference in [^{14}C]deoxyglucose autoradiographic patterns in striate cortex between Macaca and Saimiri monkeys following monocular stimulation. *Brain Res.* 170:353–358.

Hendrickson, A. E., J. R. Wilson, and M. P. Ogren, 1978. The neuroanatomical organization of pathways between the dorsal lateral geniculate nucleus and visual cortex in Old World and New World primates. *J. Comp. Neurol.* 182:123–136.

Henry, G. H., A. R. Harvey, and J. S. Lund, 1979. The afferent connections and laminar distribution of cells in the cat striate cortex. *J. Comp. Neurol.* 187:725–744.

Hubel, D. H., and T. N. Wiesel, 1968. Receptive fields and functional architecture of monkey striate cortex. *J. Physiol.* 196:215–243.

Hubel, D. H., and T. N. Wiesel, 1972. Laminar and columnar distribution of geniculocortical fibers in the Macaque monkey. *J. Comp. Neurol.* 146:421–450.

Hubel, D. H., and T. N. Wiesel, 1974. Sequence regularity and geometry of orientation columns in the monkey striate cortex. *J. Comp. Neurol.* 158:267–294.

Hubel, D. H., T. N. Wiesel, and M. P. Stryker, 1978. Anatomical demonstration of orientation columns in Macaque monkey. *J. Comp. Neurol.* 177:563–584.

Jones, E. G., 1975. Varieties and distribution of non-pyramidal cells in the somatic sensory cortex of the squirrel monkey. *J. Comp. Neurol.* 160:205–268.

Kennedy, C., M. H. Des Rosiers, O. Sakurada, M. Shinohara, M. Reivich, H. W. Jehle, and L. Sokoloff, 1976. Metabolic mapping of the primary visual system of the monkey by means of the autoradiographic [^{14}C]deoxyglucose technique. *Proc. Nat. Acad. Sci. USA* 73:4230–4234.

LeVay, S., 1973. Synaptic patterns in the visual cortex of the cat and monkey. Electron microscopy of Golgi preparations. *J. Comp. Neurol.* 150:53–86.

Lorento de Nó, R., 1949. Cerebral cortex: Architecture, intracortical connections, motor projections. In *Physiology of the Nervous System.* J. Fulton, ed. Oxford: Oxford University Press, pp. 288–330.

Lund, J. S., 1973. Organization of neurons in the visual cortex, area 17, of the monkey (*Macaca mulatta*). *J. Comp. Neurol.* 147:455–496.

Lund, J. S., and R. G. Boothe, 1975. Interlaminar connections and pyramidal neuron organization in the visual cortex, area 17, of the Macaque monkey. *J. Comp. Neurol.* 159:305–334.

Lund, J. S., and R. D. Lund, 1970. The termination of callosal fibers in the paravisual cortex of the rat. *Brain Res.* 17:24–45.

Lund, J. S., R. G. Boothe, and R. D. Lund, 1977. Development of neurons in the visual cortex (area 17) of the monkey (*Macaca nemestrina*): A Golgi study from fetal day 127 to postnatal maturity. *J. Comp. Neurol.* 176:149–188.

Lund, J. S., G. H. Henry, C. L. MacQueen, and A. R. Harvey, 1979. Anatomical organization of the primary visual cortex (area 17) of the cat. A comparison with area 17 of the Macaque monkey. *J. Comp. Neurol.* 184:599–618.

Lund, J. S., R. D. Lund, A. E. Hendrickson, A. H. Bunt, and A. F. Fuchs, 1975. The origin of efferent pathways from the primary visual cortex, area 17, of the Macaque monkey as shown by retrograde transport of horseradish peroxidase. *J. Comp. Neurol.* 164:287–304.

McLaughlin, B. J., J. G. Wood, K. Saito, R. Barber, J. E. Vaughn, E. Roberts, and T. Y. Wu, 1974. The fine structural localization of glutamate decarboxylase in synaptic terminals of rodent cerebellum. *Brain Res.* 76:377–391.

Mates, S., and J. S. Lund, 1979. Development of somal synapses in visual cortex (area 17) of the macaque monkey. *Neurosci. Abst.* 5:795.

Michael, C. R., 1978a. Color vision mechanisms in monkey striate cortex: Dual opponent cells with concentric receptive fields. *J. Neurophysiol.* 41:572–588.

Michael, C. R., 1978b. Color vision mechanisms in monkey striate cortex: Simple cells with dual opponent-color receptive fields. *J. Neurophysiol.* 41:1233–1249.

Michael, C. R., 1978c. Color-sensitive complex cells in monkey striate cortex. *J. Neurophysiol.* 41:1250–1266.

Nauta, H. J. W., A. B. Butler, and J. A. Jane, 1973. Some observations on axonal degeneration resulting from superficial lesions of the cerebral cortex. *J. Comp. Neurol.* 150:349–360.

Ogren, M. P., and A. E. Hendrickson, 1977. The distribution of pulvinar terminals in visual areas 17 and 18 of the monkey. *Brain Res.* 137:343–350.

O'Leary, J. L., 1941. Structure of the area striate of the cat. *J. Comp. Neurol.* 75:131–161.

Palmer, L. A., and A. C. Rosenquist, 1974. Visual receptive fields of single striate cortical units projecting to the superior colliculus in the cat. *Brain Res.* 67:27–42.

Peters, A., and A. Fairén, 1978. Smooth and sparsely-spined cells in the visual cortex of the rat: A study using a combined Golgi-electron microscope technique. *J. Comp. Neurol.* 181:129–172.

Peters, A., S. L. Palay, and H. de F. Webster, 1976. *The Fine Structure of the Nervous System: The Neurons and Supporting Cells.* Philadelphia: Saunders, pp. 148–149.

Poggio, G. F., and B. Fischer, 1977. Binocular interaction and depth sensitivity in striate and prestriate cortex of behaving rhesus monkey. *J. Neurophysiol.* 40:1392–1405.

Poggio, G. F., R. W. Doty, and W. H. Talbot, 1977. Foveal striate cortex of behaving monkey: Single neuron responses to square-wave gratings during fixation of gaze. *J. Neurophysiol.* 40:1369–1405.

Ramón y Cajal, S., 1911. *Histologie du système nerveux de l'homme et des vertèbrés*, Vol. 2, Paris: Maloine. (Madrid: Reimpress, Institio Cajal, 1955.)

Ribak, C. E., 1977. The immunocytochemical localization of GAD within stellate neurons of the rat visual cortex. *Anat. Rec.* 187:692.

Ribak, C. E., J. E. Vaughn, and K. Saito, 1978. Immunocytochemical localization of glutamic acid decarboxylase in neuronal somata following colchicine inhibition of axonal transport. *Brain Res.* 140:315–332.

Ruiz-Marcos, A., and F. Valverde, 1969. The temporal evolution of the distribution of dendritic spines in the visual cortex of normal and dark reared mice. *Exp. Brain Res.* 8:284–294.

Schiller, P. H., B. L. Finlay, and S. F. Volman, 1976a. Quantitative studies of single-cell properties in monkey striate cortex. I. Spatiotemporal organization of receptive fields. *J. Neurophysiol.* 39:1288–1319.

Schiller, P. H., B. L. Finlay, and S. F. Volman, 1976b. Quantitative studies of single-cell properties in monkey striate cortex. II. Orientation specificity and ocular dominance. *J. Neurophysiol.* 39:1320–1333.

Somogyi, P., 1977. A specific axo-axonal interneuron in the visual cortex of the rat. *Brain Res.* 136:345–350.

Somogyi, P., 1978. The study of Golgi stained cells and of experimental degeneration under the electron microscope: A direct method for the identification in the visual cortex of three successive links in a neuron chain. *Neuroscience* 3:167–180.

Spatz, W. B., 1975. An efferent connection of the solitary cells of Meynert. A study with horseradish peroxidase in the marmoset *Callithrix. Brain Res.* 92:450–455.

Spatz, W. B., 1977. Topographically organized reciprocal connections between areas 17 and MT (visual area of superior temporal sulcus) in the marmoset *Callithrix jacchus. Exp. Brain Res.* 27:559–572.

Szentágothai, J., 1975. The module-concept in cerebral cortex architecture. *Brain Res.* 95:475–496.

Szentágothai, J., and M. A. Arbib, 1974. Conceptual models of neural organization. *Neurosci. Res. Prog. Bull.* 12:307–310.

Uchizono, K., 1965. Characteristics of excitaory and inhibitory synapses in the central nervous system of the cat. *Nature* 207:642–643.

Valverde, F., 1971. Short axon neuronal subsystems in the visual cortex of the monkey. *Int. J. Neurosci.* 1:181–197.

Van Essen, D. C., 1979. Visual areas of the mammalian cerebral cortex. *Ann. Rev. Neurosci.* 2:227–264.

Wiesel, T. N., D. H. Hubel, and D. Lam, 1974. Autoradiographic demonstration of ocular dominance columns in the monkey striate cortex by means of transsynaptic transport. *Brain Res.* 79:273–279.

Zeki, S. M., 1974. Functional organization of a visual area in the posterior bank of the superior temporal sulcus. *J. Physiol.* 236:549–573.

J. S. Lund

6

The Electron-Microscopic Analysis of the Neuronal Organization of the Cerebral Cortex

M. Colonnier

ABSTRACT This chapter reviews the contribution of electron microscopy to the understanding of the neuronal organization of the neocortex. It discusses estimates of the number of synapses in normal adult neocortex, and describes different synaptic types and their distribution on the soma, dendritic shafts, spines, and initial segments of pyramidal, spiny stellate, and sparsely spinous stellate cells. It deals with recent data on the histochemistry of the neurotransmitters of intracortical neurons, and on the presence and distribution of gap junctions and dendrodendritic contacts. Finally it reviews the mode of termination of thalamic, associational, and commissural afferents.

The importance of electron microscopy in the understanding of the neuronal organization of the cerebral cortex is primarily that it permits the visualization of the structural details of synaptic contacts. Not only did this technique give the definitive anatomical proof of the neuron theory by demonstrating the separateness of pre- and postsynaptic elements, it is still the only one which allows us to see all synapses in a section of tissue, to classify them into morphological groups, and in many instances to identify with confidence the parts of the neurons involved in the contact.

Number of Synaptic Contacts in the Cerebral Cortex

Since electron microscopy permits the identification of all synapses in a section of tissue, it has been possible with this technique to determine the number of synapses per unit volume of cortex and from this to calculate the total number of synapses in the cerebral cortex of different species. Synapses have been counted in normal and experimental animals, both developing and adult, by many authors. This review will deal only with the volume density counts in normal adults, although it must be realized that "normal" here only means animals in which no deliberate environmental manipulation was imposed for the sake of affecting the development of synapses. Since, however, even relatively

M. COLONNIER Laboratoires de Neurobiologie, Hôpital de l'Enfant-Jésus, Pavillon Notre-Dame, 2075 Av. de Vitré, Québec, G1J 5B3, Canada, Member of the Department of Anatomy, Laval University

subtle environmental manipulations can affect the number and size of synapses (Møllgaard et al., 1971; West and Greenough, 1972), it is clear that the numbers given can only be a gross approximation for the species, and that they probably will vary considerably as a function of developmental factors.

Numerical density counts have usually been expressed in cubic centimeters or in cubic micrometers. For the purpose of comparing the results obtained in different species by different authors, these densities will be given here in cubic millimeters. Thus expressed, Cragg (1975a) reports that there are 0.6×10^9 synapses per mm^3 of tissue in the frontal and temporal cortex of a normal adult man. He finds a comparable density in the visual cortex of monkey and a slightly higher figure for the motor cortex of the same species in spite of a greater density of neurons in the visual area (Cragg, 1967a).

Such a high density of cortical synapses is not limited to primates. Indeed, though Cragg (1972, 1975b, c) has arrived at the lower figure of $0.4 \times 10^9/mm^3$ in the visual cortex of cat, Vrensen, DeGroot, and Nunes-Cardozo (1977) have reported a density similar to that of primates in rabbit visual cortex ($0.67 \times 10^9/mm^3$), and Jones and Cullen (1979) arrive at a nearly identical count in the molecular layer of "midcoronal sections" of rat cortex ($0.61 \times 10^9/mm^3$). Even more surprisingly, in the visual cortex of the rat, Cragg (1967b) has reported twice as great a volume density, and this is in agreement with figures given by Aghajanian and Bloom (1967) and by Armstrong-James and Johnson (1969,1970) in rat motor cortex (all about $1.25 \times 10^9/mm^3$).

In spite of the high density of synapses in nonprimates, primates do of course have a greater number of cortical synapses. This is not achieved by means of a higher packing density but by a larger amount of cortical tissue. Considering the constraints on the spatial expansion of the cortical surface, it is rather amazing that in fact the density of synapses is if anything lower in man than in rat. This suggests that there are optimal volume densities of synapses for given volumes of the nervous system. Efficient synaptic and neuronal functions probably require a certain mass of glial cells. Moreover, synaptic bias is to some extent controlled by the spatial distribution of synapses along the dendritic tree at definite distances from the initial segment (Rall, 1967; Rall et al., 1967). These critical spacings in the cortex are possibly incompatible with still greater numerical densities of synapses.

From the data and reviews of Donaldson (1895), Von Economo (1929), and Blinkov and Glezer (1968: see especially tables 182, 187, 192, 193), $200,000 \ mm^2$ seems to be a reasonable estimate of the surface area of the cerebral cortex of man (sum of both hemispheres). According to the same authors, the average thickness is not far from 2.5 mm. This gives a volume of about $500,000 \ mm^3$. With a density of 0.6×10^9 synapses/mm^3 of cortex, man would have about 3×10^{14} cortical synapses. This number corresponds to the number of *milliseconds* that have elapsed in the last 10,000 years, that is, since the beginning of the neolithic period. From the volume estimates of Smith (1934) and the cortical thickness given by Diamond, Johnson, and Ingham (1975), it can be calculated that the rat cortex has a surface measuring 400–500 mm^2 (sum of both hemispheres). At 1.25×10^9 synapses/mm^3, the rat would have $5–6 \times 10^{11}$ cortical synapses—three orders of magnitude lower than in man (the number of milliseconds in 15–20 rather than 10,000 years).

Estimates of the number of cortical neurons in the sum of both hemispheres have ranged from 1 to 2×10^{10} (Blinkov and Glezer, 1968, p. 201 and table 222). Dividing the total estimated number of synapses by the estimated number of neurons, one arrives at the average figure of 15,000–30,000 synapses per cortical neuron. Though this is only a very gross estimate based on data from many authors, it is surprisingly close to the average of 38,000 synapses per neuron calculated by Cragg (1975a) in those cortical areas in man in which he counted both synapses and neurons.

From these data it is clear that the total number of synapses in mammalian neocortex is so high that it would have been hopeless to begin their study in electron microscopy without first trying to find simple meaningful patterns, that is, patterns which would reveal some of the fundamental characteristics of the basic units around which the cortex is built. In fact we have not progressed much beyond that stage. The state of the art is such that we are only beginning in electron microscopy to observe significant cytoarchitectural or species differences. The stress has been on the study of basic common features, and this will be the emphasis of this review.

Synaptic Types

Fortunately, cortical synapses fall rather easily into distinct morphological types. The first, and one of the most important, contribution to the classification of synaptic types was that of Gray (1959), who in a now classical paper distinguished between two types of synaptic contacts on the basis of their membrane differentiations as seen on material immersed in osmium and stained with phosphotungstic acid (PTA).

His type 1 synapse is characterized by what appears to be a marked thickening of the postsynaptic membrane, usually occupying over 70% of the extent of apposed pre- and postsynaptic profiles (Figure 1A). The space between the membranes is increased in size from 20 to 30 nm and contains a line of opaque material lying a bit closer to the post- than to the presynaptic membrane.

In Gray's type 2 synapse the postsynaptic membrane is not as thick (Figure 1B). It usually occupies less than 40% of the zone of apposition. The extracellular space is not significantly increased in size at the point of contact. If it contains an opaque material, the latter is not arranged in as definite a linear array as in the type 1 synapse.

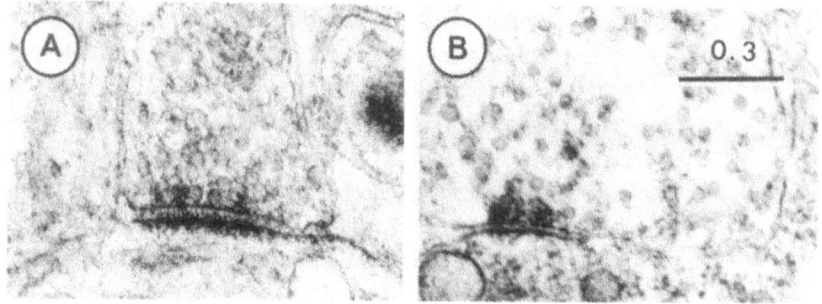

Figure 1 Synapses from cat visual cortex fixed by osmium immersion and stained with phosphotungstic acid. Calibration bar in μm. (A) Type 1 synapse of Gray (1959). (B) Type 2 synapse of Gray.

In that paper Gray was also the first to prove Ramón y Cajal's (1911a, pp. 61–67) contention that dendritic spines really are cytoplasmic extensions of dendrites and that they are the site of synaptic contacts (Figure 5A, Sp). He also showed that some of them contain a distinctive organelle made up of membranous sacs separated by dense bars, and which he called the spine apparatus (Figure 5A,B, arrowheads).

It might have been argued that the two types of membrane differentiations described by Gray did not represent different synaptic types but rather different functional states of a single type of synapse. That this is not so could be deduced from Gray's additional finding that the two types of synapses are found on different parts of neurons. Type 1 synapses are found on spines and dendritic shafts, never on somata. Type 2 synapses are found on somata and dendritic shafts, never on dendritic spines.

Subsequently Hamlyn (1963) described the same distribution of Gray's type 1 and type 2 synapses in the hippocampus, and Hamori and Szentágothai (1965) observed that the basket-cell terminals on Purkinje-cell somata were also of Gray's type 2. At about the same time axosomatic contacts were shown to be inhibitory in both these situations (Andersen, Eccles, and Løyning, 1963; Andersen, Eccles, and Voorhoeve, 1963; Andersen, 1964,1966). These were thus the first synapses to be identified both physiologically and electron microscopically in the central nervous system of vertebrates, and the observations led to the generalization that Gray's type I synapses are excitatory while type 2 are inhibitory.

With the advent of aldehyde fixation in the early 1960s, synapses were again separated into two groups, but now on the basis of the size and shape of synaptic vesicles (Uchizono, 1965). Some profiles contained vesicles which were uniform in size, averaging 50 nm in diameter and were homogeneously round in shape (Figure 2A). Others contained a mixture of smaller round vesicles and of "flattened" vesicles (Figures 2B,C). Uchizono (1967) showed that the populations of ho-

M. Colonnier

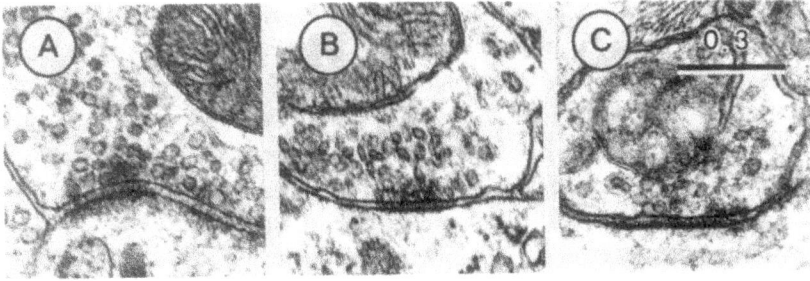

Figure 2 Synapses from cat visual cortex fixed by formaldehyde perfusion and stained with uranyl and lead. Calibration bar in μm. (A) Axon terminal containing the round-vesicle population and forming a synaptic contact with an asymmetrical membrane differentiation. (B), (C) Axon terminals containing the flat-vesicle population and forming contacts with symmetrical membrane differentiations.

mogeneously round vesicles were present in cerebellar synapses which by then were known to be excitatory, while the populations containing the flattened vesicles were present in cerebellar terminals known to be inhibitory. The tempting conclusion that the two populations thus represent excitatory and inhibitory terminals was not readily acceptable. Indeed though certain classes of neurotransmitters could conceivably be packaged in different types of vesicles, it is not the transmitter per se but the properties of the postsynaptic membrane which determines whether a synapse is excitatory or inhibitory.

In 1968, I reported that in the cerebral cortex, synapses containing populations of round vesicles are usually associated with a postsynaptic membrane bordered by a specialized dense cytoplasmic opacity which can be seen as separate from the membrane itself when the latter is cut normal to the plane of section (Figure 2A). The differentiated membranes usually occupy a wide portion of the apposed membranes. The space between the membranes is increased in size and contains a dense material, though this is never as rigidly structured as that seen in osmium-fixed, PTA-stained material. When the postsynaptic opacity is thick, these obviously correspond to Gray's type 1 synapses. When the differentiation occupies but a small portion of the apposed membranes and when the postsynaptic opacity is thin, they would probably look more like Gray's type 2 synapses in osmium-immersed, PTA-stained material.

The flat-vesicle population is usually associated with a postsynaptic membrane which is not bordered by a cytoplasmic opacity. The differentiated membranes are sometimes short as in Figure 2B and thus akin to Gray's type 2. Often, however, they occupy a wide portion of the apposed membranes as in Figure 2C. The space between the two membranes is often increased in size and contains as much dense material as that of the first group of synapses. They thus share some of the characteristics of Gray's types 1 and 2.

Synapses of the first group with the prominent postsynaptic opacity were called asymmetrical synapses, short for synapses with asymmetrical membrane differentiations, while those of the second group were referred to as symmetrical synapses, short for synapses with symmetrical membrane differentiations. These expressions were coined to "naturally call to mind one or the other group," but they are misnomers in that even in the symmetrical group the postsynaptic membrane is sometimes thicker than the presynaptic membrane, and of course in that the contents of pre- and postsynaptic profiles are different.

Thus in the cerebral cortex, terminals containing the round-vesicle population are usually associated with asymmetrical membrane differentiations, and those containing the flat-vesicle population with symmetrical membrane differentiations. The regularity of this association has since been estimated, in turtle three-layered "visual" cortex at least, to be of the order of 95%, although this is probably not as high a correlation as in mammalian neocortex (Ebner and Colonnier, 1978). Assuming that the two types of synaptic-membrane differentiations may reflect differences in membrane receptors, it was suggested (Colonnier, 1974) that the association of each vesicle type to a specific membrane type signifies that, at least in those regions where the relation holds, certain classes of transmitters packaged in round vesicles tend to be associated with receptors causing excitation, while others packaged in "flat" vesicles are usually associated with receptors giving inhibition.

This view has received strong support from studies on the localization of glutamic acid decarboxylase, the synthesizing enzyme of γ-aminobutyric acid (GABA), first in the cerebellum (McLaughlin et al., 1974) and more recently in the cerebral cortex (Riback, 1978). This transmitter, which is known to be inhibitory in both these areas, indeed has been demonstrated to be present in terminals with symmetrical membrane differentiations (Figure 3, GT, from Riback, 1978) and not in those (RT) with asymmetrical membrane differentiations. In the cerebral cortex, glutamic acid decarboxylase has been found in terminals contacting all types of postsynaptic sites where flat-symmetrical contacts are seen in material fixed and stained in the conventional manner, as discussed under the next heading.

Although one or two dense-core vesicles measuring 80–120 nm in diameter are often seen in terminals with round-or flat-vesicle populations, some vesicle-containing profiles contain large proportions of this type of vesicle (Colonnier, 1968; Ebner and Colonnier, 1978; Sloper and Powell, 1979a). According to Beaudet and Descarries (1978), varicosities labeled with norepinephrine or 5-hydroxytryptamine (5-HT) invariably contain several of these large granular vesicles. Moreover, Descarries and his collaborators (Descarries, Beaudet and Watkins, 1975; Descarries, Watkins, and Lapierre, 1977) have shown that even when viewed in two or three adjacent serial sections, less than 5% of these monoaminergic profiles are related to membrane differentiations. This

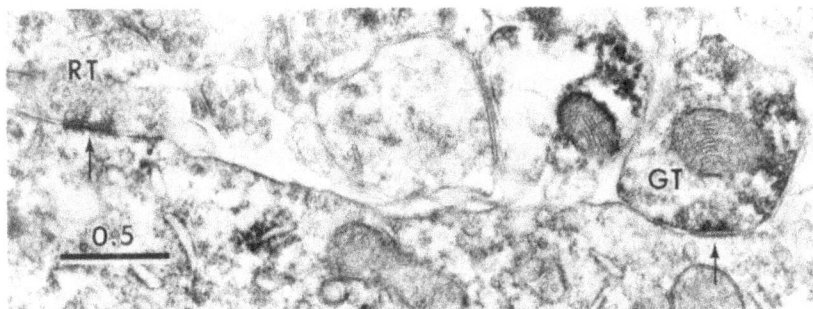

Figure 3 Synaptic contacts on glutamic acid decarboxylase-(GAD)-positive stellate cell soma from layer IV of rat visual cortex. Terminal GT contains GAD-positive reaction product and forms a symmetrical synaptic contact (arrowhead). Terminal RT lacks reaction product and forms an asymmetrical synaptic contact (arrowhead). Calibration bar in μm. (From Riback, 1978. Courtesy of Dr. Charles Riback and Chapman and Hall Ltd., London.)

is in contrast to nonlabeled vesicle-containing profiles, of which 50% relate to differentiated membranes in the same partial serial reconstructions. These authors report that when labeled profiles do relate to differentiated membranes, the latter can be either of the asymmetrical or of the symmetrical type. Similarly, Ebner and Colonnier (1978) found that in turtle cortex only one out of 146 profiles with several large granular vesicles showed a membrane differentiation in the plane of section (it was symmetrical). This is again in contrast to all other vesicle-containing profiles, of which 30% have differentiated membranes in the plane of section. Descarries has presented strong arguments that the monoamines may be released by the varicosities even in the absence of membrane differentiations, as is the case, for example, in the peripheral autonomic nervous system. He has suggested that they may act as a neurohormone or modulator of synaptic activity rather than as a classical transmitter.

On the other hand, the vesicles in those varicosities without membrane differentiations might just be backup material on their way from the cell body to a synaptic varicosity with a membrane differentiation. By using a homologous antiserum directed against dopamine-β-hydroxylase, Morrison et al. (1978) have recently demonstrated that the great number of noradrenergic fibers which can be demonstrated with this method have a distribution and orientation suggesting that fibers in layers I, II, III, and VI might be mainly fibers of passage, while terminal plexuses would be concentrated in layers IV and V. Moreover, systemic administration of 5-hydroxydopamine in newborn cats labels many terminals in the latter layers (Molliver and Krisst, 1975; Coyle and Molliver, 1977). They form numerous classical synaptic contacts of the asymmetric variety, though they are known to be largely inhibitory (for review, see the chapter by Bloom, this volume). They thus seem to invalidate, or at least to be an exception to, the generalization that all asymmetrical synapses are excitatory. It may be worth noting also that in the abdominal ganglion of *Aplysia* all synapses form symmetrical contacts (Tremblay, Colonnier, and McLennan, 1979), although of course many of them are excitatory.

Distribution of Synaptic Types on Different Parts of Different Cell Types

The different parts of cells (soma, dendritic shafts, dendritic spines, and initial segments of axons) can readily be identified in conventional electron-microscopic preparations. It is much more difficult to ascribe them to different cell types. In conventional material it is of course impossible to distinguish between the many cell types that can be identified on Golgi preparations.

When properly sectioned, however, some cell bodies do stand out clearly as pyramidal cells. Figure 4 shows a section through a small pyramidal cell in the visual cortex of cat (from Colonnier, 1968). Its nucleus (Nuc) can be seen to contain the very evenly dispersed chromatin typical of neurons. There is a sufficiently low concentration of organelles in its cytoplasm (Cyt) for the latter to appear slightly paler than the surrounding neuropil. Investigators who have studied cell bodies similar to this one (Colonnier, 1968; Peters and Kaiserman-Abramof, 1970; Jones and Powell, 1970a,b,c; Garey, 1971; LeVay, 1973; Sloper, 1973a; Tömböl, 1974; Strick and Sterling, 1974; Parnavelas et al., 1977; Sloper, Hiorns, and Powell, 1979; Sloper and Powell, 1979a; Smith and Moskovitz, 1979) have all reported, in whatever species and in whatever cytoarchitectonic area, that they receive few synaptic contacts (0 to 6 per section), always of the flat-symmetrical variety.

It would seem that this is true not only of pyramidal cells but also of spiny stellate cells. Though no one has yet defined ultrastructural characteristics to identify the latter cells in conventional material, LeVay (1973) has studied five Golgi-impregnated pyramidal and six Golgi-impregnated spiny stellate cells in the visual cortex of cat. He found that spiny stellates like the pyramidals receive few contacts on their somata, and that these synapses are all of the flat-symmetrical variety. In contrast, Parnavelas et al. (1977), in a similar study of 16 pyramidal and 2 spiny stellate cells, reported the additional presence of asymmetrical axosomatic contacts on their 2 spiny stellate somata.

Though the two studies also give a slightly different account of the synaptic surround of spiny dendrites, they do agree that the pattern is basically similar for both types of cells. Thus apart from one caveat, which will be mentioned later, the following description of spiny dendrites as seen in conventional material (Colonnier, 1968; Peters and Kaiserman-Abramof, 1969,1970; Jones and Powell, 1969b,1970a,b,c; Garey, 1971; LeVay, 1973; Strick and Sterling, 1974; Sloper, Hiorns, and

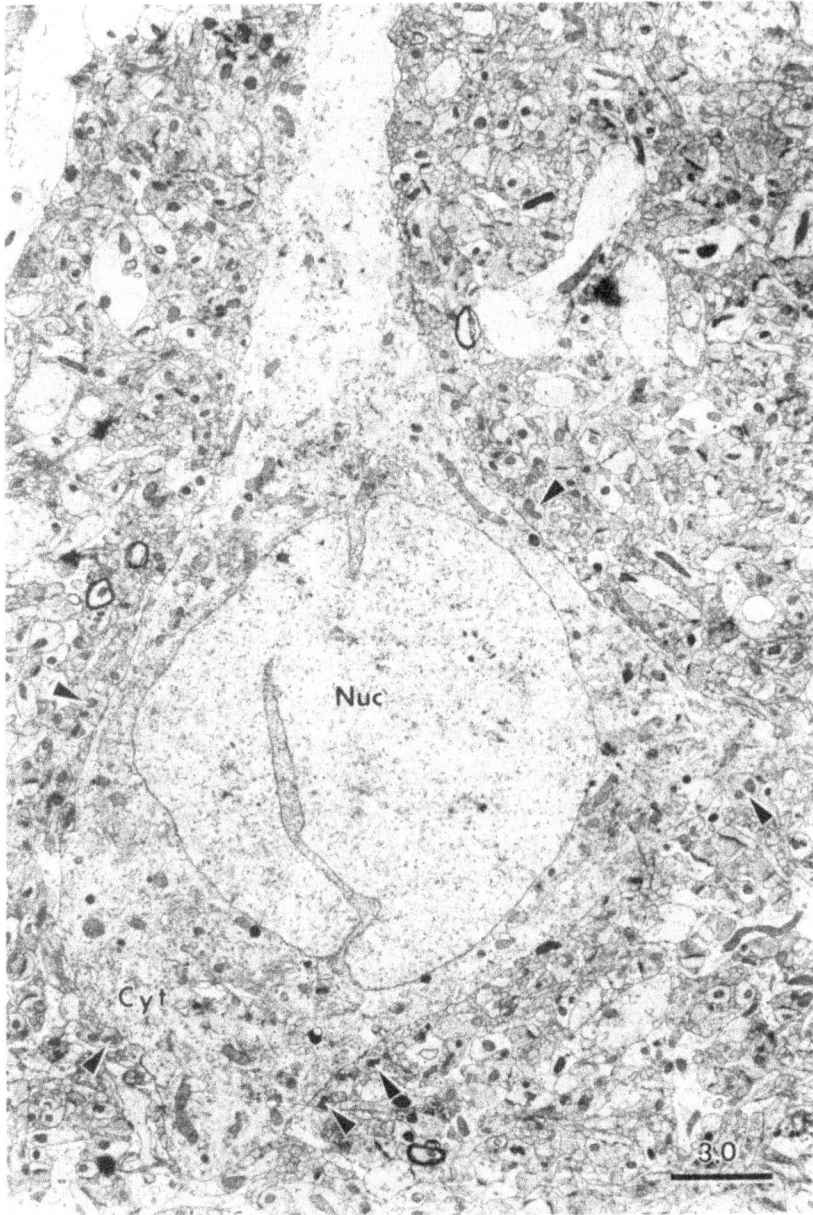

Figure 4 Pyramidal-cell body from visual cortex of cat fixed by formaldehyde perfusion and stained with uranyl and lead. Calibration bar in μm. (From Colonnier, 1968. Courtesy of Elsevier/North Holland Biomedical Press, Amsterdam.)

Powell, 1979; Sloper and Powell, 1979a; Smith and Moskovitz, 1979) applies to both types of cells.

The most striking feature of the spiny dendrites of both pyramidal and spiny stellate cells is the relative absence of synaptic contacts on their dendritic shafts. Most synapses occur on the spines. In the example illustrated in Figure 5A, no synapses are seen on the dendritic shaft, but its spine is contacted by a vesicle-containing profile.

Many of the spines contain a spine apparatus (Figure 5A,B, arrowheads). It serves as a convenient label when the plane of section severs the spine from its dendritic shaft. In individual sections some spine profiles do not contain a spine apparatus. They are usually smaller and some are probably sections through large spines, in which the plane of section has not gone through the spine apparatus. Other profiles, however, probably belong to small spines that do not contain such an organelle. In a study of intrinsic connections in area 17 of macaque, Fisken, Garey, and Powell (1975) have reported that after a perpendicular slit through the layers of the cortex, degenerating terminals of intracortical horizontal axons end largely on these small spines which do not contain a spine apparatus. This is also true in areas 17 and 18 of the squirrel monkey (personal observations).

In individual sections, spines are usually seen to receive only one synaptic contact, of the round-asymmetrical variety. The junctional sites on spines are in fact in the form of disks, many of which are perforated (Peters and Kaiserman-Abramof, 1969), so that sections passing through the perforations appear to have two (or more) separate synaptic sites on spines are in fact in the form of disks, many of which are perfoterminals, but in these cases the synapses are usually of opposite polarity, that is, the second is of the flat-symmetrical type (Figure 5C). There are few reports and few photographic documents of two axon terminals containing round vesicles and forming asymmetrical contacts on the spherule of a dendritic spine. Whether asymmetrical-symmetrical couplings are found only on pyramidals or only on spiny stellates remains an open question.

Though most contacts are on the spines, the dendritic shafts bearing the spines do receive contacts, and again all investigators agree that these are mainly of the flat-symmetrical variety. In fact LeVay (1973) has seen nothing but flat-symmetrical synapses on the dendritic shafts of his eleven Golgi-impregnated cells with spiny dendrites. Most authors, however, using the wider sampling of conventional material, have reported the presence of some round-asymmetrical contacts on the shafts of spine-bearing dendrites. They have been seen also by Parnavelas et al. (1977) on the Golgi-impregnated dendritic shafts of both pyramidal and spiny stellate cells. Jones and Powell (1969b) are of the opinion that these round-asymmetrical contacts on spine-bearing dendritic shafts are usually found at the base of the spines and are associated with sacs and dense bars identical to those of a spine apparatus.

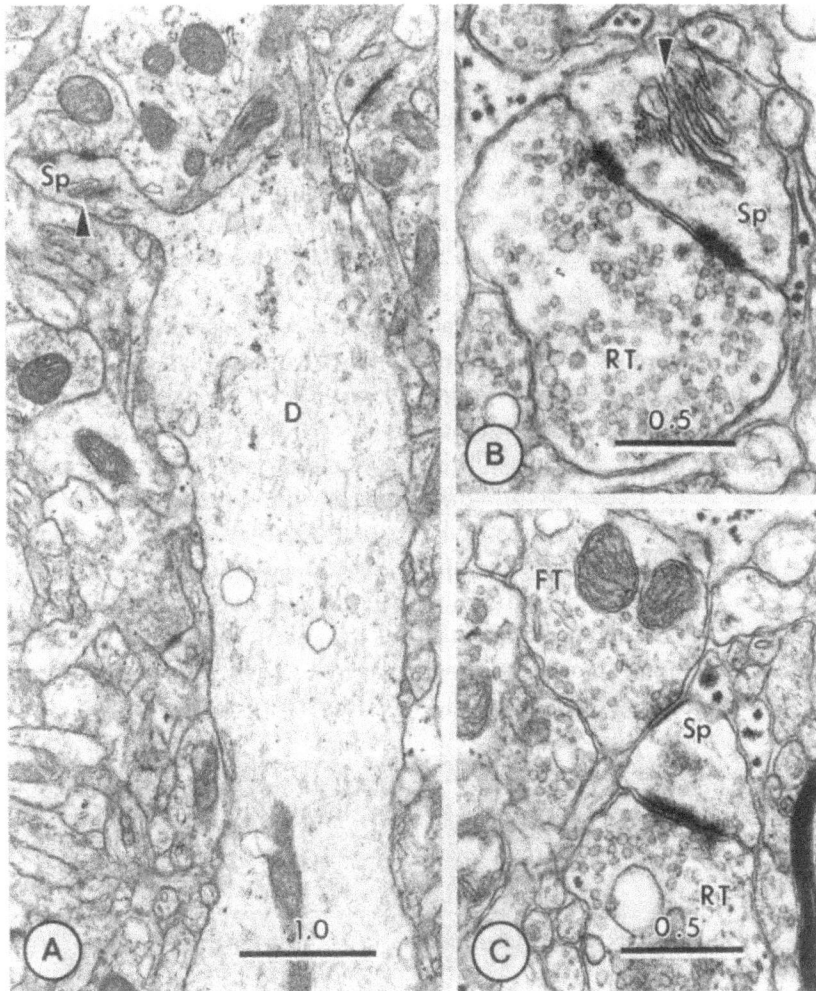

Figure 5 Synaptic contacts on dendritic spines. Calibration bars in μm. (A) Contact on dendritic spine (Sp) containing a spine apparatus (arrowhead). The spine is in continuity with a large dendritic shaft (D) characteristically filled with numerous microtubules. Note absence of contacts on dendritic shaft. (B) Contact on spine (Sp) containing a large well-defined spine apparatus. The terminal (RT) contains round vesicles and forms an asymmetrical contact. (C) Two synapses on a spine (Sp) containing an obliquely cut multivesicular body. Terminal RT contains round vesicles and forms an asymmetrical junction. Terminal FT contains the flat vesicle population and forms a symmetrical contact.

Contacts are found not only on the soma and spiny dendrites but also on the initial segment of axons. The presence of synaptic contacts on axons was first reported by Artyukhina (1965) in rat motor cortex, in the form of vesicle-containing profiles making type 1 contacts on other vesicle-containing profiles. The postsynaptic vesicle-containing profiles were probably not axon terminals but presynaptic dendrites, later shown to exist in the primate motor cortex (Sloper, 1971; Sloper and Powell, 1978a). In 1966 Westrum described type 2 synaptic contacts on axonal profiles close to their myelinated portion. These were probably not on the terminal parts of the axons but rather on their initial segments, whose ultrastructural characteristics were only subsequently identified by Palay et al. (1968) and by Peters, Proskauer, and Kaiserman-Abramof (1968). These characteristics are a fine granular undercoating of the plasma membrane, bundles of microtubules bound together by thin dark cross bars, and the presence of "cisternal organs," that is, groups of sacs separated by dense bars which look very much like well-ordered spine apparatus. Figure 6, from Peters, Proskauer, and Kaiserman-Abramof (1968), shows such a profile receiving a symmetrical synapse. The vesicles are round but Peters and his collaborators at the time were using a fixative which did not distinguish between the two types of vesicles. Authors who have used aldehyde fixatives per-

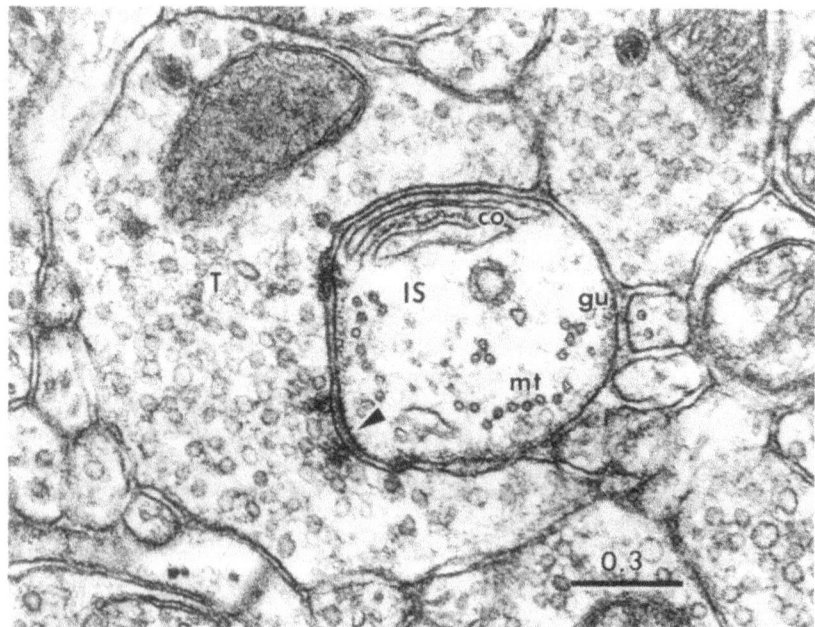

Figure 6 Transverse section of an initial segment (IS) from the cerebral cortex of rat, receiving a symmetrical contact (arrowhead) from a large axon terminal (T). The initial segment is lined by a granular undercoating (gu). It contains bundles of microtubules (mt) joined by thin cross bars, and a cisternal organ (co). Calibration bar in μm. (From Peters, Proskauer, and Kaiserman-Abramof, 1968. Courtesy of Drs. Alan Peters, Charmian Proskauer, and Ita Kaiserman-Abramof, and the Rockefeller University Press, New York.)

mitting this distinction all agree that contacts on initial segments are always of the flat-symmetrical variety (Jones and Powell, 1969a; Sloper, 1973c; Sloper and Powell, 1979b). The differentiation always seems to occupy but a small proportion of the apposed membranes. In a recent quantitative study of 13 serial reconstructions of initial segments, Sloper and Powell (1979b) have demonstrated that the cisternal organs usually lie against the nondifferentiated part of the apposition between terminal and initial segment, that the apposed membranes at the site of the cisternal organ are often dense, and that the extracellular space contains a dense material.

In summary, therefore, all pyramidal and stellate cells with spiny dendrites receive round-asymmetrical contacts on their dendritic spines. Other round-asymmetrical contacts are found on the dendritic shafts close to the base of spines. A few are probably present on the somata of some spiny stellates. Flat-symmetrical synapses are concentrated on the cell body and initial segments of axons. Some are found on dendritic shafts and still fewer are paired to round-asymmetrical contacts on the spine spherules.

The first issue raised by this distribution concerns the functional significance of dendritic spines. Ramón y Cajal (1911a, pp. 67–70) had suggested that they simply increase the surface available for synaptic contacts on dendrites. The electron-microscopic data show that this is incorrect. Though this has been known for over ten years, there is still no hard data concerning the function of spines. The best suggestive evidence derives from recordings made inside large cytoplasmic appendages of fish motoneurons, which the authors (Diamond, Gray, and Yasargyl, 1970) consider a form of spine. The observations lend themselves to the interpretation that there is a marked attenuation of the electrical signal along the fine stems of the spines, either from the dendritic shaft to the spine spherule or from the spine tip to the dendritic shaft. Changes in potentials in the parent dendrite would leave the head of the spine relatively undisturbed, and thus the potential generated by an excitatory input to the spine would be less affected by ongoing activity in the dendritic shaft. There is also evidence that the appendages may generate action potentials. It is interesting in this respect that the cells best known for their dendritic spikes are the Purkinje cells of the cerebellum (Llinas, 1975; Llinas and Nicholson, 1969) and the pyramidal cells of the hippocampus (Spencer and Kandel, 1961; Andersen and Lømo, 1966; Andersen, Holmqvist, and Voorhoeve, 1966), both of which are loaded with spines. The normal motoneuron is usually believed not to give rise to dendritic spikes (Eccles, 1960) and does not have spines.

Inhibitory contacts on the soma and on the initial segments are obviously most appropriately situated to prevent cells from firing, whatever the location of the excitatory input. Inhibitory synapses on the dendritic shafts or on the heads of spines would be more selective in their effects.

In contrast to the numerous observations on the distribution of synapses ending on pyramidal and spiny stellate cells, there is little information on the synaptic contacts formed by the axons of these cells within the neuropil. LeVay (1973) did look at the terminals of collaterals from two Golgi-impregnated pyramidal and two Golgi-impregnated spiny stellate cells and found them to end by asymmetrical membrane differentiation. Parnavelas et al. (1977) and Somogyi (1978) have confirmed this finding for the terminals of Golgi-impregnated spiny cells. White (1979) has seen a few terminals during the reconstruction of a spiny stellate and also found that they end asymmetrically. It is thus tempting to consider the spiny neurons as excitatory cells. This would not be surprising in the case of the pyramidal-cell collaterals within the cortex, since most pyramidal cells are output cells and the cortical output is excitatory. The spiny stellates would be excitatory interneurons. It is important, however, to remember that in the visual system at least some of the spiny stellates are also output cells. Ramón y Cajal (1911b, pp. 604–606) has singled out the visual cortex as being the only one in which stellate cells project to the white matter. Lund (1973) has reported the presence of spiny stellates with long axons in the visual cortex of monkey. Gilbert and Wiesel (1979a; see also their chapter in this volume) have described spiny stellates in the upper portion of layer IV of cat visual cortex projecting to the white matter. Innocenti and Fiore (1976) have labeled stellate cells in layer IV at the junction of areas 17 and 18 after the injection of HRP in the contralateral homotypic area, and Lamont and Colonnier (1978) have seen them in the upper portion of layer IV in area 17 of cat after injections in ipsilateral area 18.

The synaptic surround of smooth and sparsely spinous stellate cells (Colonnier, 1968; Jones and Powell, 1970a,b,c; Garey, 1971; Peters, 1971; LeVay, 1973; Sloper, 1973a; Tomböl, 1974; Strick and Sterling, 1974; Parnavelas et al., 1977; Peters and Fairén, 1978; Sloper, Hiorns, and Powell, 1979; Sloper and Powell, 1979a; Smith and Moskovitz, 1979) is quite different from that described for pyramids and spiny stellate cells. Sloper, Hiorns, and Powell (1979) have recently distinguished between two groups of these stellate neurons on the basis of size and of ultrastructural characteristics. The size difference is well demonstrated in the motor cortex but is not at all obvious in the somatosensory area.

The cytoplasm of the "small" cell is pale like that of a pyramidal cell, but the nucleus contains clumps of chromatin, especially under the nuclear membrane. In this respect they are reminiscent of glial cells. Dendrites seen in continuity with these somata are markedly varicose. The cell bodies are present in all layers but are especially prominent in layer II. A bipolar variety is seen in the deeper layers. Like the cell bodies of pyramidal cells, those of the small stellates receive few contacts, usually only 0 to 5 per section. They are different from the pyramids in that they receive not only flat-symmetrical but also round-asymmetrical synapses.

The "large" stellate cell has an evenly dispersed nuclear chromatin (Figure 7, Nuc), and its cytoplasm (Cyt) is so full of organelles that it appears camouflaged in the surrounding neuropil. Dendrites in continuity with these cell bodies are large and only moderately varicose (Figure 7, LD). The somata are found mainly from the bottom of layer III to the top of layer V. In somatosensory, motor (Sloper, Hiorns, and Powell, 1979), and visual (Tomböl, 1974) cortices, they represent only about 9% of all cells. The cell bodies of these stellate cells differ from that of pyramidal and small stellates in receiving many synaptic contacts, usually 4 to 12 per section, although some have been seen with up to 20–30 contacts on a single section (Colonnier, 1968). As in the case of the small stellates, the synapses are of both flat-symmetrical and round-asymmetrical types.

The nonspiny dendrites of both these types of cells receive both types of contacts on their dendritic shafts. The markedly varicose dendrites of the small cells do not have as many contacts on them (Figure 7, SD, arrowheads) as the moderately varicose dendrites of the large cells, which are densely studded with them (Figure 7, LD, arrowheads).

Moreover, Sloper and Powell (Sloper, 1972; Sloper and Powell, 1978b) have presented convincing pictorial evidence of the existence of true gap junctions between the dendrites and soma of the large stellate cells in both somatosensory and motor cortex. Smith and Moskovitz (1979) report similar junctions between somata of "granule cells" in layer IV of the auditory cortex of squirrel monkey.

Sloper and Powell do not have direct evidence identifying the specific type of cells which corresponds to these "large" stellate cells of electron microscopy. On the basis of size and distribution, they argue that they may correspond to the cortical baskets (Ramón y Cajal, 1911b, pp. 555–560; Colonnier, 1966; Marin-Padilla, 1969; Szentágothai, 1973) or Jones's (1975) type I cell. Jones has found few of these cells in layer IV, but both Ramón y Cajal and Marin-Padilla consider this layer a major site of location of the basket cells. Marin-Padilla describes their dendrites as possessing numerous spines, but this is probably due to the fact that he was using very young material. Some stellate-type cells having rather many spines in the early postnatal period do lose them with maturity (Jones, 1975; Lund, Boothe, and Lund, 1977).

In his 1973 study, LeVay examined twelve Golgi-impregnated smooth stellate cells. He was able to confirm that these do indeed receive both flat-symmetrical and round-asymmetrical synapses on their soma and dendritic shafts. He also found that their own axon terminals were all of the symmetrical type. Parnavelas et al. (1977) and Peters and Fairén (1978) subsequently confirmed these findings on Golgi-impregnated smooth stellate cells of the visual cortex of rat. The generalization that the flat-symmetrical terminals belong to cortical interneurons is further supported by the experiments of Szentágothai (1965a,b) showing that type 2 contacts on cell bodies and dendritic trunks survive after under-

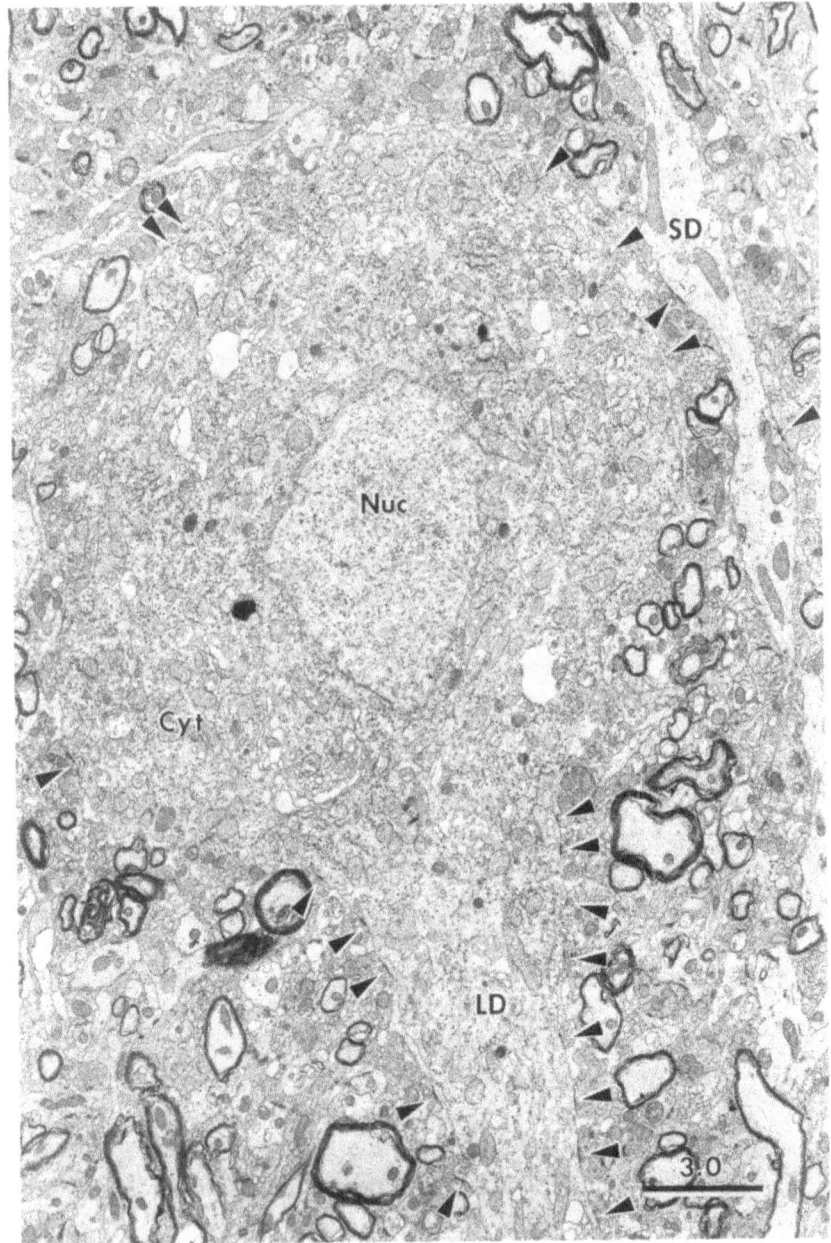

Figure 7 Large stellate cell from layer IV of cat visual cortex, with evenly dispersed nuclear (Nuc) chromatin and dense cytoplasm (Cyt), receiving 6–7 synaptic contacts. A large dendrite (LD) in continuity with the cell body is studded with contacts (arrowheads). A smaller, markedly varicose dendrite (SD) in the upper right corner receives only two contacts (arrowheads). Calibration bar in μm.

cutting the cortex. Moreover, degeneration of flat-symmetrical contacts is seen after making perpendicular slits through the cortex (Fisken, Garey, and Powell, 1975; Gatter, Sloper, and Powell, 1978) but not after lesions of afferent fiber systems (see below). Finally, in his study on the localization of glutamic acid decarboxylase, Riback (1978) found this enzyme in the cell bodies and dendrites of smooth or sparsely spinous stellate cells.

Thus the present state of the art suggests that many of the smooth stellates are GABAergic inhibitory interneurons, receiving both excitatory and inhibitory contacts on their cell bodies and dendritic shafts. Some of these surely correspond to those stellate cells whose axons terminate as baskets around the cell bodies of pyramidal cells, and these are probably the "large" stellates of electron microscopy. These large cells are linked together by gap junctions, suggesting that they would be electronically coupled (Bennet et al., 1967). A focal excitation of a group of these cells might thus result in lateral recruitment of other similar inhibitory cells within the middle and deep layers, yielding a field of inhibition wider than the excitatory input zone. This could be one of the mechanisms of the inhibitory surrounds of cortical columns.

Some smooth stellates are most probably not inhibitory. Indeed cells similar to the smooth stellate cell "à double bouquet dendritique" (Ramón y Cajal, 1911b, pp. 538–542; Colonnier, 1966; Szentágothai, 1973) or to Jones's (1975) type 3 cell have been shown in rat to contain the very powerful excitatory vasoactive intestinal polypeptide (Emson and Hunt, this volume). The axons of these cells have numerous, long, vertically oriented collaterals organized in discrete bundles and might significantly contribute to the vertical spread of excitation in the cortex responsible for the physiologically demonstrated columns. These excitatory stellates possibly belong to the group of small bipolar stellate cells of electron microscopy (White, 1978; Sloper, Hiorns, and Powell, 1979). According to Ramón y Cajal (1911b, p. 539) these cells are located mainly in layers III and IV, but Jones (1975) has seen them only in layer II and the upper part of III. This absence of Jones's type 3 cells in layer IV is probably only a reflection of the difficulty inherent in the staining of these cells by the Golgi technique. Most authors have not reported them in Golgi studies even in primates where they are most abundant. Lund (1973) specifically mentions the absence of the long, vertically arborized axons of these cells in her preparations of visual cortex of macaque.

The Site of Termination of Thalamocortical, Commissural, and Associated Connections

The site of termination of the input to the neocortex has been studied by anterograde degeneration in several architectonic areas and in several species. (1) Thalamocortical projections have been studied from the lateral geniculate nucleus to area 17 in cat (Colonnier and Rossignol, 1969; Garey, 1970; Garey and Powell, 1971; Winfield and Powell, 1976), rat (Peters and Feldman, 1976,1977; Peters, Feldman, and Salhanda, 1976; Peters and Salhanda, 1976) and monkey (Garey and Powell, 1971), and to areas 18 and 19 in cat (Garey and Powell, 1971); from the ventral lateral thalamic nucleus to the motor cortex in cat (Strick and Sterling, 1974) and monkey (Sloper, 1973b; Sloper and Powell, 1979c); and from the ventral posterior nucleus to the somatosensory cortex of cat (Jones, 1968; Jones and Powell, 1970d) and monkey (Sloper and Powell, 1979c). (2) Commissural connections have been studied in the paravisual cortex of the rat (Lund and Lund, 1970), at the junction of areas 17 and 18 in monkey (Fisken, Garey, and Powell, 1975), in the somatosensory cortex of cat (Jones, 1968; Jones and Powell, 1970d) and monkey (Sloper and Powell, 1979c), and in the motor cortex of monkey (Sloper, 1973b; Sloper and Powell, 1979c). (3) Association fibers from area 18 to area 17 (Garey and Powell, 1971) and from SII to SI (Jones, 1968; Jones and Powell, 1970d) have been studied in cat, and from area 3b and area 6 to area 4 (Sloper, 1973b; Sloper and Powell, 1979c) in monkey.

The site of termination of geniculocortical fibers has also been studied by anterograde transport of labeled amino acids in the cat (LeVay and Gilbert, 1976).

All those who have used anterograde degeneration methods agree that one of the most striking features of all these projections is the small percentage of boutons seen to degenerate after each and every such lesion. The highest estimates are of the order of 5 to 10%, even where they are most numerous, that is, within layer IV after thalamic lesions. In their autoradiographic study, however, LeVay and Gilbert (1976) report that as many as 20% of terminals in layer IV of cat area 17 are labeled from the geniculate nucleus. The low percentage found after lesions is thus most probably an expression of differences in the speed of degeneration of individual terminals coupled with a relatively short survival time in the state of "opaque degeneration" in which they are recognizable (Colonnier, 1964). It is interesting that in a recent study of turtle thalamic-recipient cortex (Smith, Ebner, and Colonnier, 1979) it has been reported that degenerating thalamocortical terminals represent as many as 25% of those present within the superficial 100 μm of cortex where they terminate. Although this may indicate a greater proportion of thalamocortical endings in that species, it probably also reflects a more sluggish catabolism of degenerating terminals in this cold-blooded vertebrate even when it is maintained at a relatively high ambient temperature.

All degenerating terminals of all the inputs have been reported to make asymmetrical contacts (Figure 8A). When the vesicles are still recognizable, they appear to be of the spheroidal variety. This has been demonstrated by autoradiography for the thalamocortical projection

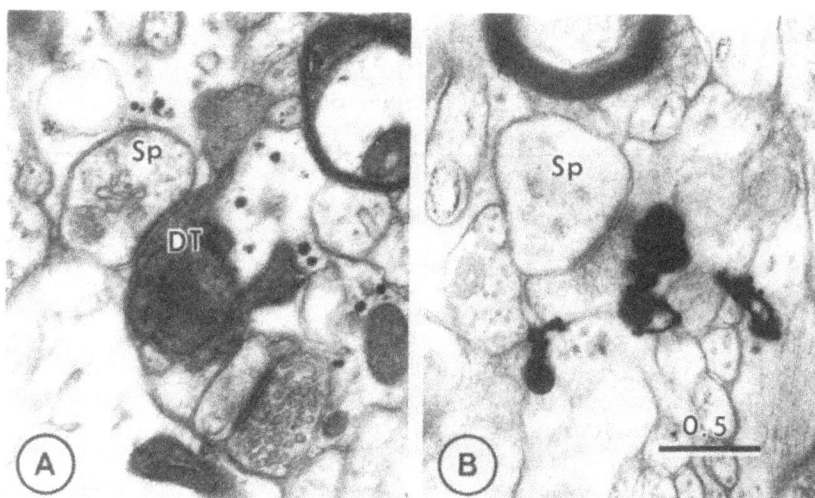

Figure 8 Thalamocortical terminals synapsing on dendritic spines in cat visual cortex. Calibration bar in μm. (A) Degenerating terminal (DT) forming an asymmetrical contact on a dendritic spine (Sp) containing a spine apparatus, in layer IV after lesion of the dorsal lateral geniculate nucleus. (From Colonnier and Rossignol, 1969. Courtesy of Little Brown and Co., Boston.) (B) Labeled terminal contacting spine (Sp) in layer VI after injection of radioactive proline in dorsal lateral geniculate nucleus. (From LeVay and Gilbert, 1976. Courtesy of Drs. Simon LeVay and Charles Gilbert, and Elsevier, New York.)

(Figure 8B, from LeVay and Gilbert, 1976). As most authors comment, this correlates with the fact that these afferents are excitatory.

Most afferent fibers end on dendritic spines (Figure 8A). Usually there is only one degenerating terminal on the spine. It is rare to find another contact on the same spine, and when one is present, it is normal and usually of the flat-symmetrical variety.

Many authors have given quantitative data (Table I, modified from Peters and Feldman, 1976). Estimates of the percentage of afferent degenerating terminals ending on spines range from 62 to 97%. These contacts on spines have been reported at 90% for the thalamocortical projection to motor cortex in cat (Strick and Sterling, 1974) and in monkey (Sloper, 1973b; Sloper and Powell, 1979c); at 83% for that to area 17 in rat (Peters and Feldman, 1976), cat and monkey (Garey and Powell, 1971); and at 75% for the somatosensory cortex of cat (Jones and Powell, 1970d). Surprisingly, contacts on spines also form 86% of the thalamocortical projection in turtle (Smith, Ebner, and Colonnier, 1979).

The next most frequent postsynaptic site of input terminals is on the dendritic shafts. Since there are few round-asymmetrical synapses on the shafts of spine-bearing dendrites, these degenerating terminals, as expected, are found mainly on synapse-studded dendritic shafts, that is, on those of smooth stellate cells. Quantitative estimates range from 8

Table I Degenerating Terminals (Percentage)

	Thalamocortical Spine–Shaft–Soma	Commissural Spine–Shaft–Soma	Associational Spine–Shaft–Soma
Motor Cortex			
Monkey: Sloper (1973b), Sloper & Powell (1979c)	89.5–9–1.5	96–3– <1	(from SI) 82–18– (from area 6) 76–24
Cat: Strick & Sterling (1974)	91–8–1		
Visual Cortex			
Area 17			
Cat: Garey & Powell (1971)	83–14–3		
Monkey: Garey & Powell (1971)	84–14–2		
Monkey: Fisken, Garey, and Powell (1975)		(Junction 17/18) 76–24	(17 to 18) 62–38
Rat: Peters & Feldman (1976)	83–15–2		
Area 18			
Cat: Garey & Powell (1971)	70–20–10		
Area 19			
Cat: Garey & Powell (1971)	85–14– <1		
Somatosensory Cortex			
Cat: Jones & Powell (1970d)	75–25		
Monkey: Sloper & Powell (1979c)	89–11– <1	(area 3b) 97–3–	

to 25% for the thalamocortical projection, from 3 to 24% for the commissural afferents, and from 18 to 38% for fibers of association.

Finally, a few terminals end on the somata of smooth stellate cells. Authors give 0 to 3% for endings on somas, with the notable exception of the thalamocortical projection to area 18 of the cat, where Garey and Powell report as many as 10% on soma.

There thus seems to be little doubt that the majority of terminals of cortical afferents contain round vesicles and form asymmetrical contacts on dendritic spines; fewer terminate on dendritic shafts, and fewer still directly on the cell soma. There is also little doubt that dendritic shafts and soma receiving 8 to 25% of the thalamocortical endings are those of smooth stellate cells, many of which are probably GABAergic inhibitory interneurons. Spines receive 75 to 90% of the thalamocortical terminals. Whether these spines belong to pyramidal cells, which are the main output cells of the cerebral cortex, or to spiny stellates, which are best interpreted for the moment as excitatory interneurons, was only recently determined in the serial reconstruction studies of Peters, White, and Fairén (1977), White (1978), and Somogyi (1978), using combined degeneration-Golgi electron-microscopic methods. These authors have shown that for the thalamocortical projection at least, incoming afferents terminate directly on the spines of both types of cells (for full discussion, see the chapter by White, this volume).

Thus it can be concluded that incoming thalamocortical afferents terminate directly on output cells, on excitatory interneurons, and on inhibitory interneurons. Some of the excitatory interneurons with long vertical axons containing the powerful vasoactive intestinal polypeptide would spread the focus of excitation in a columnar fashion through the layers of the cortex. Some of the inhibitory interneurons have horizontal axonal arborizations ending as baskets around the pyramidal-cell bodies, contain GABA, and are electronically coupled. This suggests that they are the source of the inhibitory fields, spreading more widely across columns than the excitatory input.

This is as far as electron microscopy has gone and as far as one dares conjecture from the data it has offered. The groundwork is done. Very little more can be expected from simple observation of conventional material. Progress will come, rather, from further quantitative studies of normal and experimental material, from the examination of physiologically identified and morphologically labeled neurons, and especially from the development of new histochemical electron-opaque markers. The study of the circuitry of the cortex has been extremely difficult and seemingly hopeless, mainly because the axons of its neurons lack the morphologically differentiated terminals which reveal the circuitry in other regions of the brain. The new labeling techniques now allow a useful differentiation between neurons and a fine dissection, which, allied with electron microscopy, can be expected within the foreseeable future to increase significantly our knowledge of cortical circuitry.

Acknowledgments

The author wishes to thank Dr. Michel Filion for his invaluable comments on the manuscript, and Mr. Jacques Rodrigue for his technical and photographic assistance. Work supported by a grant from the Medical Research Council of Canada.

References

Aghajanian, G. K., and F. E. Bloom, 1967. The formation of synaptic junctions in developing rat brain: A quantitative electron microscopic study. *Brain Res.* 6:716–727.

Andersen, P., 1964. Location of postsynaptic inhibitory synapses in hippocampal pyramids. *J. Neurophysiol.* 27:592–607.

Andersen, P., 1966. Correlation of structural design with function in the archicortex. In *Brain and Conscious Experience*. J. C. Eccles, ed. New York: Springer-Verlag, pp. 59–84.

Andersen, P., and T. Lømo, 1966. Mode of activation of hippocampal pyramidal cells by excitatory synapses on dendrites. *Exp. Brain Res.* 2:247–260.

Andersen, P., J. C. Eccles, and Y. Løyning, 1963. Recurrent inhibition in the hippocampus with identification of the inhibitory cells and its synapses. *Nature* 198:541–542.

Andersen, P., J. C. Eccles, and P. E. Voorhoeve, 1963. Inhibitory synapses on somas of Purkinje cells in the cerebellum. *Nature* 199:655–656.

Andersen, P., B. Holmqvist, and P. E. Voorhoeve, 1966. Excitatory synapses on hippocampal apical dendrites activated by entorhinal stimulation. *Acta Physiol. Scand.* 66:461–472.

Armstrong-James, M. A., and F. R. Johnson, 1969. Post-natal development of synapses in the cerebral cortex of the rat. *J. Anat.* 104:590.

Armstrong-James, M., and R. Johnson, 1970. Quantitative studies of post-natal changes in synapses in rat superficial motor cortex: An electron microscopical study. *Z. Zellforsch.* 110:559–568.

Artyukhina, N. I., 1965. Structure of synapses in rat motor cortex. *Fed. Proc.* 25:559–564.

Beaudet, A., and L. Descarries, 1978. The monoamine innervation of rat cerebral cortex: Synaptic and nonsynaptic axon terminals. *Neuroscience* 4:851–860.

Bennett, M. V. L., G. D. Pappas, M. Giménez, and Y. Nakajima, 1967. Physiology and ultrastructure of electrotonic junctions. IV. Medullary electromotor nuclei in gymnotid fish. *J. Neurophysiol.* 30:236–300.

Blinkov, S. M., and I. I. Glezer, 1978. *The Human Brain in Figures and Tables. A Quantitative Handbook.* New York: Plenum Press.

Colonnier, M., 1964. Experimental degeneration in the cerebral cortex. *J. Anat.* 98:47–53.

Colonnier, M., 1966. The structural design of the neocortex. In *Brain and Conscious Experience*. J. C. Eccles, ed. New York: Springer-Verlag, pp. 1–23.

Colonnier, M., 1968. Synaptic patterns on different cell types in the different laminae of the cat visual cortex. *Brain Res.* 9:268–287.

Colonnier, M., 1974. Spatial interrelationships as physiological mechanisms in the central nervous system. In *Essays on the Nervous System*. R. Bellairs, and E. G. Gray, eds. Oxford: Clarendon Press, pp. 344–366.

Colonnier, M., and S. Rossignol, 1969. Heterogeneity of the cerebral cortex. In *Basic Mechanisms of the Epilepsies*. H. Jasper, A. Ward, and A. Pope, eds. Boston: Little Brown, pp. 29–40.

Coyle, J. T., and M. E. Molliver, 1977. Major innervation of newborn rat cortex by monoaminergic neurons. *Science* 196:444–447.

Cragg, B. G., 1967a. The density of synapses and neurones in the motor and visual areas of the cerebral cortex. *J. Anat.* 101:639–654.

Cragg, B. G., 1967b. Changes in visual cortex on first exposure of rats to light. *Nature* 215:251.

Cragg, B. G., 1972. The development of synapses in cat visual cortex. *Invest. Ophthal.* 11:377–385.

Cragg, B. G., 1975a. The density of synapses and neurons in normal, mentally defective and ageing human brains. *Brain* 98:81–90.

Cragg, B. G., 1975b. The development of synapses in kitten visual cortex during visual deprivation. *Exp. Neurol.* 46:445–451.

Cragg, B. G., 1975c. The development of synapses in the visual system of the cat. *J. Comp. Neurol.* 160:147–166.

Descarries, L., A. Beaudet, and K. C. Watkins, 1975. Serotonin nerve terminals in adult rat neocortex. *Brain Res.* 100:563–588.

Descarries, L., K. C. Watkins, and Y. Lapierre, 1977. Noradrenergic axon terminals in the cerebral cortex of rat. III. Topometric ultrastructural analysis. *Brain Res.* 133:197–222.

Diamond, J., E. G. Gray, and G. M. Yasargyl, 1970. The function of the dendritic spine: An hypothesis. In *Excitatory Synaptic Mechanisms*. P. Andersen and J. K. S. Jansen, eds. Oslo: Universitetsforlaget, pp. 213–222.

Diamond, M. C., R. E. Johnson, and C. A. Ingham, 1975. Morphological changes in the young, adult and aging rat cerebral cortex, hippocampus and diencephalon. *Behav. Biol.* 14:163–174.

Donaldson, H. H., 1895. *The Growth of the Brain*. London: Walter Scott.

Ebner, F. F., and M. Colonnier, 1978. A quantitative study of synaptic patterns in turtle visual cortex. *J. Comp. Neurol.* 179:263–276.

Eccles, J. C., 1960. The properties of dendrites. In *Structure and Function of the Cerebral Cortex*. D. B. Tower, and J. P. Schadé, eds. Amsterdam: Elsevier, pp. 192–202.

Fisken, R. A., L. J. Garey, and T. P. S. Powell, 1975. The intrinsic, association, and commissural connections of area 17 of the visual cortex. *Phil. Trans. Roy Soc. B* 272:487–536.

Garey, L. J., 1970. The termination of thalamo-cortical fibres in the visual cortex of cat and monkey. *J. Physiol. (London)* 210:15–17P.

Garey, L. J., 1971. A light and electron microscopic study of the visual cortex of cat and monkey. *Proc. Roy. Soc. B* 179:21–40.

Garey, L. J., and T. P. S. Powell, 1971. An experimental study of the termination of the lateral geniculo-cortical pathway in the cat and monkey. *Proc. Roy. Soc. Lond. B* 179:41–63.

Gatter, K. C., J. J. Sloper, and T. P. S. Powell, 1978. An electron microscopic study of the termination of intracortical axons upon Betz cells in area 4 of the monkey. *Brain* 101:543–553.

Gilbert, C. D., and T. N. Wiesel, 1979a. Morphology and intracortical projections of functionally characterized neurones in the cat visual cortex. *Nature* 280:120–125.

Gray, E. G., 1959. Axo-somatic and axo-dendritic synapses of the cerebral cortex: An electron microscope study. *J. Anat.* 93:420–433.

Hamlyn, L. H., 1963. An electron microscope study of pyramidal neurones in the Ammon's horn of the rabbit. *J. Anat.* 97:189–201.

Hamori, J., and J. Szentágothai, 1965. The Purkinje cell baskets: Ultrastructure of an inhibitory synapse. *Acta Biol. Hung.* 15:465–479.

Innocenti, G. M., and L. Fiore, 1976. Morphological correlates of visual field transformation in the corpus callosum. *Neurosci. Lett.* 2:245–252.

Jones, E. G., 1968. An electron microscopic study of the termination of afferent fiber systems within the somatic sensory cortex of the cat. *J. Anat.* 103:595–597.

Jones, E. G., 1975. Varieties and distribution of non-pyramidal cells in the somatic sensory cortex of the squirrel monkey. *J. Comp. Neurol.* 160:205–267.

Jones, D. G., and A. M. Cullen, 1979. A quantitative investigation of some presynaptic terminal parameters during synaptogenesis. *Exp. Neurol.* 64:245–259.

Jones, E. G., and T. P. S. Powell, 1969a. Synapses on the axon hillocks and initial segments of pyramidal cell axons in the cerebral cortex. *J. Cell Sci.* 5:495–507.

Jones, E. G., and T. P. S. Powell, 1969b. Morphological variations in the dendritic spines of the neocortex. *J. Cell Sci.* 5:509–529.

Jones, E. G., and T. P. S. Powell, 1970a. Electron microscopy of the somatic sensory cortex of the cat. I. Cell types and synaptic organization. *Phil. Trans. Roy. Soc. B* 257:1–11.

Jones, E. G., and T. P. S. Powell, 1970b. Electron microscopy of the somatic sensory cortex of the cat. II. The fine structure of layers I and II. *Phil. Trans. Roy. Soc. B* 257:13–21.

Jones, E. G., and T. P. S. Powell, 1970c. Electron microscopy of the somatic sensory cortex of the cat. III. The fine structure of layers III to VI. *Phil. Trans. Roy. Soc. B* 257:23–28.

Jones, E. G., and T. P. S. Powell, 1970d. An electron microscopic study of lamination pattern and mode of termination of afferent fibre pathways in the somatic sensory cortex of the cat. *Phil. Trans. Roy. Soc. B* 257:45–62.

Lamont, P., and M. Colonnier, 1978. Cortico-cortical projections to area 18 in the cat. *Neurosci. Abst.* 4:76.

LeVay, S., 1973. Synaptic patterns in the visual cortex of the cat and monkey. Electron microscopy of Golgi preparations. *J. Comp. Neurol.* 150:53–86.

LeVay, S., and C. D. Gilbert, 1976. Laminar patterns of geniculocortical projection in the cat. *Brain Res.* 113:1–19.

Llinas, R., 1975. Electroresponsive properties of dendrites in central neurons. In *Advances in Neurology*, Vol. 12. G. W. Kreutzberg, ed. New York: Raven Press, pp. 1–13.

Llinas, R., and C. Nicholson, 1969. Electrophysiological analysis of alligator cerebellum: A study of dendritic spikes. In *Neurobiology of Cerebellar Evolution and Development*. R. Llinas, ed. Chicago: American Medical Association, pp. 431–456.

Lund, J. S., 1973. Organisation of neurons in the visual cortex, area 17, of the monkey (*Macaca mulatta*). *J. Comp. Neurol.* 146:455–495.

Lund, J. S., and R. D. Lund, 1970. The termination of callosal fibres in the paravisual cortex of the rat. *Brain Res.* 17:25–45.

Lund, J. S., R. G. Boothe, and R. D. Lund, 1977. Development of neurons in the visual cortex (area 17) of the monkey (*Macaca mulatta*): A Golgi study from fetal day 127 to postnatal maturity. *J. Comp. Neurol.* 176:149–187.

McLaughlin, B., J. G. Wood, K. Saito, R. Barber, J. E. Vaughn, E. Roberts, and J.-Y. Wu, 1974. The fine structural localization of glutamate decarboxylase in synaptic terminals of rodent cerebellum. *Brain Res.* 76:377–391.

Marin-Padilla, M., 1969. Origin of the pericellular baskets of the pyramidal cells of the human motor cortex: A Golgi study. *Brain Res.* 14:633–646.

Møllgaard, K., M. C. Diamond, E. L. Bennett, M. R. Rosenzweig, and B. Lindner, 1971. Qualitative synaptic changes with differential experience in rat brain. *Int. J. Neurosci.* 2:113–128.

Molliver, M. E., and D. A. Krisst, 1975. The fine structural demonstration of monoaminergic synapses in immature neocortex. *Neurosci. Lett.* 1:305–310.

Morrison, J. H., R. Grzanna, M. E. Molliver, and J. T. Coyle, 1978. The distribution and orientation of noradrenergic fibers in neocortex of the rat: an immunofluorescence study. *J. Comp. Neurol.* 181:17–40.

Palay, S. L., C. Sotelo, A. Peters, and P. M. Orkand, 1968. The axon hillock and the initial segment. *J. Cell Biol.* 38:193–201.

Parnavelas, J. G., K. Sullivan, A. R. Lieberman, and K. E. Webster, 1977. Neurons and their synaptic organization in the visual cortex of the rat. Electron microscopy of Golgi preparations. *Cell Tiss. Res.* 183:499–517.

Peters, A., 1971. Stellate cells of the rat parietal cortex. *J. Comp. Neurol.* 141:345–374.

Peters, A., and A. Fairén, 1978. Smooth and sparsely-spined stellate cells in the visual cortex of the rat: A study using a combined Golgi-electron microscope technique. *J. Comp. Neurol.* 181:129–172.

Peters, A., and M. L. Feldman, 1976. The projection of the lateral geniculate nucleus to area 17 of the rat cerebral cortex. 1. General description. *J. Neurocytol.* 5:63–84.

Peters, A., and M. L. Feldman, 1977. The projection of the lateral geniculate nucleus to area 17 of rat cerebral cortex. IV. Terminations upon spiny dendrites. *J. Neurocytol.* 6:669–689.

Peters, A., and I. R. Kaiserman-Abramof, 1969. The small pyramidal neuron of the rat cerebral cortex. The synapses upon dendritic spines. *Z. Zellforsch.* 100:487–506.

Peters, A., and I. R. Kaiserman-Abramof, 1970. The small pyramidal cell of the rat cerebral cortex. The perikaryon, dendrites and spines. *Amer. J. Anat.* 127:321–356.

Peters, A., and J. Salhanda, 1976. The projection of the lateral geniculate nucleus to area 17 of rat cerebral cortex. III. Layer VI. *Brain Res.* 105:533–537.

Peters, A., M. Feldman, and J. Salhanda, 1976. The projection of the lateral geniculate nucleus to area 17 of rat cerebral cortex. II. Terminations upon neuronal perikarya and dendritic shafts. *J. Neurocytol.* 5:85–107.

Peters, A., C. C. Proskauer, and I. R. Kaiserman-Abramof, 1968. The small pyramidal neuron of the rat cerebral cortex. The axon hillock and initial segment. *J. Cell Biol.* 39:604–619.

Peters, A., E. L. White, and A. Fairén, 1977. Synapses between identified neuronal elements. An electron microscopic demonstration of degenerating axon terminals synapsing with Golgi impregnated neurons. *Neurosci. Lett.* 6:171–175.

Rall, W., 1967. Distinguishing theoretical synaptic potentials computed for different soma-dendritic distributions of synaptic input. *J. Neurophysiol.* 30:1138–1168.

Rall, W., R. E. Burke, T. G. Smith, P. G. Nelson, and K. Frank, 1967. Dendritic location of synapses and possible mechanisms for the monosynaptic EPSP in motoneurons. *J. Neurophysiol.* 30:1169–1193.

Ramón y Cajal, S., 1911a. *Histologie du système nerveux de l'homme et des vertébrés*, Vol. 1. Consejo Superior de Investigaciones Cientificas. (Madrid 1954: Instituto Ramón y Cajal.)

Ramón y Cajal, S., 1911b: *Histologie du système nerveux de l'homme et des vertébrés*, Vol. 2. Consejo Superior de Investigaciones Cientificas. (Madrid 1954: Instituto Ramón y Cajal.)

Riback, C. E., 1978. Aspinous and sparsely-spinous stellate neurons in the visual cortex of rats contain glutamic acid decargoxylase. *J. Neurocytol.* 7:461–478.

Sloper, J. J., 1971. Dendro-dendritic synapses in the primate motor cortex. *Brain Res.* 34:186–192.

Sloper, J. J., 1972. Gap junctions between dendrites in primate neocortex. *Brain Res.* 44:641–646.

Sloper, J. J., 1973a. An electron microscopic study of neurons of the primate motor and somatic sensory cortices. *J. Neurocytol.* 2:351–359.

Sloper, J. J., 1973b. An electron microscopic study of the termination of afferent connections to the primate motor cortex. *J. Neurocytol.* 2:361–368.

Sloper, J. J., 1973c. The relationship of subsurface cisternae and cisternal organs to symmetrical axon terminals in the primate sensorimotor cortex. *Brain Res.* 58:478–483.

Sloper, J. J., and T. P. S. Powell, 1978a. Dendro-dendritic and reciprocal synapses in the primate motor cortex. *Proc. Roy. Soc. B* 203:23–38.

Sloper, J. J., and T. P. S. Powell, 1978b. Gap junctions between dendrites and somata of neurons in primate sensori-motor cortex. *Proc. Roy. Soc. B* 203:39–47.

Sloper, J. J., and T. P. S. Powell, 1979a. Ultrastructural features of the sensori-motor cortex of the primate. *Phil. Trans. Roy. Soc. B* 285:123–139.

Sloper, J. J., and T. P. S. Powell, 1979b. A study of the axon initial segment and proximal axon of neurons in the primate motor and somatic sensory cortices. *Phil. Trans. Roy. Soc. B* 285:173–197.

Sloper, J. J., and T. P. S. Powell, 1979c. An electron microscopic study of afferent connections to the primate motor and somatic sensory cortices. *Phil. Trans. Roy. Soc. B* 285:199–226.

Sloper, J. J., R. W. Hiorns, and T. P. S. Powell, 1979. A qualitative and quantitative electron microscopic study of the neurons in the primate motor and somatic sensory cortices. *Phil. Trans. Roy. Soc.* 285:141–171.

Smith, C. G., 1934. The volume of the neocortex of the albino rat and the changes it undergoes with age after birth. *J. Comp. Neurol.* 60:319–347.

Smith, D. E., and N. Moskovitz, 1979. Ultrastructure of layer IV of the primary auditory cortex of the squirrel monkey. *Neuroscience* 4:349–359.

Smith, L. M., F. F. Ebner, and M. Colonnier, 1979. The thalamocortical projection in *Pseudemys* turtles: A quantitative electron microscopic study. *J. Comp. Neurol.* (in press).

Somogyi, P., 1978. The study of Golgi stained and of experimental degeneration under the electron microscope: A direct method for the identification in the visual cortex of three successive links in a neuron chain. *Neuroscience* 3:167–180.

Spencer, W. A., and E. R. Kandel, 1961. Electrophysiology of hippocampal neurons. IV. Fast prepotentials. *J. Neurophysiol.* 24:272–285.

Strick, P. L., and P. Sterling, 1974. Synaptic termination of afferents from the ventrolateral nucleus to the thalamus in the cat motor cortex. A light and electron microscope study. *J. Comp. Neurol.* 153:77–106.

Szentágothai, J., 1965a. The use of degeneration methods in the investigation of short neuronal connections. In *Degeneration Patterns in the Nervous System. Progress in Brain Research*, Vol. 14. M. Singer, and J. P. Schadé, eds. Amsterdam: Elsevier, pp. 1–32.

Szentágothai, J., 1965b. The synapses of short local neurons in the cerebral cortex. In *Modern Trends in Neuromorphology. Symp. Biol. Hung.*, Vol. 5. J. Szentágothai, ed. Budapest: Akadémiai Kiado, pp. 251–276.

Szentágothai, J., 1973. Synaptology of the visual cortex. In *Handbook of Sensory Physiology, Vol. VII/3: Central Processing of Visual Information. Part B, Visual Centers of the Brain.* R. Jung, ed. Berlin: Springer-Verlag, pp. 269–324.

Tomböl, T., 1974. An electron microscope study of the neurons of the visual cortex. *J. Neurocytol.* 3:525–531.

Tremblay, J. P., M. Colonnier, and H. McLennan, 1979. An electron microscope study of synaptic contacts in the abdominal ganglion of *Aplysia californica. J. Comp. Neurol.* 188:367–390.

Uchizono, K., 1965. Characteristics of excitatory and inhibitory synapses in the central nervous system of the cat. *Nature* 207:642–643.

Uchizono, K., 1967. Synaptic organization of the Purkinje cells in the cerebellum of the cat. *Exp. Brain Res.* 4:97–113.

von Economo, C., 1929. *The Cytoarchitectonics of the Human Cerebral Cortex.* Oxford: Oxford University Press.

Vrensen, G., D. DeGroot, and J. Nunes-Cardozo, 1977. Postnatal development of neurons and synapses in the visual and motor cortex of rabbits: A quantitative light and electron microscopic study. *Brain Res. Bull.* 2:405–416.

West, R. W., and W. T. Greenough, 1972. Effect of environmental complexity on cortical synapses of rats: Preliminary results. *Behav. Biol.* 7:279–284.

Westrum, L. E., 1966. Synaptic contacts on axons in the cerebral cortex. *Nature* 210:1289–1290.

White, E. L., 1978. Identified neurons in mouse Sm1 cortex which are postsynaptic to thalamocortical axon terminals: A combined Golgi-electron microscopic and degeneration study. *J. Comp. Neurol.* 181:627–662.

Winfield, D. A., and T. P. S. Powell, 1976. The termination of thalamo-cortical fibres in the visual cortex of the cat. *J. Neurocytol.* 5:269–281.

7 Thalamocortical Synaptic Relations

Edward L. White

ABSTRACT It has long been known that the thalamus projects to mammalian sensory cortex, but the identity of those cortical neurons which directly receive thalamic input is largely unknown. Recent studies have shown that a variety of cell types in rodent somatosensory and visual cortex synapse with thalamocortical afferents. These findings and their implications for current concepts of the functional organization of the cerebral cortex will be discussed.

It has been known for more than a century (Gudden, 1870) that the thalamus projects to the neocortex; however, the identity of the cortical neurons which synapse with thalamic axon terminals is largely unknown. The importance of identifying the elements postsynaptic to thalamocortical axon terminals is perhaps best illustrated by considering how this information might help refine current concepts of the functional organization of the cerebral cortex. For example, Hubel and Wiesel (1962, 1968) proposed that the responses of different electrophysiologically defined cell types in cat and monkey visual cortex could best be explained by a hierarchical neuronal sequence whereby cells with simple receptive fields directly receive thalamic input and then project to cortical neurons which possess more complex receptive-field properties. "Complex" cells, which would represent some later stage in the cortical processing of thalamic input, would then project to cortical cells with even more complex, that is, hypercomplex, receptive fields. A strict interpretation of this hierarchical model would predict that only simple cells directly receive thalamic input. If we knew which neurons in the cortex were involved in thalamocortical synapses, we could then determine whether a morphological correlate exists for the electrophysiologically defined hierarchy proposed by Hubel and Wiesel, or whether, in fact, alternative modes of processing occur. For instance, Dow (1974) has described several classes of cells in visual cortex which, he concluded, process different but complementary aspects of visual information in parallel within the separate layers of the cortex. This implies that thalamic axons synapse with several different kinds of

EDWARD L. WHITE Department of Anatomy, Boston University School of Medicine, Boston, Massachusetts 02118

cortical neurons. A partial answer to the question of whether cortical cells process thalamic input by serial or parallel processing sequences could be obtained by identifying the specific neuronal types in cortex which receive input directly from the thalamus. The following is a brief account of the successful efforts to identify neurons involved in thalamocortical synapses in two primary receptive areas of the mammalian neocortex.

Layer IV of mammalian primary sensory cortex is characterized by a high concentration of small stellate cells whose dendrites, for the most part, occur within this layer, and by a dense axonal plexus containing large numbers of thalamocortical afferents. The juxtaposition of these two neuronal elements has led to the notion that layer IV stellate cells are the sole, or principal, recipients of thalamic input. However, layer IV contains many dendrites of neurons whose cell bodies occur in other layers of the cortex, and, as Peters and Feldman (1976) suggested, any of these neurons is thus in a position to receive input directly from the thalamus. In retrospect, we may well appreciate the prophetic nature of this suggestion, for it has recently been shown in both rat VI (Peters, White, and Fairén, 1977; Peters et al., 1979) and in mouse SmI cortex (White, 1978,1979; Hersch and White, 1979) that dendrites in layer IV which synapse with thalamocortical axon terminals belong to a variety of cell types whose somata occur in cortical layers III through VI. The approach used in these studies was to label both the pre- and postsynaptic elements of the thalamocortical synapse so that each could be identified with the electron microscope. Presynaptic, thalamocortical axon terminals were labeled by lesion-induced degeneration. In this procedure, a lesion of the appropriate thalamic nucleus induces degenerative changes in thalamocortical axon terminals which enable these terminals to be identified in thin sections of the cortex. The Golgi–electron-microscope technique of Fairén, Peters, and Saldanha (1977) was used to identify neurons postsynaptic to degenerating thalamic afferents. In this method, Golgi-impregnated neurons are identified by light-microscopic examination and then chemically treated to replace the dense Golgi precipitate with a deposit of fine gold particles. The treated neurons are still visible with the light microscope because of their content of gold. In the electron microscope, the gold particles are usually so distributed that the cytological details and synaptic relationships of the gold-treated neurons can be determined. The application of these methods to elucidate thalamocortical synaptic relationships is illustrated in Figures 1 and 4 (inset), which show examples of synapses between degenerating thalamocortical axon terminals and identified postsynaptic elements in mouse SmI cortex.

Results to date indicate that every neuron which sends a dendrite into layer IV of mouse SmI cortex receives synapses from thalamocortical afferents. These results are summarized in Figure 2, which shows that nonspiny and spiny stellate cells of layer IV and pyramidal cells of layers

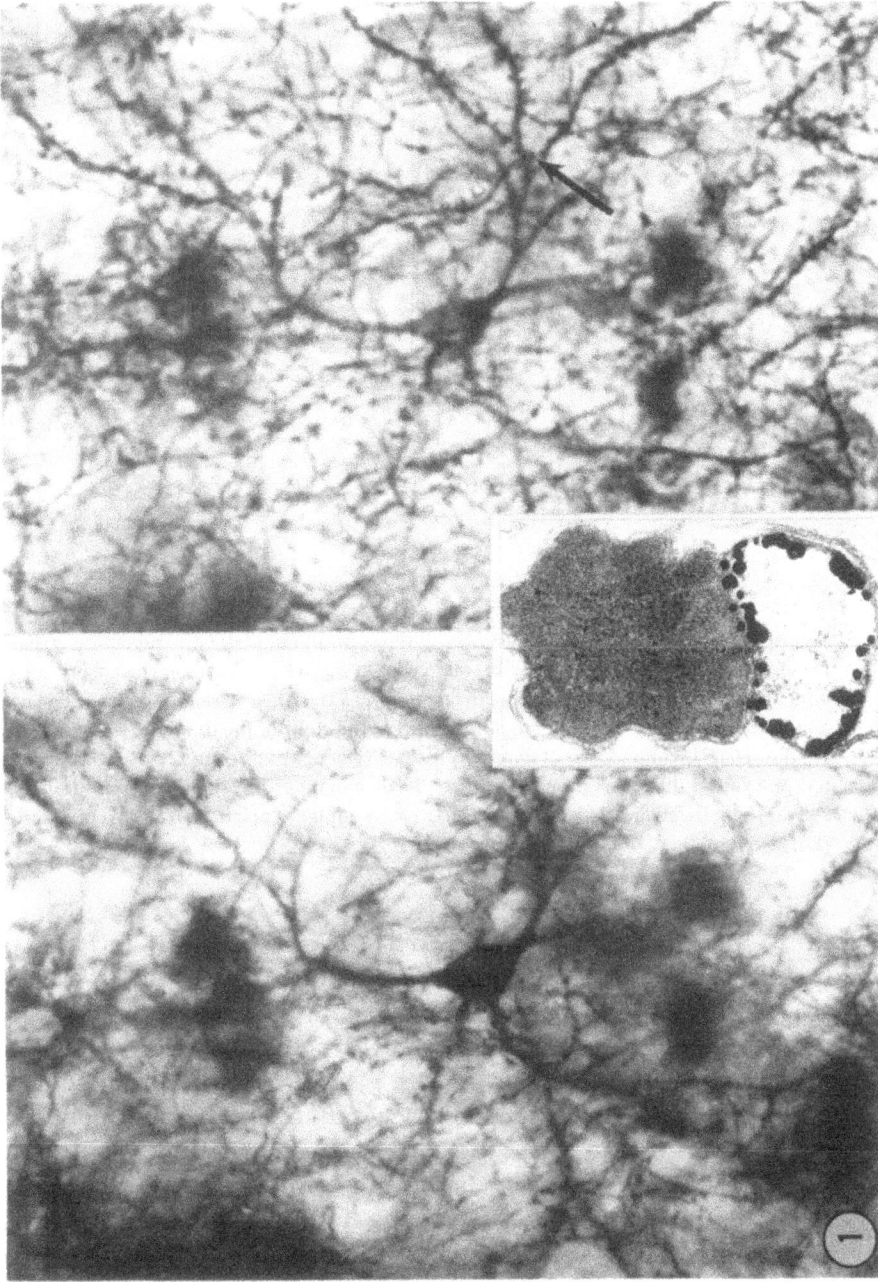

Figure 1 Light micrographs showing (on the left) a Golgi-impregnated layer III pyramidal cell and (on the right) a light micrograph of the same neuron following treatment with gold. Note the increased translucency of the cell body and dendrites following gold treatment. The arrow points to a spine which is shown in inset (×930). Inset: electron micrograph of a thin section through the spine designated by the arrow at the right of the figure, showing its synapse with a degenerating thalamocortical axon terminal (×55,800).

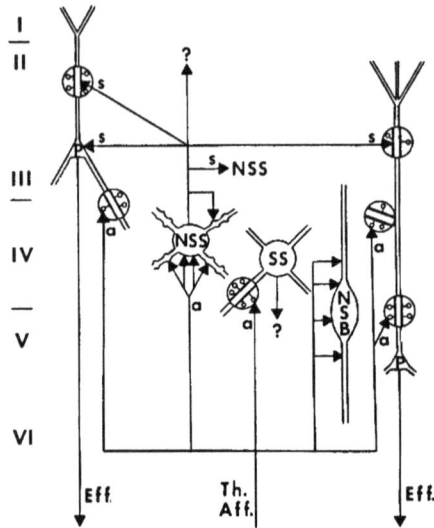

②

Figure 2 Diagram showing the various cell types (P, pyramidal; NSS, nonspiny stellate; SS, spiny stellate; NSB, nonspiny bipolar cells) in mouse primary somatosensory cortex which are postsynaptic to thalamocortical afferents (Th. Aff.). Pyramidal cells in layers V and VI are represented by the single pyramid at the right of the diagram. Also included are the synaptic connections of nonspiny stellate cells as observed in rat visual cortex (Peters and Fairén, 1978; Peters and Proskauer, 1980). Synaptic junction types are indicated by "a" (asymmetrical) and "s" (symmetrical). Roman numerals at left indicate layers of cortex (Eff., efferent).

III, V, and VI all receive input directly from the thalamus. Included in the diagram are data (Peters and Fairén, 1978; Peters and Proskauer, 1980) which indicate that the axons on nonspiny stellate cells synapse with dendrites of layer III and layer V pyramidal cells, with other nonspiny stellate cells and even with their own dendrites. These findings imply that neurons in the cortex which receive thalamic input project to other cortical neurons which also receive thalamic input. Does this mean that hierarchical neuronal sequences are invalid to describe higher brain function? Perhaps, but although the anatomy indicates that there is not a strict hierarchy with regard to the processing of thalamocortical input, preliminary data (see White, 1978) suggest that there might be a hierarchy in the quantitative sense such that some neurons—those whose cell bodies occur in layer IV—receive many thalamocortical synapses and then project to other neurons, which apparently receive a smaller proportion of their input from the thalamus. In fact, a comparison of these results with electrophysiological studies (Simons and Woolsey, 1979) of mouse somatosensory cortex suggests that the higher a neuron is in a functional hierarchy, that is, the more complex its receptive-field properties, the less direct thalamic input it receives.

The important point, though, is that if hierarchical arrangements do occur, it would seem that neurons at all levels of the hierarchy receive input directly from the thalamus. Indeed, if the thalamocortical projections to layers I and VI were to terminate on dendrites irrespective of their cell type of origin, as apparently occurs in layers IV, then neurons with cell bodies throughout the full thickness of the neocortex would receive input directly from the thalamus. Presumably, thalamocortical input could then directly and quickly alter the functional state of nearly every neuron in a specified region of cortex. Perhaps this widespread thalamic input might serve to lower the threshold of a number of neurons, so that in effect, neurons at several levels of a functional hierarchy are activated and in this sense selected out to receive and process afferent thalamic input. Carried a step further, a selection process could be envisioned whereby the threshold of many cortical neurons is altered by direct thalamic input to facilitate the transmission and processing of this input by neurons which might not always act in concert, but which by virtue of common thalamic input are drawn into a functional unit. Whether this unit is considered to be a hierarchical processing sequence or a functional column does not matter; the principle of selection by afferent input would apply to either. The proposed selection mechanism would allow each cortical neuron, which likely receives many different kinds of input and projects to various targets, to participate in more than one kind of functional unit. The relationship of a neuron at any particular time to a hierarchical processing sequence or functional column would depend on such factors as the distribution of the different synapses it receives and on the timing of synaptic events.

Information on the numbers and locations of synapses a neuron receives can only be obtained from extensive serial thin-section reconstructions. Figure 3 is a drawing of a layer IV spiny stellate cell which is being reconstructed by Michael P. Rock and the author to elucidate the numbers and arrangements of the thalamocortical and other synapses it receives. Briefly, the steps in the reconstruction procedure were as follows. A Golgi-impregnated layer IV spiny stellate cell was selected from the SmI cortex of a mouse which earlier had sustained a lesion of the ventrobasal thalamus. This neuron was treated with gold (Fairén, Peters, and Saldanha, 1977), embedded in plastic, and sectioned into about 350 serial thin secretions. Electron micrographs—about 5,000 in all—were then taken of each part of the cell as it appeared on every thin section of the series. The outlines of each profile of the neuron on every second section were traced and the tracings cut out of wooden sheets whose thickness corresponded to the average thickness of two thin sections times the final magnification of the electron micrographs.

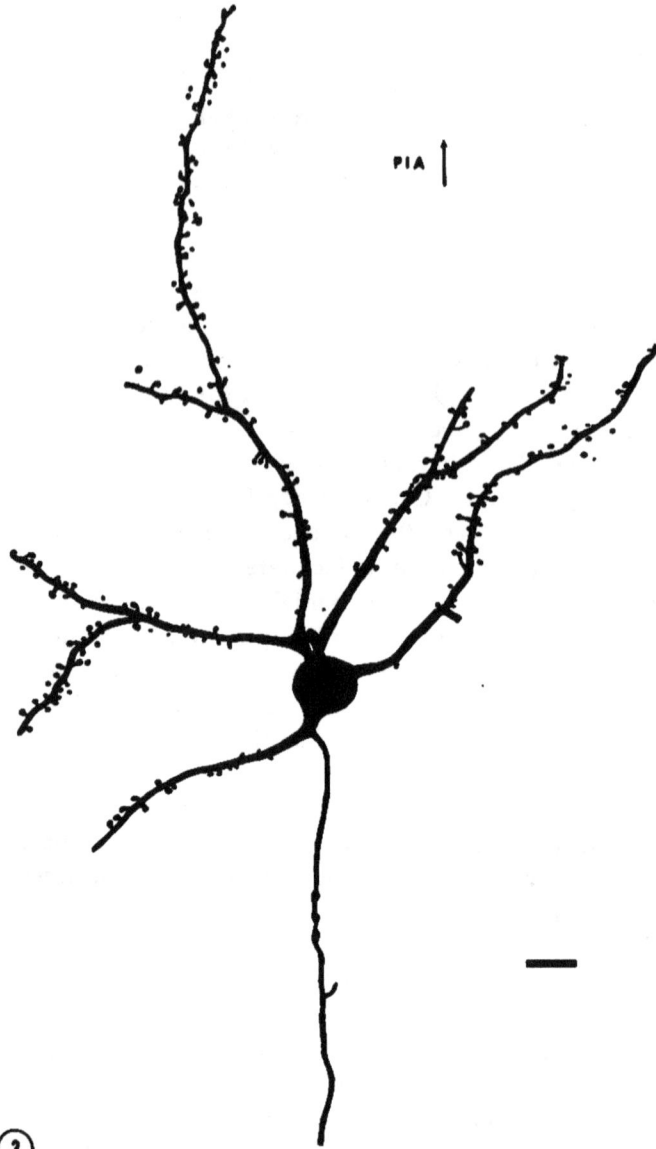

PIA ↑

③

Figure 3 Drawing made from photographs of the layer IV spiny stellate cell from mouse SmI cortex which is being reconstructed from serial thin sections. Scale is 10 μm.

Edward L. White

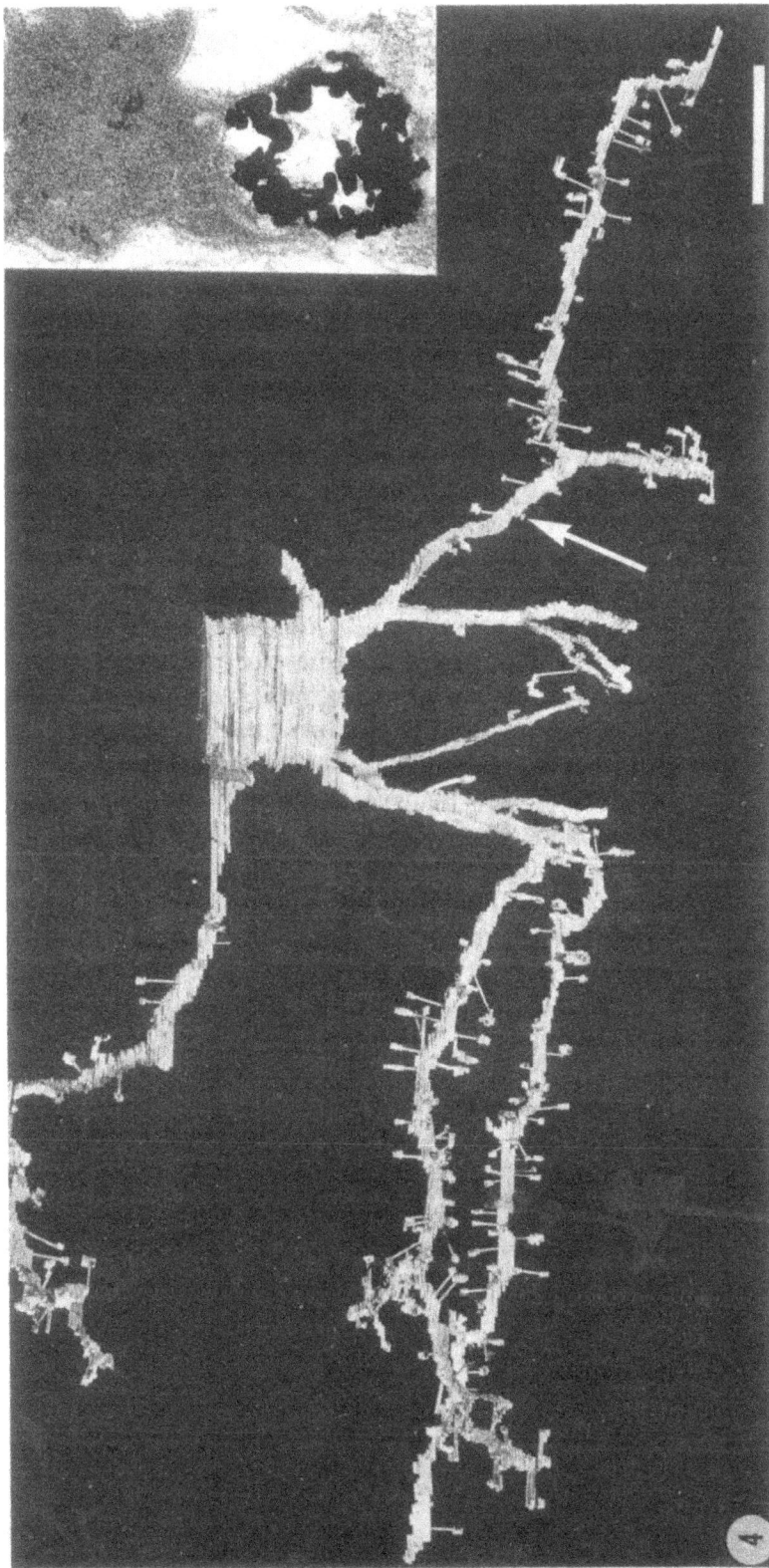

Figure 4 Nearly complete reconstruction from serial thin sections of the layer IV spiny stellate cell shown in Figure 3. Arrow indicates spine, shown in inset. Scale is 10 μm. Inset: synapse of a degenerating thalamocortical axon terminal with the spine indicated by the arrow (×72,800).

Synapses were marked in the appropriate places on the edges of the wooden profiles, which were then arranged in sequence to reconstruct the neuron (Figure 4). Reference points from the electron micrographs were used to obtain the "best-fit" alignment of the successive wooden profiles.

Examination of the reconstruction has enabled us to determine that approximately 10% of the spines of this spiny stellate cell are involved in thalamic synapses. An intriguing finding is that thalamic input, which apparently is distributed at random over most of the cell, is distributed in a regular, periodic fashion over some parts of the dendritic tree. For example, one primary dendrite has five spines which receive thalamocortical input. The necks of these spines attach to the dendrite at regular intervals of 4.5 to 5.5 μm. The secondary branch of another dendrite also possesses spines which receive input from the thalamus and which protrude from the dendritic shaft at approximately 5-μm intervals. Our interpretation of this periodicity is that it reflects the spacing of thalamocortical synapses which form with the dendritic shafts prior to the time of spine formation. The rationale for this suggestion is the observation that only the loci where these spine necks connect to their parent dendrites are periodically spaced, whereas the spine heads are not separated by regular intervals. A related finding is that spines involved in thalamocortical synapses are not clustered in particular regions of the dendrites, but are interspersed with synaptic inputs from other sources. Are these nonthalamic inputs periodically spaced along spiny-stellate-cell dendrites? Are thalamic inputs regularly distributed along the dendrites of other types of cortical neurons which receive input from the thalamus? We do not yet know, but it can be expected that further quantitative analyses of synaptic inputs to identified cortical neurons will answer these and other questions vital to understanding how the cortex receives and processes ascending sensory information.

Acknowledgments

The author wishes to thank Drs. V. B. Mountcastle and A. Peters for many fruitful discussions, and Mrs. Mary Alba for typing the manuscript. Support for this work provided by National Science Foundation Grant BNS 76-21720 and National Institutes of Health Grant NS-14838-01.

References

Dow, B. M., 1974. Functional classes of cells and their laminar distribution in monkey visual cortex. *J. Neurophysiol.* 37:927–946.

Fairén, A., A. Peters, and J. Saldanha, 1977. A new procedure for examining Golgi impregnated neurons by light and electron microscopy. *J. Neurocytol.* 6:311–337.

Gudden, B., 1870. Experimentaluntersuchungen über das peripherische und centrale Nervensystem. *Arch. F. Psychiat.* 2:693–723. [Reprinted 1938 in *The Primate Thalamus.* A. E. Walker, ed. Chicago University Press.]

Hersch, S. M., and E. L. White, 1979. The distribution of thalamocortical synapses on the apical dendrites of layer IV, V and VI pyramids. *Abst. 1979 Meet. Soc. for Neurosci.*, p. 116.

Hubel, D. H., and T. N. Wiesel, 1962. Receptive fields, binocular interaction and functional architecture in the cat's visual cortex. *J. Physiol.* 160:106–154.

Hubel, D. H., and T. N. Wiesel, 1968. Receptive fields and functional architecture of monkey striate cortex. *J. Physiol.* 195:215–243.

Peters, A., and A. Fairén, 1978. Smooth and sparsely-spined stellate cells in the visual cortex of the rat: A study using a combined Golgi-electron microscope technique. *J. Comp. Neurol.* 181:129–172.

Peters, A., and M. L. Feldman, 1976. The projection of the lateral geniculate nucleus to area 17 of the rat cerebral cortex. I. General description. *J. Neurocytol.* 5:63–84.

Peters, A., and C. C. Proskauer, 1980. Synaptic relationships between a multipolar stellate cell and a pyramidal neuron in the rat visual cortex. A combined Golgi-electron microscope study. *J. Neurocytol.* 9:163–183.

Peters, A., E. L. White, and A. Fairén, 1977. Synapses between identified neuronal elements. An electron microscopic demonstration of degenerating axon terminals synapsing with Golgi impregnated neurons. *Neurosci. Lett.* 6:171–175.

Peters, A., C. C. Proskauer, M. L. Feldman, and L. Kimerer, 1979. The projection of the lateral geniculate nucleus to area 17 of the rat cerebral cortex. V. Degenerating axon terminals synapsing with Golgi impregnated neurons. *J. Neurocytol.* 8:331–357.

Simons, D. J., and T. A. Woolsey, 1979. Functional organization in mouse barrel cortex. *Brain Res.* 165:327–332.

White, E. L., 1978. Identified neurons in mouse SmI cortex which are postsynaptic to thalamocortical axon terminals: A combined Golgi-electron microscopic and degeneration study. *J. Comp. Neurol.* 181:627–662.

White, E. L., 1979. Thalamocortical synaptic relations: A review with emphasis on the projections of specific thalamic nuclei to the primary sensory areas of the neocortex. *Brain Res. Rev.* 1:275–312.

8

Laminar Specialization and Intracortical Connections in Cat Primary Visual Cortex

Charles D. Gilbert and Torsten N. Wiesel

ABSTRACT   Cells in the primary visual cortex show considerable variety in their receptive-field properties, and are specialized to suit the functions of the areas to which they project. In each layer, cells share common inputs, functional properties, and sites of projection. To produce this range of functional classes, each having receptive-field features that are substantially more complicated than the cortical input, there is an intricate pattern of intracortical connections. This paper examines the neuronal structure and connectivity that underlies receptive-field construction.

The part of the cortex dealing with vision can be subdivided into a number of separate areas, each containing a representation of the visual world and each serving a particular purpose (Zeki, 1978). Throughout a given area neurons perform a stereotyped analysis on the visual environment, each part of the area dealing with only a part of the visual field (Talbot and Marshall, 1941; Daniel and Whitteridge, 1959; Bilge et al., 1967; Tusa, Palmer and Rosenquist, 1978; Van Essen and Zeki, 1978; Allman and Kaas, 1975). Single-cell recording has revealed a rich diversity of function among cortical cells, and within a given cortical area one can find a number of different cell types, each specific in the set of stimulus parameters to which it responds best. Along with this physiological diversity, there is also considerable morphological diversity (Ramón y Cajal, 1922; Lorente de Nó, 1922; O'Leary, 1941; Lund, 1973; Valverde, 1971), suggesting a possible relationship between cell structure and function. In the primary visual cortex the analysis of the visual world includes binocular interaction and the interpretation of forms in terms of line segments of particular orientations (Hubel and Wiesel, 1962). Cells sharing the same orientation specificity or the same eye preference are grouped together in cortical columns (actually parallel slabs), which run from pia to white matter (Hubel and Wiesel, 1962, 1977). Another organizing principle of the cortex, the segregation of cells into laminae, has long been held by anatomists to be important in its function (Brodmann, 1903; Campbell, 1903; Vogt and Vogt, 1903). The physiological

CHARLES D. GILBERT AND TORSTEN N. WIESEL Department of Neurobiology, Harvard Medical School, 25 Shattuck Street, Boston, Massachusetts 02115 specialization found for cells in different layers appears to be a reflection of the distinct inputs that each layer receives. Neurons in different layers in turn project to different sites and are specialized to suit the requirements of the regions to which they project. A number of receptive-field features are elaborated in the cortex and are not inherited directly from the lateral geniculate nucleus, so that the cells that project out of a cortical area are substantially more complicated in their receptive-field features than the thalamic cells that provide the major source of input to the area. It is consequently of great interest to understand the neuronal connectivity that underlies the production of different receptive-field properties from column to column, and different receptive-field types across the cortical layers.

In this chapter, we shall discuss the stages involved in the development of receptive field properties. As summarized in Figure 1, the cortical layers are specialized according to the inputs they receive (Garey and Powell, 1971; Hubel and Wiesel, 1972; Rosenquist, Edwards, and Palmer, 1975; LeVay and Gilbert, 1976), the receptive field properties of the cells within them (Hubel and Wiesel, 1962; Gilbert, 1977; Camarda and Rizzolatti, 1976; Leventhal and Hirsch, 1978), and their efferent targets (Toyama et al., 1974; Hollander, 1974; Palmer and Rosenquist, 1974; Gilbert and Kelly, 1975; Lund et al., 1975). Before discussing the intracortical connections that may be the basis for functional specialization of the cortical laminae, we shall first describe the receptive-field properties of striate cortical cells.

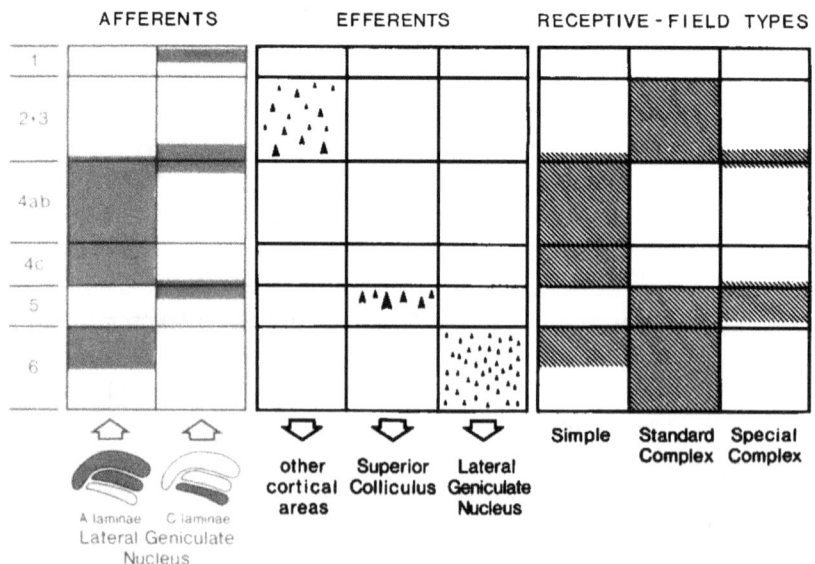

Figure 1 Schematic diagram showing the laminar distribution of the afferents from the lateral geniculate nucleus, of cells projecting to various visual areas, and of each receptive field class.

C. D. Gilbert and T. N. Wiesel

Receptive Field Classes in Primary Visual Cortex and Their Laminar Distribution

A number of different schemes have been developed for differentiating cells on electrophysiological grounds (Hubel and Wiesel, 1959, 1962; Pettigrew, Nikara, and Bishop, 1968; Henry and Bishop, 1972; Singer, Tretter, and Cynader, 1975; Schiller, Finlay, and Volman, 1976). In this chapter we shall use the scheme devised by Hubel and Wiesel (1962) and enlarged upon by others (Palmer and Rosenquist, 1974; Gilbert, 1977).

Simple Cells
The simple cell was defined by mapping its receptive field with stationary stimuli. Like most cells in area 17, it responds best to slits of a given orientation. It can be distinguished from other cell types by the presence of separate on- and off-subfields with summation within each subfield and antagonism between adjacent subfields. Simple cells respond to a slit of light swept across their fields with one or two short bursts of spikes. The peak of each burst corresponds to the slit entering or leaving one of the subfields. Simple cells are found in two levels in the cortex, one in layer IV and the other in the upper part of layer VI (Figure 1).

Complex Cells
Like simple cells, these cells respond optimally to oriented line segments, but they differ from simple cells in not having separate on- and off-subfields, and they respond continuously as a slit of light is swept across their fields (Hubel and Wiesel, 1962; Pettigrew, Nikara, and Bishop, 1968; Gilbert, 1977). For complex cells, specificity for orientation is maintained, but in comparison to simple cells they have gained some freedom in the precise position of the stimulus along the movement axis (Hubel and Wiesel, 1962). As will be discussed below, complex cells in each layer have unique properties, and there are several possible ways of breaking down the population into subclasses. It is possible, for example, to distinguish them according to their responses to different slit lengths. One type shows summation along the orientation axis, that is, it gives a stronger response as the length of the stimulating slit is increased up to the full length of the receptive field. These will be referred to as standard complex cells. They are found in all layers, but only rarely in layer IV (Figure 1). The other type (first described by Palmer and Rosenquist, 1974) responds at least as well to a very short slit (as small as $\frac{1}{8}°$) as to a slit that extends the full length of the receptive field (which for these cells averages 3°). These will be referred to as special complex cells. They are found at two levels, one at the bottom of layer III and the other in layer V (Figure 1).

For many simple and complex cells a slit that is longer than the receptive field elicits a smaller response than does a slit equal to the field in length. This property, which we refer to as end inhibition, is present in varying strengths for different cells, and makes these cells optimally responsive to oriented lines of a defined length. Originally thought to exist only for complex cells, the presence of end inhibition in both simple and complex cells (Dreher, 1972; Rose, 1977; Gilbert, 1977; Kato, Bishop, and Orban, 1978) makes a simplification of terms possible. Cells originally named hypercomplex will be referred to as complex cells with end inhibition. There are other ways of characterizing receptive fields, including field size and shape, ocular dominance, response rate, spontaneous activity, directionality, velocity tuning, and disparity sensitivity (the neuronal mechanism for stereoscopic depth perception). Some of these distinctions correlate with laminar position. Superficial-layer complex cells, for example, have smaller receptive fields than those in the deep layers. In layer VI many cells show summation for increased slit length up to very large values, some reaching 16° in length (Gilbert, 1977). The cortical machinery is therefore involved in generating an extensive set of receptive-field properties, and one must look to the intracortical connections and cell morphology to understand how these properties are produced.

Tracing Intracortical Pathways with Intracellular Recording and Marking Techniques

The characterization of receptive fields and the determination of the laminar distribution of each cell type were originally done through extracellular recording. Intracellular marking techniques can extend these findings by showing the detailed structure and intracortical wiring of cells with known response properties. Comparing the receptive-field properties of marked cells with those of cells in the layers to which they project can then provide evidence for the manner in which receptive fields are constructed. Intracellular marking techniques were first employed in the visual system by Kelly and Van Essen (1974), who used the fluorescent dye procion yellow as the marker. The development of the method of intracellular injection of the enzyme horseradish peroxidase (HRP) (Muller and MacMahan, 1976; Jankowska, Rasted, and Westman, 1976; Light and Durkovic, 1976; Kitai et al., 1976) enabled us to trace the intracortical projections of functionally identified neurons in different layers (Gilbert and Wiesel, 1979).

Functional Characterization and Labeling of Visual Cortical Neurons

Recordings were made in cats maintained on sodium thiopental anesthesia, paralyzed with succinylcholine and artificially respired. The animals' EKG, EEG, temperature, and expired CO_2 concentration were monitored. A small hole was drilled in the skull above the visual cortex, and the dura and pia were opened. Half-micrometer beveled-tip electrodes were filled with a solution of 4% HRP (Boehringer-Mannheim, grade I) in 0.2 M KAc, pH 7.6. After penetration of the brain surface with the electrode, the hole in the skull was filled with agar to reduce pulsations. The electrodes were advanced through the brain with a stepping microdrive (AB transvertex, Sweden) until a cell or process was penetrated, as judged by a sudden change in the resting potential, the appearance of large action potentials, and often synaptic activity. The cell's receptive-field properties were determined using either a hand-held projector or an optical bench. In the early part of this series of experiments cells were injected with HRP by pulses of pressure ranging from 0.5 to 5 atm, but we shifted to iontophoretic application as a more reliable technique, using pulses of positive current ranging from 1 to 2 nA in a 50-ms on–50-ms off duty cycle. At the end of the experiment each animal was perfused with a short buffer rinse followed by a long perfusion with 2% glutaraldehyde in the same buffer. After the brain was blocked, 150-μm coronal sections were cut on a Vibratome (Oxford Instruments), and then treated with a combination of the diaminobenzidine reaction at acid pH (Malmgren and Olsson, 1978) and cobalt intensification (Adams, 1977). The injected cells were reconstructed from serial sections by using a microscope equipped with a drawing tube. Subsequently, the sections were counterstained with cresyl violet, and the laminar position of cells and their processes were determined using the criteria of Otsuka and Hassler (1962).

The long projections of cortical cells and the distribution of the thalamic afferents were determined by tracing techniques that make use of anterograde transport of [^{3}H]-proline and both anterograde and retrograde transport of HRP, injected extracellularly. The detailed methods are described elsewhere (Gilbert and Kelly, 1975; LeVay and Gilbert, 1976). The HRP tracing technique has been improved by enhancing its uptake (Frank, Harris, and Kennedy, 1980) and the sensitivity of the staining procedure (Mesulam, 1976). The experiments of Gilbert and Kelly (1975) were therefore repeated (the results are shown in Figure 7, 9, and 11, below).

Cortical Afferents

Different morphological and physiological classes of retinal ganglion and geniculate cells are known to exist (Kuffler, 1953; Enroth-Cugell and Robson, 1966; Guillery, 1966; Cleland, Dubin, and Levick, 1971; Hoffman, Stone, and Sherman, 1972; Boycott and Wassle, 1974; Stone and Fukuda, 1974; Wilson, Rowe, and Stone, 1976). Chief among these are the X and Y cells. These are defined by the linearity of spatial summation within their receptive fields (Enroth-Cugell and Robson, 1966), and also have been found to differ in their firing properties and axon

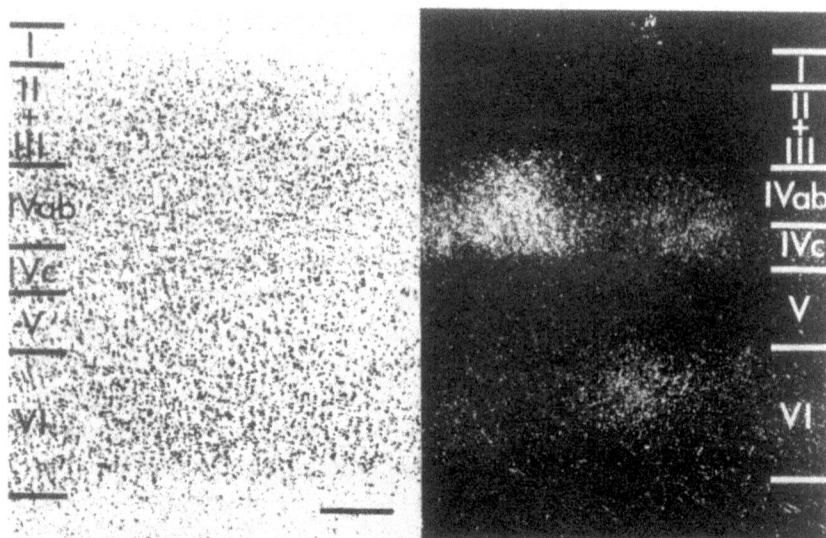

Figure 2 Projection of lamina A1 to area 17 (medial bank of lateral gyrus). Thionin-stained section in bright-field illumination (left) and autoradiograph in dark field (right). Terminals were found at two levels, in layer IV and upper part of layer VI. Because lamina A1 receives input from only the ipsilateral eye, it is possible to make out clusters of grains representing the ipsilateral ocular dominance columns. Bar = 250 μm. (From LeVay and Gilbert, 1976.)

conduction velocities. The dorsal geniculate laminae, which contain a mixture of X und Y cells (Wilson, Rowe, and Stone, 1976), project to layers IV and VI in the primary visual cortex (Rosenquist, Edwards, and Palmer, 1975; LeVay and Gilbert, 1976). In Figure 2, the injection site was restricted to an individual geniculate lamina, A1, and consequently represents the projection pattern of both X and Y cells. The autoradiographic technique for tracing connections shows the terminal distribution of large groups of neurons. Since the group in any geniculate lamina is inhomogeneous, one can only determine the combined terminal distribution of a mixture of cell types.

Using intracellular recording and marking, it is possible to penetrate and inject individual axons coming from the lateral geniculate nucleus either before or after they enter the cortex, and therefore determine the projection pattern of an individual cell type. We used the criteria of spatial summation to classify X and Y afferents (Enroth-Cugell and Robson, 1966; Hochstein and Shapley, 1976). A reconstruction of each type is shown in Figure 3. The Y afferent (Figure 3A) had off-center–on-surround organization, showed nonlinear summation, had a relatively large field center ($1\frac{1}{2}°$), and gave a transient response to a stationary flashing spot of light. It ended in layer IVAB in a rich arbor distributed in two patches separated by a terminal-free gap. The patches presumably correspond to ocular-dominance columns driven by one eye, and

C. D. Gilbert and T. N. Wiesel

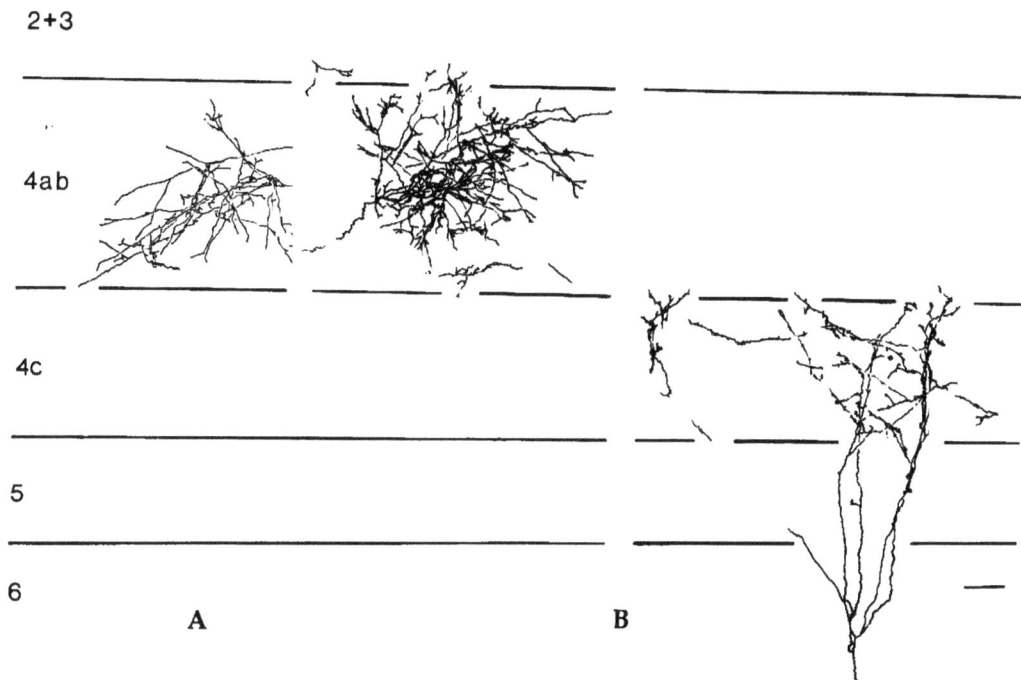

A   B

Figure 3 Two afferents from the lateral geniculate nucleus, injected within the cortex. The one on the left (A) was an off-center Y cell (center size 1½°, located 5° from the area centralis), and ramified entirely within layer IVAB. The axon on the right (B) was an off-center X cell (center size 1°, located 3° from the area centralis), which ramified entirely within layer IVC. Bar = 100 μm.

the intervening gap to the column driven by the opposite eye (Hubel and Wiesel, 1972; Shatz, Lindstrom, and Wiesel, 1977; Ferster and LeVay, 1978). Some of the injected Y afferents sent collaterals to the upper half of layer VI as well.

In contrast, the X afferent showed linear summation and arborized entirely within layer IVC (Figure 3B). No afferents were found to arborize in both sublayers of layer IV. This demonstrates, in agreement with Ferster and LeVay (1978), that the dorsal geniculate layers, which contain a mixture of at least two principal cell types, keep the input from the two types segregated upon their arrival in the cortex.

Layer IV Cells

Cells in layer IV lie in the terminal field of the geniculate afferents, and consequently represent the first level of processing in the cortex. From extracellular recordings it is known that the overwhelming majority of the cells in layer IV have simple receptive fields (Hubel and Wiesel, 1962; Kelly and Van Essen, 1974; Gilbert, 1977; Shatz and Stryker, 1978). An example of a simple cell in layer IVAB is shown in Figure 4. It was a spiny stellate cell. The axon branched a number of times soon after

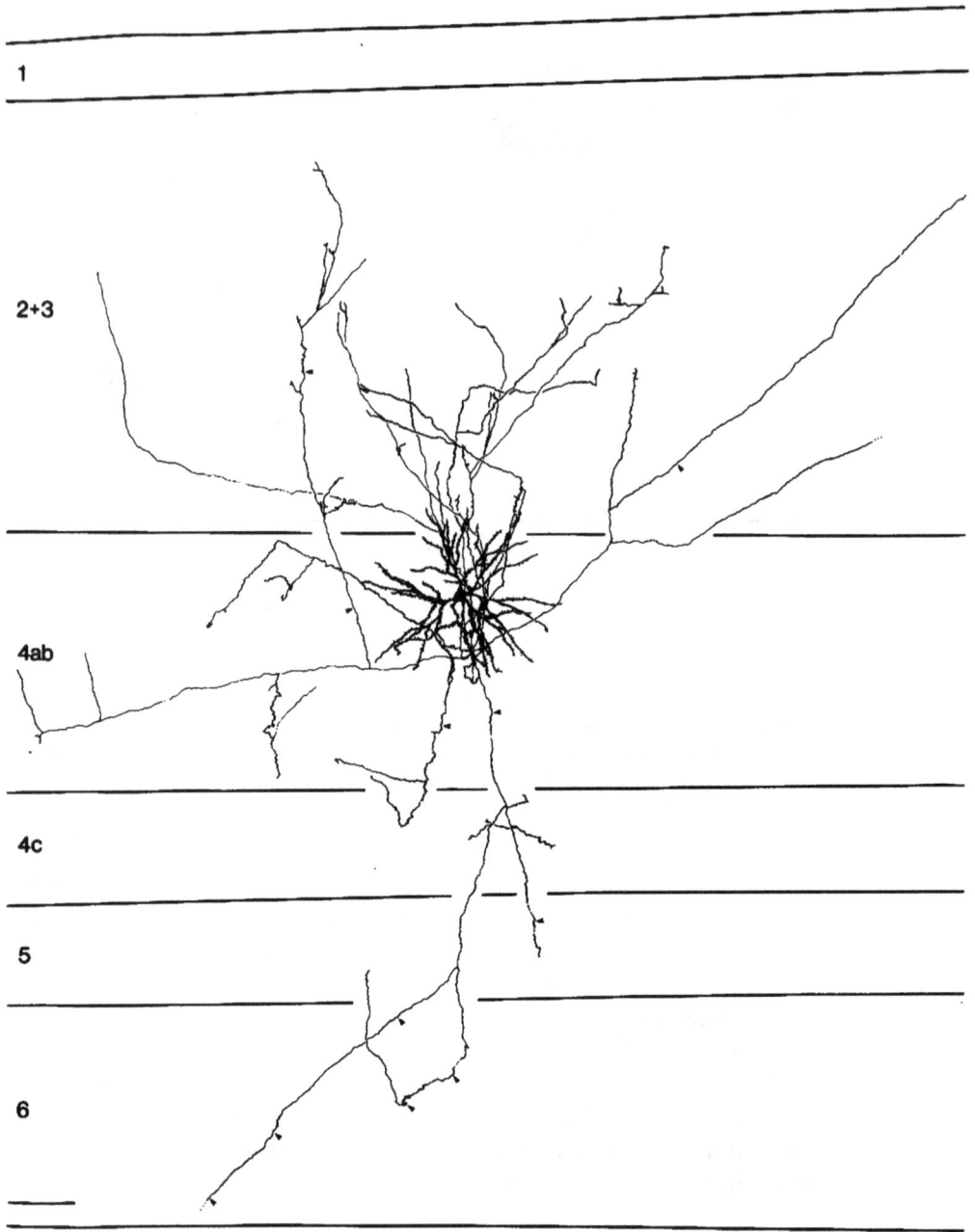

Figure 4 A spiny stellate cell in layer IVAB having a simple receptive field with an on-center and off-flanks, and showing no end inhibition. The field size was 3° × 4°, and it was located 10° from the area centralis. The arrows indicate the positions of nodes of Ranvier. Bar = 100 μm.

leaving the soma, with a number of collaterals innervating layer IVAB and then giving off a rich terminal arborization in layer II + III. The axon proceeded out of the cortex into the white matter, sending a few collaterals into the lower layers in its downward course. This general projection pattern was seen for all injected IVAB spiny cells and has also been observed with Golgi stains (Ramón y Cajal, 1922; Lorente de Nó, 1922; O'Leary, 1941; Lund, 1973). The horizontal extent of the axonal arborization was much larger than that of the dendritic arborization. This divergence could produce a further mixing in the input from the two eyes onto layer II + III cells, and could account for the higher proportion of binocularly driven cells in that layer than in layer IV (Hubel and Wiesel, 1962; Gilbert, 1977).

Only two cells have been injected in layer IVC, one a small spiny stellate cell and the other a smooth stellate cell (Figure 5). These had very similar receptive field properties; both had simple receptive fields with small on-centers (1° × ½°). These fields were much smaller than those of the layer IVAB simple cells. The smooth stellate cell's axon ramified extensively throughout layer IV. The spiny stellate cell's axon gave off many collaterals, some remaining within layer IVC and others extending up to layer IVAB. Although the cell's axon was restricted to layer IV (which is consistent with Golgi findings; O'Leary, 1941), the existence of complex cells with very small receptive fields in layer II + III (Hubel and Wiesel, 1962; Gilbert, 1977) leads us to expect that there should be other layer IVC cells with projections to that layer. In Golgi material some of these cells have been found (Lund et al., 1979), but as yet no spiny cells have been shown to project to layer II + III from IVC.

Layer II+III Cells

The predominant intracortical projection from layer IV appears to be to layer II+III, which would then represent the second level of cortical processing. Layer II+III contains complex cells almost exclusively (Hubel and Wiesel, 1962; Gilbert, 1977).

A complex cell with a small receptive field (1°×1°), showing no end inhibition, is shown in Figure 6. It was a pyramidal cell located in the upper part of layer II+III. The basal dendrites ramified close to the soma and the apical dendrite extended into the lower part of layer I. Its axon branched richly in its layer of origin, both in a region adjacent to the cell's dendritic field and in a region somewhat more distant, perhaps to a column of cells with the same orientation preference. The axon collaterals also extended into layer I. The descending axon projected extensively within layer V, which was a common feature for pyramidal cells in this layer, in agreement with degeneration (Szentágothai, 1965; Spatz, Tigges, and Tigges, 1970; Nauta, Butler, and Jane, 1973) and Golgi (Lorente de Nó, 1922; O'Leary, 1941; Lund, 1973) studies. The

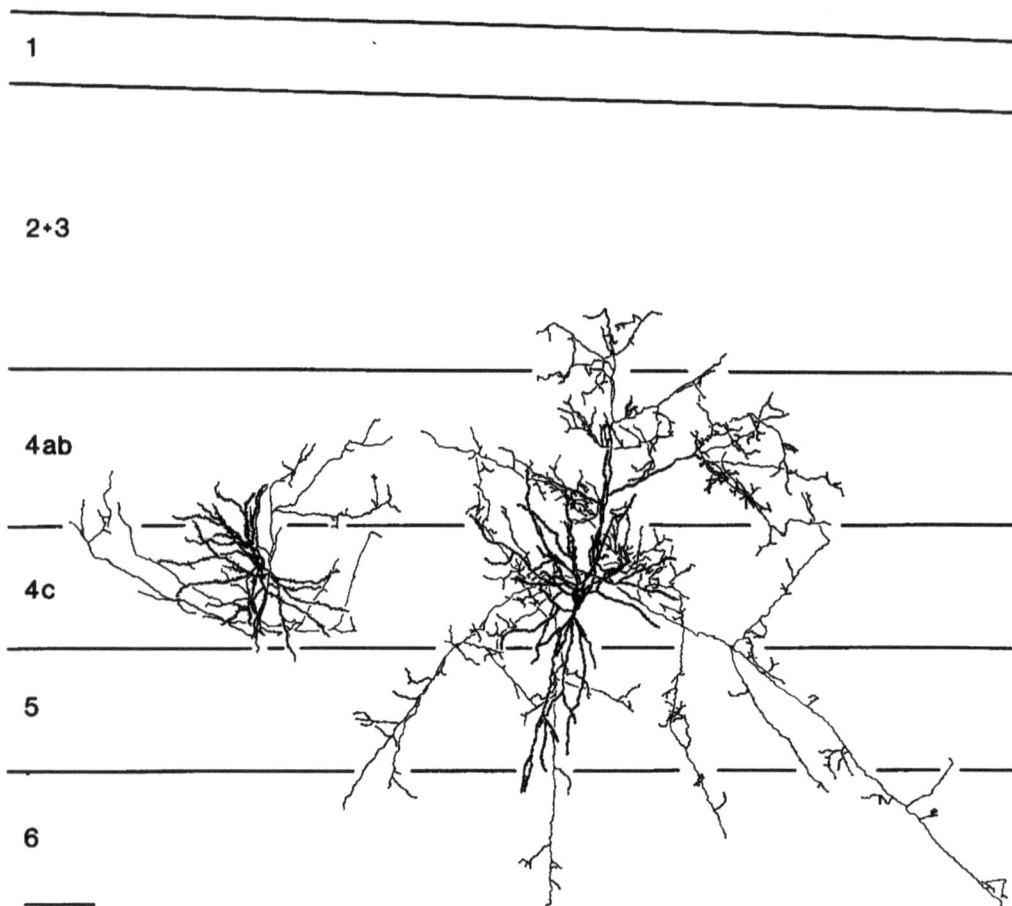

1

2+3

4ab

4c

5

6

Figure 5 A spiny stellate cell (left) and a smooth stellate cell (right) in layer IVC. Both had simple receptive fields with on-center and off-flanks, the spiny stellate cell showing no end inhibition and the smooth stellate cell showing 50% end inhibition. The size of the central on portion of the field for both cells was 1° × ½°, and both were located 2° from the area centralis. Because the plane of section was not perpendicular to the layers, this reconstruction makes it appear as if several sets of collaterals of the smooth stellate cell extend into layers V and VI, whereas in fact they remain within IVC. Bar = 100 μm.

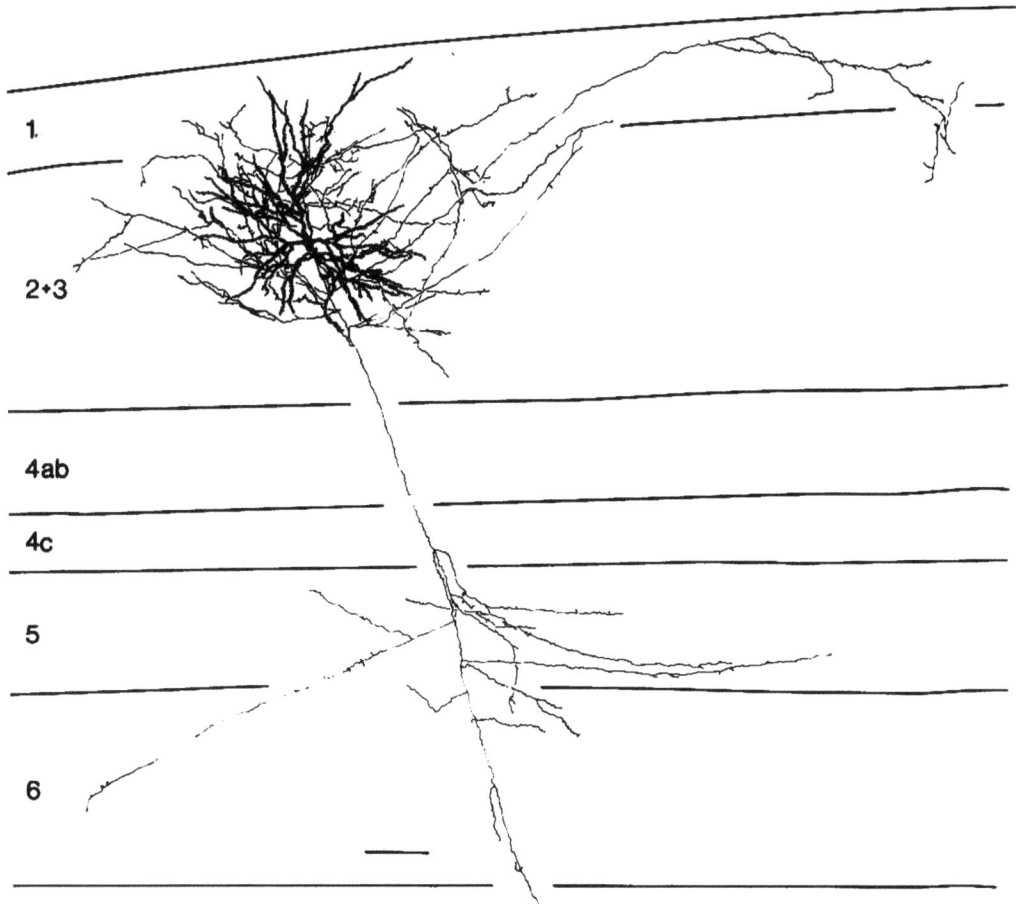

Figure 6 A pyramidal cell in the upper part of layer II + III, with a complex receptive field showing no end inhibition. The field size was 1° × 1°, and it was located 4° from the area centralis. Bar = 100 μm.

axon proceeded out of the cortex, presumably to innervate another cortical area or areas.

It is known from previous studies (Toyama et al., 1974; Gilbert and Kelly, 1975; Lund et al., 1975) that cells in layer II+III project to other areas of the visual cortex. The distribution of cells projecting to area 19, demonstrated by retrograde transport, is shown in Figure 7. They are pyramidal cells (Figure 7B), located predominantly in layer II+III (Figure 7C), with a few additional large stellate cells in the upper part of layer IVAB. These cells constitute a small proportion of the total number of cells in layer II+III, but comprise a fairly high proportion of the large cells in the layer (Figure 7C). Cells that project to area 18 or to the Clare–Bishop area have somewhat different numbers and distributions (Gilbert and Kelly, 1975), suggesting that different populations project to different areas. Figure 7A shows a dense granular terminal distribution in layer V, below the filled cells. This most likely represents collaterals of the superficial layer cells in layer V shown by the intracellular injections (Figure 6) and indicates the magnitude of this projection. It also demonstrates the intracortical projections of a subgroup of superficial layer cells, selected according to its long projection. Collateral filling of retrogradely filled cells was distinguished from anterograde projections by injecting [³H]-proline along with HRP, and thus demonstrating the anterograde projection autoradiographically. The autoradiography showed a distinct label in the upper layers, with no significant projection from area 19 to layer V. Another feature of corticocortical projections, originally described by Gilbert and Kelly (1975), and dramatically demonstrated in Figure 7A, is the patchiness of the population of cells projecting to the injection site. This patchiness suggests that the cortical columns, which were demonstrated originally in the ocular-dominance system and subsequently in other cortical areas (see the chapters by Goldman-Rakic and Jones in this volume), provide a framework for connectivity used at many stages of processing in the cortex.

Layer V Cells

Cells in layer V have complex receptive fields like those in layer II + III, but differ most notably in their large field sizes (Hubel and Wiesel, 1962). It has also been shown that within layer V, two cell types can be distinguished: one that shows summation for increased slit length (the standard complex cell), and one that responds optimally to a small moving slit of light placed anywhere within its relatively large field, showing no summation for increased slit length (the special complex cell).

Figure 8 shows a standard complex cell in layer V. A surprising finding was that the cell's axon sent an extensive projection to layer VI, coursing 6–8 mm down the medial bank, still remaining within area 17.

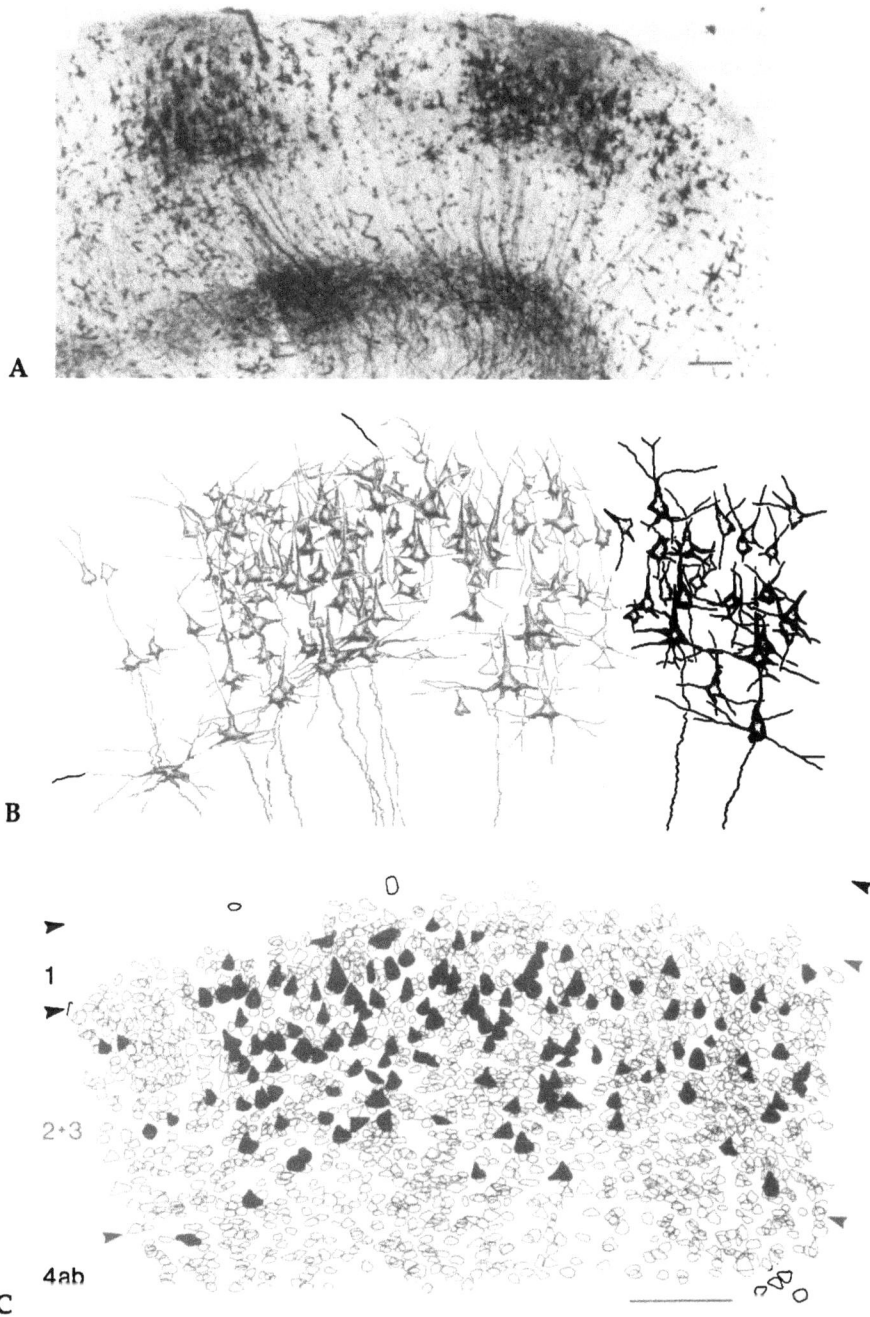

Figure 7 Cells in area 17 that project to area 19, as demonstrated by retrograde transport of HRP. (A) Photomicrograph of cells, showing their location in upper part of cortex, their distribution in two patches, and their collateral projection to layer V. (B) Camera lucida drawing of cells in right patch, showing their pyramidal morphology. (C) Outlines of labeled (black) and unlabeled (white) cells, showing size, proportion (about 20%), and distribution of layer II + III cells responsible for the projection. Bars = 100 μm.

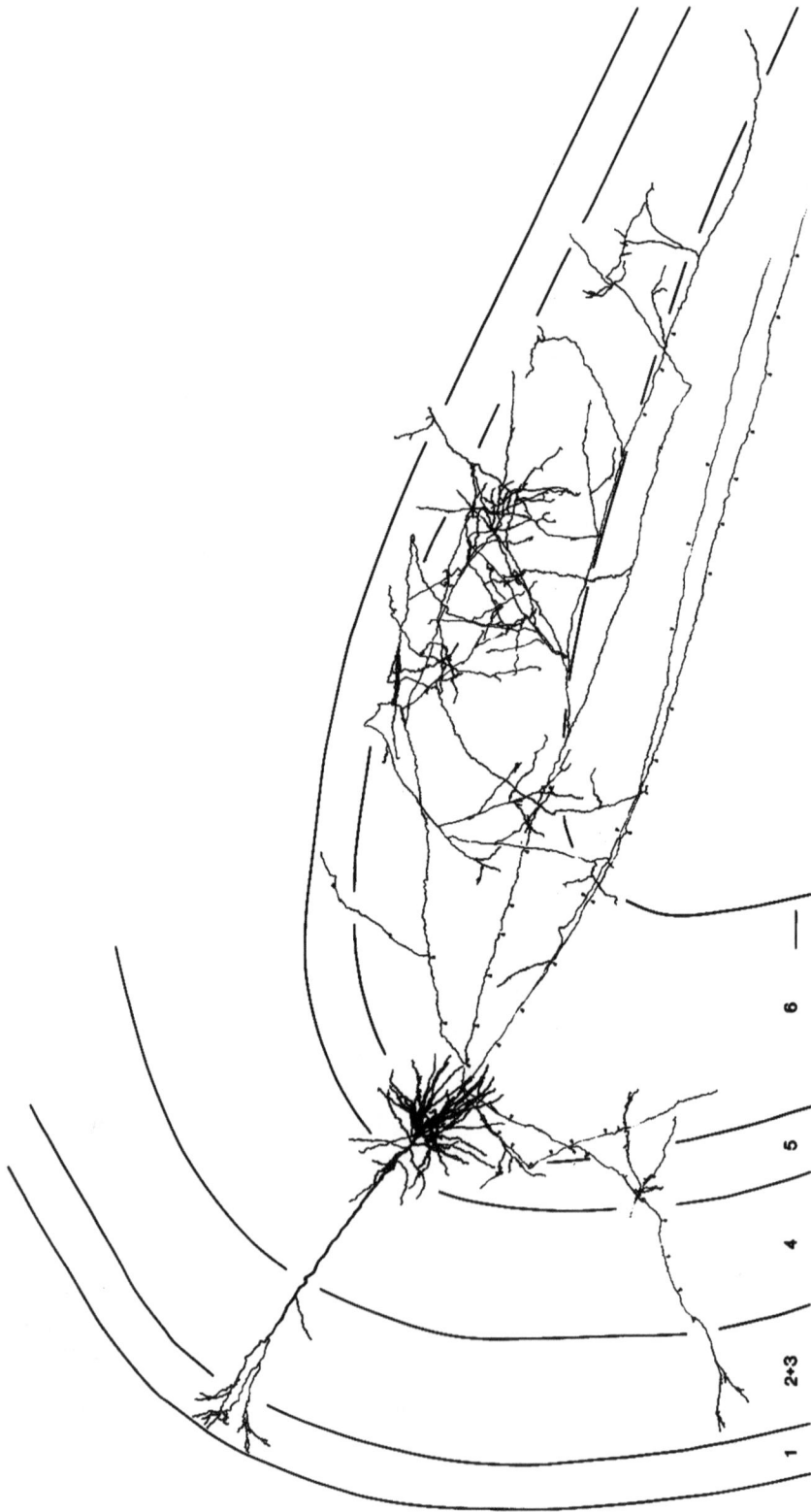

Figure 8 A pyramidal cell in layer V, with a standard complex receptive field showing no end inhibition. The field size was $2\frac{1}{4}° \times 1\frac{1}{4}°$, and it was located on the area centralis. The branches of the apical dendrite within layer I all run quite close to the pia, but this is not apparent due to the plane of section relative to the cortical layers. Bar = 100 μm.

C. D. Gilbert and T. N. Wiesel

The cell's receptive field was $2\frac{3}{4}° \times 1\frac{3}{4}°$ while its axon spanned an area of cortex representing up to 15° of visual field. Thus it reached areas that deal with parts of the field of view far outside the cell's receptive field. This projection has not been seen with Golgi stains, possibly because the axon becomes myelinated soon after leaving the cell body, and would therefore not impregnate with the Golgi technique. The distribution of the axonal field as viewed from the cortical surface was long and narrow. One might expect that the overall axis of distribution of axon should be related to the orientation axis of the cell's receptive field. This cell's axonal distribution and orientation were consistent with this view. The apical dendrite extended up into layer I, branching repeatedly there, and sent a number of processes skimming just underneath the pia. The cell had a dense dendritic arbor near its cell body, with a number of processes leaving the base of the apical dendrite at the layer IV–V border, and a set of basal dendrites extending down into the upper part of layer VI.

We have also injected special complex cells in layer V. Their axons seemed not to project as richly to layer VI as those of the standard complex cells. A large trunk projected out of the cortex, presumably to innervate the superior colliculus (Palmer and Rosenquist, 1974; Gilbert and Kelly, 1975; Lund et al., 1975; Magalhaes-Castro, Saraiva, and Magalhaes-Castro, 1975; Kawamura and Konno, 1979). Other studies have shown layer V cells also to project to the pons (Gibson et al., 1976; Kawamura and Chiba, 1979).

Figure 9 shows the layer V cells that are labeled after an injection into the superior colliculus. They are pyramidal (Figure 9B), and represent a large proportion of the largest cells in the layer, but also include a few smaller cells as well (Figure 9C). The absence of a significant amount of terminal labeling in the cortex may indicate that the corticocollicular cells are relatively poor in intracortical collateral arborization. There are clearly many pyramidal cells left unfilled after collicular HRP injection. Whether this indicates that the layer V cells projecting to different areas represent distinct populations remains to be explored.

Layer VI Cells

Layer VI is of special interest in that it receives a direct projection from the lateral geniculate nucleus (LeVay and Gilbert, 1976) and contains a mixture of simple and complex cells (Hubel and Wiesel, 1962; Kelly and Van Essen, 1974; Gilbert, 1977). Its cells have unique receptive-field properties, often requiring long slits for activation and showing summation with slit length up to very large values (16°; Gilbert, 1977). An example of a layer VI simple cell is shown in Figure 10. The basal dendrite of the cell branched in the upper part of the layer, which is precisely where the collaterals of geniculate axons end (Ferster and LeVay, 1978; see also above). Its axon projected mainly to layer IVAB, in the vi-

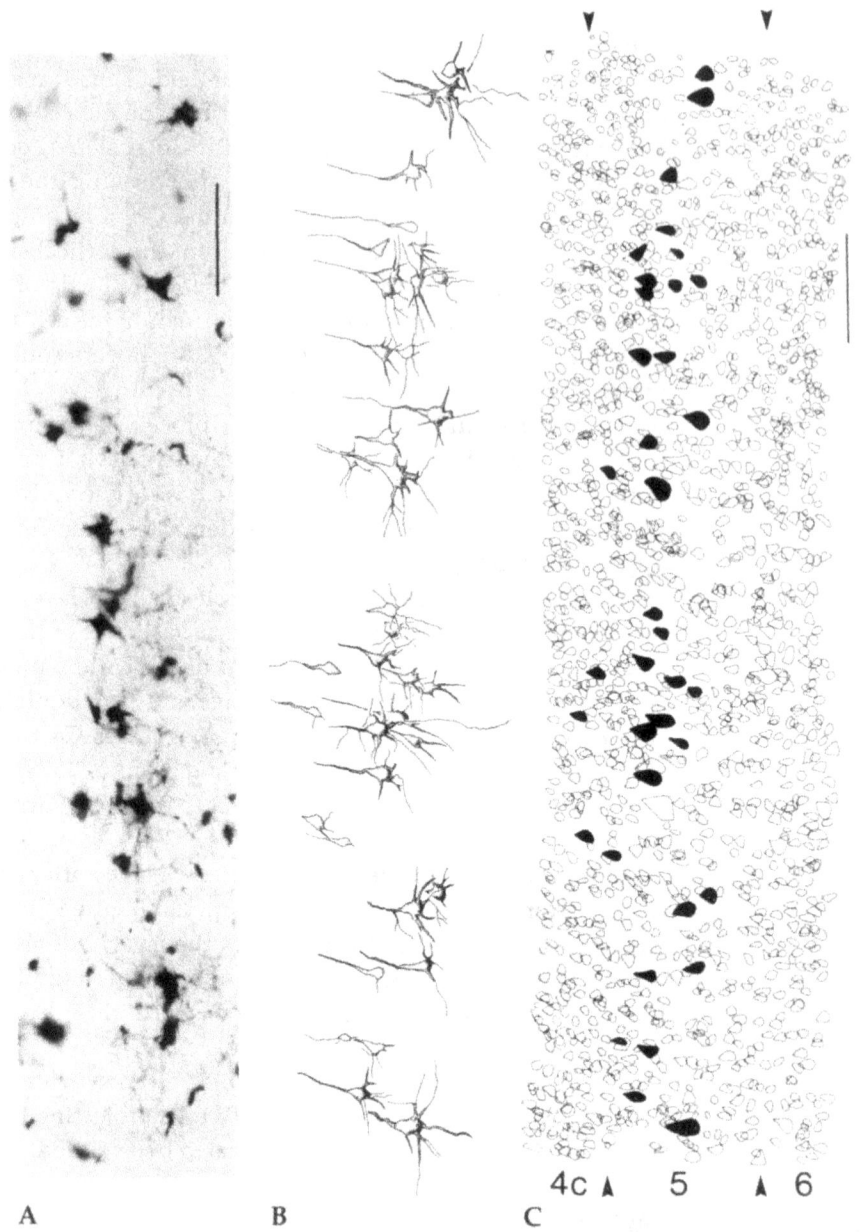

Figure 9 Cells in layer V that project to the superior colliculus. (A) Photomicrograph of cells labeled by retrograde transport of HRP from colliculus. (B) Camera lucida drawing of cells, all pyramidal in morphology. (C) Outlines of labeled (black—about 10% of the total number of layer V cells, but a higher proportion of the largest cells in the layer) and unlabeled (white) cells. Bars = 100 μm.

C. D. Gilbert and T. N. Wiesel

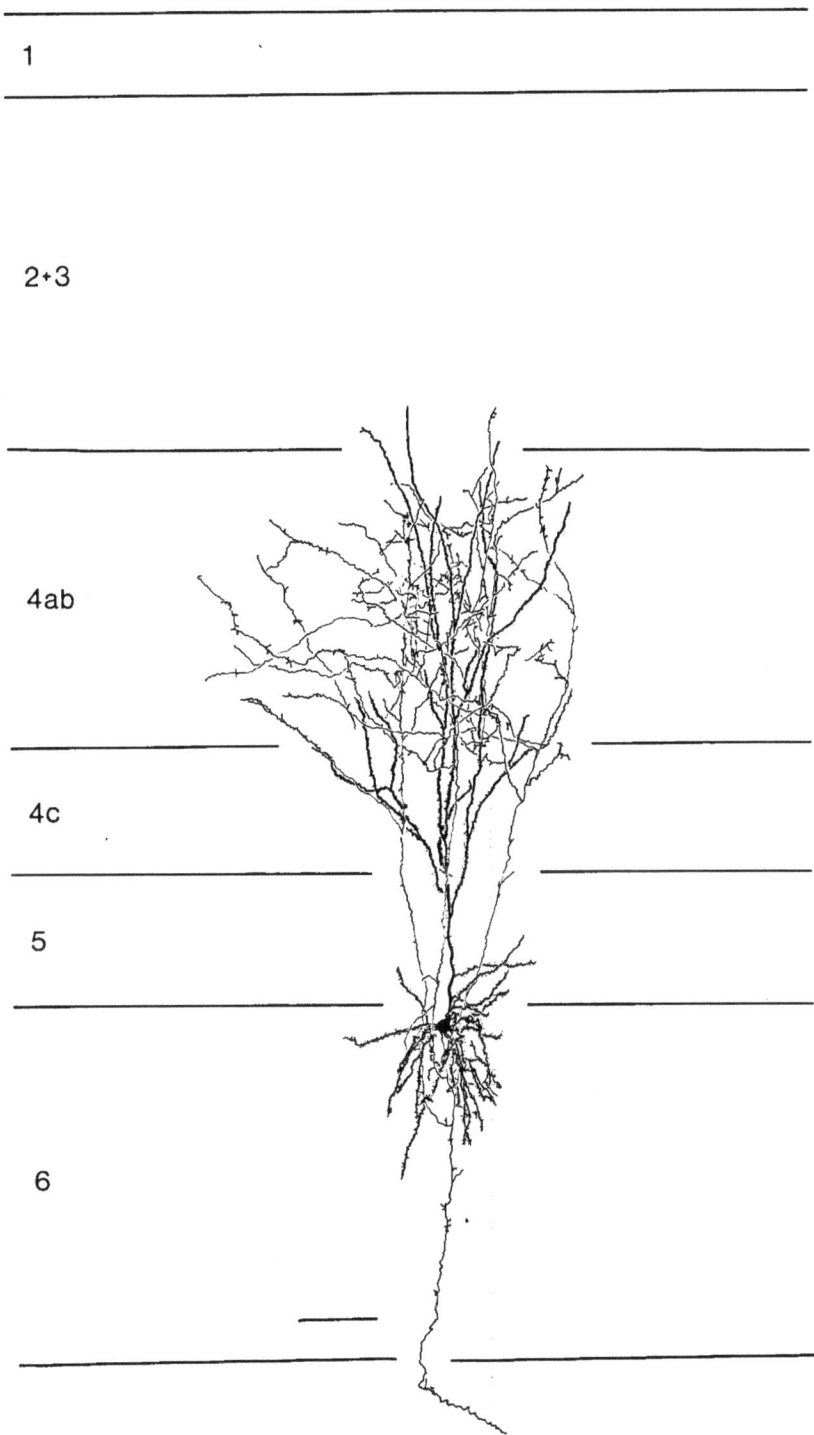

1

2+3

4ab

4c

5

6

Figure 10 A pyramidal cell in layer VI, with a simple receptive field showing the lack of end inhibition characteristic for cells in this layer. The field size was $1\frac{1}{2}° \times 2°$, centered 4° from the area centralis. It did not show obvious summation to long slits and may represent a population of layer VI cells with shorter fields. Bar = 100 μm.

cinity of its apical dendrite, which branched extensively and ended in IVAB. Other cells, both pyramidal and smooth stellate, had axonal fields that lie almost exclusively within layer VI.

Although the simple cells of layer VI were restricted to the upper half of the layer, we found complex cells throughout the layer. The apical dendrites of these cells branched at different levels within the cortex, which has been observed with the Golgi technique in the monkey by Lund and Boothe (1975) and in the cat by Lund et al. (1979). Like the cell in Figure 10, they often sent collaterals primarily to layer IV, and these were restricted either to IVAB or IVC.

Layer VI represents the source of a powerful recurrent projection from cortex to lateral geniculate nucleus. The population of cells within the layer responsible for this projection is shown in Figure 11. These cells, like those responsible for extracortical projections from layer II + III and layer V, are pyramidal (Figure 11B). They represent approximately $\frac{1}{2}$ to $\frac{2}{3}$ of all of the cells in the layer in the same overall size range (Figure 11C). The HRP filled terminals lie predominantly within layer IV, but these probably represent a mixture of the geniculocortical terminals and collateral arborization of the layer VI cells.

Intracortical Pathways and Receptive-Field Construction

Although we have not yet injected all of the morphological cell types found in the cortex (Ramón y Cajal, 1922; Lorente de Nó, 1922; O'Leary, 1941; Valverde, 1971; Lund, 1973), some patterns of projection have emerged from our present catalog of injected cells (Figure 12A). The predominant stages of information processing in the cortex appear to be as follows. The major geniculate input to the cortex arrives in layer IV, with the X input and the Y input arriving separately in layers IVC and IVAB. Both inputs also project to the upper half of layer VI. From layer IV the sequence of processing continues to the upper layers, from the upper layers to layer V, and from layer V to layer VI. Layer VI then sends output back into layer IV. The cortex is tapped for output to other regions at several stages: cortical areas from layer II + III, superior colliculus from layer V, and lateral geniculate nucleus from layer VI (Gilbert and Kelly, 1975). Also, the spread seen in the horizontal axonal projections (Figure 4) extends far beyond that expected from previous studies using the Golgi technique (Ramón y Cajal, 1922; Lorente de Nó, 1922; O'Leary, 1941; Lund, 1973).

These connections undoubtedly account for the differences in receptive-field properties seen from layer to layer and enable us to form hypotheses as to the manner in which receptive fields are constructed within the cortex. These hypotheses are derived from the receptive-field properties and the pattern of axonal arborization of the injected cells, and the receptive fields and pattern of dendritic arborization seen for the cells in the layers to which the injected cell projects. A wide-

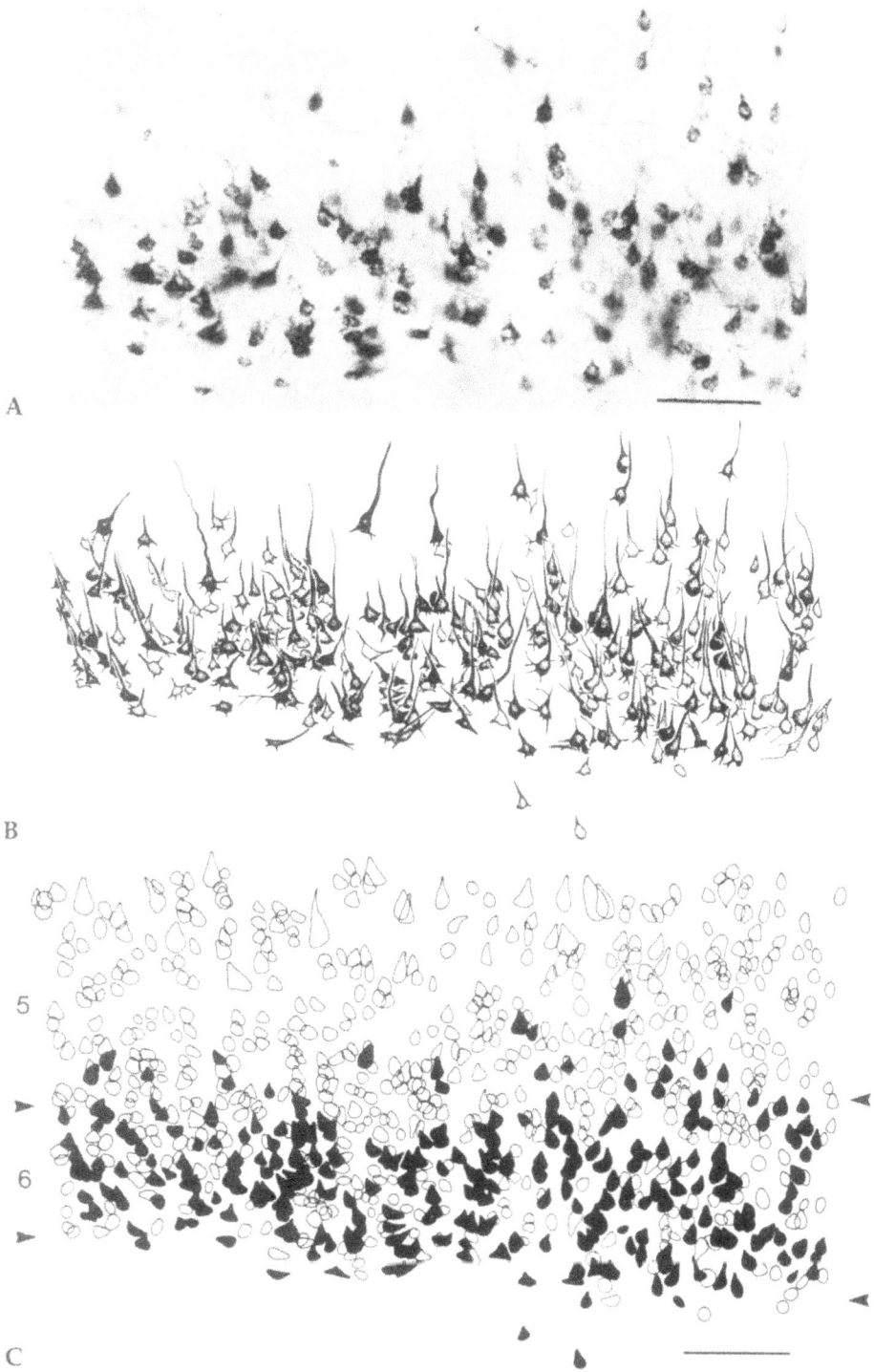

Figure 11 Cells in layer VI that project to the lateral geniculate nucleus. (A) Photomicrograph of cells labeled by retrograde transport of HRP from geniculate. (B) Camera lucida drawing of cells, all pyramidal. (C) Outlines of labeled (black—about 65% of the total number of layer VI cells) and unlabeled (white) cells. Bars = 100 μm.

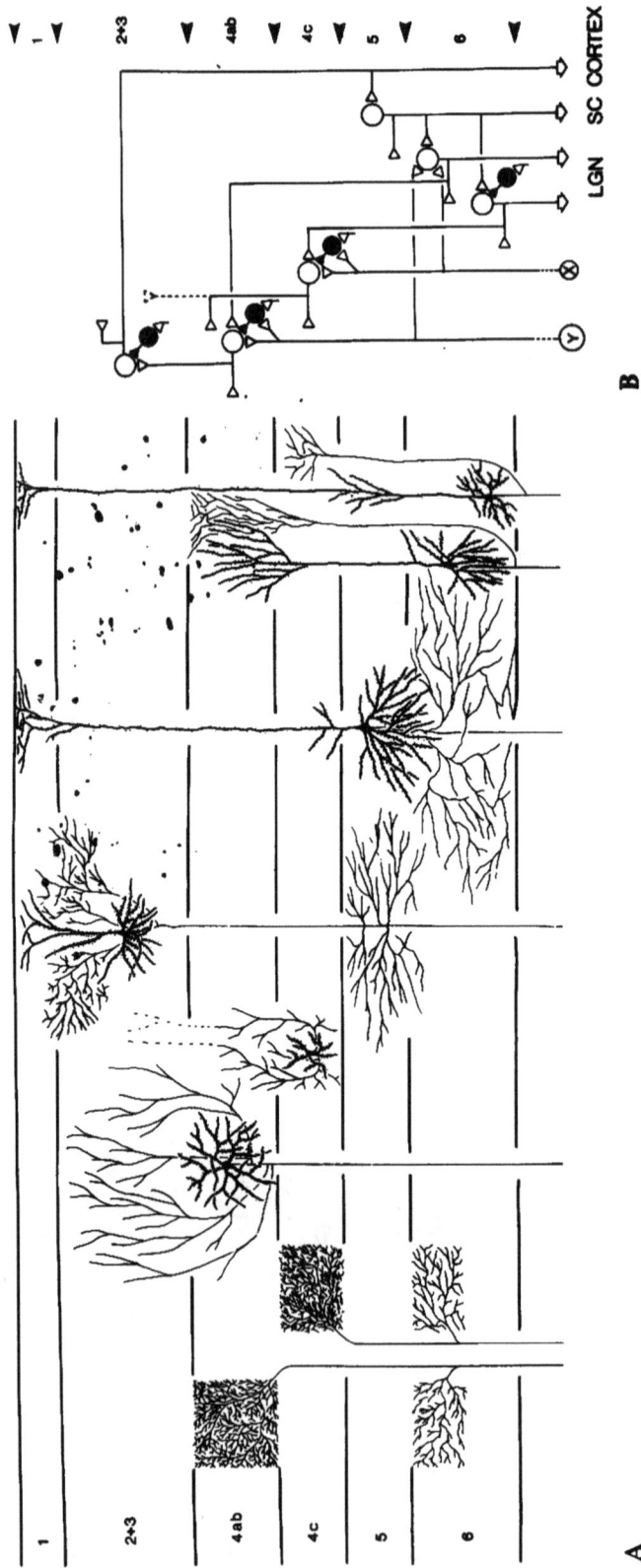

Figure 12 Schematic diagram summarizing the intracortical projection pathway. (A) Cellular elements in the pathway. (B) Suggested cortical wiring diagram. Empty circles indicate excitatory cells, filled circles inhibitory cells. See text.

C. D. Gilbert and T. N. Wiesel

spread axonal arborization, for example, demonstrates not only an extensive divergence in the projection, but also suggests that individual cells in the recipient layer receive input from a large number of cells spanning a wide area of cortex, and consequently from a larger part of the visual field than that covered by the receptive field of a single afferent cell. It is not known whether these projections are to specific cell classes. It may be, moreover, that different cell types are contacted by different parts of the terminal field, allowing, for example, for central excitation and peripheral inhibition. Also, the intracortical pathway described above does not take into account the connections that may exist between the axon of one cell and the apical dendrite of another, the emphasis being on connections between axons and basal dendrites. With these caveats in mind, we present the following model for receptive-field construction (Figure 12B).

As originally suggested by Hubel and Wiesel (1962), simple receptive fields are constructed from the fields of lateral geniculate neurons since simple cells are the predominant class in layer IV, the major geniculate afferent zone. The correspondence between simple receptive-field type and geniculate input is seen also for the cells that lie in the upper part of layer VI. While they share the same general receptive-field type, cells in layer IVC differ from those in IVAB in having smaller fields. This difference is consistent with the two features of the geniculate input to layer IV. One is that the X afferents have smaller receptive fields than the Y afferents. The other is that the IVAB afferents have a much wider terminal arborization than the IVC afferents (Ferster and LeVay, 1978). Although the receptive fields of the IVC cells were quite similar, the spiny cells are thought to be excitatory and the smooth cells inhibitory. These presumptions are based both on their synaptic morphology and transmitter neurochemistry (LeVay, 1973; Davis, Turlejski, and Sterling, 1977; Ribak, 1978). Although it has been suggested that simple cells receive X input and complex cells receive Y input (Hoffman and Stone, 1971), it is clear from our results that in both the X- and Y-geniculate afferent zones, the predominant cell class found is simple.

The superficial-layer complex cells receive their input from the layer IV simple cells. Since cells in layer IVAB project to layer II + III, and since, except for the bottom of layer III, the geniculate does not project to this layer, it is likely that the receptive fields of cells in the upper layers are generated primarily by input from layer IV. Whether the X and Y pathways are kept segregated or converge in the projection from layer IV to layer II + III remains to be worked out.

The layer V complex cells may form their fields from the concatenation of the fields of the superficial complex cells, as suggested by the extensive projection from the layer II + III cells into layer V. The lateral spread of this projection can account for the increase in receptive-field size from the superficial layers to layer V. We have no suggestions for how the inputs to standard and special complex cells differ to account for their differences in receptive-field properties. The apical dendrites of layer V cells pass through geniculate afferent zones, and evidence from combined degeneration and Golgi electromyogram (EM) studies indicates that they receive direct geniculate input (Peters et al., 1979). In distinction to cells whose basal dendrites may receive geniculate input, these cells do not have simple receptive fields.

The substantial horizontal traverse of the layer V axon in layer VI is an intriguing feature since the layer VI cells have very long receptive fields, showing summation for increased slit length up to very large values, some reaching 16° or more (Gilbert, 1977). We have seen no other inputs to layer VI or intrinsic connections within layer VI that can account for this receptive field property; the input to layer VI from the lateral geniculate nucleus is, if anything, more restricted than the geniculate input to layer IV (LeVay and Gilbert, 1976; Ferster and LeVay, 1978). Also, none of the cells within layer VI that we have injected thus far have axons that ramify within the layer over nearly as large an area as do the axons from the layer V cells. This hypothesis requires us to account for elongation in both simple and complex fields in layer VI despite the fact that the input from layer V is exclusively complex. The simple fields may be produced by an interaction between the geniculate input to the upper half of layer VI and the input from layer V.

The rich projection from layer VI to layer IV suggests that some properties manifested by layer IV cells may not depend solely on convergence of geniculate input onto layer IV cells or on connections made by those cells within the layer. It could well be that, due to their intimate involvement with layer IV through dendritic arborization and axonal projection, the layer VI cells have a role in producing orientation specificity, preference for direction of stimulus movement, and/or end inhibition.

The pattern described above emphasizes the fact that many cells in the cortex have a dual role, both in contributing to the construction of receptive fields within their own cortical area and in contributing input to other cortical areas. It is probable that their own fields are influenced in turn by the recurrent input from the areas to which they project. Once one determines the position and morphology of cells projecting to different areas, this information, together with the results from the intracellular injections, may make it possible to deduce the receptive-field properties of the cells participating in each projection.

Dendritic Morphology and Receptive Field Construction

There are several issues that are raised in considering correlations between morphology and function. As seen from our injections in layer V, for example, large neurons have large receptive fields. This is presumably due to their large dendritic fields, which enable the cells to collect input over a wide area. Another determining factor in receptive-field

C. D. Gilbert and T. N. Wiesel

size is the extent of axonal ramification of the inputs to a given cell. This is seen for the layer VI cells; although their dendritic fields are relatively small, they receive input from layer V over a very large area, due to the wide spread of the layer V cell axons. The layer V fields may derive their large area from both mechanisms: they have very wide dendritic arbors, and the layer II + III cells have widely arborizing axons in layer V.

A correlation between simple receptive-field type and stellate morphology was found by Kelly and Van Essen (1974), but, as they indicated, this correlation was not a strict one. We have injected simple cells in layers VA and VI that were pyramidal in morphology and complex cells in layer VI and layer II + III that were smooth stellate cells. Thus the simple–complex receptive-field classification seems not to be the pertinent feature in relating functional properties to the stellate–pyramidal categories. The determining factor as to whether a cell is simple or complex appears to be the position of its basal dendrites relative to the geniculate input. The function of apical dendrites remains a mystery; they may ramify at different levels within the cortex, but so far this does not seem to correlate with any receptive-field differences.

In addition to the dichotomy between stellate and pyramidal cells, there is, even for a given layer, considerable variability within each of these morphological classes. Figure 13 shows a number of superficial-layer pyramidal cells, all with complex receptive fields, which are found at different depths within the layer and which also have somewhat distinct morphologies. The manner in which this diversity is reflected in the receptive field and/or firing properties of cells is not apparent at this early stage in our study. There are certain receptive field features, such as orientation specificity and preference for direction of stimulus movement, which may ultimately be shown to correspond to particular

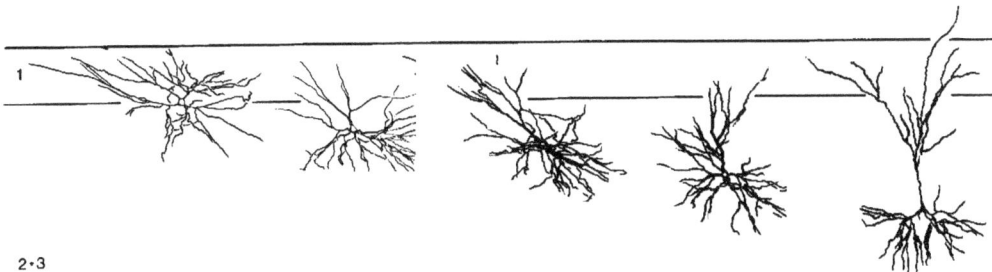

Figure 13 A series of injected pyramidal cells in layer II + III, all with complex receptive fields, to illustrate the variety of morphologies found within a single layer for a given receptive-field type.

aspects of dendritic arborization. Another functional difference between cells is the use of different transmitters, having inhibitory or excitatory postsynaptic effects which, as mentioned above, may be reflected in morphological differences, but perhaps not in differences in receptive-field properties. Pharmacological evidence suggests that inhibition is important in producing certain receptive-field features, such as orientation specificity (Sillito, 1975). Cells within a particular layer may also be differentiated according to the sites to which they project. Within an individual layer, therefore, there are a number of means by which one can distinguish cells: according to receptive-field properties, morphology, pharmacology, and sites of projection. The relationship between function and dendritic morphology remains a challenge. We expect that further analysis of, and additions to, our catalog of injected cells will reveal clues to this relationship.

Acknowledgments

We thank Lynn August for her valuable technical assistance. This work was supported by National Institutes of Health Grants EY00606 and T1EY00082.

References

Adams, J. C., 1977. Technical considerations in the use of horseradish peroxidase as a neuronal marker. *Neuroscience* 2:141.

Allman, J. M., and J. H. Kaas, 1975. The dorsomedial cortical visual area: a third tier area in the occipital lobe of the owl monkey *(Aotus Trivirgatus)*. *Brain Res.* 100:473–487.

Bilge, M., A. Bingle, K. N. Seneviratne, and D. Whitteridge, 1967. A map of the visual cortex in the cat. *J. Physiol.* 191:116P–118P.

Boycott, B. B., and H. Wassle, 1974. The morphological types of ganglion cells of the domestic cat's retina. *J. Physiol.* 240:397–419.

Brodmann, K., 1903. Beitrage zur histologischen Lokalisation der Grosshirnrinde. *J. Psychol. Neurol. Leipzig* 2:79–159.

Camarda, R. M., and G. Rizzolatti, 1976. Receptive fields of cells in the superficial layers of the cat's area 17. *Exp. Brain Res.* 24:423–427.

Campbell, A. W., 1903. Histological studies on cerebral localisation. *Proc. Roy. Soc. B* 72:488–492.

Cleland, B. G., M. W. Dubin, and W. R. Levick, 1971. Sustained and transient neurones in the cat's retina and lateral geniculate nucleus. *J. Physiol.* 217:473–496.

Daniel, P. M., and D. Whitteridge, 1959. The representation of the visual field on the calcarine cortex in baboons and monkeys. *J. Physiol.* 148:33P.

Davis, T. L., K. Turlejski, and P. Sterling, 1977. Identification by serial microscopic autoradiography of neurons in cortical area 17 that differentially accumulate exogenous 3H-gamma-aminobutyric acid. *ARVO Abst., Suppl. Invest. Ophthalm. and Vis. Sci.*:27.

Dreher, B., 1972. Hypercomplex cells in the cat's striate cortex. *Invest. Ophthal.* 11:355–356.

Enroth-Cugell, C., and J. G. Robson, 1966. The contrast sensitivity of retinal ganglion cells in the cat. *J. Physiol.* 187:517–552.

Ferster, D., and S. LeVay, 1978. The axonal arborizations of lateral geniculate neurons in the striate cortex of the cat. *J. Comp. Neurol.* 182:923–944.

Frank, E., W. A. Harris, and M. B. Kennedy, 1980. Lysophosphatidyl choline facilitates antero- and retrograde labelling of CNS projections with horseradish peroxidase. (In press.)

Garey, L. J., and T. P. S. Powell, 1971. An experimental study of the termination of the lateral geniculo-cortical pathway in the cat and monkey. *Proc. Roy. Soc. B* 179:41–63.

Gibson, A., G. Mower, J. Baker, and M. Glickstein, 1976. Corticopontine visual cells in the cat. *Ann. Meeting Soc. Neurosci., 6th, Toronto*:1,112.

Gilbert, C. D., 1977. Laminar differences in receptive field properties in cat primary visual cortex. *J. Physiol.* 268:391–421.

Gilbert, C. D., and J. P. Kelly, 1975. The projections of cells in different layers of the cat's visual cortex. *J. Comp. Neurol.* 163:81–106.

Gilbert, C. D., and T. N. Wiesel, 1979. Morphology and intracortical projections of functionally identified neurons in the cat visual cortex. *Nature* 280:120–125.

Guillery, R. W., 1966. A study of Golgi preparations from the dorsal lateral geniculate nucleus of the adult cat. *J. Comp. Neurol.* 128:21–50.

Henry, G. H., and P. O. Bishop, 1972. Striate neurons: Receptive field organization. *Invest. Ophthal.* 11:357–368.

Hochstein, S., and R. M. Shapley, 1976. Quantitative analysis of retinal ganglion cell classification. *J. Physiol.* 262:237–264.

Hoffman, K. P., and J. Stone, 1971. Conduction velocity of afferents to cat visual cortex: a correlation with cortical receptive field properties. *Brain Res.* 32:460–466.

Hoffman, K. P., J. Stone, and S. M. Sherman, 1972. Relay of receptive field properties in dorsal lateral geniculate nucleus of the cat. *J. Neurophysiol.* 35:518–531.

Hollander, H., 1974. On the origins of the corticotectal projections in the cat. *Exp. Brain Res.* 21:430–440.

Hubel, D. H., and T. N. Wiesel, 1959. Receptive fields of single neurones in the cat's striate cortex. *J. Physiol.* 148:574–591.

Hubel, D. H., and T. N. Wiesel, 1962. Receptive fields, binocular interaction and functional architecture in the cat's visual cortex. *J. Physiol.* 160:106–154.

Hubel, D. H., and T. N. Wiesel, 1972. Laminar and columnar distribution of geniculocortical fibers in the macaque monkey. *J. Comp. Neurol.* 146:421–450.

Hubel, D. H., and T. N. Wiesel, 1977. Functional architecture of the macaque monkey visual cortex. *Proc. Roy. Soc. B* 196:1–59.

Jankowska, E., J. Rasted, and J. Westman, 1976. Intracellular application of horseradish peroxidase and its light and electron microscopic appearance in spinocervical tract cells. *Brain Res.* 105:557–562.

Kato, H., P. O. Bishop, and G. A. Orban, 1978. Hypercomplex and simple/complex cell classification in cat striate cortex. *J. Neurophysiol.* 41:1071–1095.

Kawamura, K., and M. Chiba, 1979. Cortical neurons projecting to the pontine nuclei in the cat. An experimental study with the horseradish peroxidase technique. *Exp. Brain Res.* 35:269–285.

Kawamura, K., and T. Konno, 1979. Various types of corticotectal neurons of cats as demonstrated by means of retrograde axonal transport of horseradish peroxidase. *Exp. Brain Res.* 35:161–175.

Kelly, J. P., and D. C. Van Essen, 1974. Cell structure and function in the visual cortex of the cat. *J. Physiol.* 328:515–547.

Kitai, S. T., J. D. Kocsis, R. J. Preston, and M. Sugimori, 1976. Monosynaptic inputs to caudate neurones identified by intracellular injection of horseradish peroxidase. *Brain Res.* 109:601–606.

Kuffler, S. W., 1953. Discharge patterns and functional organization of mammalian retina. *J. Neurophysiol.* 16:37–68.

LeVay, S., 1973. Synaptic patterns in the visual cortex of the cat and monkey. Electron microscopy of Golgi preparations. *J. Comp. Neurol.* 150:53–86.

LeVay, S., and C. D. Gilbert, 1976. Laminar patterns of geniculocortical projection in the cat. *Brain Res.* 113:1–19.

Leventhal, A. G., and H. V. B. Hirsch, 1978. Receptive-field properties of neurons in different laminae of visual cortex of the cat. *J. Neurophysiol.* 41:948–962.

Light, A. R., and R. G. Durkovic, 1976. Horseradish peroxidase: An improvement in intracellular staining of single, electrophysiologically characterized neurons. *Exp. Neurol.* 53:847–853.

Lorente de Nó, R., 1922. La corteza cerebral del raton. *Trab. Lab. Invest. Biol. Madrid* 20:41–78.

Lund, J. S., and R. G. Boothe, 1975. Interlaminar connections and pyramidal neuron or- (*Macaca mulatta*). *J. Comp. Neurol.* 147:455–496.

Lund, J. S., and R. G. Boothe, 1975. Interlaminar connections and pyramidal neuron organization of the visual cortex, area 17, of the Macaque monkey. *J. Comp. Neurol.* 159:305–344.

Lund, J. S., G. H. Henry, C. L. Macqueen, and A. R. Harvey, 1979. Anatomical organization of the primary visual cortex (area 17) of the cat. A comparison with area 17 of the Macaque monkey. *J. Comp. Neurol.* 184:599–618.

Lund, J. S., R. D. Lund, A. E. Hendrickson, A. H. Bunt, and A. F. Fuchs, 1975. The origin of efferent pathways from the primary visual cortex, area 17, of the macaque monkey as shown by retrograde transport of horseradish peroxidase. *J. Comp. Neurol.* 164:287–304.

Magalhaes-Castro, H. H., P. E. S. Saraiva, and B. Magalhaes-Castro, 1975. Identification of corticotectal cells of the visual cortex of cats by means of horseradish peroxidase. *Brain Res.* 83:474–479.

Malmgren, L., and Y. Olsson, 1978. A sensitive method for histochemical demonstration of horseradish peroxidase following retrograde axonal transport. *Brain Res.* 148:279–294.

Mesulam, M.-M., 1976. The blue reaction product in horseradish peroxidase neurohistochemistry: incubation parameters and visibility. *J. Histochem. Cytochem.* 24:1273–1280.

Muller, K. J., and U. J. MacMahan, 1978. The shapes of sensory and motor neurones and the distribution of their synapses in ganglia of the leech: A study using intracellular injection of horseradish peroxidase. *Proc. Roy. Soc. B* 194:481–499.

Nauta, H. J. W., A. B. Butler, and J. A. Jane, 1973. Some observations on axonal degeneration resulting from superficial lesions of the cerebral cortex. *J. Comp. Neurol.* 150:349–360.

O'Leary, J. L., 1941. Structure of the area striata of the cat. *J. Comp. Neurol.* 75:131–161.

Otsuka, R., and R. Hassler, 1962. Über Aufbau und Gliederung der corticalen Sehsphare bei der Katze. *Arch. Psychiat. Nervenkrankh.* 203:212–234.

Palmer, L. A., and A. C. Rosenquist, 1974. Visual receptive fields of single striate cortical units projecting to the superior colliculus in the cat. *Brain Res.* 67:27–42.

Peters, A., C. C. Proskauer, M. L. Feldman, and L. Kimerer, 1979. The projection of the lateral geniculate nucleus to area 17 of the rat cerebral cortex. V. Degenerating axon terminals synapsing with Golgi impregnated neurons. *J. Neurocytol.* 8:331–357.

Pettigrew, J. D., T. Nikara, and P. O. Bishop, 1968. Responses to moving slits by single units in cat striate cortex. *Exp. Brain Res.* 6:373–390.

Ramón y Cajal, S., 1922. Studien über die Sehrinde der Katze. *J. Psychol. Neurol.* 29:161–181.

Ribak, C. E., 1978. Aspinous and sparsely-spinous stellate neurons in the visual cortex of rats contain glutamic acid decarboxylase. *J. Neurocytol.* 7:461–478.

Rose, D., 1977. Responses of single units in cat visual cortex to moving bars of light as a function of bar length. *J. Physiol.* 271:1–23.

Rosenquist, A. C., S. B. Edwards, and L. A. Palmer, 1975. An autoradiographic study of the projections of the dorsal lateral geniculate nucleus and the posterior nucleus in the cat. *Brain Res.* 80:71–93.

Schiller, P. H., B. L. Finlay, and S. F. Volman, 1976. Quantitative studies of single cell properties in monkey striate cortex. I. Spatiotemporal organization of receptive fields. *J. Neurophysiol.* 39:1288–1319.

Shatz, C. J., and M. P. Stryker, 1978. Ocular dominance in layer IV of the cat's visual cortex and the effects of monocular deprivation. *J. Physiol.* 281:267–283.

Shatz, C. J., S. Lindstrom, and T. N. Wiesel, 1977. The distribution of afferents representing the right and left eyes in the cat's visual cortex. *Brain Res.* 131:103–116.

Sillito, A. M., 1975. The contribution of inhibitory mechanisms to the receptive field properties of neurones in the striate cortex of the cat. *J. Physiol.* 250:305–329.

Singer, W., F. Tretter, and M. Cynader, 1975. Organization of cat striate cortex: a correlation of receptive field properties with afferent and efferent connections. *J. Neurophysiol.* 38:1080–1098.

Spatz, W. B., J. Tigges, and M. Tigges, 1970. Subcortical projections, cortical associations and some intrinsic interlaminar connections of the striate cortex in the squirrel monkey *(Saimiri). J. Comp. Neurol.* 140:155–174.

Stone, J., and Y. Fukuda, 1974. Properties of cat retinal ganglion cells: A comparison of W-cells with X- and Y-cells. *J. Neurophysiol.* 37:722–748.

Szentágothai, J., 1965. The use of degeneration methods in the investigation of short neuronal connections. In *Progress in Brain Research*, Vol. 14. M. Singer and J. P. Schadé, eds. Amsterdam: Elsevier, pp. 1–32.

Talbot, S. A., and W. H. Marshall, 1941. Physiological studies on the mechanism of visual localization and discrimination. *Amer. J. Ophthal.* 24:1255–1264.

Toyama, K., K. Matsunami, T. Ohno, and S. Takashiki, 1974. An intracellular study of neuronal organization in the visual cortex. *Exp. Brain Res.* 21:45–66.

Tusa, R. J., L. A. Palmer, and A. C. Rosenquist, 1978. The retinotopic organization of area 17 (striate cortex) in the cat. *J. Comp. Neurol.* 177:213–236.

Valverde, F., 1971. Short axon neuronal subsystems in the visual cortex of the monkey. *Int. J. Neurosci.* 1:181–197.

Van Essen, D. C., and S. M. Zeki, 1978. The topographic organization of rhesus monkey prestriate cortex. *J. Physiol.* 277:193–226.

Vogt, O., and C. Vogt, 1903. Zur anatomischen Gliederung des Cortex cerebri. *J. Psychol. Neurol.* 2:160–180.

Wiesel, T. N., D. H. Hubel, and D. M. K. Lam, 1974. Autoradiographic demonstration of ocular-dominance columns in the monkey striate cortex by means of transneuronal transport. *Brain Res.* 79:273–279.

Wilson, P. D., M. H. Rowe, and J. Stone, 1976. Properties of relay cells in cat's lateral geniculate nucleus: A comparison of W-cells with X- and Y-cells. *J. Neurophysiol.* 39:1193–1209.

Zeki, S. M., 1978. Uniformity and diversity of structure and function in rhesus monkey prestriate visual cortex. *J. Physiol.* 277:273–290.

Organization and Connections of the
Neocortex

Introduction

Ann M. Graybiel

These chapters focus on the organization of the neocortex at the level of its subdivision into groups of functionally related areas. The aim of the session that led to these chapters was to bring together anatomical and physiological studies of the neocortex in an attempt to identify aspects of the structural design of the neocortex that can be related to its functional organization. The topic was approached first by E. G. Jones, whose chapter reviews recent progress that has been made in relating the architecture of the neocortex to its input–output organization. Information on this subject has increased dramatically in the past ten years because of improvements in anatomical technique and the use of anatomical methods in combination with electrophysiological mapping. As a result, it is possible to add to conclusions about the columnar organization of the cortex a major generalization regarding the significance of cortical laminae, namely that both the afferent and the efferent connections of the neocortex are divided up according to cortical layers of origin. The outlines of this organization are already known and are summarized by Jones. Principal thalamic afferents terminate in the middle layers of the neocortex, and callosal and association fibers in the supragranular and infragranular laminae, in patterns whose precision and intricacy of detail were only first made visible by the autoradiographic axon-transport methods. The cells of origin of the efferent connections also are strictly sorted, so that the supragranular layers give rise mainly to the ipsilateral association and callosal fibers, while the projection fibers originate mainly in the infragranular layers. Within each of these major classes of efferent and afferent connections there are further subclasses having separate strata of origin or distribution; in addition, some afferents and efferents have been shown to respect columnar arrangements as well. Indeed, Jones suspects that at least some "input columns" and "output columns" in the somatic sensory cortex coincide, and much the same has been suggested for the auditory cortex. The neocortex thus comprises a horizontally and vertically organized mosaic, with the long tracts having a morphological signature in the compartments they engage.

J. H. Kaas and colleagues deal in depth with functional representation in the somatic sensory cortex. Major findings of two sorts have emerged from their analysis. The first regards the pattern of somatotopic mapping in the "primary" somatic sensory cortex in primates. Kaas and his coworkers have identified four adjoining representations of the body within the traditional primary somatic sensory cortex (SI) corresponding, respectively, to cytoarchitechtonic areas 3b and 1 (representations of the body surface) and areas 3a and 2 (representations of deep body tissues). The four body maps are parallel to one another, form thin strips with long axes running from medial to lateral, and border one another along matching somatotopic points. This last arrangement suggests that there are mirror reversals at the borders, as there are in the auditory and visual cortex. In the somatic sensory cortex the individual maps do not resemble faithful "homunculi" but contain splits and discontinuities, so that even though a general somatotopy is maintained, the topology is complex and includes apparent divisions of the map into local representations of body parts (for example, the digits). Finally, in each of the maps there is an inverse relationship between receptive field and magnification factor, as in the visual cortex.

The second set of observations by Kaas and colleagues concerns the microorganization of the cutaneous map in area 3b. By analyzing in detail the hand representation of area 3b in the Macaque, they discovered the probably somesthetic analogue of the approximately 1-mm-wide hypercolumns described by Hubel and Wiesel in the primary visual cortex of the Macaque. For each digit, rapidly adapting and slowly adapting submodalities are represented in separate strips of unequal width (800 μm for fast, 200 μm for slow). Thus each digit is doubly represented on a microscopic scale within the context of a single overall somatotopic map. Kaas and colleagues also define the smallest *topographic* unit, about 40–60 μm wide, in an ingenious nerve-regeneration experiment in which they measured cortical patches containing units with mislocated receptive fields. Kaas suggests, however, that in addition to these precise columnar organizations there may be a less finely graded somatic representation revealed upon denervation and "hidden" in the normal state.

With the presentation by E. V. Evarts, the session turned from the compartmental nature of the neocortex to the long-axon affiliations of the cortex considered in terms of neural "systems." In discussing the motor cortex Evarts brings up a long-recognized paradox of the motor system: despite the clinical distinctions between pyramidal and extrapyramidal disorders, the main outputs of the extrapyramidal system (that is, of the cerebellum and basal ganglia) lead to the pyramidal system (motor cortex, via the thalamic VA-VL complex). Evarts first reminds us that the neocortex itself constitutes another great source of input to the motor cortex. He then divides the functional influences on area 4 into two major classes that match, at least in part, its two main types of afferent connection: (1) the transcortical association fibers

(Evarts emphasizes the chains area 3b → area 1 → area 2 → motor cortex and 3b → 2 → 5 → 4); and (2) the thalamocortical radiations (cerebellum and globus pallidus → VA-VL complex → areas 4 and 6).

Evarts ascribes to the transcortical fibers the function of a closed-loop servomechanism acting to stabilize movements. As experimental evidence, he describes findings in alert trained monkeys demonstrating that almost all identified pyramidal-tract neurons in area 4 are involved in reflex afferent control of small-amplitude precision movements. The stepwise routes from area 3b to areas 1 and 2 and on to the motor cortex clearly form major conduction routes for this "cortical reflex." Physiological evidence implicates the thalamic VA-VL input to the motor cortex as a second source of short-latency somesthetic input. Evarts argues, however, that a main function of this thalamocortical projection is to convey to the motor cortex information from the cerebellum and basal ganglia regarding open-loop control of ballistic movements and, more generally, programs for voluntary movements. Work by Evarts and his colleagues and by others is consistent with this view. For example, Strick has found that the firing rates of neurons in the dentate and interposed nuclei of the cerebellum are affected by motor "set" as early as 10 msec before comparable changes in activity in cortical neurons in area 4.

Long-loop systems of the neocortex are also treated by Graybiel, who describes anatomical experiments carried out in collaboration with Berson on the multiple areas of the visual "association" cortex. Working in cats, where as many as thirteen visual areas have been demonstrated physiologically in the parieto-temporo-occipital association cortex, Graybiel and Berson have identified discrete sets of parallel pathways leading through the LP-pulvinar complex to the extrastriate cortex. On this basis they suggest that there are clusters or "families" of cortical areas in the extrastriate cortex, each related to a particular subdivision of the extrageniculate thalamus. They then compare these thalamic affiliations of the extrastriate areas to their transcortical connections and find that, in general, cortical areas related to the same thalamic subdivision tend to be interconnected, while cortical areas in different extrastriate families tend to be linked less tightly. They argue that this suggests an underlying logic governing patterns of within-family and cross-family connectivity and emphasize that the ties can be of both the direct corticocortical type and the indirect cortico-thalamo-cortical type. Graybiel and Berson cite as an example of this organization the fact that the primary visual cortex (area 17) projects to a discrete subdivision of the LP-pulvinar complex, which in turn projects back to area 17 and virtually all cortical areas that receive transcortical input from area 17. There are therefore parallel transcortical and cortico-thalamo-cortical pathways related to area 17, but a marked paucity of connections linking these regions with, for example, the tectorecipient and pretectorecipient parts of the LP-pulvinar and their cortical families. The major conclusion drawn is that there are multiple clusters of cortical areas in the visually responsive cortex rather than a single hierarchical organization depending on pathways leading out from area 17.

The final presentation of the session on the organization of the neocortex was by W. J. H. Nauta, who discussed the second great category of association cortex, the limbic cortex of the frontal lobe and its cortical affiliates in the cingulate gyrus and temporal pole. Regretfully, circumstances made it impossible for a corresponding manuscript to be prepared for this volume. Nauta's main theme was that the prefrontal cortex and its cortical affiliates are unique among subdivisions of the cerebral cortex in having at once strong direct and indirect connections with the hypothalamus and, mainly by transcortical circuits, close affiliations with the parieto-temporo-occipital association cortex. Nauta extended this conclusion in a new way by incorporating recent findings from his own and other laboratories regarding the ventral striatum. This subdivision of the striatum encompasses the nucleus accumbens septi and adjoining ventral parts of the basal forebrain and is now recognized as a limbic equivalent of the caudate-putamen complex (dorsal striatum). It is tightly linked to the septo-hypothalamo-mesencephalic continuum and to the dopamine-containing cell groups A8 and A10. Nauta emphasized the multiple connections relating this subcortical network to the frontal lobes and suggested that even without the physiological mapping studies comparable to those on the posterior association cortex, one could predict a close functional relation between the prefrontal cortex and basal forebrain mechanisms related to the ventral striatum. The session came full circle with his demonstration that despite the apparent distancing of the prefrontal cortex from the sensory and motor peripheries, its subdivision into laminar and columnar compartments is as striking as that of the primary sensory cortex.

9

Anatomy of Cerebral Cortex: Columnar Input–Output Organization

E. G. Jones

ABSTRACT   In the cerebral cortex, the search for manageable circuit elements comparable, say, to the mossy fiber–granule cell–Purkinje cell circuit of the cerebellum has been hampered by lack of knowledge regarding the meaning of cortical lamination and a lack of agreement regarding the classes and distribution of interneurons. Recent work indicates that in higher primates, each lamina of the cortex to a large extent represents an aggregation of pyramidal-cell somata whose axons project to the same cortical or subcortical site. There is even evidence for a sublaminar organization along these lines in layers III and V.

The laminar distribution of thalamic, commissural, and ipsilateral corticocortical afferents parallels the segregation of these efferent-cell somata and there are hints that some of the inputs may selectively synapse upon particular categories of efferent cell. A major problem that remains to be resolved, however, is the extent to which afferent fibers to a given layer terminate upon the apical or basal dendrites of pyramidal cells whose somata are situated in other layers.

The horizontal laminar spread of thalamic and callosal inputs appears to be composed of much smaller, punctate zones of terminations, some 0.5–1 mm wide, derived from vertical bundles of incoming fibers. These bundles may have as their basis clustered aggregations of thalamic or callosal cells receiving like inputs. In the case of thalamic cells, the input would likely specify the place and modality characteristics that their axon bundle would then impose upon the punctate cortical recipient zone. The extent to which axons of one bundle branch and contribute to other bundles has implications for the specificity of cortical "modules" based upon afferent inputs. In the somatic sensory cortex, branching outside a bundle may be minimal, so that adjacent input foci are largely independent. In the visual cortex, branching in one dimension may lead to substantial overlap within an ocular-dominance strip but not between adjacent ocular-dominance strips. Nevertheless, branching may occur to a more distant ocular-dominance strip related to the same eye. In the motor cortex, distant branching may be quite extensive, so that a thalamic axon bundle may terminate in several widely separated foci.

Focal zones based on afferent input can form highly regular and repeating patterns of organization by their alignment in rows, as in the case of thalamic foci forming ocular-dominance strips in the visual cortex and callosal foci forming mediolaterally oriented strips in the pre- and postcentral gyri.

E. G. JONES   Department of Anatomy and Neurobiology, Washington University School of Medicine, St. Louis, Missouri 63110

The focal nature of thalamic inputs to the middle layers of the cortex seems to be transmitted through other layers by a class of apparently excitatory interneurons with tight vertical bundles of axon branches 100–200 μm wide that synapse upon the apical dendrites of pyramidal cells of all layers. The effect of this is to make an input column also an output column, the dimensions of which are determined by the input bundle and the vertical interneurons with which it connects. The degree of rigidity in this kind of circuitry is, as yet, unclear for it is uncertain to what extent neurons other than the interneurons with vertical axons are the major recipients of thalamic synapses.

Several other generic classes of cortical interneurons are coming to be recognized on the basis of specific axonal distributions rather than the shapes of dendritic fields which can vary in concert with cortical folding and changes in cell packing density. Some of these must have very localized actions though their axonal ramifications in some cases may enfold several hundred other neurons. Others seem to operate over long distances within the cortex. One long-axoned class is the cortical "basket cell" described especially in the pre- and postcentral gyri. This cell and its 1–2-mm-long axon branches are preferentially arranged at right angles to the long axes of the gyri. The axon terminals seem to form the major input to pyramidal-cell somata and appear to have characteristics, including the presence of glutamic acid decarboxylase, to suggest that they are inhibitory. In this way it is assumed that inhibitory influences may operate in a preferred direction from one focal input–output zone or column to another.

Introduction

It may seem presumptuous at this time to attempt any generalized account of the intrinsic circuitry of the cerebral cortex. Though there have been many outstanding contributions to our knowledge of this structure in recent years, these new data are derived from studies in which the viewpoints of physiologist and morphologist have not always been identical, and from studies on different species and on cortical areas that may diverge considerably from a basic pattern. The significant differences in thickness, laminar pattern, cell packing density and connectional organization between, for example, the visual and the somatic sensory areas have led some to despair that any common principles of cortical organization will ever emerge. However, it is still true to say that all areas of the neocortex show a fundamental similarity of structure and it would be surprising if the truly basic functional organization of each were fundamentally different.

In what follows, I have attempted to draw up a scheme that I consider may be representative of all areas, at least in the primate. Perhaps surprisingly, this scheme adopts a viewpoint that is not necessarily constrained by knowledge of the visual cortex. Dramatic as they are, the new findings in this area seem to indicate a cortical field that has departed further than most from a common pattern. Nevertheless, it is hoped that this account will have some relevance to the visual cortex as well.

Cortical Lamination

The first scheme of cortical lamination was proposed by Meynert in 1867. Despite many years of subsequent work, the significance of lamination is still little understood. To a large extent, this is because the cortex changes its laminar pattern from area to area and with its folding into the depths of sulci and over the crowns of gyri. Any analysis is further complicated by the fact that pyramidal-cell somata situated in one lamina have dendrites that extend through several supra- and subjacent laminae. Finally, there is no agreement regarding the classes and distribution of interneurons (local-circuit neurons) within the cortex, so that some authors such as Sholl (1954) recognized but a single class whereas others such as Lorente de Nó (1922) recognized more than thirty.

All of the above contrasts with the cerebellar cortex, which has a uniform structure, a rigidly defined lamination, and in which the identification of cell types is agreed upon by all. These factors have permitted the cerebellar cortex to be analyzed with a greater degree of anatomical and physiological finesse than probably any other part of the brain, though it has to be admitted that the overall functions of the cerebellum remain rather a mystery.

Yet the cerebral cortex has a degree of laminar stereotypy in that cells of like somal size tend to be aggregated together and some of the changes that occur at areal boundaries can be abrupt and are reproduced from animal to animal. Among questions that need to be addressed, therefore, are the following: Why cortical lamination? Why does it vary? On what does it depend? Is it an aggregation of cells with like outputs, with like inputs, or both? Are all the cells of a single layer of one kind or are they different but joined by some common feature into functional groupings? If this commonality can be identified, will it enable us to unravel circuit elements comparable, for example, to the mossy fiber–granule cell–Purkinje cell circuit of the cerebellar cortex? If such circuits can be identified within the cortex, what will they tell us about communication between cells in the vertical (interlaminar) and horizontal (intralaminar) dimensions of the cortex?

None of these questions has yet been answered satisfactorily, but there is a certain amount of evidence available to justify some provisional hypotheses.

The introduction of the retrograde axonal transport method to identify the cell bodies of origin of a particular set of axons has led to a large number of studies of the cells of origin of most corticofugal pathways emanating from a variety of areas (e.g., Gilbert and Kelly, 1975; Lund et al., 1975; Jones and Wise, 1977; Catsman-Berrevoets and Kuypers, 1978). In the first place, all fairly definitely indicate that the pyramidal cell is the efferent cell of the cortex. There are few convincing examples of nonpyramidal cells sending axons outside the cortical area in which they lie. (A possible exception is a small proportion of commissurally projecting nonpyramidal cells in the cat visual cortex; Shatz, 1977). Second, though subject to certain reservations and true mainly for the primate, each cortical lamina largely represents an aggregation of pyramidal cells which send their axons to the same cortical or subcortical site (Figure 1). There is a fairly clear distinction between the supra- and infragranular layers: the former contain the somata of pyramidal cells with axons projecting to ipsi- and contralateral cortical areas, with contralaterally projecting (callosal) cell somata generally larger and situated deep to those of ipsilaterally projecting cells; in the infragranular layers, layer VI contains the somata of most cells whose axons return to the related thalamic nucleus and layer V the somata of all other corticofugal neurons. Within both layers there seems to be a moderate degree of sublaminar segregation of cell somata according to their target sites. In layer V, corticostriatal cells are the smallest and tend to be the most superficially situated; corticospinal and corticotectal cells are the largest and most deeply situated, with (in between) corticothalamic cells projecting to the intralaminar nuclei or pulvinar and, in relevant areas, corticorubral and corticobulbar cells. In layer VI of the visual cortex, corticothalamic cells projecting to the magnocellular layers of the lateral geniculate nucleus are situated deeper than those projecting to the par-

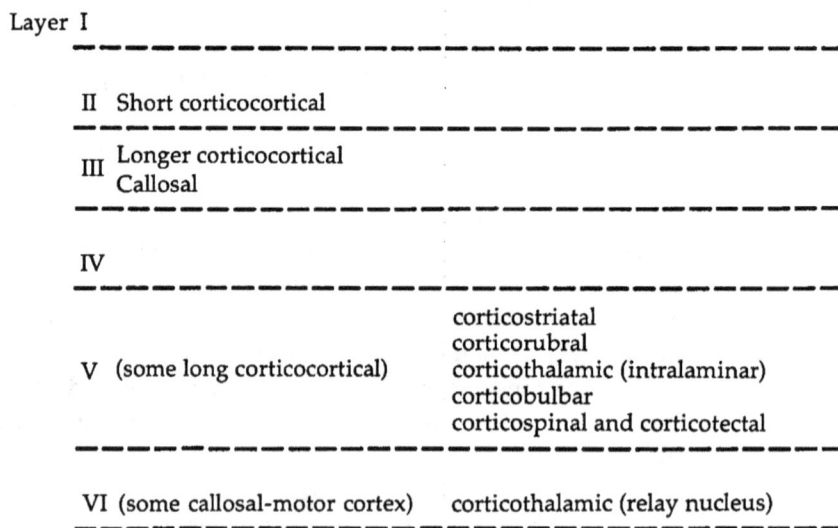

Layer I

    II Short corticocortical

    III Longer corticocortical
        Callosal

    IV

    V (some long corticocortical)   corticostriatal
                                  corticorubral
                                  corticothalamic (intralaminar)
                                  corticobulbar
                                  corticospinal and corticotectal

    VI (some callosal-motor cortex)   corticothalamic (relay nucleus)

Figure 1 Laminar distribution of somata of cortical efferent (pyramidal) cells in monkeys as determined by retrograde labeling studies (see text). Vertical lines to right indicate zones of termination in sensory cortex of thalamic (solid lines) and corticocortical (interrupted line) afferents. In areas outside the primary sensory areas, thalamic fibers do not terminate in layer IV.

vocellular layers. These findings mean that it is now unlikely that axons projecting to one site in the central nervous system are collaterals of those projecting to another.

The laminar and sublaminar segregation of efferent cells according to their target sites is less well defined in nonprimates but mainly in relation to the supra- and infragranular dissociation of cortically and subcortically projecting cells. In the rat, for example, although subcortically projecting cells are segregated in layers V and VI, callosally projecting cells are found in these layers in numbers as great as in the supragranular layers (Wise and Jones, 1976). It is conceivable that this reflects the less distinct lamination of the nonprimate cortex. Another relevant factor may be that in the developing rodent brain, neurons destined to form a particular layer are generated over a relatively longer time span than in the primate (Caviness and Sidman, 1973). It is not known, however, whether the accumulation of cells generated at a particular time in a particular layer in the primate necessarily implies that these cells are preprogrammed to form a particular type of efferent connection.

Laminar Terminations of Thalamic Fibers

There is no close developmental relationship between efferent cells and afferent fibers—at least with regard to the positioning of the efferent cells—for in newborn rats and fetal cats (Wise, Hendry, and Jones, 1977; Wise, Fleshman, and Jones, 1979) corticofugal axons have reached targets as distant as the spinal cord before the growth of thalamic and other afferents into the cortex. However, following on from the above, it seems appropriate to ask whether afferent fibers from the thalamus, which have been known for many years to be distributed in the cortex in a laminated fashion, bear any consistent relationship to the laminae of efferent cells in the adult.

The terminal portions of thalamic fibers ramify to a large extent in the middle layers of the cortex (see, e.g., Jones and Burton, 1976). This has been interpreted for years to indicate that they terminate upon the small "granule cells" of layer IV. Though there is still good reason to believe that this is, indeed, the case (evidence reviewed in Jones, 1975a), we can no longer suppose that these cells are the exclusive recipients of thalamic terminals, nor even that they form a single cell class. First, in the primary sensory areas the thalamic afferent terminals extend well upward among the large, deeply situated pyramidal cells of layer III; in areas outside the primary sensory areas (constituting some 80% of the primate cortex) they avoid layer IV and terminate mainly in the deep part of layer III (Figure 2) (Jones and Burton, 1976). Whether this implies that a relevant recipient cell has moved out of layer IV in the nonprimary areas or that there is a definite shift of terminals away from a par-

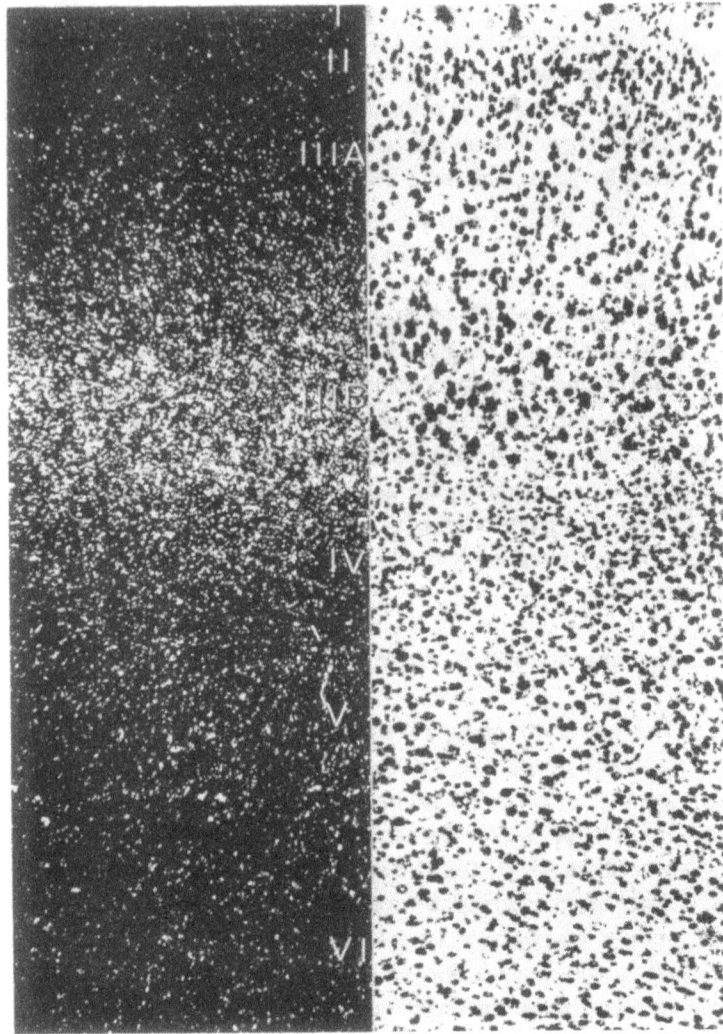

Figure 2 Bright-field and dark-field photomicrographs from the same field and at the same magnification (×110) showing labeling of terminal ramifications of thalamocortical axons in area 5 of the monkey parietal cortex. As in all areas outside the primary sensory areas, these are distributed largely among the deeper-seated pyramidal cells of layer III, rather than in layer IV. (From Jones and Burton, 1976.)

ticular cell class has not yet been determined. Nevertheless, termination on the basal dendrites of layer III pyramids, as first suggested by Valverde (1971), seems possible.

The second intimation that layer IV cells may not be the sole recipients of thalamic terminals arises from the fact that apical and basal dendrites of pyramidal cells and dendrites of nonpyramidal cells in adjacent layers traverse layer IV. The recent electron-microscopic evidence of Peters and his colleagues indicates that in rodents, at least, thalamic afferents may terminate seemingly quite indiscriminately on the dendrites of any cell type within their zone of termination (Peters, Feldman, and Saldanha, 1976; White, 1978). This, perhaps disappointing, result makes the likelihood of "hard wiring" between thalamic fiber and a particular class of cortical cell rather remote. It would, in any case, be rather surprising if thalamic inputs were to end solely on one class of cell, given the several varieties of interneuron present (Ramón y Cajal, 1911; Lund, 1973; Szentágothai, 1975, 1976; Jones, 1975a; Valverde, 1976). The situation is perhaps analogous to that in the cerebellar cortex, where mossy fibers terminate on Golgi cells as well as on granule cells, except that in the cerebral cortex there are several potential recipients. It may be necessary, therefore, to think of the circuitry in more complicated terms and with dynamic components, that is to say, of a fairly direct, and perhaps more secure transfer route from thalamic afferents to a particular class of recipient cell and thence to the output (pyramidal) cells, with subsidiary pathways via interneurons that serve to sculpt and focus the zone of excitation in much the same way that a Golgi cell focuses a zone of granule-cell excitation in the cerebellum (Eccles, Ito, and Szentágothai, 1967). There is also the potential for direct thalamic input to the output cells that may bypass any interneuronal pathways. Figure 3 indicates the cell classes with dendrites situated within the thalamic afferent plexus in the monkey sensory-motor cortex. Each of these probably receives thalamic synapses. The arrangement is typical of most cortical areas, though substantial modifications may occur in the visual cortex on account of its unique layering pattern and thalamic fiber distribution. Further details of potential interneuronal pathways will be taken up below.

A third factor to be taken into account when dealing with the terminations of thalamic afferents is that some of these or their branches may have preferential access to certain classes of pyramidal cells. Perhaps the best example of this is in the subsidiary layer of terminations at the junction of layers V and VI, now widely recognized in many species (see Jones and Burton, 1976). In the cat visual cortex, this zone of terminations, which is formed by collaterals of thalamic axons ascending to layer IV (Ferster and LeVay, 1978), has been suggested to be the basis for monosynaptic thalamic inputs to corticotectal cells. These, in turn, impose the property of direction selectivity on units in the superficial layers of the superior colliculus (Palmer and Rosenquist, 1974). If this

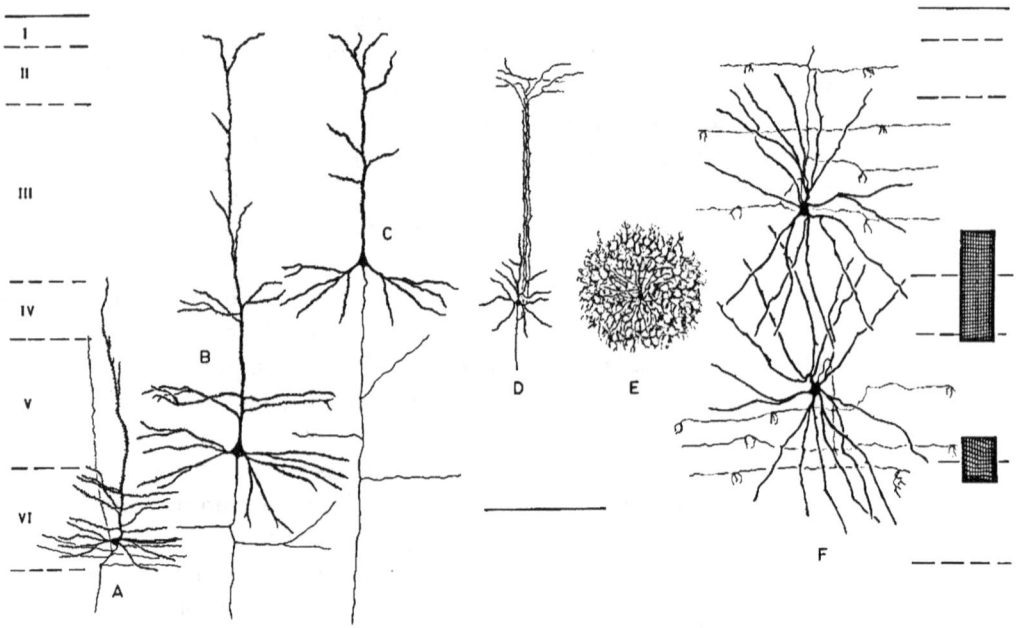

Figure 3 Semischematic drawing, mainly after Jones (1975a), showing cell classes with dendrites within the two zones of thalamic axon terminations (bars right) in monkey somatic sensory cortex. (A) Corticothalamic cell of layer VI; (B), (C) pyramidal cells of layers III and V; (D) small spiny cell with vertical axon branches; (E) Golgi type II cell; (F) basket cells. Bar represents approximately 500 μm.

suggestion should be validated, it would represent our best example yet of a tightly coupled input–output system in the cerebral cortex. It may be wondered whether there is a similar tight coupling between the corticothalamic cells of layer VI and the layer V–VI zone of thalamic terminations for, like many layer V cells, layer VI cells have pronounced dendritic branching plexuses confined to that region (Jones, 1975a; Lund and Boothe, 1975) (Figure 3). Monosynaptic thalamic terminations on corticothalamic cells (Bullier and Henry, 1979), bypassing the main region of elaboration of thalamic inputs in more superficial layers of the cortex, could provide rapid return signaling to the thalamic relay prior to the arrival of further afferent volleys.

Differential sublaminar distributions of thalamic fibers within the main (layer III–IV) zone of termination has only been identified in the visual cortex of cats and monkeys (Hubel and Wiesel, 1972; LeVay and Gilbert, 1976). Generally speaking, they represent the terminations of axons arising from different laminae in the lateral geniculate nucleus and from relay cells receiving inputs from different classes of retinal ganglion cell (see the chapter by Gilbert and Wiesel, in this volume). To date, there is no morphological evidence for their selective terminations on particular classes of cortical cell.

Diffuse cortical inputs from intralaminar and certain other classes of thalamic nuclei and from the various aminergic cell groups of the brain stem will not be considered here, though they clearly introduce another level of complexity into the system.

Laminar Terminations of Corticocortical Fibers

Apart from thalamic fibers, ipsilateral corticocortical and contralateral callosal fibers form the major inputs to a cortical area. In primates, each set of fibers, arising only in other cortical areas that are clearly specified for any particular area, terminate in layer IV and in all the supervening layers (Figure 1). Thus, although they overlap the terminal territory of thalamic fibers, they also involve more superficial layers (Jones, Burton, and Porter, 1975; Jones, Coulter, and Wise, 1979). The extent to which these sets of afferents terminate on cortical cells that are the same as or different from those receiving thalamic fibers is unknown. The more superficial extent of their terminal ramifications does not necessarily imply this for they could simply extend their terminations further along the apical dendritic systems of the same pyramidal cells.

In primates, in any particular area, ipsilateral and callosal fibers terminate in the layers (II–III) in which the cell bodies of origin of comparable fibers leaving that cortical area are mostly situated. In the callosal system there is reason to believe that commissural fibers terminate on the same class of pyramidal cells from which they arise in the opposite cortex. First, the system is organized with great topographic precision, so that in a connected area, only mirror-image points on the two sides are interconnected. Hence, double labeling involving injection of both retrograde and anterograde tracers at the same cortical point results in a focus of terminal axonal labeling exactly superimposed on a focus of retrograde labeling of deeper layer III pyramidal cells (Figure 4). Second, the shape of the focus of axonal labeling—wide in layer IV and the deeper part of layer III, narrow in upper layer III, and flaring out in layers II and I—suggests that it is conforming to the combined dendritic trees of the group of enclosed pyramidal cells (Figure 4). Electron microscopy (Jones and Powell, 1970) indicates terminations on pyramidal cells, though it does not rule out terminations on nonpyramidal cells contained within the focus or "column" of callosal axons as well.

Callosal Columns and Strips

The callosal system of fibers in the sensory-motor regions of the monkey (Jones, Burton, and Porter, 1975; Jones, Coulter, and Wise, 1979) furnishes an example of an afferent system in which the horizontal, laminar distribution that has been emphasized in all the afferent systems so far discussed is broken up into subsidiary foci in the vertical

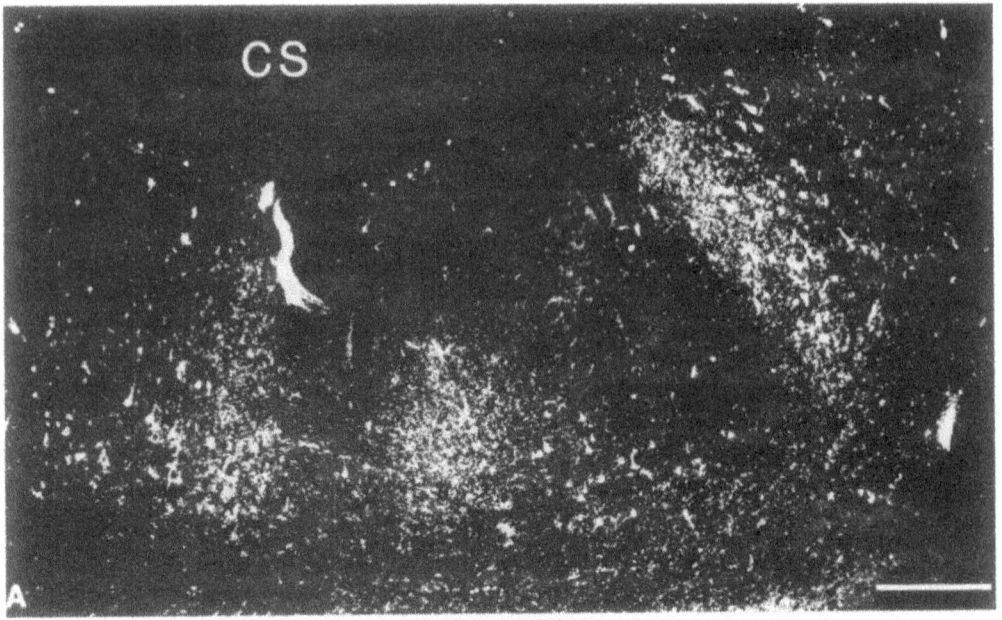

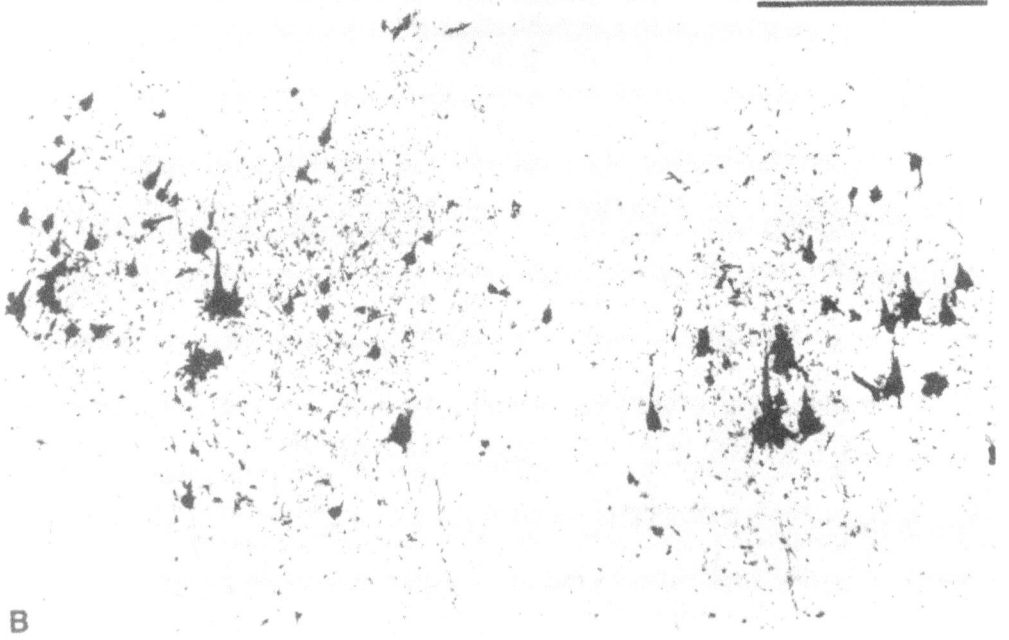

Figure 4 Dark-field (upper) and bright-field (lower) photomicrographs showing super-imposition of columns of anterograde and retrograde labeling of callosally projecting cells and axons following injection of horseradish peroxidase in a symmetrical region of the contralateral cortex. CS: central sulcus; bars represent 250 μm. (From Jones, Coulter, and Wise, 1979.)

dimension of the cortex. If the total distribution of callosal fibers is demonstrated by callosotomy, followed by staining with axonal degeneration techniques, three facts emerge: first, large parts of the hand and foot representations are free of callosal connections (Figure 5); second, within the connected regions, the callosal fibers terminate in focal bundles some 0.5–1 mm wide separated from their neighbors by less densely connected zones 0.25–0.5 mm wide (Figure 6); third, these focal bundles are aligned in register so as to form a series of strips oriented mediolaterally more or less in the long axes of the pre- and postcentral gyri (Figure 5). In view of the reciprocity of the system described above, a comparable experiment involving injection of a retrogradely transported label results in labeling of deep layer III pyramidal cells in exactly similar strips.

The disjunctive, column-like nature of callosal terminations has also been described in the auditory cortex of the cat. Here the bundles seem to impose on the cells in the column in which they terminate a particular kind of binaural interaction, different from that of cells in adjacent, unconnected columns (Imig and Brugge, 1978).

The column-like distribution, strip-like configuration, and reciprocity are also particularly well demonstrated in the somatic sensory

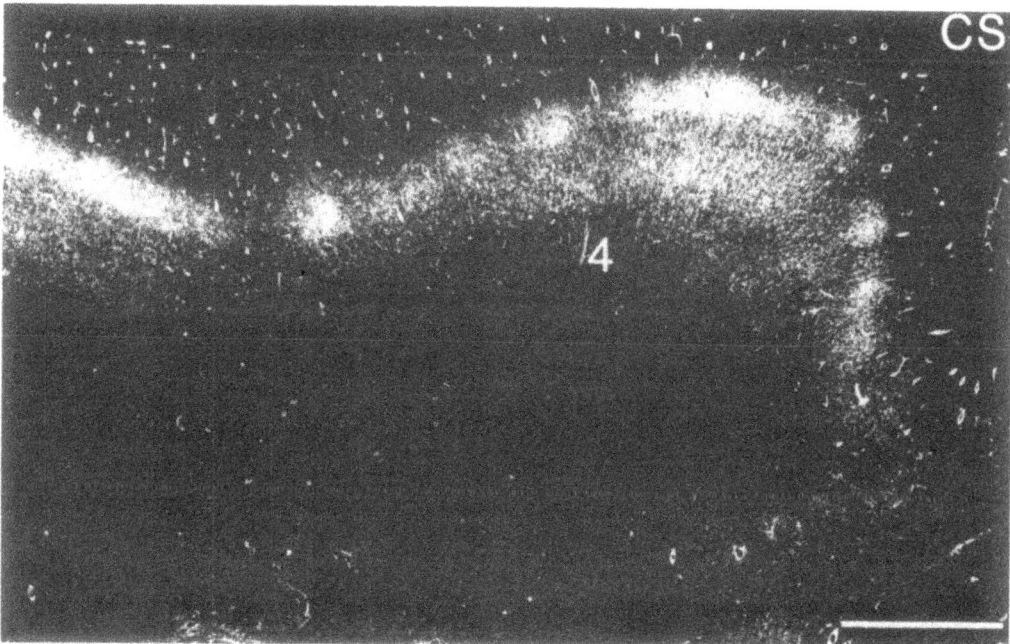

Figure 5A Dark-field photomicrograph showing multiple column-like clusters of callosal axon terminations in area 4 of monkey cortex following callosotomy and subsequent silver staining of degenerating axons. CS: central sulcus; bar represents 2 mm. (From Jones, Coulter, and Wise, 1979.)

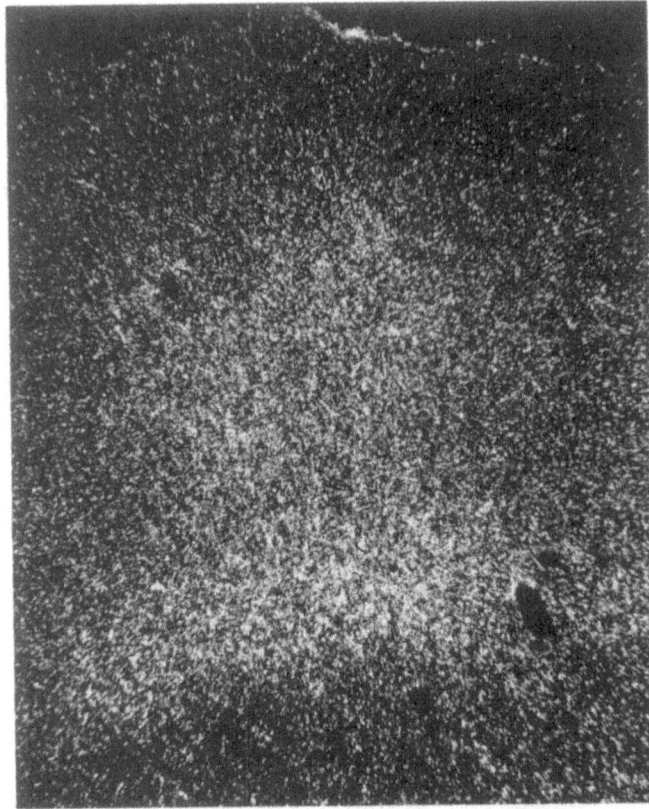

Figure 5B Column-like zone of termination of ipsilateral corticocortical fibers in granular and supragranular layers of monkey second somatic sensory area following injection of tritiated amino acids in first somatic area. Bar represents 250 μm. (From Jones, Burton, and Porter, 1975.)

cortex of species such as the rat (Wise and Jones, 1976), in which the aligned bundles serve to outline the topographic map of the body surface formed by the aggregations of granule cells in layer IV (Welker, 1976). The rat seems to be rather unusual in that there appears to be a complete dissociation of the terminal zones of callosal fibers from those of thalamic fibers arising in the ventrobasal complex (Figure 7). The thalamic fibers are distributed only to the granule-cell aggregations and the callosal fibers to the intervening and surrounding less granular zones (Wise and Jones, 1978). This has suggested some kind of competitive interaction between the two fiber systems during development, though attempts to manipulate the system experimentally so far have led to negative results (Wise and Jones, 1978). A dissociation of thalamic and callosal zones is not present in the primate, though it is clear that some parts of the sensory-motor cortex receive only thalamic inputs while others receive both thalamic and callosal inputs. To date there is

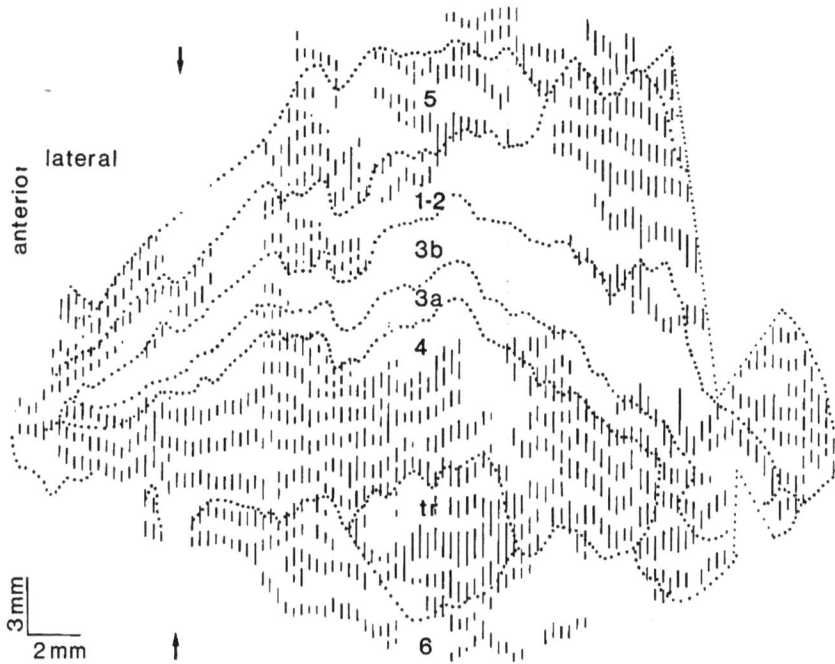

Figure 6 Unfolded surface reconstruction made from sagittal sections similar to that illustrated in Figure 5. Each line represents a column of callosal fiber terminations, which in connected regions tend to be aligned to form mediolaterally oriented strips. 1–6: fields of pre- and postcentral gyri; arrows indicate medial border of hemisphere. (From Jones, Coulter, and Wise, 1979.)

no obvious differentiation of function in terms of focal groupings of the two inputs.

The relationship between strip-like configurations of afferent fibers of different classes to one another is not yet entirely clear. In the primate visual cortex the strip-like arrangements of thalamic fiber terminations that constitute the ocular-dominance columns meet the representation of the vertical meridian of the visual field at right angles (LeVay, Hubel, and Wiesel, 1975). This would imply that the single strip of callosal fibers that runs along the vertical meridian (Zeki, 1978) crosses their ends orthogonally. In the somatic sensory cortex, thalamic-fiber strips have not been identified, so the geometric relationships, if any, of callosal and thalamic fibers in that area are not clear. Powell and Mountcastle (1959) noted that as a microelectrode traversed the posterior bank of the central sulcus dorsoventrally (anteroposteriorly) there was little change in the positions of the receptive fields of successively encountered single units. Conversely, mediolateral penetrations encountered abrupt shifts in receptive-field position. If this can be taken to imply that thalamic input fibers are aligned to form strips running anteroposteriorly across the somatic sensory cortex, then the callosal strips would

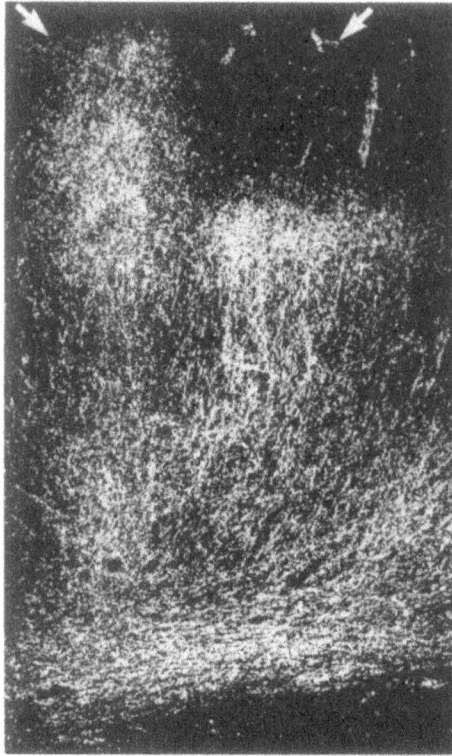

Figure 7 Double-labeling experiment showing dissociation of column of callosal fiber terminations (left) from column of thalamic fiber terminations in rat somatic sensory cortex; ×60. (From Wise and Jones, 1978.)

also cross their ends at right angles (Figure 8), but there is no anatomical confirmation of this yet. Even if the anatomical arrangements depicted in Figure 8 should prove to be correct, we still need to know what is being mapped in the mediolateral (y) dimension and what in the (x) dimension orthogonal to this.

The relationship of strip-like arrangements of callosal and ipsilateral corticocortical fibers also needs to be examined further. It is not clear whether there are distinct zones of dominance or whether there is superimposition of the terminals of these two afferent systems (Figure 5). More work also needs to be done to determine whether the axons of the two systems arise from entirely separate populations of cells, though there is evidence that shorter ipsilateral fibers arise from cells separate from those giving rise to callosal fibers (Jones and Wise, 1977).

Focal Input and Axonal Bundling—Thalamic

The evidence from the callosal system that focal aggregations of cells in one hemisphere give rise to column-like bundles of fibers that termi-

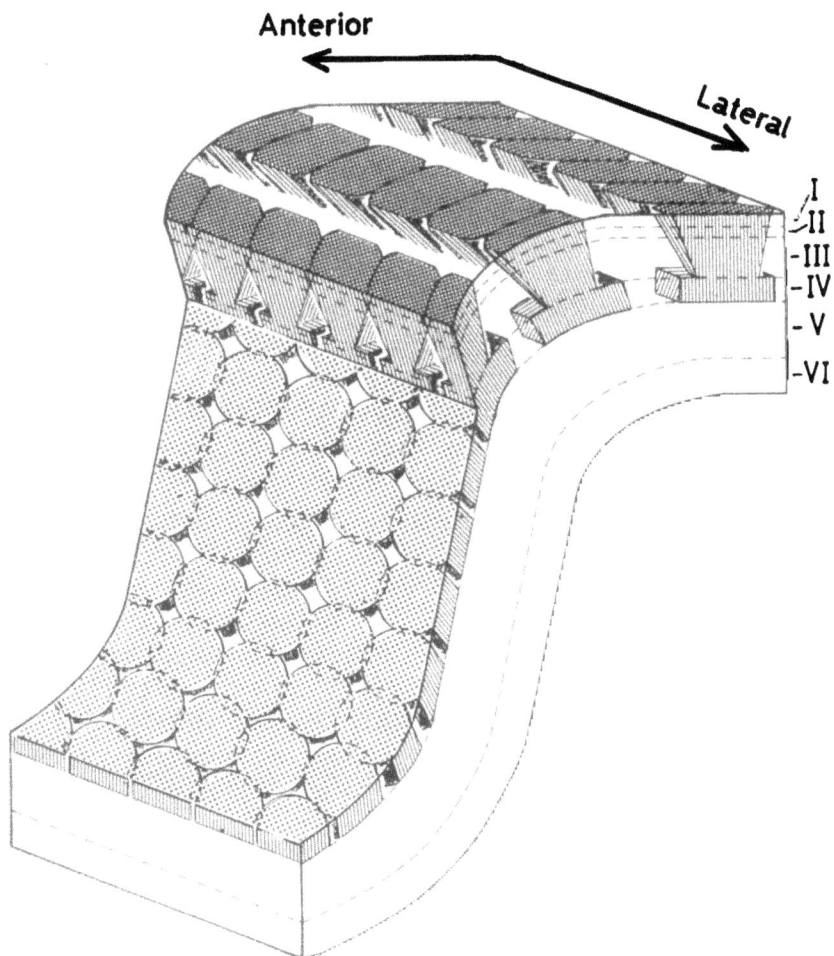

Figure 8 Hypothetical drawing, based upon observations of Powell and Mountcastle (1959), Jones, Coulter, and Wise (1979), and material illustrated in Figures 9–11, showing potential relationship between columns of thalamocortical fiber terminations (light stipple) and columns of callosal fiber terminations (heavy stipple) in postcentral gyrus of monkey.

nate in equally discrete foci in the contralateral hemisphere raises the possibility that the thalamic afferent system may be organized along similar lines. Moreover, the realization that callosal columns form strip-like configurations reproducible from animal to animal raises the question whether these have some preferred relationship to equally stereotyped configurations of thalamic fibers such as that predicted in Figure 8.

Of course, the strip-like nature of ocular-dominance "columns" in the primate visual cortex has been known for some years (Hubel and Wiesel, 1972, 1977). However, it is not known whether each of these consists of nonoverlapping focal zones of thalamic input or whether there is extensive overlap along the length of a strip.

In the first somatic sensory cortex (SI) of the monkey, recent anatomical evidence indicates that inputs from small groupings of thalamic cells may be distributed in a relatively nonoverlapping manner. The evidence is twofold: first, punctate injections of horseradish peroxidase, 1–2 mm in extent in the cortex, retrogradely label only one or two equally localized focal groupings of cells in the thalamus (Jones, Wise, and Coulter, 1979) (Figure 9); second, in the tongue representation, receiving mechanoreceptive and gustatory inputs, small isolated bundles of thalamic axons, 0.5–1 mm wide, emanating from the gustatory relay nucleus are clearly dissociated from those arising in the mechanoreceptive relay nucleus (Burton and Jones, 1976) (Figure 10). Elsewhere in the somatic sensory cortex, similar bundles appear to exist (Figure 11) but, in being aligned side by side, it is difficult to "dissect them out" in isolation. The aggregation of thalamic cells upon which the bundling of thalamocortical fibers seems to depend is particularly well seen in small mammals such as the rat, in which it is possible to label retrogradely virtually every thalamic relay cell from a single large cortical injection of horseradish peroxidase (Wise and Jones, 1978) (Figure 12). Although combined labeling of relay cells and afferent fibers has not been carried out, there is reason to believe that these aggregations of relay cells represent groupings that are the targets of incoming medial lemniscal fibers which are also distributed in focal groupings (Ramón y Cajal, 1911; Hand and van Winkle, 1977) (Figure 13). Bundling of lemniscal fibers occurs, and in the rat trigeminal system, at least, such bundles maintain the topographic relationships between peripheral structures such as sinus hairs and their central representations (Killackey and Belford, 1976). Perhaps of greater consequence is the work of Poggio and Mountcastle (1963), which indicates that the focal aggregations of thalamic cells in the monkey have the same place and modality characteristics. "Modality" in their sense is a fairly broadly based term and does not necessarily imply that each focal aggregation receives inputs from only one class of peripheral receptor situated at a particular "place" in the receptive periphery.

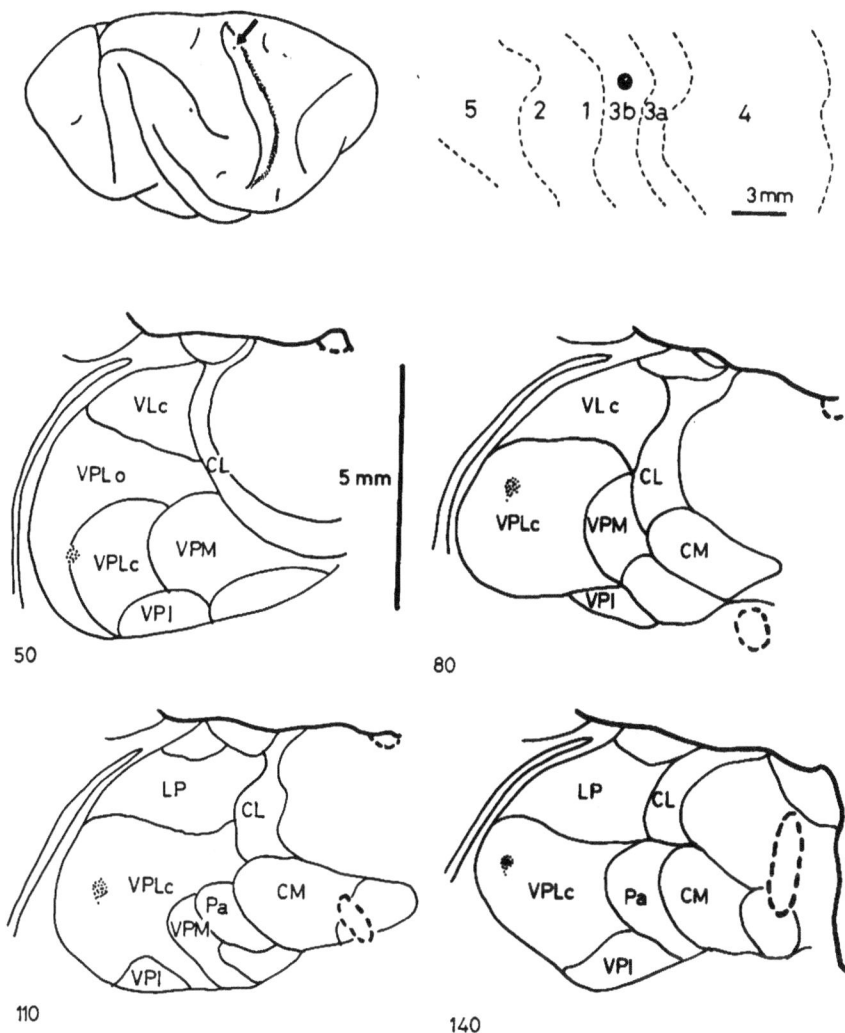

Figure 9 Projection drawings of frontal sections (lower) from thalamus of a monkey brain showing focal distribution of retrogradely labeled cells following an injection of horseradish peroxidase in posterior bank of central sulcus (top left) and involving area 3b over an extent of approximately 1 mm (top right). Numbers on sections indicate anteroposterior sequence of 50-μm-thick sections.

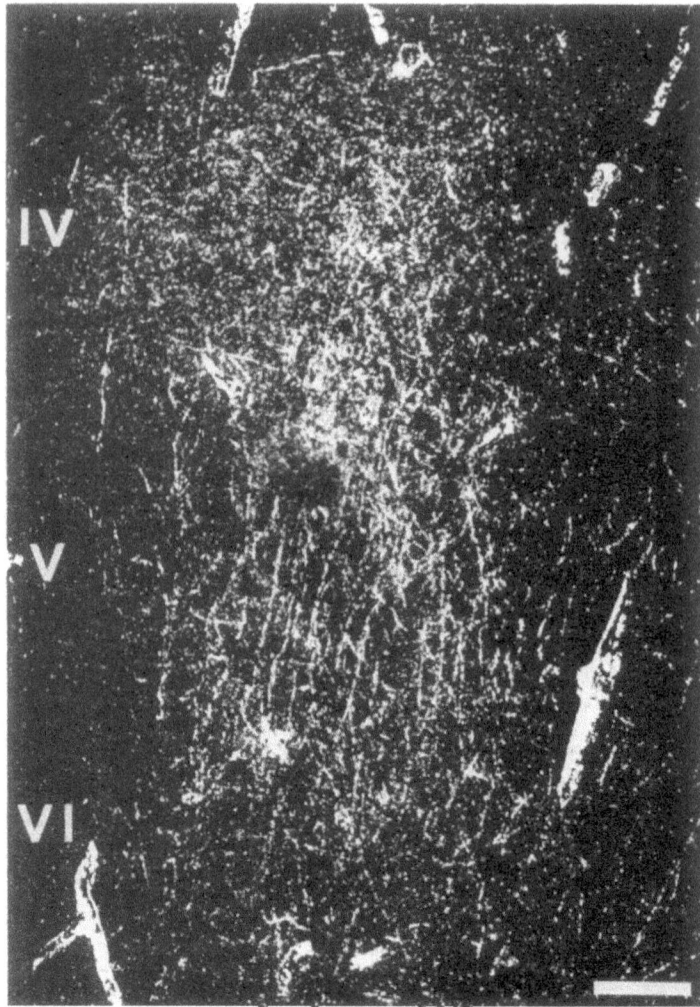

Figure 10 Small bundle of degenerating thalamocortical fibers terminating in gustatory region of somatic sensory cortex following destruction of taste relay nucleus of monkey thalamus (from material illustrated in Burton and Jones, 1976).

E. G. Jones

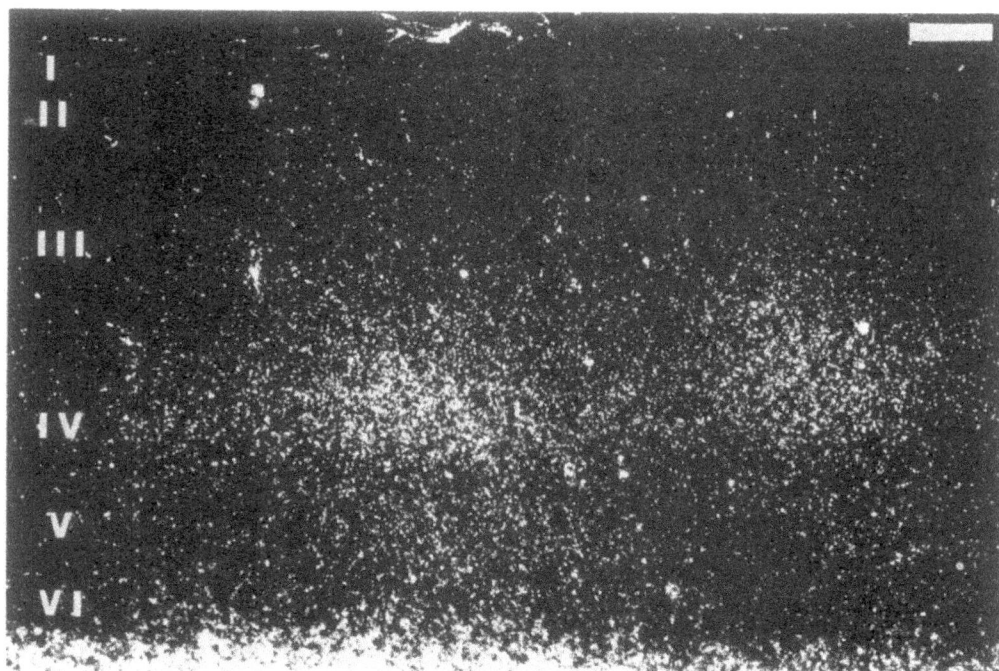

Figure 11 Two foci of autoradiographically labeled, thalamocortical terminal bundles in posterior bank of central sulcus of a monkey following injection of tritiated amino acids into a cluster of thalamic cells, comparable to that illustrated in Figure 9 and identified on the basis of a multiunit response to cutaneous stimulation of a localized region of the contralateral forearm. (From unpublished material of D. P. Friedman and E. G. Jones.)

All of the above leads up to the suggestion that an effective unit of thalamocortical input is not the single thalamocortical fiber but a bundle of such fibers arising from a small group of thalamic cells whose aggregation is determined by their input from a group of afferent fibers of like place and modality characteristics in the sense of Poggio and Mountcastle. The specificity of such a unit and, more particularly, the degree to which this specificity is imposed upon recipient cells in the cortex will obviously be determined by the degree of overlap, caused by axonal branches leaving one bundle of thalamocortical fibers to join another. In the first somatic sensory area extensive branching of this nature seems to be unusual, though there may be overlap at the edges of adjacent bundles and branching within a bundle is considerable. In the visual cortex there is minimal overlap between bundles destined for adjacent left- and right-eye ocular-dominance strips, but single fibers may send branches to two left or to two right ocular-dominance strips (Ferster and LeVay, 1978), and the degree of overlap within a strip remains unknown. Extensive branching leading to widely dissociated

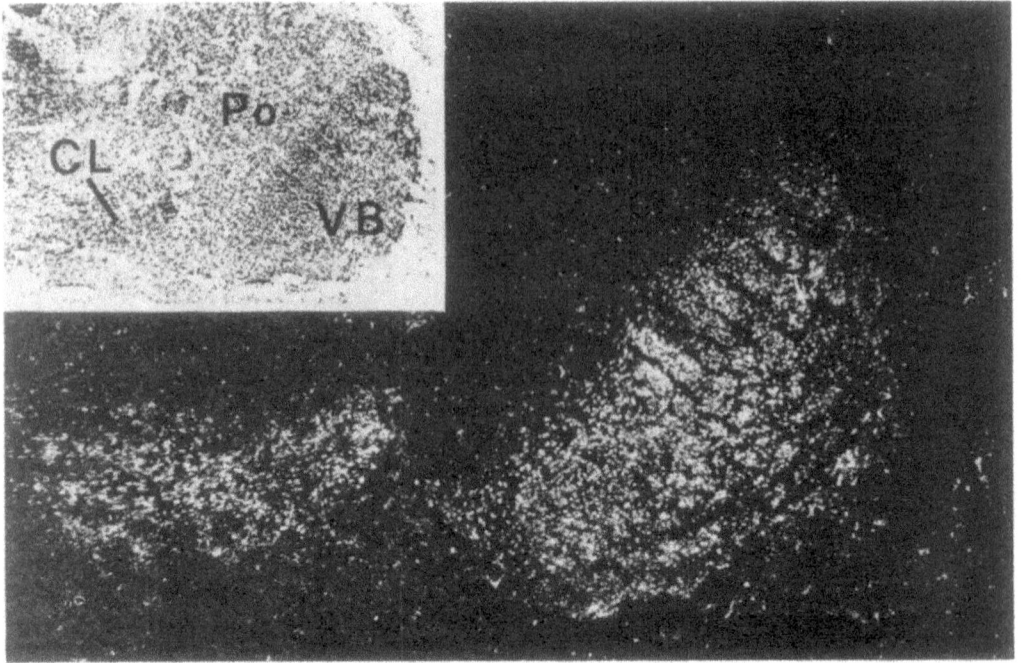

Figure 12 Retrograde labeling of focal aggregations of relay cells in thalamic ventrobasal complex (VB) of a young rat following injection of horseradish peroxidase in somatic sensory cortex. Other retrogradely labeled cells are in central lateral nucleus (CL); ×65, inset ×25. (From Wise and Jones, 1978.)

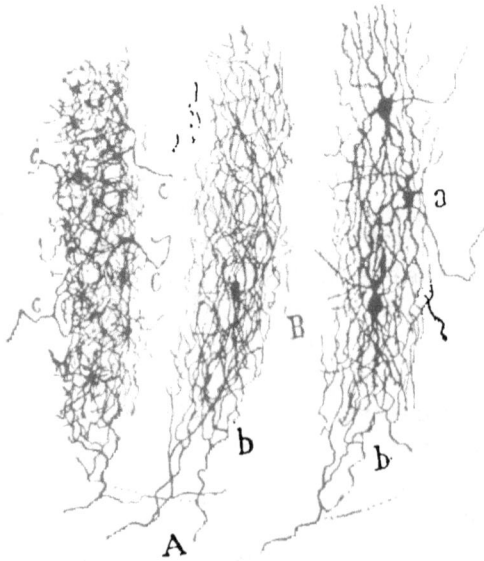

Figure 13 Clustered nature of thalamocortical relay cells and of lemniscal and corticothalamic fibers in horizontal section of mouse thalamus. (From Ramón y Cajal, 1911.)

zones dominated by a single class of afferent input has been reported in the motor cortex (Asanuma et al., 1974), but the extent of segregation of these zones from adjacent zones has been a matter of some controversy. Branching of thalamic fibers so as to give inputs to two cortical areas, such as occurs between thalamic ventrobasal cells and the first (SI) and second (SII) somatic sensory areas (Jones, 1975b), is at a different level of organization from that being considered here.

None of these known branching patterns necessarily implies a break-down in a tightly coupled system of thalamocortical bundles and recipient cells, for it would be possible for a single thalamic cell aggregation to provide multiple input bundles, each segregated from one another and from its neighbors. This would have important implications for the way in which the body-surface or other receptor sheet is represented within a single cortical area. The anatomical results in the SI cortex, however, are against multiple input bundles arising from single thalamic foci (though adjacent thalamic foci may project to divergent cortical foci).

It would probably be wrong to assume that cortical cells toward the perimeter of one focal input zone necessarily receive only axons of the input bundle to that zone, for there is probably some degree of overlap from adjacent zones. Though the anatomy, so far as it stands, would suggest that such cells should receive the majority of their inputs from the relevant bundle, a totally segregated system of this sort would be contrary to the organization known to exist in the majority of comparable neural networks. It is to be assumed, therefore, that interneuronal mechanisms, analogous for example to the case of the cerebellar Golgi cell, quoted above, may be involved in focusing and otherwise molding the focal input. A task for the future will be to decide to what extent comparable mechanisms serve to refine and focus single fiber inputs within a bundle, in other words, the extent to which separate receptor inputs can remain dissociated within the afferent bundle or maintained as separate by central mechanisms. In the somatic sensory cortex, the segregation of inputs from slowly and rapidly adapting mechanoreceptors (see the chapter by Kaas et al., this volume) would imply that convergence is not necessarily total.

Vertical Interactions Within the Cortex

One of the major effects of the previously outlined inputs to the cortex is presumably the generation of some kind of output. Outputs must be twofold: corticocortical, presumably involved in integrative aspects of cortical function, leading at the highest level to perception and the like; and corticosubcortical, leading to interactions with sensory relay centers and with motor control centers of the brain stem and spinal cord.

The relay of afferent, particularly thalamic, input to layers of cortex lying above and below the zone of thalamic terminations has been a source of interest since the first anatomical analyses of Lorente de Nó (1938), the interpretations of which were based upon excitatory mechanisms and reverberatory circuits. Since then, such study has received added impetus from the physiological observations mainly in the visual cortex (Hubel and Wiesel, 1968), but to some extent also in the somatic sensory cortex (Whitsel, Roppollo, and Werner, 1972), that cells in the heart of the thalamic afferent plexus have simple receptive fields while those in deeper and in more superficial layers have relatively more complex receptive fields. The latter implies that "simple" cells converge upon the "complex" cells. A wiring diagram for such a circuit was relatively easy to construct when it was assumed that thalamic afferents terminated on one class of cell in layer IV which then sent its axon to terminate upon immediately superficial and deep cells. Such a hypothesis formed the basis for Kelly and Van Essen's (1974) interpretation of their results when they noted that, of a small sample of cells injected with Procion yellow in the cat visual cortex, the majority with complex receptive fields were pyramidal cells and the majority with simple receptive fields were nonpyramidal.

Despite the apparently increasing complexity in their peripheral receptive fields, superficial and deep cells in narrow 0.5–1-mm-wide vertical ("columnar") groupings tend to preserve many of the spatial and modality characteristics of layer IV cells within the same grouping. This fact lies at the heart of the columnar hypothesis of sensory cortical organization, as originally proposed by Mountcastle (1957), and it implies that in the traditional circuitry, the interlaminar connections arising from layer IV should be vertical and confined to rather narrow domains no wider than a zone of focal thalamic input.

It has become increasingly difficult to accept a simple circuit diagram based upon a single thalamic recipient cell because of the evidence, outlined earlier, that thalamic afferents may end on many classes of nonpyramidal cells and also directly on pyramidal cells. The latter finding probably accounts for the observation that many cells with "simple" receptive fields in the visual cortex are pyramidal rather than nonpyramidal (see the chapter by Gilbert and Wiesel, this volume). Conversely, in the major example where a monosynaptic thalamic input to pyramidal cells seems assured—the case of lateral geniculate inputs to corticotectal cells—the relevant cells have properties that would cause them to be classified as complex cells (Palmer and Rosenquist, 1974; Bullier and Henry, 1979).

However, there is no reason why the simple circuit should not form one of several synaptic routes through the cortex. Indeed, it would seem to be the most logical to recruit, in a systematic way, pyramidal cells in all layers in order to preserve the spatial and modality characteristics and the restricted focal domain of influence of an underlying thalamic input bundle. The illustrations of Sokoloff and his colleagues (Kennedy et al., 1976) indicate by means of the 2-deoxyglucose technique that the flow of activity in the cortex following thalamic activation is in the vertical dimension: following stimulation of one eye in monkeys, the label, though maintaining the width of a typical ocular-dominance column as seen with thalamic fiber-labeling alone, now extends out of layer IV into the superficial and deep layers. Although this could still reflect activation of superficial and deep pyramidal cells by means of thalamic synapses directly upon them, this is not cause to rule out parallel and perhaps more secure circuits based upon concentrated inputs from intermediate cells.

Such an intermediate interneuron has been clearly identified in the visual and somatic sensory cortex of the primate by Szentágothai (1969, 1976), Valverde (1971), and Jones (1975a). It is spiny and appears to be a major recipient of thalamic afferents. The axon is its most distinctive feature for it has strongly recurrent branches that ascend vertically as a tight bundle enclosing, as in a sleeve, a group of pyramidal-cell apical dendrites (Figures 14A,B). Such dendrites can belong to pyramidal cells with somata in all layers, but especially layers III and V. The synapses between the axon and the apical dendrites appear to be effected upon the dendritic spines of the latter, and electron microscopy indicates that the majority of such synapses have the morphological features of excitatory synapses.

This interneuron is thus in a position to relay thalamic effects to pyramidal cells of all layers while preserving, because of its verticality, the focal nature of the thalamic input in a narrow column-like zone. Since the dendritic fields of these interneurons are only about 100 μm wide and their ascending axonal bundles even less, many can be accommodated in a 0.5–1-mm-wide zone of thalamic terminations. It is unknown whether each cell should be considered a unit subsidiary to the thalamic input bundle or whether mechanisms, based upon other interneurons, exist for focusing single thalamic-fiber inputs within a bundle onto single cells of this class.

Input Columns Are Also Output Columns

The vertical circuitry described above ensures that a focal zone of thalamic afferent terminations becomes a vertical column extending through most layers of the cortex. But this is an output as well as an input column for the pyramidal cells upon which the vertical interneuron terminates are the efferent elements of the cortex. Since pyramidal cells, because of their size, are probably the major cell class sampled in experiments in which cortical "columns" are defined in terms of single-unit responses to peripheral stimuli, it would be artificial to separate an input column from an output column. Some reflection of a column-like arrangement of efferent cells may be seen in the distribu-

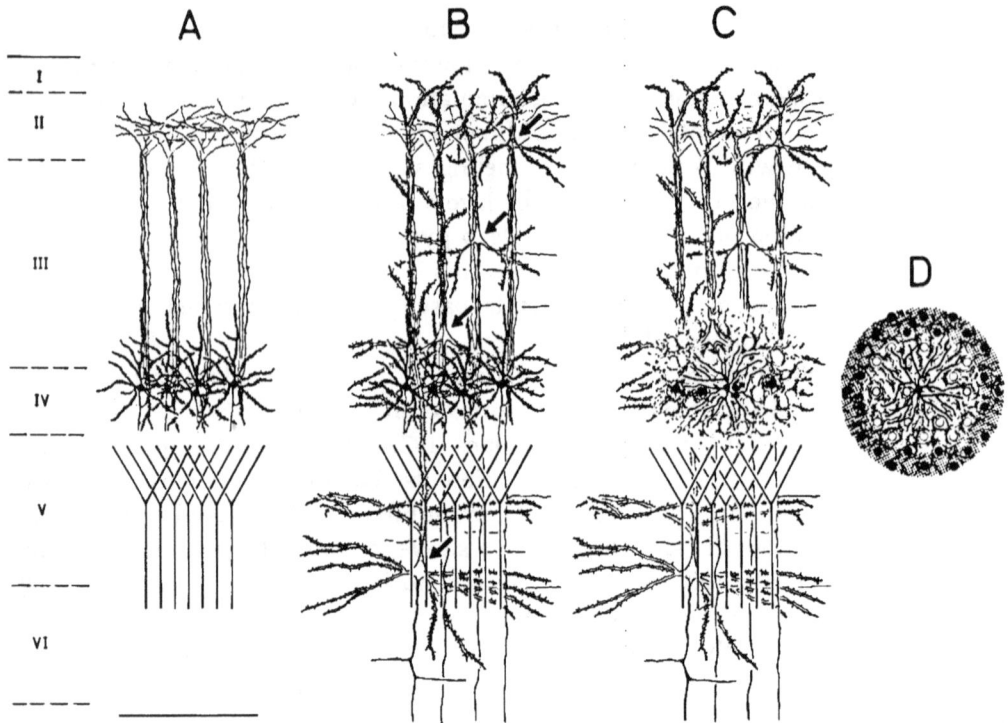

Figure 14 Semischematic figure, drawn mainly from Valverde (1971) and Jones (1975), showing postulated input–output columns based upon bundling of thalamocortical fibers. Focal nature of such input is maintained throughout thickness of cortex by small spiny cells with vertical axons (A) which receive thalamocortical synapses. Vertical axons by synapsing on pyramidal cells of all layers (B) ensure that input column is also an output column. Focal nature of inputs is thought to be maintained and "focused" by putatively inhibitory Golgi type II cells, also receiving thalamic synapses (C) and serving to inhibit (D) small spiny cells less strongly excited at perimeter of thalamic input zone (black and stipple). Note that synaptic relationships outlined do not exclude terminations of thalamic fibers on other classes of cortical interneurons nor directly on pyramidal cells (see text). Bar represents approximately 500 μm.

tion not only, as pointed out above, of callosally projecting cells, but also of many other classes of cortical efferent cell (Jones and Wise, 1977). Instead of being distributed homogeneously, these are broken up into clusters and strip-like aggregations of variable size (Figure 15). It remains to be seen whether a focal thalamic input interacts by means of the vertical interneurons with every class of efferent cell or selectively with certain classes. Because of the clumped nature of different classes of efferent cell, it is conceivable that a particular thalamic input focus might predominantly influence one or a few classes of output cell but, equally, such a focus could interact with representatives of all classes. The only situation in which there seems to be a clear dissociation of clusters of output cells from one another and from afferent inputs is in the rat somatic sensory cortex, where subcortically projecting cells lie deep to the granular aggregations that receive ventrobasal thalamic fibers and separate from the callosally connected zones (Wise, Murray, and Coulter, 1978).

One reason for believing that cortical output may be just as highly focused as the input is found in the callosal system already discussed. Groupings of callosally projecting cells give rise to axons that terminate in an exactly homotopic zone with little or no divergence. Where heterotopic callosal projections are known, such as that from SI to the contralateral SII, these, too, are precisely focused to terminate in homologous parts of the body representation (Jones, Coulter, and Wise, 1979).

A further example of precise reciprocity is found in the corticothalamic projection to the thalamic relay nucleus appropriate to a particular cortical area. Double-labeling techniques comparable to those used to demonstrate the callosal system show that a cluster of thalamic cells providing input to a focal cortical zone receive returning fibers only from layer VI cells deep to that zone and that these fibers do not distribute outside the cell cluster (Jones, Wise, and Coulter, 1979). This would again imply that there is little divergence of outputs from a cortical efferent column. Once again, of course, it must be stressed that these observations are made at a relatively gross morphological level; absolute and rigid segregation of such columns or their terminal territories is not necessarily implied.

Horizontal Interactions within the Cortex

Though once again speaking in more or less absolute terms when in reality a greater degree of dynamism is probably present, it is possible to identify interneuronal circuit elements that may provide for horizontal interactions between focal zones of activity determined by thalamic inputs (Figure 16). These are the so-called basket cells first convincingly demonstrated by Marin-Padilla (1969) in the human motor cortex and now recognized in other cortical areas as well (Jones, 1975a; Szen-

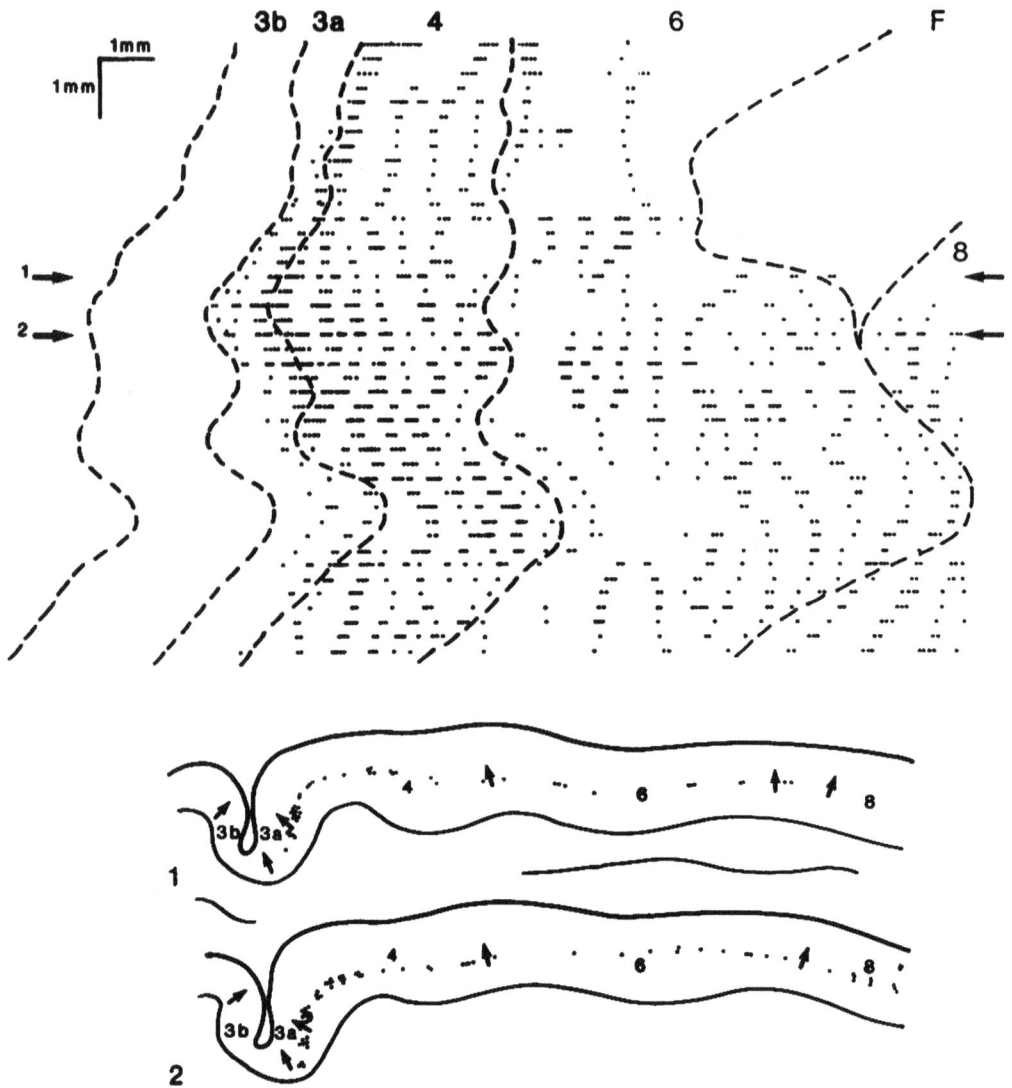

Figure 15 Surface map (upper) made from sagittal sections (lower) of a monkey brain showing clustered nature of one class of cortical efferent cell (corticorubral cells) following injection of horseradish peroxidase in the ipsilateral red nucleus. (From Jones and Wise, 1977.)

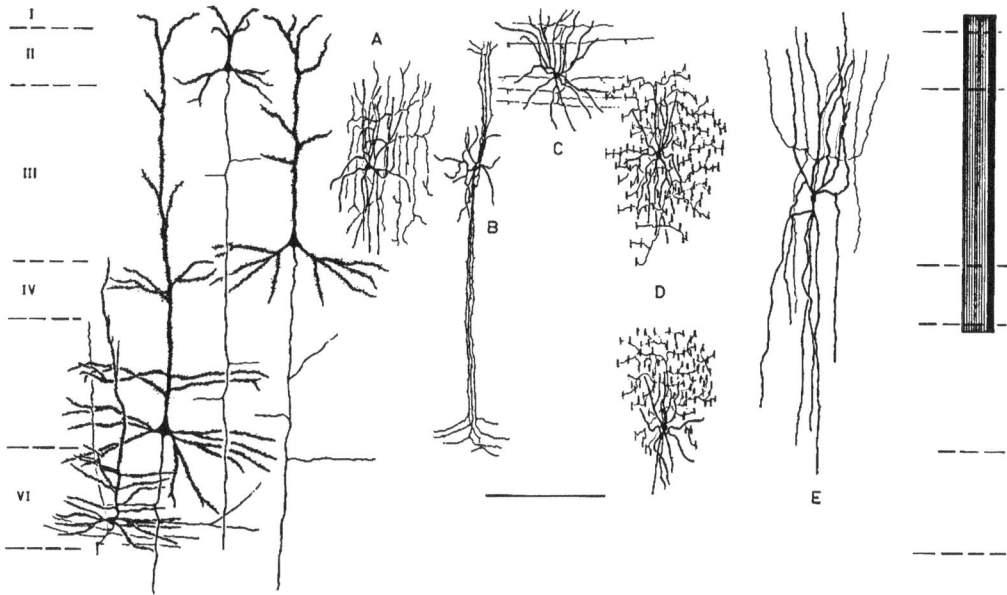

Figure 16 (A)—(E) Classes of cortical interneuron most of which do not have dendrites within the zones of thalamic fiber terminations and about which little is known, drawn after Jones (1975a). (A) Common cell with local axonal arcades; (B) double bouquet cell; (C) small basket cell of layer II; (D) chandelier cells; (E) large, possibly peptide-containing cell. Large bar at right indicates laminar distribution of corticocortical fiber terminals in monkey. Small horizontal bar represents approximately 500 μm.

tágothai, 1976). There is reason to believe that the terminal configurations generated by the axons of these large cells on pyramidal-cell somata are less dense and less basket-like than those generated by cells of the same name on Purkinje cells in the cerebellum. Nevertheless, they provide an example of a very precisely ordered interneuronal system, for in the pre- and postcentral gyri they are oriented as flattened disks in a plane at right angles to the long axes of the gyri. Their axons have horizontal branches which extend for long distances (1–2 mm) in the same plane and in most layers of the cortex. Such cells are sufficiently large to have at least some of their dendrites in layer IV and, thus, may well receive thalamic inputs. There seems little doubt that they should be considered a class of large inhibitory interneuron, for not only do their axon terminals on pyramidal-cell somata have the morphological characteristics of inhibitory synapses, but a comparison with the work of Ribak (1978) in the rat would suggest that they are one class of cell showing immunocytochemical labeling with antibodies to glutamic acid decarboxylase (Figure 17).

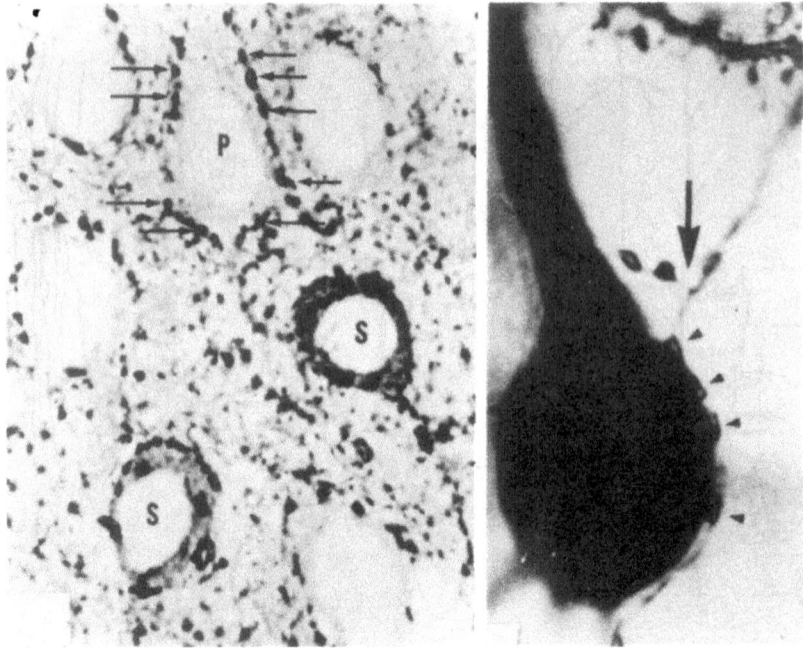

Figure 17 (Left) Immunocytochemical labeling of large cortical interneurons (S) and their axon terminals (arrows) with labeled antibodies to glutamic acid decarboxylase in rat visual cortex. (From Ribak, 1978, by courtesy of Dr. Charles Ribak.) Labeled terminals on pyramidal cell somata (P) are thought to correspond to those of basket cells (Figures 3, 18) demonstrable by Golgi impregnation on pyramidal cell somata (right) in monkey sensory-motor cortex; left ×1250, right ×725. (From Jones, 1975.)

Given these facts, it is likely that in the sensory-motor cortex, the basket cells could provide inhibitory interactions operating at preferred orientations and in all cortical layers between vertical groupings of cortical cells dependent upon focal thalamic inputs (Figure 18). This would have implications for the observations of Powell and Mountcastle (1959) that excitation of one place- and modality-specific column in the somatic sensory cortex is accompanied by inhibition in adjacent columns. Unfortunately, no comparable inhibition-based effect has been demonstrated in the visual cortex. However, the intracortical mechanisms responsible for the generation of columns or slabs of cells responding to particularly oriented visual stimuli and which seem to have a preferred orientation with respect to the ocular-dominance strips (Hubel, Wiesel, and Stryker, 1978), would seem to require the activities of interneurons with stereotyped axonal arborizations of this type.

The only other cortical axons that are consistently oriented in the horizontal dimension are the axon collaterals of pyramidal cells. It prob-

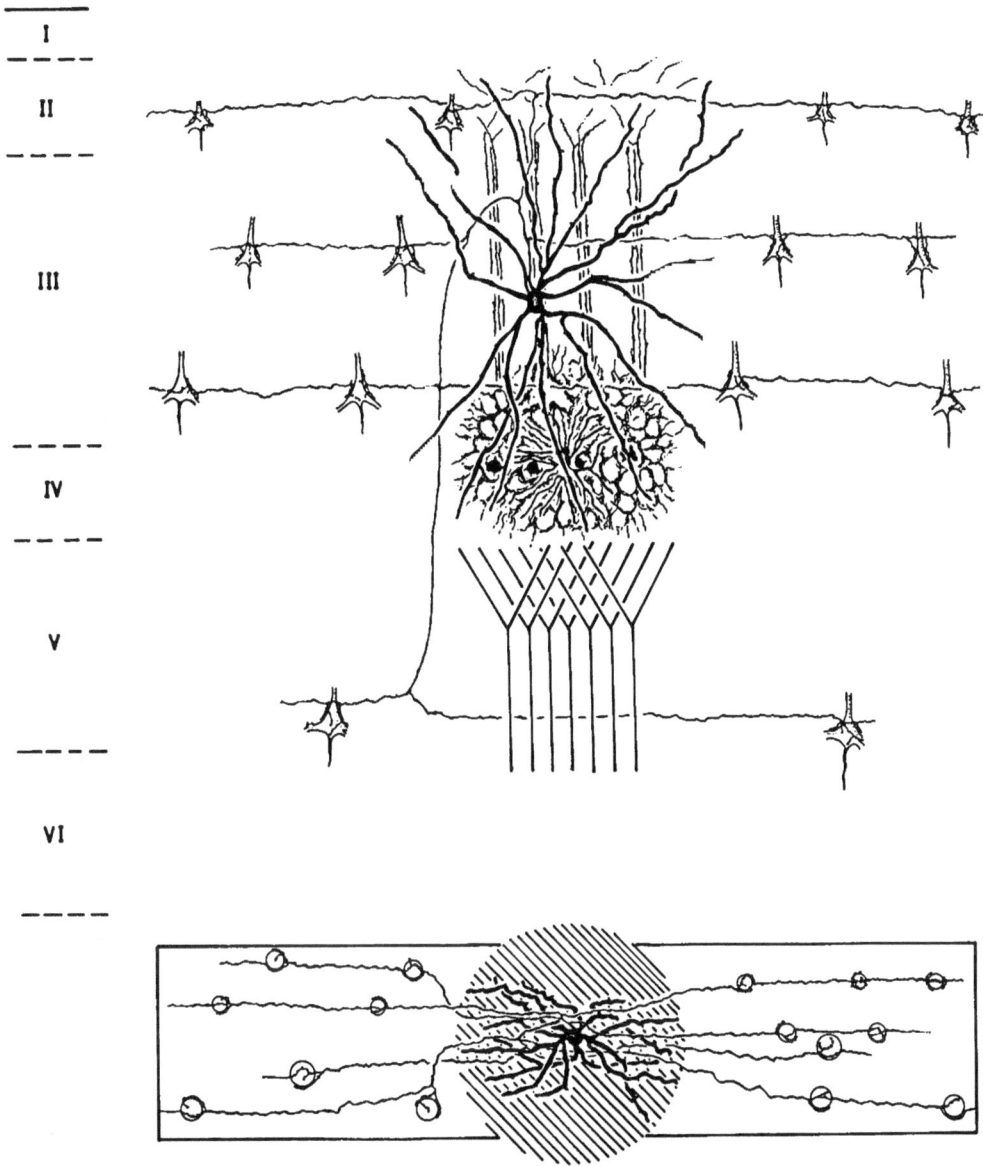

Figure 18 Semischematic drawing after Marin-Padilla (1969) and Jones (1975a), showing (upper) a large basket cell of the monkey sensory-motor cortex, its relation to the vertical input–output bundles illustrated in Figure 14, its long axon branches and their terminations (Figure 17) in all layers. Lower figure indicates preferred orientation of cell and its axon branches as a flattened slab or disk with the axon branches extending across several input–output columns and probably serving to inhibit the pyramidal cells of those on each side of a focal zone of excitation (hatching).

ably can be safely assumed now that pyramidal cells of all layers have a long axon that leaves the cortex either to reach a subcortical destination or to reenter another cortical area. Collateral branches, on the other hand, tend to remain within the cortical area in which the parent cell lies, being particularly concentrated in layers III and V (Figures 3, 16). Though some workers have emphasized the recurrent nature of such collaterals, others have been more impressed by their largely horizontal or oblique orientation. Irrespective of this, too little is known of their distribution or their preferred orientations, if any, and apart from the interesting predictions of Gilbert and Wiesel (this volume), there is virtually no indication of their physiological effects. Since all efferent connections of the cortex appear to be excitatory, the collaterals, too, would presumably have such an effect, as originally suggested by Phillips (1959); but its relative efficacy upon cortical cells cannot be predicted.

Other Cortical Interneurons

After the vertical and horizontal interneurons just described, several other classes can be distinguished on the basis of their axonal ramifications. This seems to be the only way of successfully distinguishing morphological classes of nonpyramidal cells, for their dendritic configurations can be very similar. One cell class which seems to invite speculation is the classical Golgi type II cell of layer IV (called a "spider-web" cell by Ramón y Cajal, 1911) with a densely but locally ramifying unmyelinated axon (Figures 3, 14C). These ramifications in the monkey somatic and visual areas (Valverde, 1971; Jones, 1975a), spread over territories approximately 500 μm $\times$ 500 μm, and Valverde considers that they may each be preferentially distributed to 300–500 of the interneurons with vertical axons, for these make up the bulk of the rest of the population of layer IV and their somata seem to fill the interstices of the Golgi type II plexus. The Golgi type II cells have dendrites like those of glutamic acid decarboxylase containing cells (Ribak, 1978) and have a strong resemblance to known inhibitory neurons elsewhere. If we assume that they are inhibitory and that they also receive thalamic inputs, their effect could well be to selectively inhibit vertical axon cells weakly excited at the perimeter of a focal zone of thalamic input. In this way, they would tend to focus the input zone (Figure 14C) and maintain its individuality, much as Golgi cells are postulated to do with mossy fiber inputs in the cerebellum, as mentioned in an earlier section.

Other interneurons whose physiological effects cannot be readily predicted are the so-called "chandelier cells" of Szentágothai (1976) that dominate layer III (Figure 16) (Jones, 1975a). Their axons are definitely very locally ramifying and seem to be selectively oriented depending upon the depth of the cell in layer III. They seem to terminate in presumed inhibitory synapses on the initial axon segments of pyramidal cells (Somogyi, 1977). Other rather common cells with loosely ramifying axons (Figure 16), concentrated in layer III (Jones, 1975a) and thought by Szentágothai to be inhibitory, may prove to be comparable to the stellate cells of the cerebellar cortex that are weakly inhibitory to Purkinje cells. Perhaps as in the cerebellar cortex, they serve to further focus column-like zones of input onto output cells by inhibiting weakly excited output cells at the perimeter of a vertical zone dependent on focal thalamic input.

Several other classes of cortical interneuron have been described at various times. A synthesis of the recent work of Lund (1973), Szentágothai (1976), Jones (1975a) and Valverde (1976) would seem to indicate that only four types additional to those already mentioned are consistently recorded (Figure 16). These include a rare giant cell of layer II and of unknown provenance (not illustrated), a large fusiform or tufted cell of layer III but with long dendrites, (perhaps corresponding to the peptide containing cells, described in the chapter by Emson and Hunt in this volume), a small cell with basket-type axon confined to layer II, and a cell of layers II and III with a tightly bundled system of vertical axon branches corresponding to the major type of "double bouquet" cell of Ramón y Cajal (1911). These descending axon branches resemble the ascending axons of the spiny cells described above and terminate upon apical dendrites of pyramidal cells as the branches descend to ramify with pyramidal-cell collaterals in the inner band of Baillarger (Jones, 1975a). Unfortunately, we know very little about the inputs to all the cell classes illustrated in Figure 16. Since their somata and dendrites are concentrated in superficial layers, they may receive corticocortical rather than thalamic afferents, but it is not yet possible to weld them into any particular connectional scheme of the cortex.

Though this conclusion and much else that has been said here may seem disappointing, we have advanced a considerable distance since Ramón y Cajal described the cortex as "a kind of unfathomable physiological sea." Now that the output cells are clearly defined and there is some measure of agreement regarding the classes of interneurons, the next steps needed for a satisfactory wiring diagram are (1) clear identification of the cell types upon which afferent fibers terminate; (2) more data on the geometric relationships of repeating patterns of afferent fibers to one another and to the cells of the cortex; (3) further information regarding the synaptology, relative numbers, preferred distributions, and transmitter characteristics of the different classes of interneurons; (4) together with some understanding of the anatomy of pyramidal-cell axon collaterals. It may be unreasonable to hope that the cerebral cortex will ever yield totally to the kind of analysis, both qualitative and quantitative, that has been so fruitful in a far more stereotyped structure like the cerebellum. It is also unreasonable to assume that a structure of its level of functional complexity will ever be understood in terms of a rigidly wired set of connections, for dynamic influences leading to ever changing patterns of activity must be inherent. Nevertheless, some fundamental circuit elements do seem to be detectable and offer the hope of further developments.

Summary

A generalized view of cortical organization is presented, drawing primarily upon data from the sensory-motor areas of monkeys.

It is shown that fibers forming the two major inputs to a cortical area—thalamic and corticocortical—arise from focal clusters of cells and enter the cortex in aggregated bundles that terminate in small focal zones, often with relatively little overlap. Such focal zones can be aligned in register to form strip-like configurations, but the relationships of strips formed by one class of input to those formed by another are incompletely known.

It is suggested that a manageable unit of thalamocortical input in the sensory cortex is not the single thalamocortical fiber but a bundle of such fibers arising from a focal cluster of thalamocortical relay cells representing the same "place" and "modality" and terminating in a relatively discrete zone of cortex. Further units of organization, perhaps based upon inputs from single receptor types, may lie within such a broad unit.

Review of recent evidence indicates that in the majority of cortical areas, thalamocortical fibers end largely or exclusively outside layer IV (in layers III and V–VI). Furthermore, they terminate on at least three classes of cortical interneuron, and even on certain pyramidal cells. Therefore, it becomes necessary to consider several parallel synaptic circuits for transmission of sensory impulses through the cortex.

One such pathway, forming the potential basis for the well-known vertical processing within the cortex, consists of a small, spiny, thalamic recipient cell with vertically directed axon branches that synapse upon the apical dendrites of pyramidal cells with somata in all layers. This tends to preserve the focal nature of the bundled thalamic input across all layers. In addition, because pyramidal cells are the output cells of the cortex, such an input "column" is also an output "column." Pyramidal cells projecting to different sites are aggregated in different layers and sublayers, but it is unknown whether a column based upon focal thalamic input contains representatives of all pyramidal-cell classes.

A focal column of the type outlined above could be "focused" by thalamic-recipient, Golgi type II inhibitory interneurons that would serve to inhibit weakly excited, vertical interneurons at the periphery of a focal thalamic input zone. Other large inhibitory interneurons (basket cells), potentially also receiving thalamic inputs and with preferred axonal distributions, may selectively inhibit adjacent columns.

Five or six other classes of cortical interneuron with dendrites largely outside the layers of termination of thalamic inputs are consistently recognized in all areas and by most authors. These, together with the axon collaterals of pyramidal cells, may serve to further refine and focus column-like input–output zones in the cortex by selective excitation and inhibition.

Acknowledgments

Personal work described here was supported by Grant NS 10526, from the National Institutes of Health, United States Public Health Service. I am also grateful for support provided by the Josiah Macy Jr. Foundation and by the Department of Physiology, Monash University, Melbourne, Australia.

References

Asanuma, H., J. Fernandez, M. E. Scheibel, and A. B. Scheibel, 1974. Characteristics of projections from the nucleus ventralis lateralis to the motor cortex in cats: an anatomical and physiological study. *Exp. Brain Res.* 20:315–330.

Bullier, J., and G. H. Henry, 1979. Laminar distribution of first order neurons and afferent terminals in cat striate cortex. *J. Neurophysiol.* 42:1271–1281.

Burton, H., and E. G. Jones, 1976. The posterior thalamic region and its cortical projection in new world and old world monkeys. *J. Comp. Neurol.* 168:249–302.

Catsman-Berrevoets, C. E., and H. G. J. M. Kuypers, 1978. Differential laminar distribution of corticothalamic neurons projecting to the VL and the centermedian. An HRP study in the cynomolgus monkey. *Brain Res.* 154:359–365.

Caviness, V. S., Jr., and R. L. Sidman, 1973. Time of origin of corresponding cell classes in the cerebral cortex of normal and mutant mice: An autoradiographic analysis. *J. Comp. Neurol.* 148:141–152.

Eccles, J. C., M. Ito, and J. Szentágothai, 1967. *The Cerebellum as a Neuronal Machine.* Berlin: Springer.

Ferster, D., and S. LeVay, 1978. The axonal arborization of lateral geniculate neurons in the striate cortex of the cat. *J. Comp. Neurol.* 182:923–944.

Gilbert, C. D., and J. P. Kelly, 1975. The projection of cells in different layers of the cat's visual cortex. *J. Comp. Neurol.* 163:81–105.

Hand, P. J., and T. van Winkle, 1977. The efferent connections of the feline nucleus cuneatus. *J. Comp. Neurol.* 171:83–110.

Hubel, D. H., and T. N. Wiesel, 1968. Receptive fields and functional architecture of monkey striate cortex. *J. Physiol. (London)* 195:215–243.

Hubel, D. H., and T. N. Wiesel, 1972. Laminar and columnar distribution of geniculo-cortical fibers in the macaque monkey. *J. Comp. Neurol.* 146:421–450.

Hubel, D. H., and T. N. Wiesel, 1977. Functional architecture of macaque monkey visual cortex. *Proc. Roy. Soc. B* 198:1–59.

Hubel, D. H., T. N. Wiesel, and M. Stryker, 1978. Anatomical demonstration of orientation columns in macaque monkey. *J. Comp. Neurol.* 177:361–379.

Imig, T. J., and J. F. Brugge, 1978. Sources and terminations of callosal axons related to binaural and frequency maps in primary auditory cortex of the cat. *J. Comp. Neurol.* 182:637–660.

Jones, E. G., 1975a. Varieties and distribution of non-pyramidal cells in the somatic sensory cortex of the squirrel monkey. *J. Comp. Neurol.* 160:205–268.

Jones, E. G., 1975b. Possible determinants of the degree of retrograde neuronal labeling with horseradish peroxidase. *Brain Res.* 85:249–253.

Jones, E. G., and H. Burton, 1976. Areal differences in the laminar distribution of thalamic afferents in cortical fields of the insular, parietal and temporal regions of primates. *J. Comp. Neurol.* 168:197–248.

Jones, E. G., and T. P. S. Powell, 1970. An electronmicroscopic study of the laminar pattern and mode of termination of the afferent fibre pathways to the somatic sensory cortex. *Phil. Trans. Roy. Soc. B* 257:45–62.

Jones, E. G., and S. P. Wise, 1977. Size, laminar and columnar distribution of efferent cells in the sensory-motor cortex of monkeys. *J. Comp. Neurol.* 175:391–438.

Jones, E. G., H. Burton, and R. Porter, 1975. Commissural and cortico-cortical "columns" in the somatic sensory cortex of primates. *Science* 190:572–574.

Jones, E. G., J. D. Coulter, and S. P. Wise, 1979. Commissural columns in the sensory-motor cortex of monkeys. *J. Comp. Neurol.* 188:113–136.

Jones. E. G., S. P. Wise, and J. D. Coulter, 1979. Differential thalamic relationships of sensory-motor and parietal cortical fields in monkeys. *J. Comp. Neurol.* 183:833–883.

Kelly, J. P., and D. C. Van Essen, 1974. Cell structure and function in the visual cortex of the cat. *J. Physiol. (London)* 238:515–547.

Kennedy, C., M. H. des Rosiers, O. Sakurada, M. Shinohara, M. Reivich, J. W. Jehle, and L. Sokoloff, 1976. Metabolic mapping of the primary visual system of the monkey by means of the autoradiographic (^{14}C) deoxyglucose technique. *Proc. Nat. Acad. Sci. USA* 73:4230–4234.

Killackey, H. P., and G. R. Belford, 1976. Discrete afferent terminations in the trigeminal pathway of the neonatal rat. *Anat. Rec.* 184:446.

LeVay, S., and C. D. Gilbert, 1976. Laminar patterns of geniculocortical projection in the cat. *Brain Res.* 113:1–20.

LeVay, S., D. H. Hubel, and T. N. Wiesel, 1975. The pattern of ocular dominance columns in monkey visual cortex revealed by a reduced silver stain. *J. Comp. Neurol.* 169:559–576.

Lorente de Nó, R., 1922. La corteza cerebral del ratón. (Primera contribucion-La corteza acústica). *Trab. Lab. Invest. Biol. Madrid* 20:41–78.

Lorente de Nó, R., 1938. Cerebral cortex: Architectonics, intracortical connections. In *Physiology of the Nervous System.* J. F. Fulton, ed., 2nd ed. New York: Oxford University Press, pp. 288–313.

Lund, J. S., 1973. Organization of neurons in the visual cortex area 17 of the monkey *(Macaca mulatta). J. Comp. Neurol.* 147:455–496.

Lund, J. S., and R. G. Boothe, 1975. Interlaminar connections and pyramidal neuron organization in the visual cortex, area 17, of the macaque monkey. *J. Comp. Neurol.* 159:305–334.

Lund, J. S., R. D. Lund, A. E. Hendrickson, A. H. Bunt, and A. F. Fuchs, 1975. The origin of efferent pathways from the primary visual cortex, area 17, of the macaque monkey as shown by retrograde transport of horseradish peroxidase. *J. Comp. Neurol.* 164:287–304.

Marin-Padilla, M., 1969. Origin of the pericellular baskets of the pyramidal cells of the human motor cortex: A Golgi study. *Brain Res.* 14:633–646.

Mountcastle, V. B., 1957. Modality and topographic properties of single neurons of cat's somatic sensory cortex. *J. Neurophysiol.* 20:408–434.

Palmer, L. A., and A. C. Rosenquist, 1974. Visual receptive fields of single striate cortical units projecting to the superior colliculus in the cat. *Brain Res.* 67:27–42.

Peters, A., M. L. Feldman, and J. Saldanha, 1976. The projection of the lateral geniculate nucleus to area 17 of the rat visual cortex. II. Terminations upon neuronal perikarya and dendritic shafts. *J. Neurocytol.* 5:85–107.

Phillips, C. G., 1959. Actions of antidromic pyramidal volleys on single Betz cells in the cat. *Quart. J. Exp. Physiol.* 44:1–25.

Poggio, G. F., and V. B. Mountcastle, 1963. The functional properties of ventrobasal thalamic neurons studied in unanesthetized monkeys. *J. Neurophysiol.* 26:775–806.

Powell, T. P. S., and V. B. Mountcastle, 1959. Some aspects of the functional organization of the cortex of the postcentral gyrus of the monkey: a correlation of findings obtained in a single unit analysis with cytoarchitecture. *Bull. Johns Hopkins Hosp.* 105:133–162.

Ramón y Cajal, S., 1911. *Histologie du système nerveux de l'homme et des vertébrés*, Vol. 2. Trans. S. Azoulay. Paris: Maloine.

Ribak, C. E., 1978. Aspinous and sparsely-spinous stellate neurons in the visual cortex of rats contain glutamic acid decarboxylase. *J. Neurocytol.* 7:461–478.

Shatz, C., 1977. Anatomy of interhemispheric connections in the visual system of Boston siamese and ordinary cats. *J. Comp. Neurol.* 173:497–518.

Sholl, D. A., 1954. *Anatomy of the Cerebral Cortex*. London: Methuen.

Somogyi, P., 1977. A specific axo-axonal interneuron in the visual cortex of the rat. *Brain Res.* 136:345–350.

Szentágothai, J., 1969. Architecture of the cerebral cortex. In *Basic Mechanisms of the Epilepsies*. H. H. Jasper, A. A. Ward, and A. Pope, eds. Boston: Little Brown, pp. 13–28.

Szentágothai, J., 1975. The module-concept in cerebral cortex architecture. *Brain Res.* 95:475–496.

Szentágothai, J., 1976. Basic circuitry of the neocortex. *Exp. Brain Res., Suppl.* 1:282–287.

Valverde, F., 1971. Short axon neuronal systems in the visual cortex of the monkey. *Int. J. Neurosci.* 1:181–197.

Valverde, F., 1976. Aspects of cortical organization related to the geometry of neurons with intra-cortical axons. *J. Neurocytol.* 5:509–529.

Welker, C., 1976. Receptive fields of barrels in the somatosensory neocortex of the rat. *J. Comp. Neurol.* 166:173–190.

White, E. L., 1978. Identified neurons in mouse SmI cortex which are postsynaptic to thalamocortical axon terminals: A combined Golgi-electron microscopic and degeneration study. *J. Comp. Neurol.* 181:627–662.

Whitsel, B. L., J. R. Ropollo, and G. Werner, 1972. Cortical information processing of stimulus motion on primate skin. *J. Neurophysiol.* 35:691–717.

Wise, S. P., and E. G. Jones, 1976. Organization and postnatal development of the commissural projection of the rat somatic sensory cortex. *J. Comp. Neurol.* 168:313–343.

Wise, S. P., and E. G. Jones, 1978. Developmental studies of thalamocortical and commissural connections in the rat somatic sensory cortex. *J. Comp. Neurol.* 178:187–208.

Wise, S. P., J. W. Fleshman, Jr., and E. G. Jones, 1979. The maturation of pyramidal cell form in relation to developing afferent and efferent connections of the rat somatic sensory cortex. *Neuroscience* 4:1275–1297.

Wise, S. P., S. H. C. Hendry, and E. G. Jones, 1977. Prenatal development of sensorimotor cortical projections in cats. *Brain Res.* 138:538–544.

Wise, S. P., E. H. Murray, and J. D. Coulter, 1978. Somatotopic organization of cortico-spinal and corticotrigeminal neurons in the rat. *Neuroscience* 4:65–78.

Zeki, S. M., 1978. The cortical projections of foveal striate cortex in the rhesus monkey. *J. Physiol. (London)* 277:227–244.

10 Organization of Somatosensory Cortex in Primates

J. H. Kaas, R. J. Nelson, M. Sur, and M. M. Merzenich

ABSTRACT The traditional primary somatosensory cortex SI of higher primates contains as many as four separate, complete, and parallel representations of the body rather than one. Separate body surface representations are found in cortical fields 3b and 1. Area 2 contains an orderly representation of predominantly "deep" body tissues. Area 3a may constitute a fourth representation of largely muscle afferents. Preliminary experiments on the microorganization of one of the representations suggests repeating modules of "minicolumns" and "macrocolumns." The organizations of the cutaneous representations can be experimentally altered by inactivating part of the sensory input.

Introduction

For the last several years, we have been using electrophysiological mapping methods, anatomical studies of connections, and recordings from single neurons to investigate the organization of parietal somatosensory cortex in primates and other mammals. Most of what we have discovered relates to the somatotopic organization of the region of postcentral cortex in monkeys that has been traditionally described as SI or primary somatosensory cortex, and these discoveries will be emphasized here. To briefly summarize, we hypothesize that (1) each of the four distinct architectonic bands of parietal cortex that is responsive to somatosensory stimuli, namely, areas 3a, 3b, 1, and 2, constitutes a separate and complete representation of the body; (2) the representations are parallel with each other, so that they roughly correspond in medial to lateral organization; (3) matched body locations are represented along the common borders of adjoining architectonic fields, so that a mirror reversal of organization occurs at the border (such borders are called congruent); (4) each of the representations differs from the others in the details of its organization, the response properties of the contained neurons, connections with other structures, the behavioral

J. H. KAAS, R. J. NELSON, M. SUR, and M. M. MERZENICH Department of Psychology, Vanderbilt University, Nashville, Tennessee 37240; Department of Anatomy, Vanderbilt University, Nashville, Tennessee 37232; Department of Psychology, Vanderbilt University, Nashville, Tennessee 37240; Coleman Laboratory, University of California, San Francisco, California 94143

consequences of removal or inactivation, and therefore functional role; (5) representations are composites of somatotopically organized regions with lines of discontinuity that cut across dermatomes; the representations are not accurately depicted by simple continuous homunculi, and they cannot be explained as a simple consequence of the pattern of sensory organization in the spinal cord; (6) representations have a microorganization that is compatible with a concept of repeating basic modules of "minicolumns" and "macrocolumns"; (7) the obvious or dominant organization of each representation masks a hidden organization which can be revealed by experimentally inactivating the dominant input; (8) representations differ in minor ways from individual to individual and in more significant ways from species to species; these differences suggest constraints and rules of somatotopic organization; and (9) the representation in area 3b of primates is homologous with SI of other mammals. All of these tenets are supported by the available data to varying extents. Some conclusions are strongly supported, others are presently more speculative. The reasons why we have postulated these tenets are given below.

A Brief History of the Multiple-Representations Hypothesis

The first detailed information about the organization of postcentral somatosensory cortex in monkeys came from the landmark studies of Woolsey, Marshall, and Bard, first published in 1937 and then more completely in 1942. These investigators recorded potentials from the surface of the brain evoked by sensory stimuli to restricted body locations. By removing the anterior bank of the central sulcus, they were also able to explore the posterior bank. The results led to the important conclusions that (1) the tactile sensory system projects to parietal areas 3, 1, and 2 of Brodmann; (2) the medial to lateral sequence of sensory representation basically follows a tail-to-tongue sequence along the body (see Woolsey, Marshall, and Bard, 1942, for details); (3) there are obvious discontinuities in the cortical representation of the skin surface (for example, the face is separated from the rest of the head, and anterior and posterior aspects of the leg are separated; (4) cutaneous surfaces with the greatest tactile acuity have the largest cortical projection areas and vice versa; and (5) with the exception of the mouth region, the projection is from the contralateral half of the body. These basic conclusions have been repeatedly supported by the results of subsequent studies.

The possibility that the postcentral responsive region might contain several representations of the body was not addressed in these early studies, and the concept of a single representation, often in the form of a homunculus, later became established in reviews and textbook simplifications. However, there were observations even in these first mapping studies that were more compatible with a multiple-rep-

J. H. Kaas, R. J. Nelson, M. Sur, and M. M. Merzenich

resentations than a single-representation hypothesis. Most notably, Woolsey, Marshall, and Bard (1942) described separate foci within the responsive zone, but some distance apart, as activated by stimuli to the thumb.

A second important advance resulted from the single-unit study of Powell and Mountcastle (1959), which showed that neurons in area 3 (3b) were predominantly activated by cutaneous receptors, those in area 1 by stimulation of the skin or deep tissues of the body, and neurons in area 2 were responsive almost exclusively to noncutaneous receptors. These results require the conclusion that either different body regions are subserved by quite different receptor populations, or that the concept of a single body-surface representation across all three architectonic zones is invalid. Although Powell and Mountcastle (1959) did not attempt to determine the somatotopic organization of postcentral parietal cortex, they did observe that the same restricted body region could activate neurons at a number of rostrocaudal locations across areas 3, 1, and 2. As a result, Powell and Mountcastle concluded that "it is difficult to fit our observations with the idea that the cortical projection pattern is a distorted figure of the animal."

The next major advance was made by Werner and Whitsel (1968) with later refinements by Whitsel and coworkers (Whitsel, Dreyer, and Roppolo, 1971; Dreyer et al., 1974, 1975). These investigators also observed that neurons at several rostrocaudal locations across areas 3a, 3b, 1, and 2 could be activated by the same body region, and recognized that such observations were incompatible with the concept of a single topographic homunculus across these architectonic fields. Instead, they proposed a complex representation in which some body parts were found twice, once rostrally and once caudally, and other body parts extended rostrally and caudally to include two or more architectonic areas.

The understanding of the organization of somatosensory cortex progressed further when Paul, Merzenich, and Goodman (1972) found that the hand of macaque monkeys was represented "in its entirety" once in surface cortex of the postcentral gyrus and again in the posterior bank of the central sulcus. Paul and coworkers acknowledged that they did not resolve whether the entire body surface is partially or wholly represented twice in postcentral cortex, but they did conclude that in either case "the classical view of SI as constituting a single, simple whole body representation must be modified."

With the discoveries of these previous investigators in mind, we set out systematically to map somatosensory cortex in primates in order to test the hypothesis that each of the architectonic strips of postcentral parietal cortex (areas 3a, 3b, 1, and 2) constitutes a separate representation of the body, and a functional entity. In order to simplify the mapping procedure, initial investigations were in the owl monkey, where the central sulcus is either missing or a shallow dimple (Kaas et al., 1976; Merzenich et al., 1978; Kaas et al., 1979). Later investigations were extended to include squirrel monkeys (Nelson, Sur, and Kaas, 1978), cebus monkeys (Felleman et al., 1979), and macaque monkeys (Kaas et al., 1979; Nelson et al., 1980). In addition, prosimian galagos (Sur, Nelson, and Kaas, 1980), tree shrews (Weller, Sur, and Kaas, 1979), and grey squirrels (Sur, Nelson, and Kaas, 1978) were considered for comparative purposes. Most of the formulations discussed below are based on these studies.

The Microelectrode Multiunit Mapping Method

Our microelectrode multiunit mapping procedure is a modification of the basic approach developed and used so productively by Wally Welker and coworkers (see Krishnamurti, Sanides, and Welker, 1976) in comparative studies of somatosensory cortex organization in a wide range of mammals. The procedure is both simple and more effective than the alternatives of macroelectrode surface recordings of evoked potentials or single-unit mapping. In brief, a large area of the brain (to reduce brain movements) including the region of interest is exposed in an anesthetized animal, and covered with a silicone pool held within a plastic dam bonded to the skull. The exposed brain surface is photographed and a highly magnified print is produced. A low-impedance microelectrode is inserted vertically into the cortex with a micromanipulator and the penetration is cited on the photograph. Recordings are usually from the middle layers of cortex, and as many as 300 to 500 electrode penetrations in a closely spaced grid in the region of interest are commonly produced. Deep penetrations are made to explore buried fissures and nuclei.

The essential feature of the microelectrode mapping method is the large number of closely spaced recordings at identified sites in the same animal. Surface-recording methods, which have been used so productively in the pioneering studies of Woolsey and colleagues (see Woolsey, 1952, 1958), have the advantage of allowing the receptive fields for a large number of cortical sites to be defined, but the surface electrode simply records the activity of too large a region of cortex to provide the detail and the precise relation of recording sites to cortical architecture needed in many studies. Investigators sometimes think that single-neuron recordings would be a further improvement in the mapping procedure. This mistake is often the result of confusing the goal of characterizing the response properties of neurons, which can vary greatly, with the goal of determining receptive-field locations, which are overlapping and similar for adjacent neurons. Thus, both single-unit and multiunit procedures should produce identical maps. However, single-unit mapping often introduces serious time delays that are inherent in electrophysiologically isolating neurons and determining the stimulus parameters specific to the isolated neurons. Because of the time delays, the number of cortical sites that can be sam-

J. H. Kaas, R. J. Nelson, M. Sur, and M. M. Merzenich

pled in a single experiment is greatly reduced in comparison with multiunit methods. Thus, single-unit-mapping studies compromise the detail or completeness of the derived maps. Finally, if there are reasons to believe that some neurons in a representation will have displaced or unusual receptive fields, it is easier to detect the existence and frequency of these neurons in multiunit recordings since some of the neurons are likely to have usual receptive fields for comparison at any given recording site. This advantage has been especially important in our nerve-regeneration experiments, where displaced receptive fields are commonly observed.

Mapping Evidence for the Multiple-Representations Hypothesis

We have argued that each of areas 3a, 3b, 1, and 2 is a functionally distinct subdivision of somatosensory cortex with a separate map of the body (Merzenich et al., 1978; Kaas et al., 1979). The most compelling evidence for this hypothesis comes from recordings within areas 3b and 1. Neurons throughout both of these areas respond to light cutaneous stimuli and therefore receptive-field locations can be defined accurately and quickly, so that the organization of large regions of cortex can be determined within single experiments. Neurons in both areas 3a and 2 are activated predominantly by receptors in deep body tissues (muscles and joints), and it is difficult and time consuming to accurately localize their receptor sources and "receptive fields." For this reason, we have a detailed knowledge of the organizations of areas 3b and 1 in a number of primates, but only limited understanding of the organizations of areas 3a and 2.

The Representations in Areas 3b and 1
The organizations of areas 3b and 1 are most easily determined and illustrated in a relatively smooth-brained monkey like the owl monkey, and for this reason initial experiments concentrated on this primate. The locations and overall somatotopic organizations of areas 3b and 1 are shown for an owl monkey in Figure 1. The central fissure, which buries most of area 3b in the majority of monkeys, is absent or only a shallow dimple in owl monkeys. Therefore, all but the small portion of 3b and 1 on the medial wall of the cerebral hemisphere and laterally in the sylvian fissure is directly accessible and easily explored. Figure 1 illustrates our major conclusion that all or nearly all of the body surface is represented in a systematic manner once in area 3b and again in area 1. The figure also summarizes some of the details of the two organizations. The summary was reconstructed by outlining regions of cortex activated by stimuli to particular body parts using receptive fields for 486 recording sites in a single owl monkey. For example, all recording sites within the lateral unshaded regions marked D_1 in area 3b and in area 1 were activated by lightly touching the glabrous surface of the first

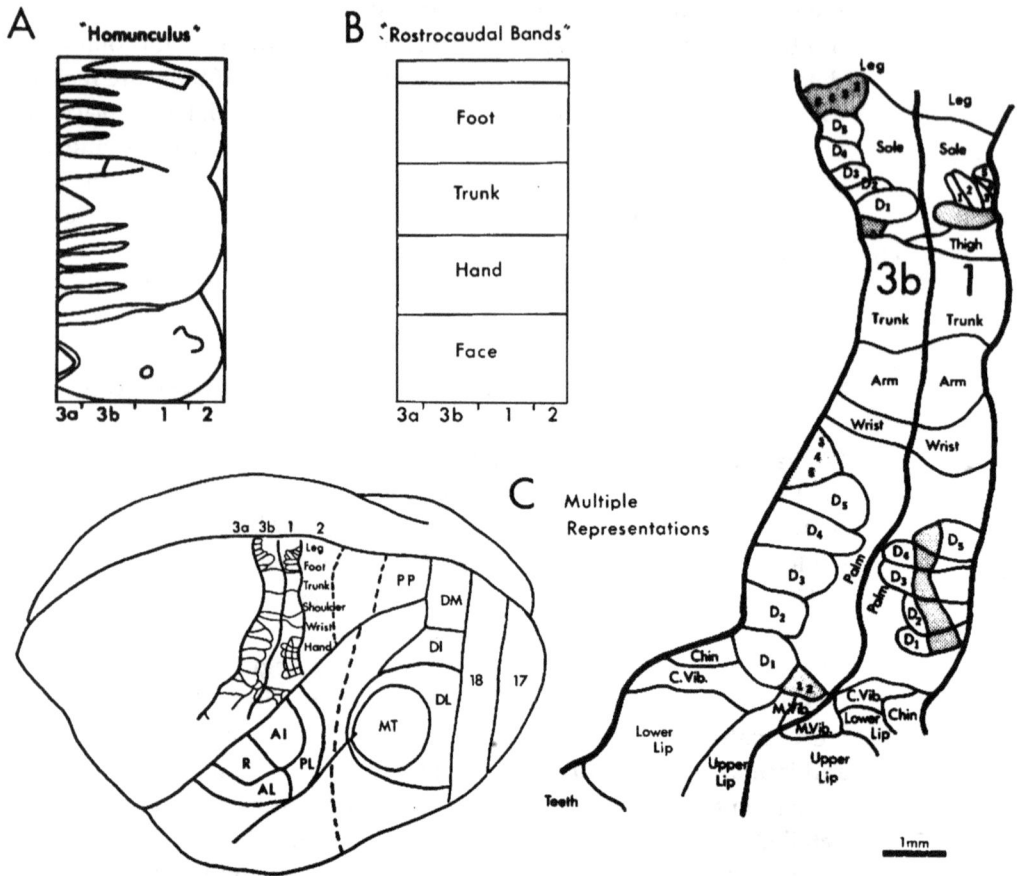

Figure 1 Three conceptions of the organization of postcentral parietal somatosensory cortex SI of monkeys, and some details of the two cutaneous representations in owl monkeys. (A) The traditional concept has been that a single body representation occupies four architectonic fields. (B) A modification of the traditional concept is that major body parts are represented across all architectonic fields in rostrocaudal bands. (C) Our microelectrode mapping experiments indicate that the SI region contains multiple representations. Some of the features of the two cutaneous representations in areas 3b and 1 of the owl monkey are shown on a dorsolateral view of the brain on the lower left and in more detail on the right. Portions of cortex activated by given body parts are outlined. The representations of hairy surfaces of the foot and hand are shaded. The digits of the hand and foot are numbered. C. vib. = chin vibrissae; M. vib. = mandibular vibrissae. The parallel organization of area 2, predominantly activated by joint receptors, is also indicated. Visual and auditory areas are from studies of Allman and Kaas (1976), and Imig et al. (1977). (From Kaas et al., 1979. By permission, copyright 1979 by the American Association for the Advancement of Science.)

digit of the hand. Stimuli to any particular body surface activated a
similar restricted location within area 3b and a second restricted location within area 1. Maps generated by data for one owl monkey were
basically similar to those from other owl monkeys, and all species of
monkeys showed this double representation related to areas 3b and 1.

The procedure for generating summary maps is shown for parts of
areas 3b and 1 in Figure 2. Each dot on the surface diagram indicates the
site of a perpendicular electrode penetration. The clusters of sites activated by particular body parts are outlined. Obviously, some of the
lines are artificial in the sense that they only separate recording sites
with receptive fields *centered* on one body region from those *centered* on
an adjoining body region. Some receptive fields centered on the distal
phalange of digit 2, for example, extended onto the middle phalange of
digit 2, and vice versa. Other lines mark real borders. The line between
digit 1 and 2, for example, is such a border, for receptive-field sites on
one side of the line were on digit 1 and for the other side, on digit 2, and
receptive fields did not overlap the two digits.

The evidence for separate representations in areas 3b and 1 is best
appreciated by considering receptive-field locations for rows of recording sites selected from the total sample, since illustrations showing

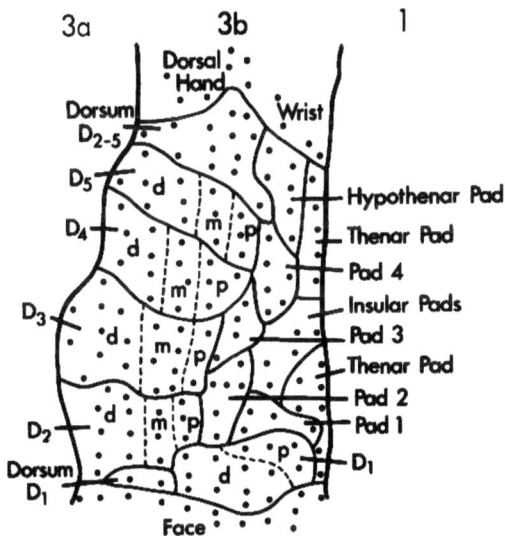

Figure 2 Recording-site locations for a map of the hand representation in area 3b of an
owl monkey. See Figure 1 for the location of the hand portion of area 3b in the owl
monkey brain. Each dot marks the site of an electrode penetration. All penetrations with a
receptive field centered on a particular glabrous digit (D_1–D_5), pad of the palm, or dorsum
of the digits are outlined. Dashed lines separate electrode penetrations centered on the
distal (d), middle (m), or proximal (p) phalanges. Similar data were used to construct the
maps of area 3b and area 1 shown in Figure 1. Note the similarities and differences in the
hand representation of area 3b in the monkey illustrated here and the monkey shown in
Figure 1.

all of the recording sites and all of the receptive fields are confusingly complex. Rostrocaudal rows of recording sites conveniently demonstrate the dual nature of the representations, since the representations are parallel and roughly mirror image in organization (Figure 1). Thus, receptive fields for selected recording sites in roughly rostrocaudal rows (varying slightly with position in the maps) progress across a restricted body region once for area 3b, and reverse and cross the same body region again in area 1. This observation can be demonstrated for any body region, and is shown for glabrous digits 2 and 4 and adjoining palm in Figure 3.

The Representations in Areas 3a and 2

All our observations on the locations of receptive fields for recording sites in areas 3a and 2 are consistent with the concept of separate and complete representations of predominantly deep body tissues in these two architectonic strips. However, the evidence is limited and details are lacking. Relatively few recordings were obtained in area 3a. Our usual procedure was to make rostrocaudal rows of recording sites across areas 3b and 1, which were consistently responsive to cutaneous stimuli. The rostral border of this tactile zone was sharp, and the one or two recording sites per row across the border in area 3a did not respond to light stimulation of the skin. Instead, manipulation of muscles and other subcutaneous tissues were usually effective stimuli (although responses were sometimes poor or absent). In every case where the tissue of effective stimulation was at least roughly defined, it corresponded in general location to the receptive fields on the skin for the immediately caudal recording sites in area 3b. For example, recording sites in area 3a responsive to manipulation of the hand were rostral to recording sites in area 3b responsive to lightly touching the hand. While further details of the organization of area 3a are not available, it is apparent that the mediolateral sequence of representation parallels that in area 3b.

Observations on the organization of area 2 were somewhat more extensive. Recording sites in this cortical strip were predominantly activated by stimulating deep body tissues. Often, recording sites were strongly activated by moving one or more joints. At other times, the nature of the effective stimulus was less clear. Because it is difficult precisely to define the deep locations of the effective receptors for these recording sites without dissection, these data allowed only a crude idea of cortical organization. Nonetheless, as in area 3a, it was obvious that the "deep-body" representation in area 2 again closely parallels those in areas 3b and 1. Moving the joints in digit 1 of the hand, for example, activated the portion of area 2 just caudal to the portion of area 1 activated by the skin on digit 1.

While neurons in area 2 of owl monkeys were almost exclusively activated by stimulating deep body tissues, recording sites in at least part of area 2 of macaque monkeys often responded to cutaneous as well as

J. H. Kaas, R. J. Nelson, M. Sur, and M. M. Merzenich

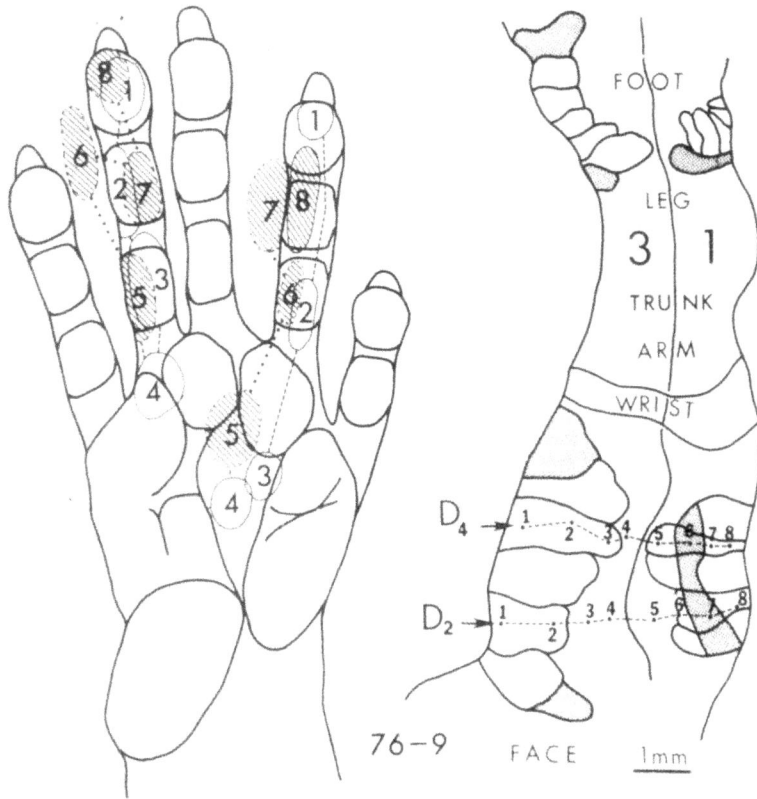

Figure 3 Receptive fields for two rows of recording sites across the separate hand representations in areas 3b and 1 of an owl monkey. Both anterior to posterior rows produced similar progressions of receptive fields from digit tip to the palm and back again to the digit tip. The point of reversal is at the 3b–1 border. These results show that the digits are systematically represented once in area 3b and again in area 1 in roughly a mirror-image fashion. However, an important difference in the two representations is in the locations of the dorsal hairy surfaces of the digits. The displaced receptive fields for recording-site 7 for row D_2 and for recording-site 6 for row D_4 were actually on the dorsal surfaces of the digits. Thus, the representations of the hairy digits interrupt the glabrous digits in area 1. In area 3b, the representations of the dorsal hairy surfaces of the digits are displaced medially and laterally (shaded) as shown in Figure 2. (Previously unpublished illustration from the studies of Merzenich et al., 1978.)

Organization of Somatosensory Cortex in Primates

deep stimuli. (This responsiveness may reflect a difference in the susceptibility of cortically relayed cutaneous input to anesthetics; neurons within area 2 in squirrel monkeys were also sometimes responsive to cutaneous stimuli.) When recording sites in area 2 were activated by cutaneous stimuli, receptive fields could be defined more precisely, and further details of the organization of area 2 were revealed. As is shown in Figure 4, progressions of receptive fields for rows of recording sites across areas 1 and 2 indicate a mirror reversal of somatotopic organization across the border. Thus, the available evidence suggests that area 2 is somatotopically organized not only in parallel with the organization of area 1, but also approximately as a mirror reversal.

Other Evidence for the Multiple-Representations Hypothesis

The concept that each of areas 3a, 3b, 1, and 2 constitutes a separate and functionally distinct representation of the body is supported by anatomical studies of connections, studies of the properties of single units, and the behavioral effects of restricted cortical lesions. This large body of observations is more readily explained by the postulate that separate representations occupy separate architectonic fields than the traditional alternative of a single body representation occupying three or four architectonic fields. The anatomical evidence indicates that each of the four architectonic fields has its own distinct pattern of extrinsic connections. Most significantly, areas 3a, 3b, 1, and 2 are connected or reciprocally interconnected (Vogt and Pandya, 1978; Jones, Coulter, and Hendry, 1978; Shanks, Pearson, and Powell, 1978) in patterns that might be expected between homotopic regions of parallel representations but would be surprising between parts of a single representation. In addition, these fields project differentially to motor cortex (area 4) and area 5 of parietal cortex (Vogt and Pandya, 1978; Jones, Coulter, and Hendry, 1978; Pearson and Powell, 1978). Other observations better explained by the concept of multiple representations include differential input from the thalamus to the four architectonic zones (Lin et al., 1979; Jones, Wise, and Coulter, 1979), commissural connections from one architectonic zone to more than one in the other hemisphere (Shanks, Rockel, and Powell, 1975), and different projection zones in the spinal cord (Coulter and Jones, 1977) for separate architectonic fields.

The electrophysiological properties of neurons in the four fields need to be further characterized, but elsewhere we have reviewed the evidence that muscle afferents feed into area 3a, inputs from several types of cutaneous receptors into 3b and 1, and joint and other deep-receptor inputs into area 2 (Merzenich et al., 1978). Furthermore, Pacinian receptor influences appear to be limited to neurons in area 1 (Paul, Merzenich, and Goodman, 1972; Merzenich et al., 1978), and neurons in

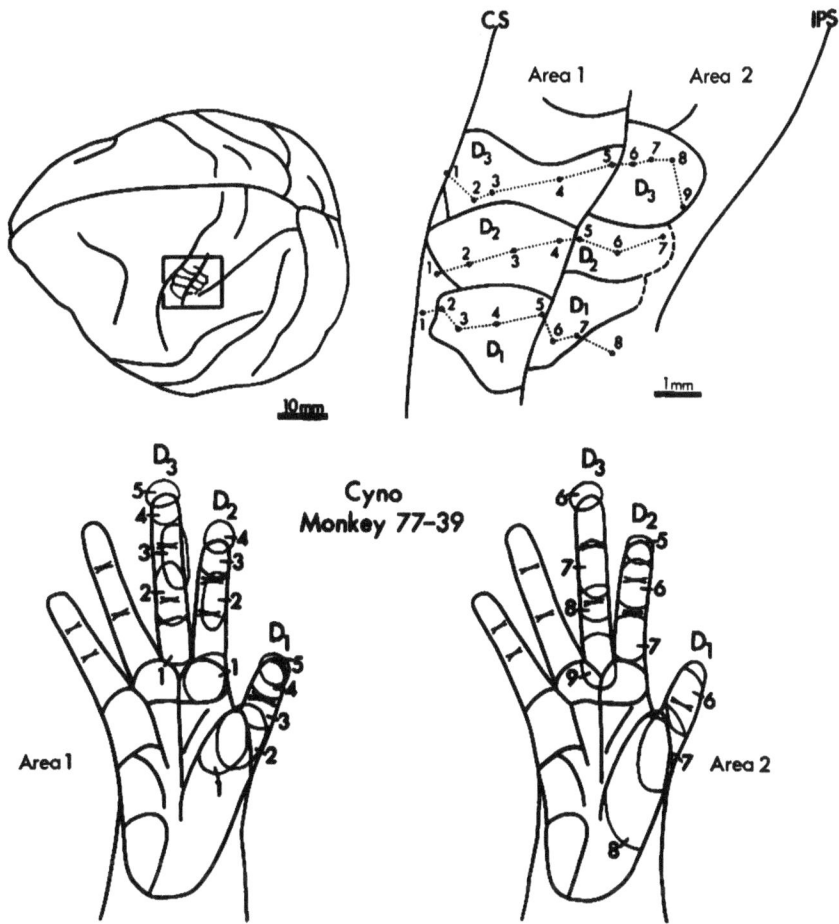

Figure 4 Receptive fields for rows of recording sites across the representations of the digits in area 1 and area 2 of a macaque monkey. Data for digits 1–3 are shown. Note that these digits are represented separately in each architectonic field, and that the two representations are joined at the finger tips so that the representations are roughly mirror images of each other. (Modified from Kaas et al., 1979.)

area 1 have complex center–surround receptive-field organizations not found for neurons in area 3b (Sur, 1979).

A particularly useful test of functional distinctiveness would be to selectively ablate parts of single architectonic zones of somatosensory cortex and test for behavioral alterations. In one such study, Randolph and Semmes (1974) trained macaque monkeys on tactile discrimination tasks and found that lesions of the hand region of area 2 were followed by impairments on tasks involving the discrimination of angles, lesions of area 1 disrupted discriminations of texture, while lesions of area 3b affected both tasks. Thus, there is limited evidence from ablation–behavior experiments that the separate architectonic zones are functionally distinct.

Principles of Organization of the Parietal Somatosensory Fields

Besides the evidence for multiple representations in parietal cortex, our experiments have provided evidence on the organization of individual fields, and the relation of fields to each other. In particular, we have been struck with the observations that representations are regionally somatotopic but contain discontinuities, adjoining representations have matched or congruent borders, the implications of the inverse relation of receptive field size to magnification factor, and the evidence for modular and microorganization within fields.

Representations as Somatotopic Composites

In somatosensory representations, complete topological equivalency of the skin surface and the cortical map does not seem possible, and splits and discontinuities are seen in detailed maps. If, for example, the cutaneous representations in areas 3b and 1 of owl monkeys are considered, it is apparent that neither representation corresponds to a simple unfolding of the contralateral skin surface. Both representations have splits or tears and displacements so that neither representation is topologically equivalent to the skin surface. Yet, restricted regions within the representation are topologically equivalent to restricted regions of the body surface, and each representation can be accurately described as a composite of somatotopic regions (Merzenich et al., 1978). An example of a split in the representation is shown in Figure 5, where the adjoining skin fields in the thenar and hypothenar pads of the palm activate separate regions of cortex in area 3b (and area 1). Such splits are common within each of the cutaneous fields, and are more pronounced in some monkey species than in others. Thus, one feature of the maps is that some adjacent body locations are nonadjacent or separate in cortex (Figure 6). Another feature of the maps is that widely separated skin surfaces such as the thumb and the chin occupy adjoining zones of cortex, so that some nonadjacent or separated body locations are adjacent in cortex (Figure 6).

J. H. Kaas, R. J. Nelson, M. Sur, and M. M. Merzenich

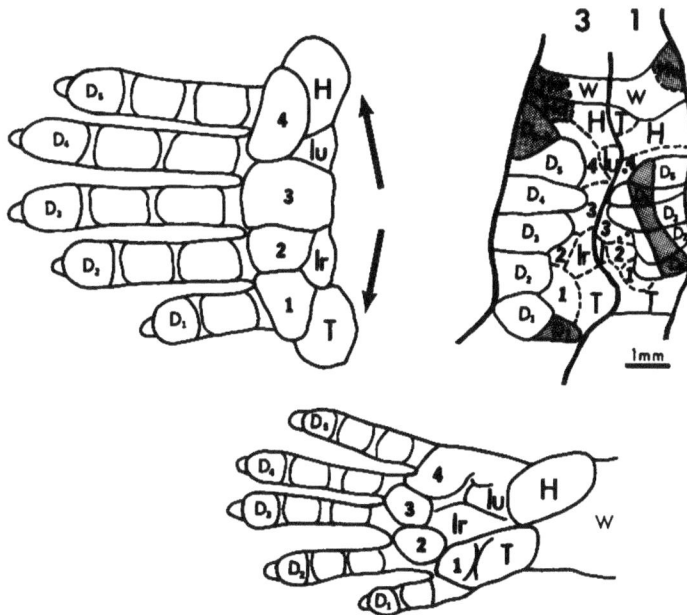

Figure 5 The representations of the glabrous hand in areas 3b and 1 of the owl monkey. The hand surface (below) is split between the pads of the palm and distorted (upper left) to fit the confines of area 3b in the cortical representation (upper right). The representation in area 1 is roughly a mirror image of the representation in area 3b. (From Merzenich et al., 1978.)

While splits and approximations seem necessary in cortical maps in order to fit the complexities of the body surface on a 2-dimensional sheet, there may be functional reasons for the particular locations of these features. There is, for example, a notable tendency to preserve topological equivalence for important sensory surfaces. Thus, the glabrous digits are topologically represented in order for both the foot and hand in all maps of area 3, while the hairy dorsal surfaces of the digits are discontinuously represented in a number of ways. Thus, certain consistencies may be related to functional needs. In addition, differences in the maps of area 3b and area 1 in the same animal are likely to reflect the differing functional roles of the two representations. It is difficult to imagine why the dorsal surfaces of the digits of the hands are represented in such different ways in areas 3b and 1, if not for functional reasons.

Parallel Representations with Congruent Borders
We believe that the evidence indicates that the four architectonic fields constitute four representations of the body, each organized from tail to tongue from medial to lateral in the cortex in a parallel fashion. Moreover, areas 3b and 1 form mirror-image reversals of each other at the common border, and areas 1 and 2 reverse at least at the border in

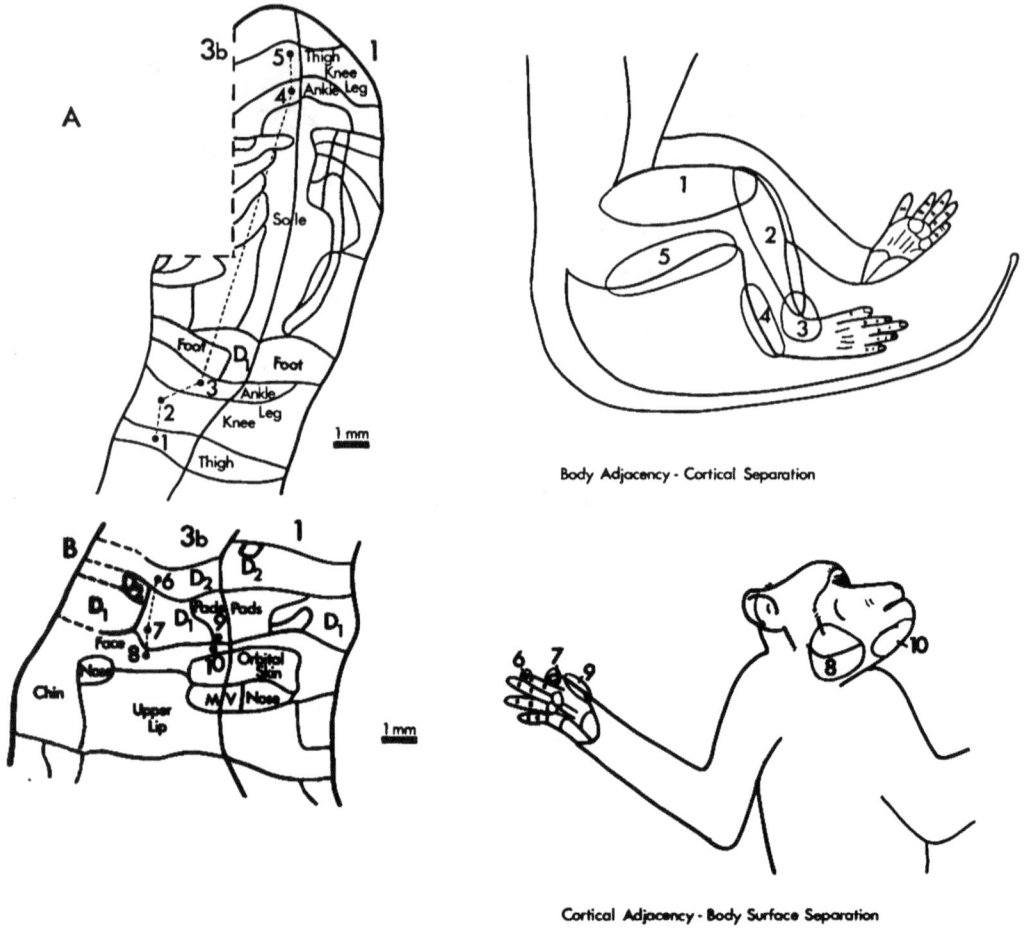

A

3b

B

Body Adjacency - Cortical Separation

Cortical Adjacency - Body Surface Separation

Figure 6 Examples of the cortical map failing to conform to the skin surface. Numbered recording sites are shown for parts of the flattened map of area 3b of macaque monkeys on the left and the corresponding receptive fields are on the right. (See Nelson et al., 1980, for complete maps and location on the brain surface.) In medial cortex (A), recording sites 1 and 5 are widely separated in the brain and have adjacent receptive fields. In more medial cortex, recording sites 9 and 10 are adjacent and have widely separate receptive fields. (From Nelson et al., 1980.)

the hand region. These observations suggest that mirror reversals or "congruent borders" (see Kaas, 1977) between representations are important for developmental or functional reasons. In nonprimates, SI and SII also have a congruent border (Nelson, Sur, and Kaas, 1979), and there are no known exceptions for somatosensory cortex. Congruent borders between adjoining sensory representations are also common both in the cortex and in the thalamus in the visual and auditory systems (see Kaas, 1977).

The power of the mirror-reversal "rule" is seen most dramatically in squirrel and cebus monkeys, both members of the cebus family, where parts of the 3b representation are reversed from that normally found (Felleman et al., 1979; Nelson, Sur, and Kaas, 1978). Where the organization is reversed in area 3b, it is also reversed in area 1. Thus, variation in organization within a representation is possible, but a change in the organization of one representation is coupled with a change in the other.

Representations May Contain Relatively Independent Subdivisions

The observation that parts of the representations in the cebus family of monkeys are reversed in orientation relative to that of other monkeys, and that other parts are not reversed (Felleman et al., 1979; Nelson, Sur, and Kaas, 1978), suggests that at least in these monkeys the representations can be divided into relatively independent sectors or "blocks." The large glabrous foot and hand representations form medial and lateral blocks that do not reverse, while the middle trunk–leg–arm block does reverse. It is possible that the greatly enlarged representations of the hand and foot in monkeys have served to subdivide the cortical maps by reducing the overall continuity.

Cortical Magnification, Receptive-Field Size, and the Cortical Processing Unit

There are two obvious observations in any mapping study of somatosensory cortex. First, receptive fields for some recording sites are much larger than others; and second, the amount of cortex devoted to any given area of body surface varies greatly. These two factors are related; large receptive fields are found on body parts with little cortical representation, and vice versa. Because our cortical maps were done in great detail, it was possible to quantify the relation between cortical magnification and receptive field size (Sur, Merzenich, and Kaas, 1980). When this was done, it appeared that the amount of cortex activated by stimuli within any given receptive field is approximately the same for all parts of the body. This given amount of cortex is a basic processing unit in the sense that within the representation it contains all of the information available from stimulation within a given receptive field.

This "processing unit" is conceptually similar to the "hypercolumn" of Hubel and Wiesel (1974).

More specifically, measurements from areas 3b and 1 in the owl monkey (Sur, Merzenich, and Kaas, 1980) indicated that the cortical magnification (cortical area per unit body surface area) for the glabrous digits is about 100 times that of the trunk (magnifications differ for the same body parts in areas 3b and 1, but they are roughly similar). However, the receptive fields for the trunk are about 100 times larger than those on the glabrous hand. Detailed measurements of receptive-field size and cortical magnification for different body regions show that the two are inversely related. As a consequence of this inverse relationship, recording sites within 500 to 600 μm of each other have overlapping receptive fields, while those separated by a greater distance do not. Because overlap can occur for pairs of recording sites in all directions, it is necessary to assume that an area 1–1.5 mm in diameter anywhere in area 3b or area 1 would receive the projections of all receptors within a receptive field anywhere on the body surface.

The "hypercolumn" for somatosensory cortex is basically a theoretical construct, and it does not require that area 3b be subdivided into discrete 1.5-mm processing units. Instead, it provides a basis for thinking concretely about cortical microorganization, for it specifies the approximate size of the cortical region within a representation processing all input from a given body locus.

Modular and Microorganization

Our observations on the organization of areas 3b and 1 in monkeys lead to the conclusion that these representations do contain discrete processing subunits or divisions. One type of processing unit is basically consistent with the concept of a vertical column of cells of similar response features and receptive-field locations as originally proposed by Mountcastle (1957). The dimensions or even the reality of such columns have been difficult to demonstrate since cells in adjoining columns may have similar properties, and may differ little in overall receptive-field locations. However, Paul, Goodman, and Merzenich (1972) introduced a powerful approach to the study of cortical columns when they studied the receptive-field locations for cortical cells after section and regeneration of peripheral cutaneous nerves. In such preparations, some of the nerve fibers regenerated to wrong locations. Thus, some cortical neurons have receptive fields that were displaced from those of adjoining neurons, or had both displaced and normal receptive fields. Furthermore, when neurons were discovered with displaced receptive fields, all neurons within the vertical electrode penetration had displaced receptive fields, thus demonstrating that an error in input affects a vertically aligned row of cells.

We have extended the observations of Paul, Goodman, and Mer-

J. H. Kaas, R. J. Nelson, M. Sur, and M. M. Merzenich

zenich (1972) by asking, what is the width of the vertical array of cells that is altered by an error in input? In areas 3b and 1 of owl and squirrel monkeys, tangential electrode penetrations were used to record from cells and determine receptive-field locations (M. Merzenich, J. Kaas, M. Sur, and R. Nelson, unpublished observations). The logic of the approach is shown in Figure 7. Normally it would be difficult to detect adjacent cortical columns by changes in receptive-field locations because the locations would be similar. However, if some nerve fibers regenerate to wrong locations, the change from one cortical column to another might be indicated by a sudden shift in receptive-field locations. The results of such experiments seem to support the concept of discrete cortical columns. Over a significant electrode-penetration distance, all neurons typically had a given set of normal and abnormal receptive fields. After a given horizontal distance a sudden change occurred, so that neurons over a second width had a new set of receptive fields. While our experiments are incomplete, the preliminary results suggest that the width of the basic processing unit or cortical column is on the order of 40–60 μm.

Other experiments have revealed a larger processing unit or module

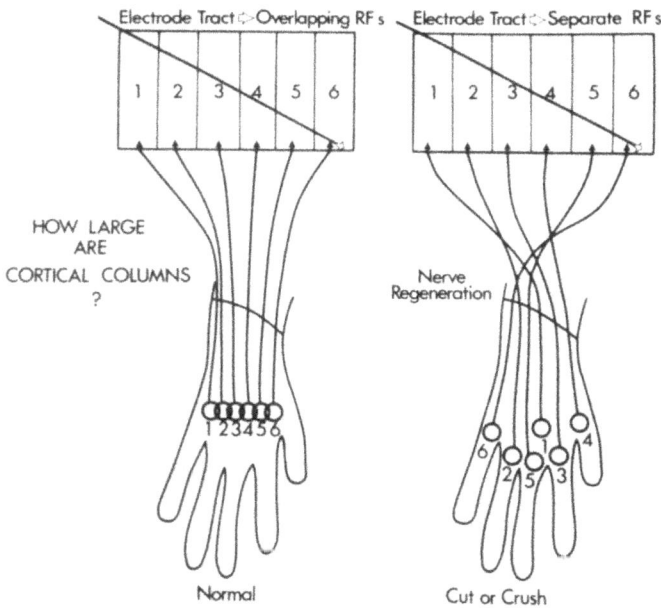

Figure 7 How nerve-regeneration experiments can be used to estimate the sizes of cortical columns. Normally, adjacent columns have adjoining and overlapping receptive fields. An electrode penetration across the columns would reveal a progression of receptive fields, but there would be no jumps in receptive-field location when the electrode crossed column boundaries. If peripheral nerve fibers regenerate to wrong locations, then jumps in receptive-field location would be expected at the borders of adjacent columns.

in area 3b of macaque monkeys (Sur, 1979). Within area 3b, neurons can be characterized as being activated by slowly adapting (SA) or rapidly adapting (RA) inputs. The spatial distribution of these inputs was investigated for neurons within or close to cortical layer IV (SA input was difficult to detect away from layer IV) in closely spaced grids of perpendicular electrode penetrations, and in tangential penetrations in the part of area 3b representing the digits. These single-unit studies indicate that the SA and RA inputs are segregated into blocks of "columns" rather than being mosaically related. The two types of inputs were separated in layer IV in a way that related very specifically to the cortical map (Figure 8). From lateral to medial in the map of the glabrous hand in area 3b, the digits are represented in order from thumb to little finger. SA input was usually found at the margins of each digit representation, where SA input activated a narrow band of layer IV only 200 μm or so wide, but apparently several millimeters long. A *central core* of neurons some 800 μm or so wide was activated by RA input. The receptive fields for neurons in the central 800-μm RA core covered the complete finger, and the receptive fields for neurons in the 200-μm SA fringe overlapped those for the RA core, thus forming a second map of the finger.

The segregation of SA and RA inputs into separate bands or modules, each representing the same body part, is a complication of the body-surface map in area 3b that is not apparent unless the organization is considered in great detail. If the segregation observed in the representation of the glabrous hand occurs in other parts of area 3b, then we

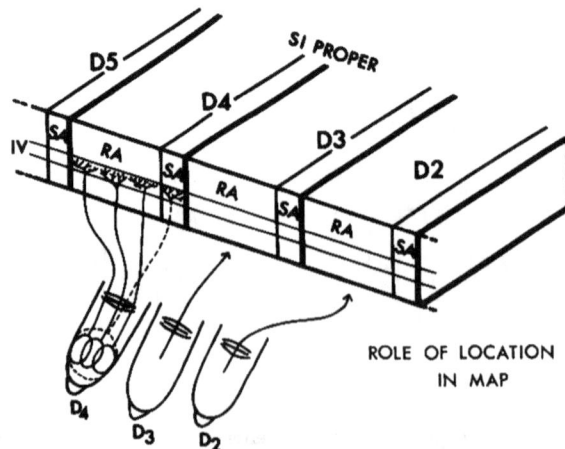

Figure 8 Modular distribution of slowly (SA) and rapidly (RA) adapting inputs in the region of cortex representing the digits in area 3b of macaque monkeys. Each digit is represented by a central core of RA input and flanked on one or both sides by sidebands of SA input. Other configurations are also possible. (Based on Sur, 1979.)

J. H. Kaas, R. J. Nelson, M. Sur, and M. M. Merzenich

must conclude that in some sense there are two interrelated body-surface maps within area 3b.

Amount of Convergence in Areas 3b and 1

The nerve-regeneration experiments also provide information on another aspect of cortical organization. Both cutaneous representations in monkeys receive input from the same thalamic nucleus, the ventroposterior nucleus, and there is even indirect evidence that some thalamic neurons project to both fields (Lin et al., 1979). The receptive fields for recording sites in area 1 are generally larger than the receptive fields for matched recording sites in area 3b (Merzenich et al., 1978), suggesting a greater convergence of receptor inputs in area 1. In the normal animal, it is difficult to determine the number of peripheral units feeding into a cortical recording site because receptive fields overlap (Figure 9). However, in a nerve-regeneration experiment where errors in locations have been induced, the relative amount of convergence, at least, can be compared between two areas by noting differences in the numbers of distinctly separate receptive fields for given recording sites. Our preliminary nerve-regeneration studies indicate that neurons in area 3b typically have from one to three normal and abnor-

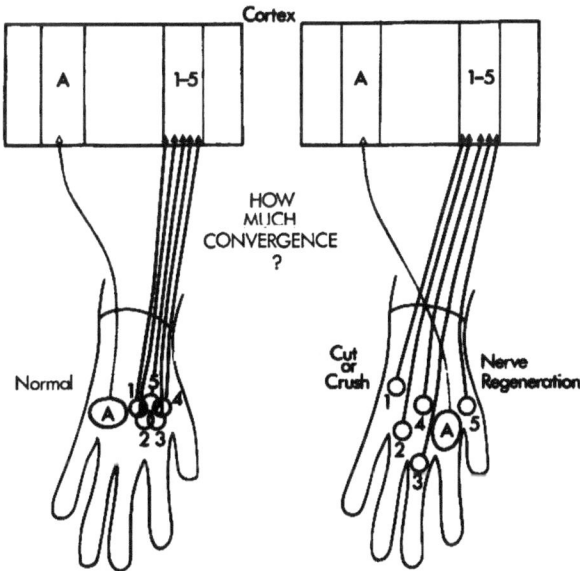

Figure 9 How nerve-regeneration experiments can be used to detect convergence. In the normal animal, converging inputs from the same location (1–5) are difficult to distinguish from a single input (A). If there have been errors in regeneration, then cortical neurons with converging inputs will have separate receptive fields.

mal receptive fields, while neurons in area 1 have from two to five and as many as seven (M. Merzenich, J. Kaas, M. Sur, and R. Nelson, unpublished observations).

Dynamic Features of Cortical Maps

The topographic organization of a cortical field is stable throughout the length of a recording session. Thus, the receptive field for any cortical recording site, when defined repeatedly during an experiment, remains basically the same in skin position and in size. However, it also appears that this stable organization is a result of balancing dynamic influences. When this balance is disrupted by inactivating part of the peripheral sensory input, the organizations of the cortical maps are immediately altered and continue to change over time.

In recent experiments (Merzenich et al., 1980) we have examined the maps of the hand in area 3b and in area 1 before and at various times after cutting and suturing the central stump of the median nerve. Since the median nerve provides the central input from cutaneous receptors located on much of the palm and the glabrous portions of digits 1–3, one expected outcome of this surgical inactivation of the median nerve might be the consequent inactivation of the portions of the cortical maps subserved by the median nerve. This expected outcome was only partially and temporarily observed. When the hand representation was mapped, followed by a nerve cut, and the cortex was immediately remapped, the result was that only part of the cortical median nerve field was inactivated. For the majority of the "deafferented" regions of these two cortical representations, neurons could not be appreciably activated by cutaneous stimuli anywhere on the hand. However, neurons over a significant part of the cortical median-nerve field now could be activated by stimulating parts of the hand outside the peripheral distribution of the median nerve, and these neurons had restricted definable receptive fields. The new receptive fields were not randomly located, but formed a remarkable pattern. Recording sites that were formerly activated from receptive fields on the glabrous surface of the fingers, for example, now became activated from receptive fields with similar locations but on the hairy dorsum of the corresponding fingers. Thus, a fragmentary map of the hairy dorsum of the fingers immediately replaced the map of the glabrous surface.

These results show that the organizations revealed by mapping experiments in normal animals reflect only part of the total anatomical pattern of connections that must exist (also see Wall and Egger, 1971; Kalaska and Pomeranz, 1979). Some pathways must be responsible for the dominant organization that is revealed under the usual recording conditions. Other highly ordered pathways are not revealed by patterns of minimal excitory receptive fields unless the "dominant" pathways are inactivated. However, the "hidden," as well as the patent, features

J. H. Kaas, R. J. Nelson, M. Sur, and M. M. Merzenich

of the cortical maps are probably important in the normal cortical processing of somatosensory information.

The cortical map found immediately after cutting the median nerve changes further over time, even though the nerve is not allowed to regenerate. Over a period of a few weeks, the large silent sectors of cortical tissue gradually become active, and these are activated by adjacent normally innervated parts of the hand in a pattern suggesting that there is constant competition for cortical sites by adjacent skin surfaces. Thus, cortical maps even in adults are probably subject to constant modifications based on the use or activity of the peripheral sensory pathways.

The end result of inactivating the input from part of the hand is that other parts of the hand have a greatly expanded cortical representation. Some body parts, such as the dorsal surfaces of the digits, retain their original small orderly cortical representation, and also acquire a second orderly and greatly expanded representation. One wonders what the consequences of these cortical changes are, if any, for sensory perception!

What Is SI?

The clear evidence in monkeys for two highly ordered maps of the body surface in areas 3b and 1 and a third map of deep body tissues with some cutaneous input in area 2 raises the obvious question, how do these three fields compare to the single cutaneous map SI that has been described in a range of nonprimates and in prosimian primates? Since the multiple maps within the classical SI have been recognized only recently in monkeys, it seems reasonable to start to answer this question by considering the possibility that multiple maps will also be revealed within the presently described SI of prosimians and most nonprimates. Recently, microelectrode mapping techniques have been used to carefully explore the traditional SI regions in a number of mammals, and it now seems certain that where SI has been related to a single architectonic field, this single field constitutes a single representation of the skin surface. Thus, in the rat (Welker, 1971), grey squirrel (Sur, Nelson, and Kaas, 1978), tree shrew (Weller, Sur, and Kaas, 1979), galago (Sur, Nelson, and Kaas, 1980), and slow loris (Krishnamurti, Sanides, and Welker, 1976), to cite a few examples, the existence of a single cutaneous representation within the traditional SI field has been confirmed by microelectrode mapping techniques and related to a single architectonic field. (As an interesting variation the glabrous digits and palm are replicated within the otherwise single SI representation in the squirrel). The situation is less clear in domestic cats, where SI has traditionally included several architectonic fields, designated 3a, 3b, 1, and 2 as in monkeys. It has been reported that area 3b (or part of it) alone contains a complete body surface map and that other cutaneous representations exist (Rasmussen, Dykes, and Hoeltzell, 1979).

Applying the term SI to a single representation in some mammals and a collection of representations in others is confusing. We believe that the 3b field in monkeys is the homolog of SI as it has been defined in at least most other mammals, and therefore we suggest the term "SI proper" for the 3b fields (Merzenich et al., 1978; Kaas et al., 1979) in order to both make it clear that we are not using SI in the old sense for monkeys, and emphasize the identity of the 3b field with SI as it is defined in most mammals.

There are two main reasons for considering the representation in area 3b to be the homolog of SI in other mammals. First, the positions of the two representations are comparable. Both SI and area 3b are the first cutaneous fields behind motor cortex. Second, the somatotopic organizations of SI and area 3b are basically the same. As an important example, the glabrous digits of the hand have been consistently described as pointing rostrally in SI, and they point rostrally in area 3b. Other similarities between the SI and 3b fields are in cytoarchitecture, and in connections with the ventroposterior nucleus of the thalamus. Given these observations, it seems necessary to conclude that the 3b field of higher primates is the same field as SI as it is defined in many mammals.

The conclusion that area 3b (SI proper) and SI are homologous, raises the question of the existence of the 3a, 1, and 2 fields in nonprimates and in prosimians. There is architectonic evidence for a narrow field with both sensory and motor characteristics between motor cortex and SI in a range of mammals that is similar to the primate 3a field. It is not known whether or not this intermediate field is activated by muscle afferents or is organized like area 3a in monkeys except in cats, where a 3a field has been identified and related to muscle-receptor inputs (see Rasmussen, Dykes, and Hoeltzell, 1979; Oscarsson and Rosen, 1966). Separate fields for area 1 and area 2 have been postulated in some mammals, and not in others. However, systematic body maps have not been found in these postulated fields in mammals other than monkeys. Given the uncertainty of conclusions based solely on cortical architecture, there is no compelling evidence for or against the existence of homologs of areas 1 and 2 in nonsimian mammals (in cats, areas 1 and 2 are responsive to cutaneous stimuli, and apparently are interconnected with area 3b, but separate maps have not yet been established). Thus, both the possibilities that the number of sensory representations has increased in primate evolution and that some or all of the 3a, 1, and 2 fields (in addition to 3b) are basic to several or all lines of mammalian evolution need to be considered in future research.

Acknowledgments

Research by the authors was supported by National Science Foundation Grant BNS-81824.

J. H. Kaas, R. J. Nelson, M. Sur, and M. M. Merzenich

References

Allman, J. M., and J. H. Kaas, 1976. Representation of the visual field on the medial wall of occipital-parietal cortex in the owl monkey. *Science* 191:572–575.

Coulter, J. D., and E. G. Jones, 1977. Differential distribution of corticospinal projections from individual architectonic fields in the monkey. *Brain Res.* 129:335–340.

Dreyer, D. A., P. R. Loe, C. B. Metz, and B. L. Whitsel, 1975. Representation of head and face in postcentral gyrus of the macaque. *J. Neurophysiol.* 38:714–733.

Dreyer, D. A., R. J. Schneider, C. B. Metz, and B. L. Whitsel, 1974. Differential contributions of spinal pathways to body representation in postcentral gyrus of *Macaca mulatta*. *J. Neurophysiol.* 37:119–145.

Felleman, D. J., R. J. Nelson, M. Sur, and J. H. Kaas, 1979. Organization of the somatosensory cortex in cebus monkeys. *Neurosci. Abst.* 5:706.

Hubel, D. H., and T. N. Wiesel, 1974. Uniformity of monkey striate cortex: A parallel relationship between field size, scatter, and magnification factor. *J. Comp. Neurol.* 158:295–306.

Imig, T. J., M. H. Ruggero, L. M. Kitzes, E. Javel, and J. F. Brugge, 1977. Organization of auditory cortex in the owl monkey *(Aotus trivirgatus)*. *J. Comp. Neurol.* 171:111–128.

Jones, E. J., J. D. Coulter, and S. H. Hendry, 1978. Intracortical connectivity of architectonic fields in the somatic sensory, motor, and parietal cortex of monkeys. *J. Comp. Neurol.* 181:291–348.

Jones, E. G., S. P. Wise, and J. D. Coulter, 1979. Differential thalamic relationships of sensory-motor and parietal cortical fields in monkeys. *J. Comp. Neurol.* 183:833–882.

Kaas, J. H., 1977. Sensory representations in mammals. In *Function and Formation of Neural Systems*. G. S. Stent, ed. Berlin: Dahlem Konferenzen, pp. 65–80.

Kaas, J. H., M. M. Merzenich, C.-S. Lin, and M. Sur, 1976. A double representation of the body in "primary somatosensory cortex" ('SI') of primates. *Neurosci. Abst.* 2:914.

Kaas, J. H., R. J. Nelson, M. Sur, and M. M. Merzenich, 1979. Multiple representations of the body within the primary somatosensory cortex of primates. *Science* 204:521–523.

Kalaska, J., and B. Pomeranz, 1979. Chronic paw denervation causes an age-dependent appearance of novel responses from forearm in "paw cortex" of kittens and adult cats. *J. Neurophysiol.* 42:618–633.

Krishnamurti, A., F. Sanides, and W. I. Welker, 1976. Microelectrode mapping of modality-specific somatic sensory cerebral neocortex in slow loris. *Brain Behav. Evol.* 13:367–383.

Lin, C.-S., M. M. Merzenich, M. Sur, and J. H. Kaas, 1979. Connections of areas 3b and 1 of the parietal somatosensory strip with the ventroposterior nucleus in owl monkey *(Aotus trivirgatus)*. *J. Comp. Neurol.* 185:355–372.

Merzenich, M. M., J. H. Kaas, M. Sur, and C.-S. Lin, 1978. Double representation of the body surface within cytoarchitectonic Areas 3b and 1 in "SI" in the owl monkey (*Aotus trivirgatus*). *J. Comp. Neurol.* 181:41–74.

Merzenich, M. M., R. J. Nelson, M. Sur, J. T. Wall, D. J. Felleman, and J. H. Kaas, 1980. Plasticity in somatosensory cortex in monkeys: Progressive reorganization within somatosensory fields 3b and 1 following peripheral deafferentation. (In preparation.)

Mountcastle, V. B., 1957. Modality and topographic properties of single neurons of cat's somatic sensory cortex. *J. Neurophysiol.* 20:408–434.

Nelson, R. J., M. Sur, and J. H. Kaas, 1978. Multiple representations of the body surface in postcentral cortex ("SI") of the squirrel monkey. *Neurosci. Abst.* 4:556.

Nelson, R. J., M. Sur, and J. H. Kaas, 1979. The organization of the second somatosensory area (SmII) of the grey squirrel. *J. Comp. Neurol.* 184:473–490.

Nelson, R. J., M. Sur, D. J. Felleman, and J. H. Kaas, 1980. Representations of the body surface in postcentral parietal cortex of *Macaca fascicularis*. *J. Comp. Neurol.* (in press).

Oscarsson, O., and I. Rosen, 1966. Short-latency projections to the cat's cerebral cortex from skin and muscle afferents in the contralateral forelimb. *J. Physiol.* (*London*) 182:164–184.

Paul, R. L., H. Goodman, and M. M. Merzenich, 1972. Alterations in mechanoreceptor input to Brodmann's Areas 1 and 3 of the postcentral hand area of *Macaca mulatta* after nerve section and regeneration. *Brain Res.* 39:1–19.

Paul, R. L., M. M. Merzenich, and H. Goodman, 1972. Representation of slowly and rapidly adapting cutaneous mechanoreceptors of the hand in Brodmann's Areas 3 and 1 of *Macaca mulatta*. *Brain Res.* 36:229–249.

Pearson, R. C. A., and T. P. S. Powell, 1978. The cortico-cortical connections to Area 5 of the parietal lobe from the primary somatic sensory cortex of the monkey. *Proc. Roy. Soc. B* 200:103–108.

Powell, T. P. S., and V. B. Mountcastle, 1959. Some aspects of the functional organization of the cortex of the postcentral gyrus of the monkey. A correlation of findings obtained in a single unit analysis with cytoarchitecture. *Bull. Johns Hopkins Hosp.* 105:133–162.

Randolph, M., and J. Semmes, 1974. Behavioral consequences of selective subtotal ablations in the postcentral gyrus of *Macaca mulatta*. *Brain Res.* 70:55–70.

Rasmussen, P. D., R. W. Dykes, and P. B. Hoeltzell, 1979. Segregation of modality and submodality information in SI cortex of the cat. *Brain Res.* 166:409–412.

Shanks, M. F., R. C. A. Pearson, and T. P. S. Powell, 1978. The intrinsic connections of the primary somatic sensory cortex of the monkey. *Proc. Roy Soc. B* 200:95–101.

Shanks, M. F., A. J. Rockel, and T. P. S. Powell, 1975. The commissural connections of the primary somatic sensory cortex. *Brain Res.* 98:166–171.

Sur, M., 1979. Somatosensory cortex in macaque monkeys: Columnar organization of slowly and rapidly adapting neurons and receptive field organization. *Fed. Proc.* 38:898.

Sur, M., M. M. Merzenich, and J. H. Kaas, 1980. Some quantitative features of the body surface representations in areas 3b and 1 in owl monkeys: Magnification, receptive field area and "hypercolumn size." *J. Neurophysiol.* (in press).

Sur, M., R. J. Nelson, and J. H. Kaas, 1978. The representation of the body surface in somatosensory area 1 of the grey squirrel. *J. Comp. Neurol.* 179:425–450.

Sur, M., R. J. Nelson, and J. H. Kaas, 1980. The representation of the body surface in somatic koniocortex in the prosimian, *Galago. J. Comp. Neurol.* 189:381–462.

Vogt, B. A., and D. N. Pandya, 1978. Cortico-cortical connections of somatic sensory cortex (Areas 3, 1, and 2) in the rhesus monkey. *J. Comp. Neurol.* 172:179–192.

Wall, P. D., and M. D. Egger, 1971. Formation of new connections in adult rat brains after partial deafferentation. *Nature* 232:542–545.

Welker, C., 1971. Microelectrode delineation of fine grain somatotopic organization of SmI cerebral neocortex in the albino rat. *Brain Res.* 26:259–275.

Weller, R. E., M. Sur, and J. H. Kaas, 1979. Representation of the body surface in SI of the tree shrew. *Anat. Rec.* 133:716.

Werner, G., and B. L. Whitsel, 1968. Topology of the body representation in somatosensory area I in primates. *J. Neurophysiol.* 31:856–869.

Whitsel, B. L., D. A. Dreyer, and J. R. Roppolo, 1971. Determinants of body representation in postcentral gyrus of macaques. *J. Neurophysiol.* 34:1018–1034.

Woolsey, C. N., 1952. Patterns of localization in sensory and motor areas of the cerebral cortex. In *The Biology of Mental Health and Disease.* New York: Milbank Memorial Fund, Hoeber.

Woolsey, C. N., 1958. Organization of somatic sensory and motor areas of the cerebral cortex. In *Biological and Biochemical Bases of Behavior.* H. F. Harlow and C. N. Woolsey, eds. Madison, WI: University of Wisconsin Press.

Woolsey, C. N., W. H. Marshall, and P. Bard, 1942. Representation of cutaneous tactile sensibility in the cerebral cortex of monkeys as indicated by evoked potentials. *Bull. Johns Hopkins Hosp.* 70:399–441.

11 Functional Studies of the Motor Cortex

Edward V. Evarts

ABSTRACT The laws of reflex action, long known to operate at the level of the spinal-cord motoneuron, also operate at the level of the cerebral motor cortex in the course of volitional movements. Motor-cortex neurons are impinged upon by afferent inputs which constitute the incoming limb of a transcortical servo loop. Thus, the phylogenetically new motor cortex of the primate is subject to the same laws of reflex action that characterize phylogenetically older components of mammalian motor-control systems. But in addition to being driven by a servo system that stabilizes movement and posture, motor cortex can be driven by a second major set of inputs, and it is this second set of inputs that underlies internally generated motor programs. These programs are themselves a product of activity in other cortical areas and in basal ganglia and cerebellum.

Of the two major classes of inputs impinging upon the cerebral motor cortex and generating the stream of impulses passing to the spinal cord, that class of inputs which operates automatically and constitutes the afferent limb of the transcortical servo loop seems less difficult to understand. This transcortical servo operates according to Sherringtonian principles of reflex action. The second set of inputs passing to motor cortex via the thalamus depends upon basal ganglia and cerebellum, and is much more complicated. In order to understand voluntary movement we need to comprehend the sorts of information processed by cerebellum and basal ganglia, and to discover the way in which the outputs of cerebellum and basal ganglia interact in the thalamus. It is these problems which stand at the forefront of studies on brain mechanisms of movement.

Introduction

The concept of a "motor cortex" arose as a result of the discovery by Fritsch and Hitzig (1870) that electrical stimulation of a localized area of the cerebral cortex of one hemisphere elicits contractions of muscles on the opposite side of the body. These findings provided experimental confirmation for conclusions already reached by Hughlings Jackson (1931) on the basis of the clinical observation that an irritative lesion of the cerebral cortex of one side of the brain could cause epileptic move-

E. V. EVARTS Laboratory of Neurophysiology, National Institute of Mental Health, Bethesda, Maryland 20205

ments affecting the opposite side of the body. The experiments of Fritsch and Hitzig, carried out on dogs, were confirmed in the monkey by Ferrier (1873).

Discovery that electrical stimulation of the cerebral cortex could evoke movements had a remarkable impact on neurological thinking in the late nineteenth century. To fully understand this impact, one must realize that prior to 1870 it was widely believed that *ideas* (and not movements) were the items represented in the cerebral cortex. Thus, Walshe (1943) points out that "a study of Jackson's early papers reveals what strength of opposition his inferences encountered and how firmly rooted in the contemporary view was the notion that the cerebral convolutions were 'for mentation' only."

As described in the historical treatise by Clarke and O'Malley (1968), in 1874 the Russian anatomist Betz discovered some extraordinarily large nerve cells (now known as Betz cells) in motor cortex of man and subhuman primates. The axons of these Betz cells have now been shown to descend to make direct connections with spinal-cord motoneurons—especially the motoneurons controlling muscles which are used in the precise movements of speech and manipulation, and it is in connection with these movements that motor cortex is particularly important. The special role of motor cortex in such movements is reflected in the fact that a disproportionately large part of the motor cortex is devoted to control of that very small proportion of the body musculature which participates in speech and manipulation.

There is a marked increase both in size of motor cortex and in direct (monosynaptic) control of motoneurons by motor cortex from monkey to chimpanzee to man. Phillips and Porter (1977) have noted that the major differences between the hand movements of man and monkey lie not so much in the movements which it is anatomically possible for either to perform, but rather in the purposive nature of the volitional movements which are performed. In Old World monkeys, apes, and man, the thumb becomes truly opposable, and with this opposability the precision grip of the index finger evolves. Independent movement of the fingers is acquired in higher primates in parallel with motor-cortex enlargement, reaching its fullest development in man. Kuypers (1964, 1973) has shown that along with this increase in individual finger-movement control there is an increase in direct monosynaptic projections from motor cortex to motoneurons. In man, some of these monosynaptic connections occur in the thoracic spinal cord in regions containing motoneurons innervating respiratory muscles. One might at first wonder why motor-cortex neurons supposed to control precise skilled movements should terminate on motoneurons controlling muscles which participate in an act as automatic and primitive as respiration, but Phillips and Porter (1977) point out that these terminations are probably related to use of respiratory muscles in speech and song rather than in breathing: the motor-cortex projection provides for control of old muscles in new patterns, and as Hughlings Jackson recognized almost a century ago, loss of the corticospinal projection does not paralyze muscles per se, but eliminates their use in the context of certain movements. Destruction of the corticospinal projection to thoracic motoneurons does not impair the utilization of respiratory muscles in the context of respiration, though these same muscles may be useless in the context of speech.

The Activity of Brain Cells during Voluntary Movement

Within the past decade much information concerning the function of motor cortex has been provided by techniques which make it possible to introduce microelectrodes into the brains of experimental animals carrying out skilled movements. These techniques have made it possible to study the functional properties of motor cortex underlying its critical role in precise manual control—the type of precise control which allows a surgeon peering through a dissecting microscope accurately to move a scalpel a fraction of a millimeter. The critical role of motor cortex in such precise motor control has been amply reflected in the nature of the deficits resulting from motor-cortex lesions. Denny-Brown (1960) observed that the most obvious immediate deficit resulting from destruction of the precentral gyrus on one side in the monkey is a paralysis of the lower part of the face and the limbs of the opposite side. There is considerable recovery of function with the passage of time, but the type of movement that is completely and permanently abolished by ablation of the precentral gyrus involves orientation of the hand or foot or lips on the basis of somatosensory information.

The special role of motor cortex in precise movement controlled by somatosensory inputs led to studies (Evarts and Fromm, 1977, 1978; Fromm and Evarts, 1977) of the responsiveness of motor-cortex neurons to afferent input under conditions in which monkeys made small, precisely controlled arm movements. It seemed that if motor cortex output were to control precise fine movements, then its neurons would be strongly modulated even with the most minute changes of activity of peripheral musculature occurring with small volitional movements. Furthermore, since precise manual control is highly dependent upon sensory feedback from the hand, it seemed that motor-cortex activity during fine, precisely controlled movements should be under continuous closed-loop negative-feedback control by sensory input. To see whether motor cortex exhibited intense modulation with small volitional movements, we trained monkeys to make precise movements of a handle whose rotation controlled a visual display, with reward being given to the monkeys according to the precision of their performance. To see whether sensory feedback from the hand exercised automatic servo control over this motor cortex output, we delivered sensory stimuli to the monkey's hand in the course of these movements.

The two hypotheses referred to above were studied in a visual pursuit paradigm (Figure 1) which involved several features:

(1) A *holding period* of 1.5 to 2.5 sec during which the monkey held a handle vertically to align a "track" lamp with a "target" lamp.

(2) *Small movements* of 1–2° were carried out by the monkey when a misalignment of track and target lamps resulted either from the monkey's failure to keep the handle within the narrow hold zone or from a shift of the track display from the center lamp to the one on its right or left. In the latter case the shift was caused by adding an error signal to the output of the potentiometer. Figure 2 shows a series of such small pronation (top left) and supination (bottom left) corrective movements carried out by the monkey in order to realign the track and target lamps.

(3) *Large movements* (20°) (marked "unperturbed ballistic" in Figure 2) were triggered by a jump of the target to the extreme right or left of the display panel. For the special case of such large target jumps the criterion of success was movement velocity: the monkey was rewarded with a drop of juice if the handle was rotated in the direction of the target jump with a movement time less than 150 msec (movement velocity >300°/sec). The monkey's "ballistic" movements were not precisely controlled as to termination, since target zones at both extreme positions were stopped by a physical barrier.

(4) Immediately after a ballistic movement, the target jumped back to the center and the monkey returned the handle to the central hold zone to initiate a new cycle (step 1).

(5) The handle was coupled to the axle of a dc torque motor (Colburn and Evarts, 1978) which produced a constant torque during steady holding. This torque required either steady supinator or pronator force and resulted in an effective force of 90 g applied to the monkey's hand. Units were usually tested under both load conditions. In addition, 50-msec rectangular *torque pulses* could be delivered to the handle via the motor to study unit sensitivity to peripheral inputs. Randomly alternated pronating and supinating torque pulses were applied (a) after 700 msec of *steady holding*, (b) at a fixed delay of 120 msec after a target jump and thus immediately *preceding the ballistic movement*, (c) *at the start* of a ballistic movement, and (d) at the start of a small movement. The latter pulses [(c) and (d)] were triggered at the time the handle left the central hold zone.

Precentral single-unit activity associated with movements of the contralateral arm was recorded in monkeys in whom pyramidal-tract neurons (PTNs) were antidromically identified by stimulation of the medullary pyramid. Figure 2 shows data displays generated in this paradigm, where each raster row corresponds to a trial, with dots representing individual spikes. The central vertical line in each raster repre-

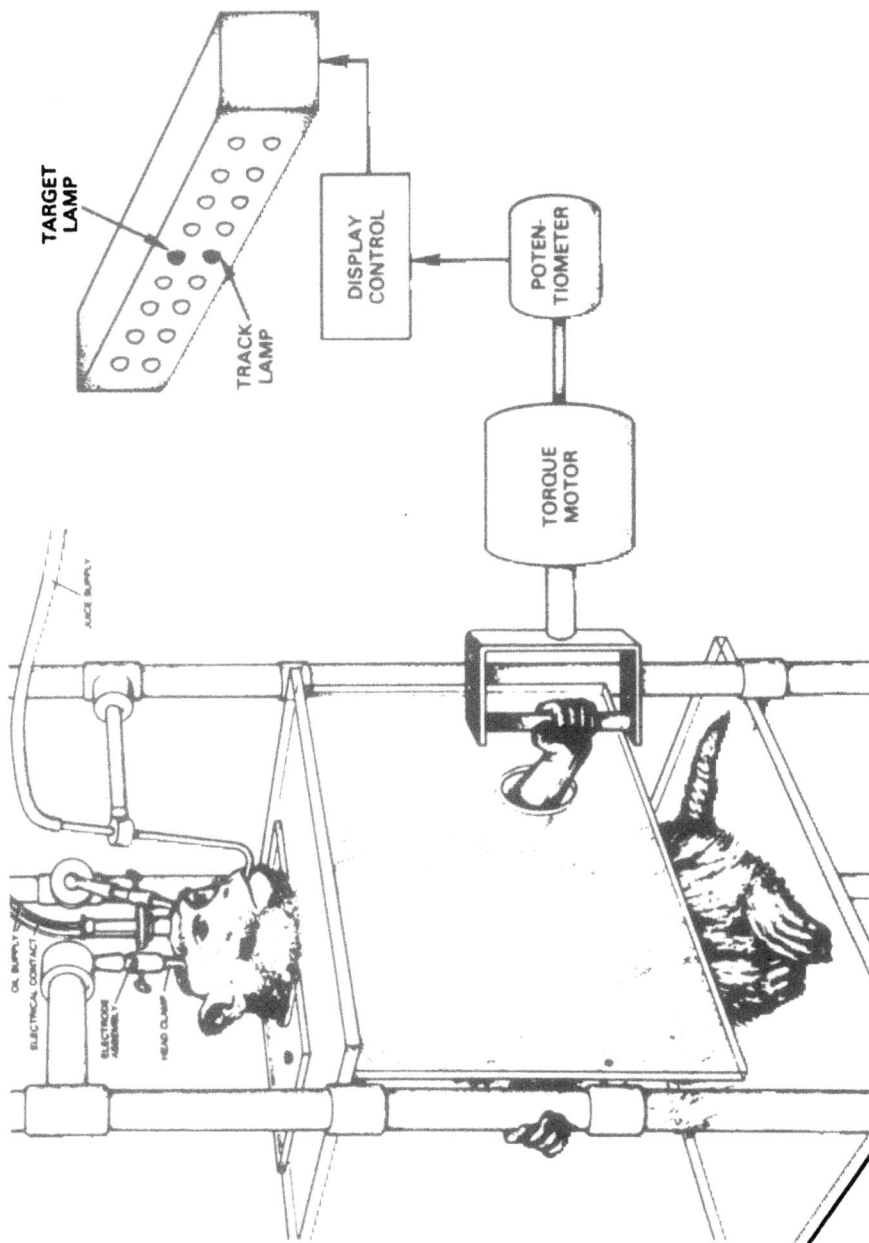

Figure 1 Visual-pursuit tracking paradigm. The movements of the handle grasped by the monkey changed a potentiometer output which controlled the position of the track lamp. Displacements of the hand could be produced by the torque motor. The monkey was required to maintain alignment between track lamp and target lamp. (From Evarts, 1980.)

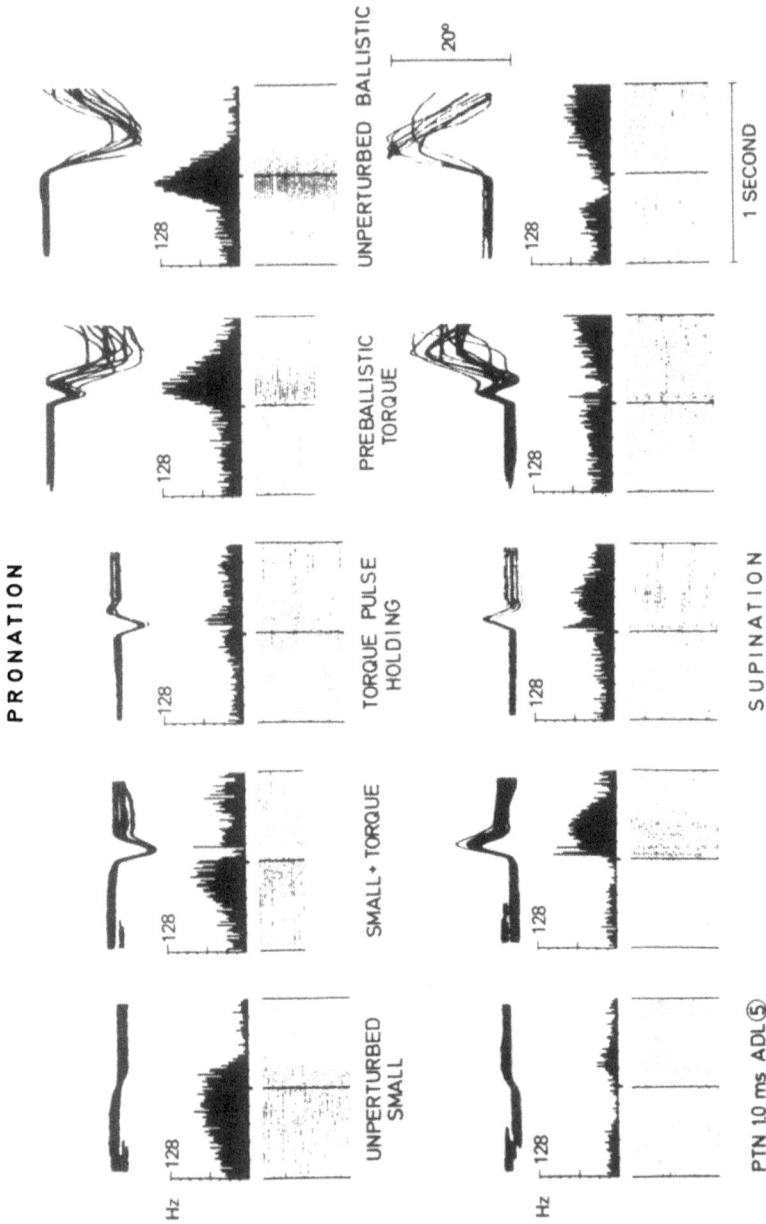

Figure 2 Three sorts of displays are shown: (1) superimposed position traces; (2) histograms of unit discharge; and (3) rasters of unit discharge. Attention is directed to several points: (1) unperturbed small pronation (top left) is preceded by more prolonged unit discharge than is the case for unperturbed ballistic movement (top right); (2) the inhibitory effect of the torque pulse is greater when it is delivered during a small pronation (top row marked "small + torque") than when it is delivered during holding (top, marked "torque pulse holding"); (3) there is a corresponding accentuation of the excitatory effects of the supinating torque pulse when this is delivered during small movement (bottom, marked "small + torque") as compared to holding (bottom, marked "torque pulse holding"). For further details, see text. (From Evarts and Fromm, 1978.)

sents the event with respect to which raster rows are aligned. In the torque pulse rasters (Figure 2, center) this central vertical line marks the onset of the torque pulse. For the ballistic movements the central line shows when the handle leaves the hold zone (Figure 2, right column). For the small movements (Figure 2, left column) the central line corresponds to the handle entering the correct zone to realign track and target lamps. In each case the event occurring at the vertical central lines is taken as the reference point for the superimposed position traces. In this figure, upward deflection of the position record indicates supination, while downward deflection indicates pronation.

Of 280 PTNs studied in two monkeys, 124 were not related to any of the movements performed in this paradigm. Of the 156 PTNs which were related, 85 exhibited significant changes in association with both small and large movements, while the remaining 71 PTNs changed their firing rates exclusively in relation to the large, ballistic movements. Within this entire group of 156 PTNs related to small and/or large movements, there was a clear tendency for PTNs discharging most intensely with the smallest movements to be most sensitive to limb displacements produced by torque pulses (Figure 2, center). These torque pulses produced a handle displacement of about 5°, as shown in Figure 2, and elicited reflex responses which occurred at 20 msec. Of 85 PTNs which showed significant changes of discharge frequency with small controlled movements, 94% were clearly influenced by the perturbation. In contrast, only 31% of 71 PTNs which were recruited solely with the large, rapid movements exhibited significant responses to the kinesthetic input. The point to stress from these results is the finding of almost invariable reflex driving of those units most involved in control of small, precise movements. This appears analogous to the great sensitivity to segmental reflex inputs in those alpha motoneurons first to be recruited in the course of movement (Henneman, 1974).

The existence of PTNs discharging with small movements and sensitive to afferent feedback is consistent with Phillips's (1969) proposal that there is a transcortical loop functioning to automatically sense errors occurring during precisely controlled movement. But do the PTN responses to afferent feedback have properties consistent with servo control? To answer this question, let us begin by noting that in closed-loop negative-feedback control systems a disturbance of the controlled output generates nerve impulses whose central connections elicit outputs that tend to overcome the disturbance and thereby tend to nullify the nerve activity that was generated by the disturbance. What are the a priori expectations which one might have for PTN discharges elicited by afferent negative feedback occurring during movement? For PTNs in such a servo loop, the movement resulting from their discharge should tend to reduce (i.e., to inhibit) their discharge, whereas a displacement opposing such a movement should tend to increase (i.e., excite) discharge. This is a restatement of Phillips's (1969) hypothesis as to the effect of "match" and "mismatch" on corticomotoneuronal discharge. A familiar neuronal circuit exhibiting these properties is the loop involving muscle receptors and alpha motoneurons. Within this loop, the consequences of alpha-motoneuron discharge (decreased muscle length and/or increased muscle tension) feed back onto the alpha motoneuron so as to reduce alpha motoneuron discharge:

↓ muscle length → ↓ muscle spindle discharge → ↓ alpha motoneuron discharge;
↑ muscle tension → ↑ tendon organ discharge → ↓ alpha motoneuron discharge.

The motor-cortex PTN shown in Figure 2 appears to be in a loop analogous to the one impinging on spinal-cord alpha motoneurons, a loop carrying information such that externally induced (i.e., passive) movement corresponding to the active movement called for by the PTN inhibits the PTN's discharge. By analogy with the model of negative feedback presented for the alpha motoneuron, an external "assist" which helps to realize the movement "commanded" by the discharge of the PTN will inhibit its discharge, whereas application of a force which opposes this movement will excite the PTN.

Anatomical Pathways for Afferent Feedback to Motor Cortex

There are two major classes of anatomical pathways whereby motor cortex PTNs discharging with precisely controlled fine movements might receive the afferent feedback which modulates their discharge. These two classes are corticocortical and thalamocortical. The studies of Pandya and Kuypers (1969) and Jones and Powell (1970) using silver impregnation of degenerating terminals established the general principle that there is extensive corticocortical interconnection between the subareas of the sensorimotor cortex: areas 6, 4, 3, 1, 2, and 5. Current studies using degeneration staining methods as well as injections of HRP and isotopically labeled amino acids are now providing detailed information concerning these projections. The results of studies using small lesions and small injections localized within subsectors of SI (areas 3a, 3b, 1, or 2) have been of increasing interest with the demonstration that rather than containing a single body representation, SI contains a series of representations of the body. As summarized in the recent paper by Merzenich et al. (1978), there is a large systematic representation of the body surface coextensive with area 3b and another systematic representation in area 1. In addition, all or part of area 2 may contain a systematic representation of deep body structures. It furthermore is speculated that the part of area 3a receiving short-latency muscle afferent input may constitute a fourth "representation." These results are the outgrowth of the initial observations of Paul, Merzenich, and Goodman (1972) showing that there were two distinct maps of the digits within SI, and are consistent with the results of the prior anatomical studies of Jones and Powell (1970), who had suggested that the body surface might be represented more than once in SI. This suggestion of Jones and Powell was based on their finding that there were segregated anatomical pathways from the somatosensory thalamus to cortical areas 3, 1, and 2.

In considering the projections into motor cortex from the subdivisions of SI, it will be useful to summarize the different sorts of receptor modalities projecting to the subdivisions of SI as well as the different patterns of thalamocortical inputs to the SI subsectors: area 3a responds to stimulation of group-I muscle afferents; area 3b is activated by slowly adapting mechanoreceptors in the skin; area 1 is activated by rapidly adapting cutaneous mechanoreceptors; and area 2 is primarily activated by joint movements.

While all divisions of SI receive a thalamic input from the ventrobasal complex, the density of the thalamic input is not uniform across the different divisions. This lack of uniformity was demonstrated in the work of Jones (1975) in studies using the Nauta technique following lesions of the thalamus and also in autoradiographs following injections of tritiated proline into various divisions of the ventrobasal complex. There were obvious qualitative and quantitative differences between the thalamic terminations in area 3b on the one hand and those in areas 1 and 2 on the other, with the concentration of thalamic terminals being much less in areas 1 and 2 than in area 3b. As Jones pointed out, the concept that certain cortical areas receive fewer thalamic afferent fibers than others is not a new one and can be inferred from the number of granule cells in the fourth layer of the cortex. Thus, the relative lack of thalamic input to areas 1 and 2 as compared to area 3b is correlated with a relatively thin internal granular layer in these cytoarchitectonic areas.

Given this rather striking difference between thalamic inputs to area 3b versus areas 1 and 2, one wonders how the regions contrast in terms of corticocortical inputs. The recent work of Vogt and Pandya (1978) and of Jones, Coulter, and Hendry (1978) shows that there is in fact an inverse relationship between the strength of thalamocortical inputs to the subsectors of SI and the input of corticocortical projections to these subsectors. Vogt and Pandya studied corticocortical connections of somatosensory cortex (areas 3b, 1, and 2) in the rhesus monkey using ablation-degeneration techniques. In commenting on the finding of Jones and Powell (1970) and Jones (1975) showing a heavy projection from thalamus to area 3b and weaker projection to areas 1 and 2, Vogt and Pandya point out that, conversely, area 3 receives a relatively small projection from areas 1 and 2, while outgoing connections from areas 3 to 1 and 1 to 2 are quite massive. The authors go on to interpret these findings as follows: "The relative influence of thalamic and SI afferents on each of these areas, therefore, is quite different. Thus, cellular activity in area 3b may be dominated by peripheral stimulation entering via the thalamus while areas 1 and 2 which also respond to peripheral stimulation may be influenced to a greater degree by cortically processed somatic information which is mediated via cortical connections."

One negative finding in the study of Vogt and Pandya is of particular significance: area 3 did not project forward into MI. While having strong projections caudally, into area 1 and to a lesser extent into area 2, area 3b failed to project to the motor cortex. Thus, the somatosensory information reaching area 3b (skin mechanoreceptor information) must be further processed in areas 1 and 2 and cannot directly influence activity in motor cortex. In an overall sense, the Vogt and Pandya findings provided strong support for a hierarchical sequential system of information processing from receipt of afferent input to control of motor output. Vogt and Pandya concluded that "thus, the projections of these three subdivisions of the postcentral gyrus indicate that there is a strong and sequential outflow of connections from area 3b to areas 1 and 2, then from area 1 to area 2 and finally from area 2 to area 5 and rostral area 7. Each of these connections originates to a large extent from the supragranular layers. In contrast, connections of these areas in the opposite direction toward the central sulcus are less pronounced."

The work of Jones, Coulter, and Hendry (1978) used tracer techniques to study this same problem of corticocortical connections of SI cortex, and obtained findings virtually identical to those which Vogt and Pandya obtained using degeneration staining. Thus, Jones, Coulter, and Hendry (1978) found that area 3b, which receives the strongest thalamocortical input, receives virtually no corticocortical input from areas 1, 2, or 4. It is thus apparent that area 3b is dominated by primary afferent input from the thalamus with relatively little admixture of signals arising from other cortical areas. The output of area 3b via corticocortical projections is not directed to the immediately adjacent motor cortex, but instead projects heavily back into area 1 and 2, *but the projection from area 3b to areas 1 and 2 is not reciprocated*: instead of projecting back to area 3b, areas 1 and 2 project to motor cortex. Thus, the cutaneous mechanoreceptor information reaching area 3b is not sent directly on to MI, but is instead subjected to further processing in area 2 which, while lacking the intense thalamic input reaching area 3b, has instead a very strong corticocortical input from areas 3b and 1. Just as area 2 receives from area 3b but fails to project back to area 3b, so area 5 receives from area 2 but fails to project back to area 2. It seems possible that the successive hierarchically organized somatosensory areas generate complex and hypercomplex signals which are then relayed to MI from area 5.

Consistent with these anatomical findings on a hierarchical organization are the results of single-unit recordings from the parietal lobe in monkeys. Thus, Sakata and Iwamura (1978) have presented evidence for "a hierarchical order of processing within SI," with integrative processes being more important in areas 1 and 2 than in area 3b. Even more complicated processing was found in area 5.

Thalamocortical Pathways for Afferent Feedback to Motor Cortex

In addition to the corticocortical pathways referred to above, there are pathways which can bring afferent input to motor cortex directly from the thalamus. Independent studies by Lemon and van der Burg (1979) and by Horne and Tracey (1979) have shown that neurons in thalamic nucleus VPL_O (ventralis posterolateralis, pars oralis) receive short-latency (6–10 msec) inputs from muscle and joint nerves of the arm and transmit these signals to the arm area of the motor cortex. In these studies, motor cortex was electrically stimulated to allow antidromic activation of the VPL_O neurons projecting to motor cortex, and it was found that many of the neurons projecting to motor cortex were activated at short latency by peripheral inputs. Injections of HRP into motor cortex confirmed the location of antidromically activated neurons within the region of VPL_O projecting to motor cortex.

The short latency of the sensory responses in VPL_O ruled out a transcerebellar pathway for the sensory inputs to VPL_O, pointing to a lemniscal pathway, and Lemon and van der Burg concluded that the "neurones in VPL_O both receive a clear peripheral input and project to the motor cortex, and that these neurones may be partly responsible for the short-latency transmission of information from the moving limb to the motor cortex."

Combining the evidence on thalamic and corticocortical projections to motor cortex, it seems clear that both sorts of pathways have the capacity to control motor-cortex output on the basis of sensory input. Thus, just as areas 2 and 5 of the postcentral gyrus receive sensory inputs both from thalamus and from other cortical areas, so too motor cortex receives sensory inputs both from thalamus and from other cortical areas. The relative strengths and physiological roles of these dual systems remain to be worked out.

Open-loop Control

The anatomical and physiological data which have now been reviewed, together with the additional physiological evidence of projections from area 3a into motor cortex, point to pathways whereby negative feedback may reach motor cortex to allow servo regulation of precise movement. But closed-loop negative-feedback systems have the inherent disadvantage of involving a delay for return of the feedback signal and the resultant phase shifts which may generate oscillations. In contrast, open-loop control systems have a great speed advantage. Arbib (1980) has contrasted open- and closed-loop control in the case of a person making a large arm movement to reach out and grasp an object. At the start, when a large arm displacement must be made to get near to the object, there is an initial ballistic movement and then, when the hand is near the object, final adjustments in hand position are made on the basis of feedback. The ballistic phase of the movement is based on open-loop control, while final adjustments use feedback. Open-loop control is brought into play when the error is large, and if well calibrated, the open-loop controller will, with a single brief time pattern of control, return the system to nearly the correct position, making the error small enough for feedback to function effectively. Arbib's notion of open-loop control implies a strategy that generates large control signals to rapidly bridge large discrepancies in desired output at too great a velocity for long-latency feedback paths to play a major part. The results of a number of studies indicate that both of these two strategies are utilized during movements of human subjects.

Though the term open loop is relatively new, the idea of open-loop control was inherent in the term "ballistic movement" as used by the nineteenth-century neurologist Richer in reference to very fast movements, where a brief initial contraction of the agonist muscle was rapidly followed by a complete relaxation *before* the end of the movement. Such ballistic preprogrammed movements may be contrasted with "continuously controlled" movements during which sensory input from the moving part allows continuous adjustment. As implied by the name "ballistic," such movements have been thought of as analogous to the flight of an object whose trajectory is determined by a brief initial application of energy, without the possibility of modification thereafter. Thus, a ballistic movement is thought of as being predetermined, just as the flight of a projectile is predetermined by the initial forces applied to it. Some of the classical early experiments on ballistic movements were carried out by Woodworth (1899). In these experiments subjects were instructed to touch a target perceived visually as soon as this target appeared. Woodworth then systematically displaced the target at varying intervals following its appearance. It was found that displacements of the target occurring less than 100 msec prior to the start of the movement were ineffective in modifying the course of the movement. These unmodifiable movements were said to be ballistic since they were not subject to modification on the basis of visual input during their occurrence.

But now with this brief introduction to open-loop control, let us return to consider PTN discharges during large ballistic movements of the monkey, movements for which optimal performance would require open-loop control rather than the negative feedback characterizing the small precisely controlled movements of the sort which our monkeys made in the visual-pursuit tracking paradigm, where they sought to make 1° pronating or supinating arm movements. Fromm and I compared (1) the reflex responses of precentral neurons to limb displacements during steady holding with (2) the reflex responses to the same displacements occurring at the start of a ballistic movement. The responses to afferent input in these two conditions are illustrated in Figure 2, showing a PTN which exhibited excitation in response to the supinating arm displacement (center column, bottom). When torque pulses were delivered immediately prior to ballistic movement (Figure 2, "preballistic torque"), there was attenuation of the excitatory effects of the supinating displacement and also attenuation of the inhibitory effects of the pronating torque pulse. Discharge of the PTN shown in Figure 2 increased with active pronation and decreased with active supination (either small or large).

In addition to delivery of displacements prior to ballistic movement, we have delivered such stimuli upon detection of the start of the ballistic movement. We analyzed 87 non-PTNs and 36 PTNs which showed significant ($p < 0.01$ in the poststimulus histogram) responses to at least one direction of torque pulse applied during holding and for which complete raster plots for all four movement–perturbation combinations were obtained. In 28 PTNs and 60 non-PTNs (about 70% of the combined group), there was no difference between discharge pattern with the unperturbed control and the perturbed ballistic movement. Sixteen non-PTNs and 6 PTNs were significantly affected by the kinesthetic input during the ballistic movement, but the response was less than the response elicited by the same torque pulse during steady holding. Only 11 non-PTNs and 2 PTNs showed equal reflex responses for both modes of torque-pulse application. This attenuation of PTN responses during ballistic movement and enhancement of PTN responses during precise fine movement is illustrated in Figure 2. In this figure the column marked "small +torque" shows enhanced torque pulse responses compared to the control torque pulse responses marked "torque pulse holding." Heightened sensitivity to displacements occurring during fine movements—particularly obvious for the excitatory reflex—is reflected not only in the increased magnitude and duration of discharge but also by a discharge pattern which shows fluctuations which are very tightly time locked to the torque pulses delivered during precise small movement. Moreover, it should be noted that both the inhibitory and excitatory sensory responses during precise movement had to override the oppositely directed change of unit activity called for by the "movement program." This result indicates that alterations of PTN excitability (membrane polarization) at the time the somesthetic input reaches motor cortex during a perturbed movement can hardly account for the differential responsiveness to disturbances during fine movements as compared to postural stability.

What are the implications of these observations for the events which occur in our brains when we make precisely controlled fine movements? To answer this question, let us consider the output of motor cortex under conditions in which the movement which we seek to perform becomes smaller and smaller and smaller. A good example would be a movement of the index finger under a microscope, where the actual displacement of the finger tip is 50 or 100 μm. Given visual feedback, such a movement is not difficult to carry out. Using peripheral electromyogram (EMG) recording, it would be rather difficult to locate the few motor units which are in fact responsible for the very slight muscle activity associated with a 50-μm flexion of the tip of the index finger. But recordings of PTN activity in cerebral motor cortex reveal that even for very small peripheral EMG changes there is intense motor-cortex discharge: it is easier to detect the motor-cortex activity preceding discharge of a few alpha motoneurons than it is to detect the EMG activity set up by this alpha-motoneuron discharge. The finding that many motor-cortex PTNs utilize their full frequency range regardless of how small a movement becomes is in accord with the observation that maximum cortical motor potentials accompany precisely controlled changes in the firing of even a single motor unit or a single EMG spike in man (Tanji and Kato, 1971; Kristeva and Kornhuber, 1979).

Modulation of Motor-Cortex Discharge with "Readiness" and "Set"

But in addition to discharging with large and small movements and being responsive to sensory inputs, motor-cortex PTNs also show relations to "intentions" and to preparatory "motor sets" occurring in the absence of any movement at all. Indeed, it seems likely that changes of "spontaneous activity" of PTNs in the absence of any alpha-motoneuron discharge may reflect changes in readiness to move—changes which are also reflected in "readiness potentials." Studies on effects of readiness and preparatory set on PTNs (Tanji and Evarts, 1976) were carried out in monkeys trained to react to limb displacement according to prior cues, where the prior cues sometimes called for muscular contractions opposite to those which would have resulted from servo controls. To clarify the monkey's task in such a paradigm, let us consider the case of a person who is standing upright and who is instructed to lean forward (without moving his feet) when the experimenter subsequently displaces him. In this situation the subject will first get set to move forward and then await the impending displacement. If the displacement is then one which by itself moves the subject forward, the subject's reflex postural response (necessary for maintenance of equilibrium) will be to lean backward rather than forward as instructed. In order to lean forward as instructed, the subject would have to shift out of the closed-loop mode necessary for maintenance of the stable, upright posture—and shift into an open-loop mode to generate the antireflex centrally programmed movement of leaning forward (into a net or the waiting arms of someone who will catch him when he falls).

To study motor-cortex discharges in association with "antireflex" pre-programmed movements, monkeys were trained to begin by positioning a handle precisely and holding it immobile for a few seconds. Then a red or green lamp was illuminated, this lamp being the cue which instructed the monkey how to react to a subsequent displacement of the handle. The red lamp was an instruction to get ready to pull (INS-PULL), and when the red lamp was on a handle displacement (regardless of its direction) was a signal to pull backward. Green was an instruction to get ready to push (INS-PUSH), so that with the green lamp on a handle displacement (regardless of its direction) was a signal to push forward. The monkey was rewarded for reacting to handle displacement according to the red or green cue.

An important control in this experiment was to establish that the warning signal to the monkey (the red or green light) did not itself cause a motor response. This was done by monitoring electromyographic activity and also by comparing the response to a given displacement of the handle in conditions in which the preset of the monkey involved preparation to move in a direction opposite to or the same as the direction of the displacement. These EMG and displacement records showed that warning signals which set up preparatory states for a particular direction of centrally programmed movement did so without generating detectable motor responses.

Figure 3 shows a motor-cortex PTN response to the pull (red) as compared to the push (green) "get ready" instruction. Two sorts of displays are presented in this figure: rasters show the raw data for 25 individual trials, with the instruction occurring at the center of the raster; and histograms represent summation of data in the rasters. For the PTN repre-

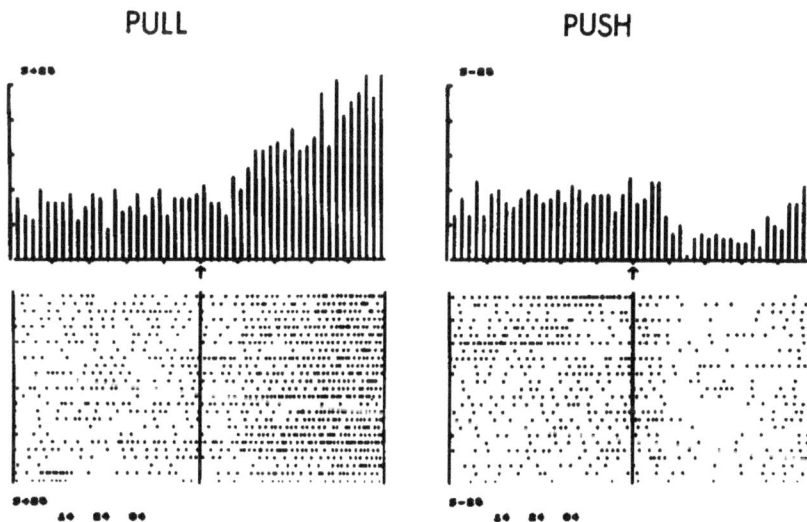

PULL   PUSH

Figure 3 Discharge of a pyramidal tract neuron for 1 sec before and 1 sec after the appearance of the red signal (pull) and the green signal (push). The activity of this PTN is displayed in two different formats. At the top are histograms with bins representing summation of activity in successive 40-msec periods. Below are rasters where each row is a trial, with dots representing individual single-unit discharges. Details of this analysis are described in the text. (From Tanji and Evarts, 1976.)

sented in Figure 3, inspection of the rasters shows that the "get ready to pull" instruction caused an increase, and the "get ready to push" instruction caused a decrease, in discharge frequency.

Monkeys rarely pushed when they were supposed to pull or vice versa, but those instances in which mistakes did occur provided information concerning the extent to which a cell's "correct" response to the "get ready" instruction was a necessary precondition for the monkey's correct motor response to the triggering displacement. Consider the case of a neuron which normally exhibited increased discharge following the push instruction and decrease discharge following the pull instruction. If this cell showed the "wrong" response to the prior instruction, would the monkey then make the wrong response to the displacement? An instance of such an occurrence is shown in Figure 4. Normally this cell became more active for the "get ready to push" instruction and less active for the "get ready to pull" instruction. For one trial with the "get ready to pull" instruction, however, the cell failed to become less active but instead became more active. On this occasion, when the cell had responded to the INS-PULL as if it had been INS-PUSH, the perturbation elicited the wrong movement. Thus, the response of the cell to the "get ready" instruction reliably predicted the subsequent motor response.

In order to determine the time required by monkeys to "get ready," short intervals were occasionally inserted between "get ready" instruction and triggering perturbation in a series of otherwise normal trials. For these short intervals, the perturbation arrived (calling for a push or pull response) during a period when the monkey was not yet set to respond. The delivery of the perturbation within 300 msec or less after the "get ready" instruction, before the effect of the instruction became manifest in motor-cortex neuron discharge, was associated with a grossly impaired motor response. Thus, when motor-cortex discharge associated with preparatory set had not been allowed to occur, the following movement was delayed in onset and/or incorrect in direction.

Central Programs That Override the Servo

During the period after the "get ready" signal but before the displacement which triggered movement, the monkey was seeking to maintain immobility and motor cortex was in the closed-loop mode of control. How quick was the shift from closed- to open-loop control when such a shift was required in cases where the reflex effects of the triggering displacement were opposite to the movement that the monkey had preprogrammed? Recall that monkeys had been trained to react to limb displacements according to prior cues which sometimes called for muscular contractions opposite to those which would have resulted from servo controls. In records of PTN discharge obtained in this paradigm, it was seen that servo control of motor-cortex output was cut off within 40

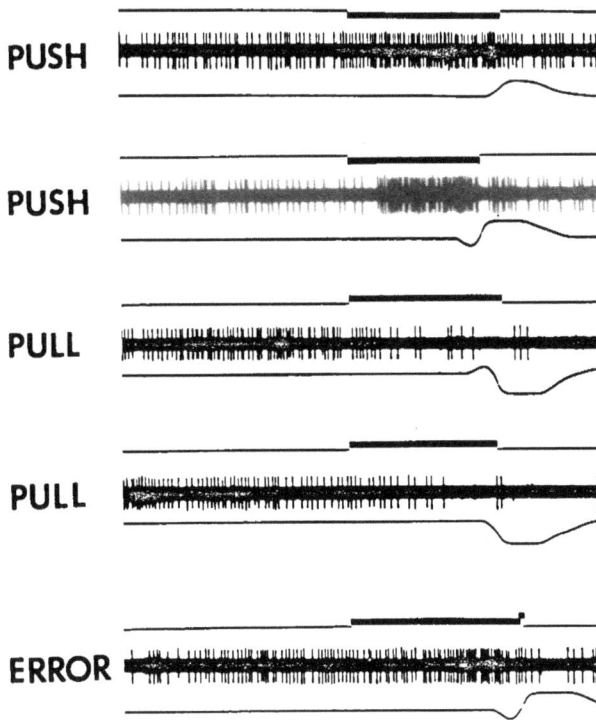

Figure 4 Relationship between the neuronal response to an instruction and the occurrence of an error of performance. Neuronal activity is shown for five trials. Corresponding to each trial there is a set of three traces: the solid black line in the top trace indicates the onset of the instruction; the middle trace in each group of three shows PTN discharge; and the bottom trace is the potentiometer output. In the upper two sets of traces the instruction was push, and shortly following the push instruction (but before the perturbation) there was an increase in neuronal-discharge frequency. For the uppermost push trial the perturbation was in the same direction as the required response, whereas in the next push trial the perturbation was in the opposite direction. In both cases the monkey made the correct response, moving the handle into the push zone. Pushing is indicated by an upward deflection of the potentiometer trace. For the two sets of traces marked "pull" the opposite instruction was given, and a reduction of neuronal discharge followed the instruction. Thus, pull responses were preceded by a decrease of neuronal discharge frequency and push responses were preceded by an increase. In the bottom trace (marked "error") the instruction was pull but the activity of the neuron increased instead of decreasing. The response of the monkey to the perturbation on this trial was pushing, which was incorrect, rather than pulling, which had been called for by the pull instruction. (From Tanji and Evarts, 1976.)

msec of the handle-displacement signal which triggered a "prepro-grammed" pull or push movement that the monkey had got set to perform upon receiving the red or green cue. Within this brief 40-msec period, the control of motor-cortex PTNs was abruptly shifted from the mode involving negative feedback and underlying postural stability to the open-loop mode appropriate for control of the preprogrammed movement.

Subcortical Origins of Motor Programs

What inputs control motor-cortex discharges which underlie centrally programmed movements occurring *in spite of* rather than *because of* the reflex consequences of sensory input? Evidence that the cerebello-thalamocortical pathway is involved in such centrally programmed open-loop control has been provided by the work of Strick (1978), who recorded activity of single nerve cells in dentate and interposed nuclei of the cerebellum of the monkey in the same paradigm which Tanji and I had used—the paradigm in which preprogrammed arm movements were triggered by displacements of the arm which was to move. Strick found that motor set (as established by the red or green cue) had profound effects upon the responses of most cerebellar dentate neurons, with the "set-dependent" activity beginning as early as 30 msec after the signal to move. Such dentate activity, dependent upon prior instruction and occurring at 30 msec, has time to traverse the thalamus and generate centrally programmed activity beginning at 40 msec in the motor cortex.

Strick's results on the role of cerebellar neurons in preprogrammed movements were consistent with those of Thach (1970a,b; 1975), who had demonstrated that cerebellar neurons discharged well in advance of visually triggered volitional movement. The role of cerebellar signals in generating motor-cortex output has been further demonstrated by Meyer-Lohmann, Hore, and Brooks (1977) in experiments involving reversible cooling of the cerebellum. In these experiments the activity of motor-cortex neurons was recorded before, during, and after cerebellar cooling, and it was shown that the initiation of motor-cortex discharge (and of movement) was delayed when the cerebellum was cooled. This delay implied that the cerebellar output (by its projection to motor cortex via the thalamus) was instrumental in activating motor cortex in centrally programmed movements. In addition to transmitting cerebellar outputs to motor cortex, the thalamus relays signals from a large set of subcortical cell groups which are collectively referred to as "the basal ganglia." DeLong (1974) showed that basal-ganglia-cell discharge occurs in advance of volitional movements. His findings were consistent with the evidence from neurological disorders in man that the basal ganglia are of critical importance in the earliest stages of movement initiation—the stages in which an abstract idea is translated by as yet unknown processes into a concrete motor act.

ˡReferences

Arbib, M. A., 1980. Perceptual structures and distributed motor control. In *Handbook of Physiology, Section, Vol. III: Motor Control*. V. B. Brooks, ed. Bethesda: American Physiological Society (in preparation).

Clarke, E., and C. D. O'Malley, 1968. *The Human Brain and Spinal Cord*. Berkeley: University of California Press.

Colburn, T. R., and E. V. Evarts, 1978. Use of brushless DC torque motors in studies of neuromuscular function. In *Progress in Clinical Neurophysiology, Vol. 4: Cerebral Motor Control in Man: Long Loop Mechanisms*. J. E. Desmedt, ed. Basel: Karger, pp. 153–166.

DeLong, M. R., 1974. Motor functions of the basal ganglia: single unit activity during movement. In *The Neurosciences: Third Study Program*. F. O. Schmitt and F. G. Worden, eds. Cambridge, MA: MIT Press, pp. 319–325.

Denny-Brown, D., 1960. Motor mechanisms—introduction: the general principles of motor integration. In *Handbook of Physiology. Section 1, Vol. II: Neurophysiology*. J. Field, ed. Bethesda: American Physiological Society, pp. 781–796.

Evarts, E. V., 1980. Brain mechanisms in voluntary movement. In *Neural Mechanisms in Behavior: A Texas Symposium*. D. McFadden, ed. New York: Springer-Verlag (in press).

Evarts, E. V., and C. Fromm, 1977. Sensory responses in motor cortex neurons during precise motor control. *Neurosci. Lett.* 5:267–272.

Evarts, E. V., and C. Fromm, 1978. The pyramidal tract neuron as summing point in a closed-loop control system in the monkey. In *Progress in Clinical Neurophysiology, Vol. 4: Cerebral Motor Control in Man: Long Loop Mechanisms*. J. E. Desmedt, ed. Basel: Karger, pp. 56–69.

Ferrier, D., 1873. Experimental researches in cerebral physiology and pathology. *West Riding Lun. Asyl. Med. Rep.* 3:30–96.

Fritsch, G., and E. Hitzig, 1870. Über die elektrische Erregbarkeit des Grosshirns. In *The Cerebral Cortex*. G. von Bonin, ed. Springfield, IL: Charles C. Thomas, pp. 73–96.

Fromm, C., and E. V. Evarts, 1977. Relation of motor cortex neurons to precisely controlled and ballistic movements. *Neurosci. Lett.* 5:259–265.

Henneman, E., 1974. Principles governing distribution of sensory input to motor neurons. In *The Neurosciences: Third Study Program*. F. O. Schmitt and F. G. Worden, eds. Cambridge, MA: MIT Press, pp. 281–291.

Horne, M. K., and D. J. Tracey, 1979. The afferents and projections of the ventroposterolateral thalamus in the monkey. *Exp. Brain Res.* 36:129–141.

Jackson, H., 1931. *Selected Writings of John Hughlings Jackson*, Vol. I. J. Taylor, ed. London: Staples Press.

Jones, E. G., 1975. Lamination and differential distribution of thalamic afferents in the sensory-motor cortex of the squirrel monkey. *J. Comp. Neurol.* 160:167–204.

Jones, E. G., and T. P. S. Powell, 1970. An anatomical study of converging sensory pathways within the cerebral cortex of the monkey. *Brain* 93:793–820.

Jones, E. G., J. D. Coulter, and S. H. C. Hendry, 1978. Intracortical connectivity of architectonic fields in the somatic sensory, motor and parietal cortex of monkeys. *J. Comp. Neurol.* 181:291–348.

Kristeva, R., and H. H. Kornhuber, 1979. Cerebral potentials related to the smallest human finger movement. In *Motivation, Motor and Sensory Processes of the Brain: Electrical Potentials, Behavior and Clinical Use. Prog. Brain Res.*

Kuypers, H. G. J. M., 1964. The descending pathways to the spinal cord, their anatomy and function. *Prog. Brain Res.* 11:178–200.

Kuypers, H. G. J. M., 1973. The anatomical organization of the descending pathways and their contributions to motor control especially in primates. In *New Developments in Electromyography and Clinical Neurophysiology*, Vol. 3. J. E. Desmedt, ed. Basel: Karger, pp. 38–68.

Lemon, R. N., and J. van der Burg, 1979. Short-latency peripheral inputs to thalamic neurones projecting to the motor cortex in the monkey. *Exp. Brain Res.* 36:445–462.

Merzenich, M. M., J. H. Kaas, M. Sur, and C.-S. Lin, 1978. Double representation of the body surface within cytoarchitectonic areas 3b and 1 in "SI" in the owl monkey (*Aotus trivirgatus*). *J. Comp. Neurol.* 181:41–74.

Meyer-Lohmann, J., J. Hore, and V. B. Brooks, 1977. Cerebellar participation in generation of prompt arm movements. *J. Neurophysiol.* 40:1038–1050.

Pandya, D. N., and H. G. J. M. Kuypers, 1969. Cortico-cortical connections in the rhesus monkey. *Brain Res.* 13:13–36.

Paul, R. L., M. Merzenich, and H. Goodman, 1972. Representation of slowly and rapidly adapting cutaneous mechanoreceptors of the hand in Brodmann's areas 3 and 1 of *Macaca mulatta. Brain Res.* 36:229–249.

Phillips, C. G., 1969. Motor apparatus of the baboon's hand. *Proc. Roy. Soc. B* 173:141–174.

Phillips, C. G., and R. Porter, 1977. *Corticospinal Neurones, Their Role in Movement.* New York: Academic Press.

Sakata, H., and Y. Iwamura, 1978. Cortical processing of tactile information in the first somatosensory and parietal association areas in the monkey. In *Active Touch.* G. Gordon, ed. Oxford: Pergamon, pp. 55–72.

Strick, P. L., 1978. Cerebellar involvement in 'volitional' muscle responses to load changes. In *Progress in Clinical Neurophysiology, Vol. 4: Cerebral Motor Control in Man: Long Loop Mechanisms.* J. E. Desmedt, ed. Basel: Karger, pp. 85–93.

Tanji, J., and E. V. Evarts, 1976. Anticipatory activity of motor cortex neurons in relation to direction of an intended movement. *J. Neurophysiol.* 39:1062–1068.

Tanji, J., and M. Kato, 1971. Volitionally controlled single motor unit discharges and cortical motor potentials in human subjects. *Brain Res.* 29:343–346.

Thach, W. T., 1970a. Discharge of cerebellar neurons related to two postures and movements. I. Nuclear cell output. *J. Neurophysiol.* 33:527–536.

Thach, W. T., 1970b. Discharge of cerebellar neurons related to two postures and movements. II. Purkinje cell output and input. *J. Neurophysiol:* 33:537–547.

Thach, W. T., 1975. Timing of activity in cerebellar dentate nucleus and cerebral motor cortex during prompt volitional movement. *Brain Res.* 88:233–241.

Vogt, B. A., and D. N. Pandya, 1978. Cortico-cortical connections of somatic sensory cortex (areas 3, 1 and 2) in the rhesus monkey. *J. Comp. Neurol.* 177:179–192.

Walshe, F. M. R., 1943. On the mode of representation of movements in the motor cortex, with special reference to "convulsions beginning unilaterally" (Jackson). *Brain* 66:104–139.

Woodworth, R. S., 1899. The accuracy of voluntary movement. *Psychol. Monogr.*, Vol. III.

12 On the Relation between Transthalamic and Transcortical Pathways in the Visual System

Ann M. Graybiel and David M. Berson

ABSTRACT The anatomical connections of the visual association cortex have been studied in the cat by anterograde and retrograde axon-transport techniques. The findings suggest that clusters of areas in the extrastriate cortex are systematically related to particular subdivisions of the nucleus lateralis posterior-pulvinar complex of the thalamus and therefore to distinct lines of vision-related conduction separate from the main retino-geniculo-cortical pathway. Only one of the families of cortical areas, the set of areas receiving input from the striate-recipient zone of the thalamus, is heavily interconnected with the striate cortex by direct transcortical pathways. Nor are the different extrastriate families tightly linked by cortical association pathways. Instead, there is a tendency for high within-family connectivity and restricted cross-family connectivity. Conclusions of two types are drawn from these results. First, the visual cortex is not organized according to a single striate-to-extrastriate hierarchy but according to a more intricate plan that takes into account, as one determinant of transcortical connectivity, the thalamic affiliations of each cortical zone. Second, a highly systematic logic appears to govern the configurations of transthalamic and transcortical circuits and their relationships to one another.

Introduction

The neocortex is characterized by a unique plan of organization of its extrinsic long-axon connections. First, the input routes to the neocortex are sharply limited in type. With the exception of monoamine-containing cell groups, only regions of the forebrain can project directly to the neocortex, and for the great majority of ascending pathways there is even a more restrictive rule, namely, that the thalamus is an obligatory stopping point *en route*. In contrast to this afferent plan, the range of efferent connectivity of the neocortex is the greatest of any subdivision of the brain. Again excepting the amine pathways, the neocortex is the only subdivision of the brain with access to all other parts of the central nervous system. These two characteristics serve to maximize the inter-

ANN M. GRAYBIEL AND DAVID M. BERSON Department of Psychology and Brain Science, Massachusetts Institute of Technology, Cambridge, Massachusetts 02139

nal connectivity of the forebrain and to emphasize as its main distribution mechanism the cerebral cortex, and especially the neocortex.

Dramatic recent progress has been made in relating the intrinsic structure of the neocortex to the main classes of its input and output pathways. We now know that both thalamocortical and corticocortical afferents are organized into columns or slabs as well as into layers; that cortical efferents destined for different regions of the neuraxis arise in different neuronal layers or sublayers; and that the patterns of layering hold with relatively few variations for all parts of the neocortex. The fundamental question raised by these new findings is how functional heterogeneity is engrafted on this basic ground plan. To approach this question we must learn more about the specific synaptic relations between different types of afferent and efferent neurons and learn what principles of organization determine the different types of afferent and efferent connections characterizing a particular cortical region. It is our purpose in this chapter to discuss the second of these two problems, taking the visual cortex as an example. The key conclusions we wish to draw are first, that functional diversity is achieved in the neocortex in part by virtue of connectional rules that tend to segregate families of cortical areas; and second, that the family members are themselves multiply interlocked by a highly systematic set of transthalamic and transcortical circuits.

Multiple Representation in the Visual Association Cortex

Three related findings are crucial starting points for this discussion.

(1) Recent electrophysiological mapping studies of the visual cortex have demonstrated the presence of as many as thirteen retinotopically ordered areas in the posterior association cortex (Allman and Kaas, 1975; Palmer, Rosenquist, and Tusa, 1978; Tusa, Palmer, and Rosenquist, 1975; van Essen, 1979; Zeki, 1978; see Figure 1).

(2) The transcortical association pathways leading out from the primary visual cortex terminate in some but not all of these extrastriate visual areas (Kawamura, 1973; van Essen, 1979; Zeki, 1978).

(3) There are, in addition to these transcortical routes, multiple lines of ascending conduction that reach the extrastriate cortex by way of transthalamic pathways synapsing in the nucleus lateralis posterior-pulvinar (LP-pulvinar) complex (Berson and Graybiel, 1978a; Glendenning et al., 1975; Graybiel, 1972b).

It is still a mystery how the electrophysiologically definable maps in the extrastriate cortex relate to behaviorally defined classes of visual function. Only in a few instances have the findings in physiological experiments suggested functional specialization at this level of analysis (participation of area 18 in coarse stereopsis being one; Hubel and

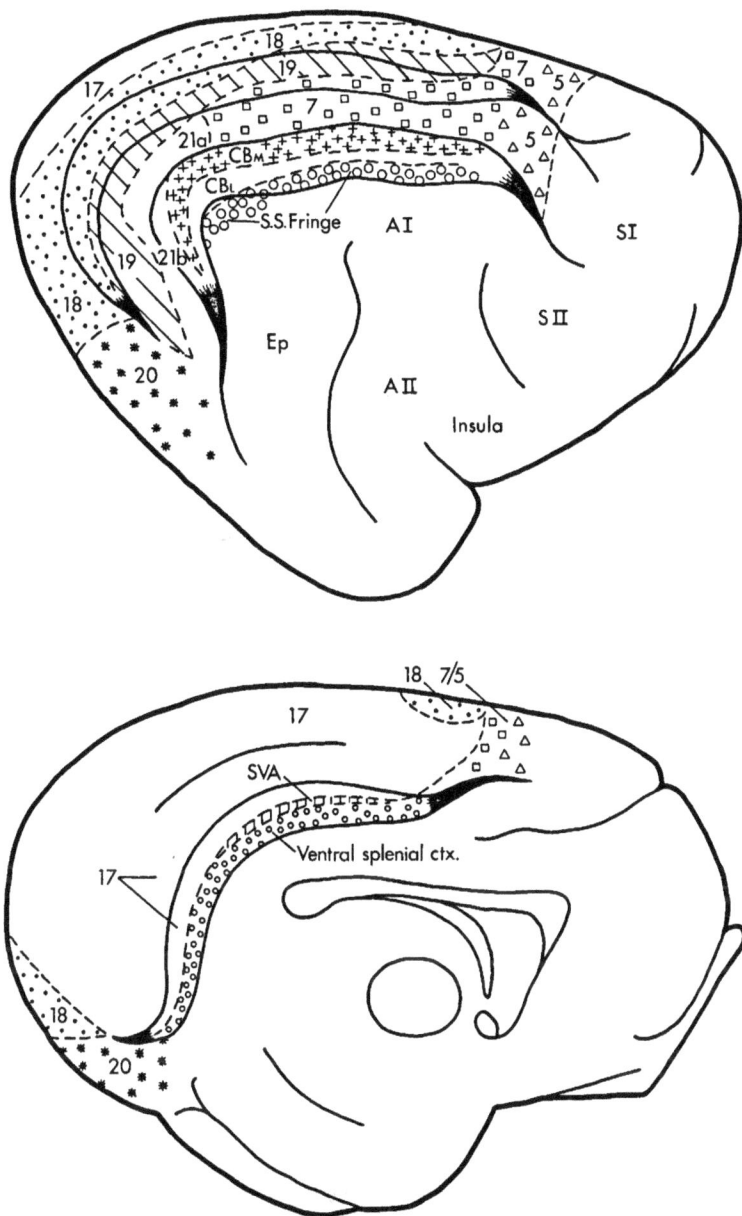

Figure 1 Lateral (top) and medial views of the cerebral hemisphere in the cat illustrating subdivisions of the posterior association cortex. The delineation of areas in the visually responsive extrastriate cortex is largely based on the work of Tusa, Palmer, and Rosenquist (1975), Palmer, Rosenquist, and Tusa (1979), and Kalia and Whitteridge (1973), although slight modifications have been made on the basis of anatomical findings discussed in the text. CBm and CBl refer to the medial and lateral subdivisions of the Clare–Bishop complex. The medial subdivision is roughly equivalent to the medial group of LS (lateral suprasylvian) areas of Palmer, Rosenquist, and Tusa; the lateral subdivision corresponds to the lateral set of LS areas of the Philadelphia group. SS Fringe: suprasylvian fringe; SVA: splenial visual area.

Wiesel, 1970). Some clues may come from the anatomy. For example, the inferotemporal cortex in the monkey appears to be peculiar among visual association areas in projecting directly to the amygdala. This fact has encouraged efforts to demonstrate a role for the inferotemporal cortex in the affective side of visual experience, as suggested originally by the Klüver–Bucy syndrome. Even where an association with one or another behavioral capacity cannot be made satisfactorily, knowledge of the anatomy may still be critical in trying to assess the degree of relatedness of the different extrastriate fields, and in turn, in attempting to grasp the organizational plan that governs their patterns of connection with other parts of the brain. As we shall emphasize in the following account, neuroanatomical findings suggest that each extrastriate field is associated with a remarkably extensive network of thalamocortical connections, not simply with a single thalamic circuit interconnecting the cortical area in question with its principal thalamic nucleus. Moreover, many of the transthalamic circuits are actually parts of cortico-thalamo-cortical loops, some reciprocal, some not. Part of understanding the integrative capabilities of the neocortex must therefore almost certainly lie in understanding the thalamus.

Multiple Representation in the Extrageniculate Thalamus

Corresponding to the extrastriate cortex at the thalamic level is a group of nuclei in the caudal thalamus that together comprise the various subdivisions of the nucleus lateralis posterior and the pulvinar. This posterior thalamic territory projects to the extrastriate cortex and, accordingly, shows in different species a development that is roughly proportional to that of the extrastriate cortex itself. The LP-pulvinar complex accounts for a considerable fraction of the thalamic mass in cats as well as in primates. In the cat, distinct subdivisions of the LP-pulvinar have been identified on the basis of their input and output connections and most recently on the basis of histochemical differences among them (Berson and Graybiel, 1978a; Graybiel, 1974; Graybiel and Berson, 1980b; Updyke, 1977). Certain of the anatomical subdivisions have been confirmed in electrophysiological mapping experiments (Kinston, Vadas, and Bishop, 1969; Mason, 1978).

A striking finding concerning the afferent organization of the LP-pulvinar region in the cat is that the terminal distributions of both ascending and descending visual pathways are arranged in a series of adjoining, roughly parallel zones (Figure 2). Two of these receive ascending fiber projections from optic-tract recipients in the mesodiencephalic region directly caudal to the LP-pulvinar: the pretectum projects to the laterally situated pulvinar, which for this reason is known as the *pretectorecipient zone*; and the superficial layers of the superior colliculus project to the medial part of the nucleus lateralis posterior (LPm), the *tectorecipient zone*. Between these two subdivisions, and ap-

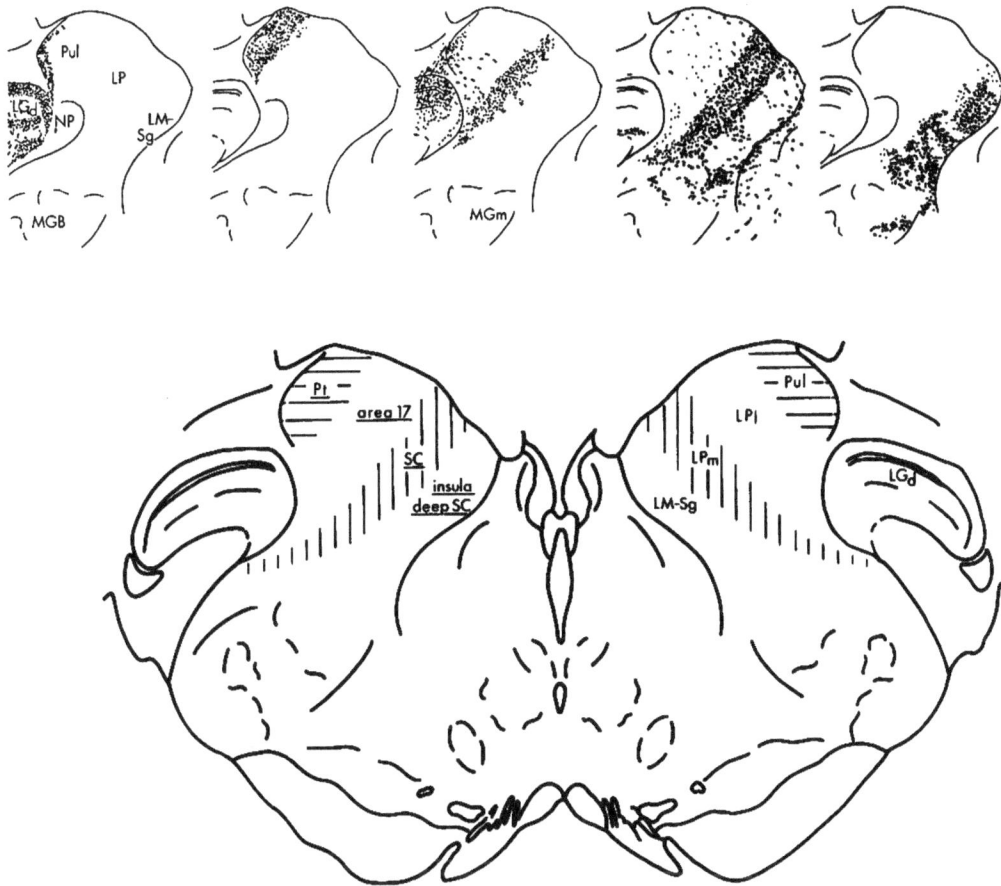

Figure 2 A schematic transverse section through the posterior thalamic region of the cat is shown to illustrate subdivisions of the LP-pulvinar complex delineated on the basis of their individually distinct afferent connections, and the adjoining LM-Sg complex, which receives afferent projections from the insula and deep layers of the superior colliculus. In the drawing at the bottom, the origins of the afferent connections are shown on the left, the name of the corresponding subdivisions on the right. At the top, single chartings show from left to right the terminal distributions of projections from the retina and pretectal region in the pulvinar, the visual cortex and superior colliculus in adjoining strips of the nucleus lateralis posterior (LP), and the insular cortex in the LM-Sg complex (nucleus lateralis medialis-suprageniculate nucleus). Other abbreviations: LGd, dorsal division of the lateral geniculate body; Pul, pulvinar; MGB, medial geniculate body; Pt, pretectal region; SC, superior colliculus.

proximately coextensive with them in the anteroposterior dimension, lies a third region that receives a descending projection from the striate cortex. This middle subdivision (LPl-NP, or for simplicity, LPl) is called the *striate-recipient zone* because it is the only one of the three to receive a direct projection from the primary visual cortex. Recent evidence suggests that there may also be a sparse ascending projection to this zone, probably from the superficial part of the superior colliculus.

Within the limits of accuracy of the anterograde tracer and degeneration techniques employed in identifying these districts, there seems to be little overlap between neighboring zones. They are roughly 1–3 mm wide in cross section, and from available Golgi-impregnated material it seems unlikely that the dendritic trees of the thalamic neurons would extend through more than one or at most two of them. This suggests that at the initial input stage at least, both ascending and descending extrageniculate visual pathways are carefully segregated in the caudal thalamus. Moreover, each of the three main afferent zones of the LP-pulvinar can be identified histochemically by virtue of its particular content of acetylcholinesterase (Figures 3 and 5). It remains to be seen whether this means that the different afferent pathways employ different neurotransmitters in the thalamus, but the histochemistry has already proven helpful in recognizing the zones and crucial in trying to relate them to regions having different efferent connections.

It is important to point out that some cortical regions in the extrastriate visual system project to more than one zone of the LP-pulvinar. For example, there are fiber projections from area 19 to the pulvinar and LPl, and from the crown of the middle suprasylvian gyrus to the pulvinar and LIc, the caudal part of the intermediate subdivision (Figure 5C). There also is a double-band pattern in the ascending projections traced from the pretectotectal border zone to LIc and the pulvinar (Figure 5B), but this may represent parallel rather than branched pathways. The apparent "doubling" of the corticothalamic projection is a pattern to which we shall return below.

Two other thalamic subdivisions shown in Figure 2 should briefly be mentioned. At the lateral edge of the LP-pulvinar triad there is a thin marginal strip that is notable because it receives direct input from the retina. This narrow zone, to which the striate cortex and pretectal region also project, appears to represent a differentiated lateral part of the pulvinar. A thin dorsal extension of this zone is reported to receive input from the deep cerebellar nuclei (Itoh and Mizuno, 1979). On the medial side of the LP-pulvinar triad, separating it from the pretectum and intralaminar nuclei, lies the thalamic complex formed by the nucleus lateralis medialis and the suprageniculate nucleus (the LM-Sg complex). This zone may be related to the auditory or somatic sensory modalities or to some mixture of auditory, somatic sensory, and visual processing: it receives input from the insular cortex and from the deep layers of the superior colliculus (Figure 2). Not shown in the figure is a

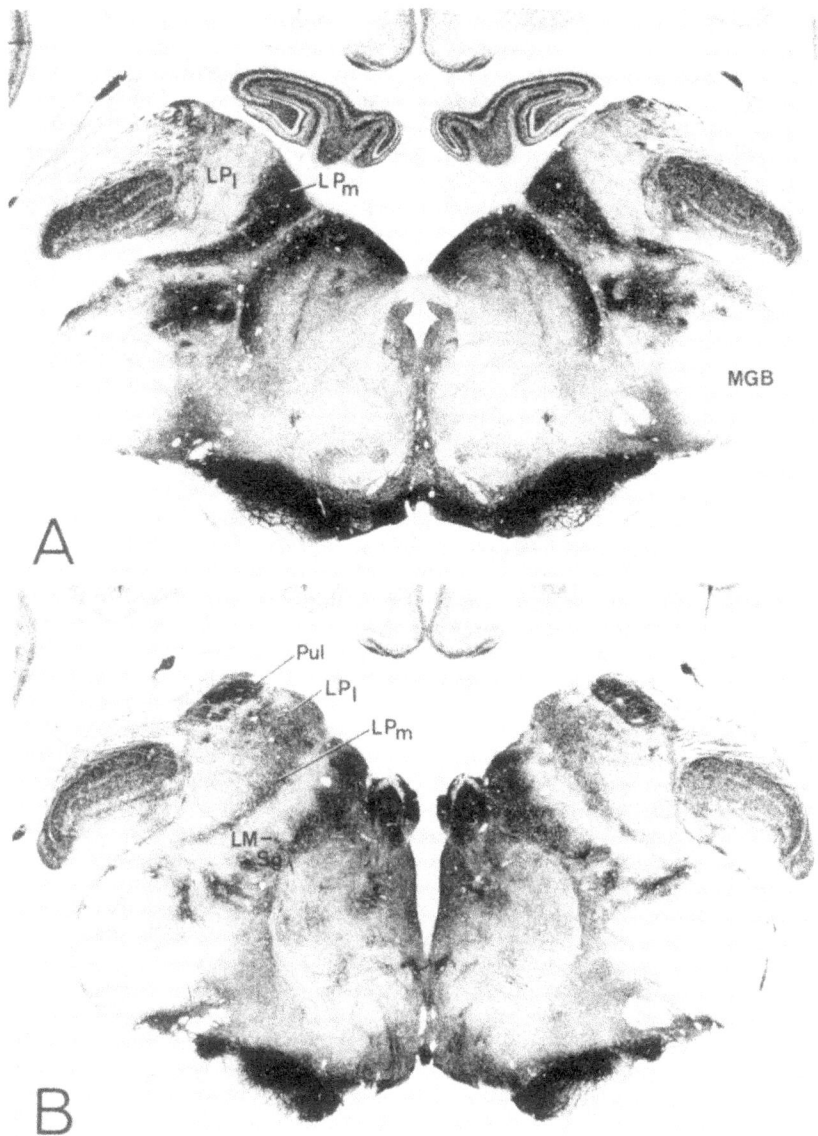

Figure 3 Transverse sections through caudal (A) and more rostral (B) levels of the LP-pulvinar complex in the cat. The sections were stained by the thiocholine method for demonstrating the activity of acetylcholinesterase (Graybiel and Berson, 1980b). (A) shows that the tectorecipient zone (LPm) is darkly stained, the striate-recipient zone is lightly stained. The section is caudal to the main part of the pulvinar, but (B) illustrates the high enzyme activity in this region (the pretectorecipient zone). Also shown is the LM-Sg complex that flanks the LP-pulvinar on the medial side.

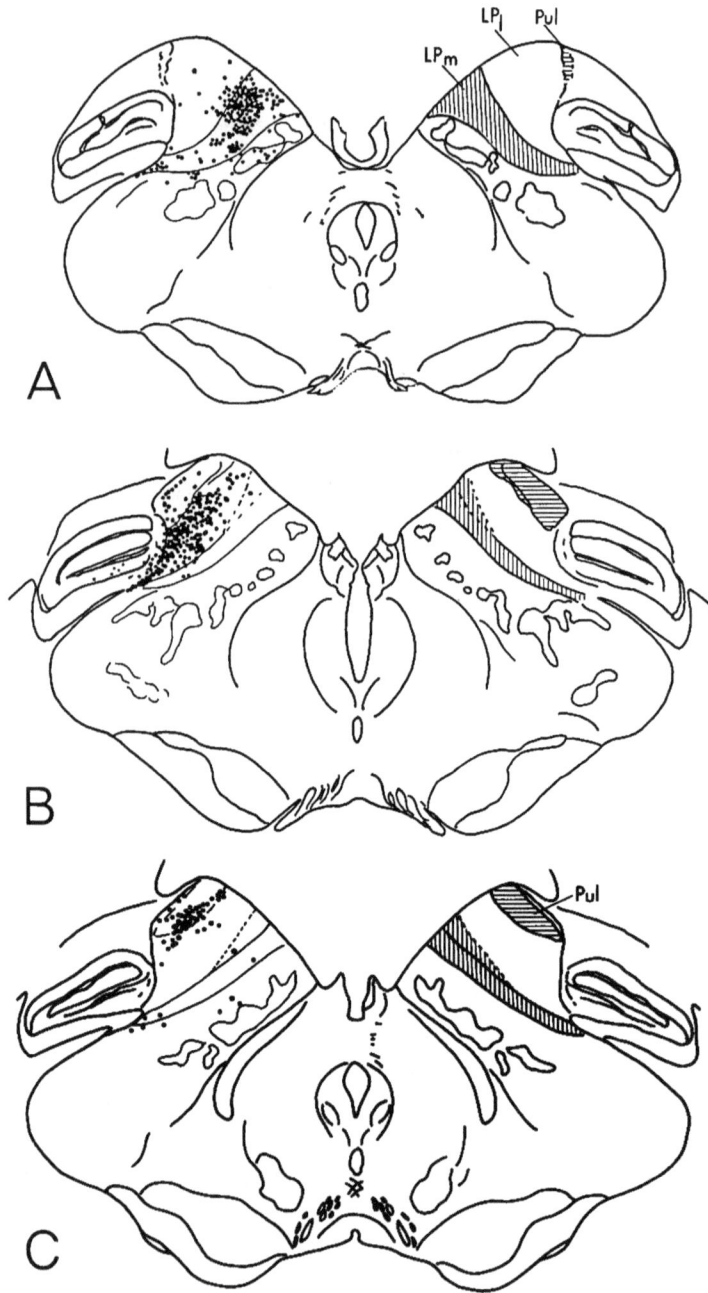

Figure 4 Chartings illustrating the distinctive patterns of retrograde labeling of neurons in the LP-pulvinar complex seen after injection of the tracer enzyme horseradish peroxidase (HRP) into three different regions of the cat's extrastriate cortex: the lateral Clare–Bishop area (A); the medial Clare–Bishop area (B); and the crown of the middle suprasylvian gyrus (C). In each chart the boundaries of the thalamic subdivisions were traced in on the left from serially adjoining sections stained for acetylthiocholinesterase and carefully aligned with the HRP sections. On the right, these same cholinesterase subdivisions were drawn in in mirror-image fashion and the dense cholinesterase staining of the tectorecipient LPm and pretectorecipient pulvinar were indicated by the hatching.

A. M. Graybiel and D. M. Berson

third very thin strip that runs along the medial part of the pulvinar at rostral levels and receives a direct projection from the hypothalamus (Fujii and Yoshii, 1979). Our own experiments suggest that neurons in this thalamic strip project to the cingulate gyrus-splenial cortex region, but we will not discuss this zone further in the present chapter.

Patterns of Thalamocortical Projection to the Extrastriate Cortex

The orderly separation of input zones in the LP-pulvinar complex demonstrates that the region is not diffusely organized, but says very little about the way the through-conduction routes to the neocortex are arranged. Work on the thalamocortical projections has progressed more slowly than work on the afferent connections, but enough is now known to say (a) that the outputs are also organized in slab-like zones, (b) that these seem to match quite closely the input zones, and (c) that each one of these thalamic districts has an individually distinct pattern of projection to extrastriate cortex involving, in all likelihood, more than one cortical area.

Evidence supporting these conclusions is summarized for the main LP-pulvinar triad in Figures 4–6. The *tectorecipient zone* (LPm) projects to the lateral part of the Clare–Bishop complex including its extension in the posterior suprasylvian sulcus (areas ALLS, PLLS, and DLS of Palmer, Rosenquist, and Tusa, 1978; cf. Hubel and Wiesel, 1969). Either LPm itself or the immediately adjoining part of the LM-Sg complex projects to part of the anterior ectosylvian sulcus. The *pretectorecipient zone* (the pulvinar) projects to the crown of the middle suprasylvian gyrus and to part of area 20, to ventral splenial cortex, and at least sparsely to area 19 and the small adjoining cortical field 21a. The *striate-recipient zone* (LPl) projects to a third group of cortical fields: to areas 19 and 21a; to the medial division of the Clare–Bishop complex and area 21b; to parts of area 20; and probably to the splenial visual area of Kalia and Whitteridge (1973). Finally, LPl projects in a special layering pattern directly to areas 17 and 18. The thalamocortical projections of the regions mentioned as flanking the LP-pulvinar triad are still under study, but the evidence so far available suggests that the LM-Sg complex, projects to the insular cortex, suprasylvian fringe and frontal cortex, and probably to part of the perirhinal cortex as well; LIc to the crown of the middle suprasylvian gyrus and probably to area 20; and the marginal retinorecipient zone that lies along the lateral edge of the pulvinar probably to area 19.

These findings strongly suggest that the strip-like arrangement of inputs and outputs in the LP-pulvinar complex is an organizational design allowing different lines of vision-related information to be channeled toward the neocortex along separate pathways. The tectorecipient zone, for example, conveys information from the superficial layers of

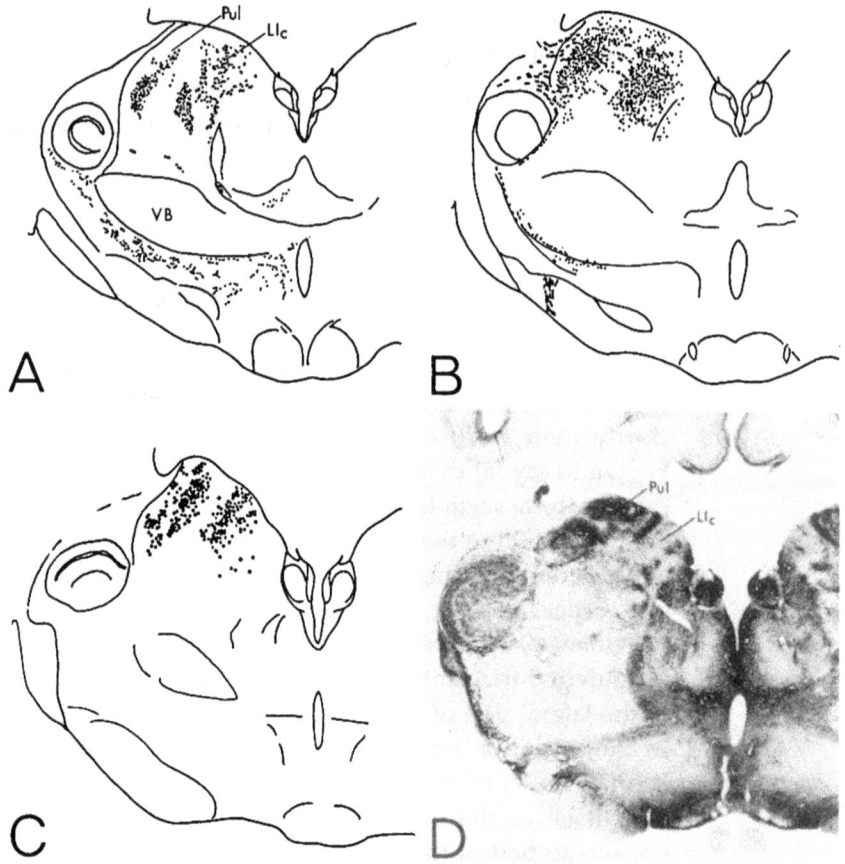

Figure 5 A comparison of the pattern of distribution of afferent connections (A,B), cells of origin of thalamocortical connections (C), and acetylcholinesterase staining (D) in the rostral part of the LP-pulvinar complex and adjoining intermediate subdivision of the lateral thalamic mass (its caudal part, LIc). (A) shows anterograde autoradiographic labeling after an injection of tritiated amino acids centered in the pretectal region; (B) shows similar distribution of terminal labeling elicited by an injection of the crown of the middle suprasylvian gyrus. In (C), black dots indicate neurons labeled by retrograde transport after an injection of HRP into the suprasylvian crown cortex. The double-band pattern of pulvinar and LIc labeling visible in the three charts should be compared with the pattern of cholinesterase distribution in (D), in which the pulvinar and LIc can be distinguished by their differing contents of the enzyme.

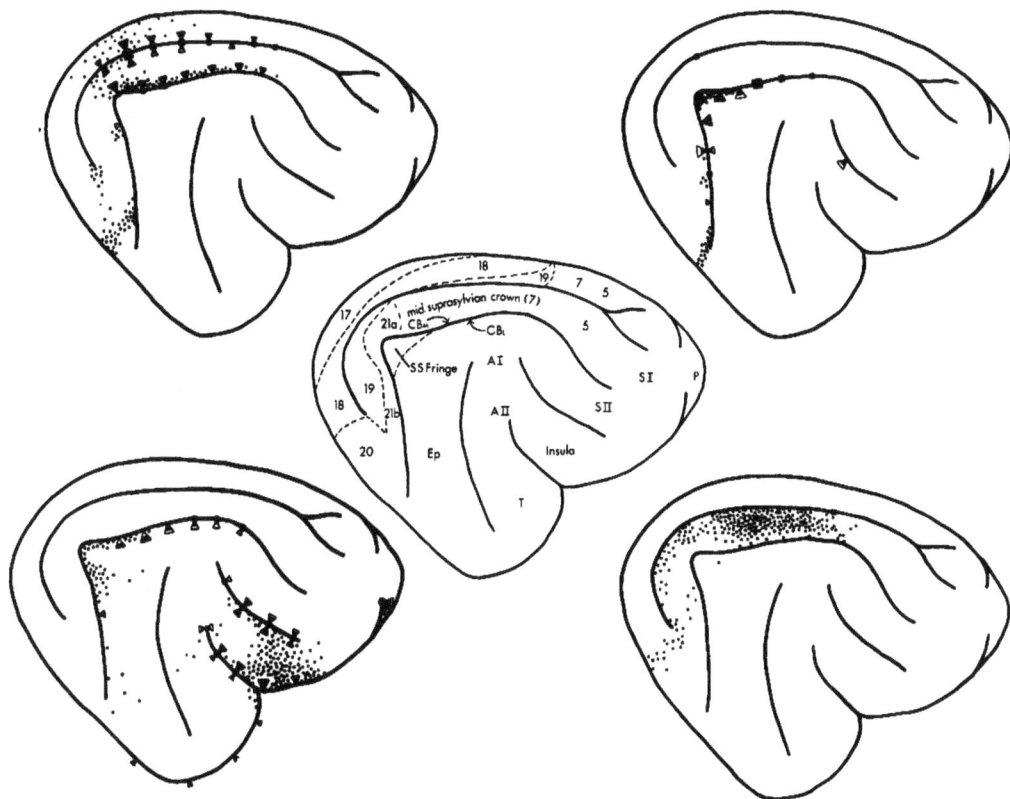

Figure 6 Side views of the cat's cerebral cortex illustrating the differential thalamocortical projections of the three main subdivisions of the LP-pulvinar complex and the adjoining LM-Sg subdivision. The figure was prepared to permit comparison of the different patterns of intracortical labeling observed in autoradiographic axon-transport experiments after injections of [³H]-amino acids in (1) the striate-recipient LPl zone (upper left); (2) the tectorecipient LPm zone (upper right); (3) the pretectorecipient pulvinar (lower right); and (4) the LM-Sg complex (lower left). Solid black dots represent labeling of cortex forming the crown of a gyrus. Labeling of sulcal cortex is indicated by triangles and squares: squares for the fundus of a sulcus, triangles for the sulcal banks. Blackening of the triangles is used to denote the position of labeling along each sulcal bank. Size of squares or triangles indicates density of cortical labeling. The central diagram summarizes the location of the main subdivisions of the extrastriate cortex (see also Figure 1).

the superior colliculus to the lateral part of the Clare–Bishop complex (CBl) and apparently keeps this communication line separate from the pretectal channel leading over the pulvinar to the crown of the suprasylvian gyrus. Other pathways form cortico-thalamo-cortical loops. For example, area 17 projects to the striate-recipient zone, which in turn projects to the medial part of the Clare–Bishop complex (CBm). From the same observations, however, it can also be concluded that most if not all of the thalamic strips are related to more than one input and to more than one output; and in some cases the multiple associations suggest that the extrageniculate pathways are at least partly interlocked. In the remainder of this paper we wish to develop the hypothesis that the patterns of interlocking of these channels are indicative of an ordered set of relationships governing the connections of extrastriate cortex at both thalamic and cortical levels.

Organization of the Visual Cortex into Family Clusters: The Geniculate Family and Striate-Recipient Cortex

The hypothesis that extrastriate cortex is divided into families of cortical areas rests on evidence for highly systematic correlations between the thalamocortical and corticocortical connections of family members. Knowledge of the anatomical pathways is most complete for the networks linking the extrastriate with striate cortex, understandably so because still by far the most extensive efforts to analyze the central visual pathways have been devoted to the principal conduction route of the visual system, the retino-geniculo-striate pathway. A key advantage of starting with the geniculocortical system is that we can with considerable confidence identify geniculorecipient cortex (in the primate this appears to be limited to the striate cortex) and in turn define the extrastriate cortical areas receiving input from the striate cortex as striate-recipient cortex. If we next consider the pathways linking these areas with the extrageniculate thalamic subdivisions of the LP-pulvinar complex, we find (in the cat) that striate-recipient regions of the thalamus project almost exclusively to striate-recipient areas of the neocortex.

This pattern of anatomical connections is a crucial starting point for our argument that there is an underlying logic that governs sets of fiber connections in the striate and extrastriate visual systems. We are far from being able to specify the rules adequately, but we can at least point to observations suggesting a startling systematicity of connectional patterns. Some of these are summarized in the sequence of flow diagrams shown in Figures 7–10. Although the figures refer exclusively to experimental findings in the cat, we suspect that the general nature of the organization by family cluster holds true also in other species, including those of the primate order.

A. M. Graybiel and D. M. Berson

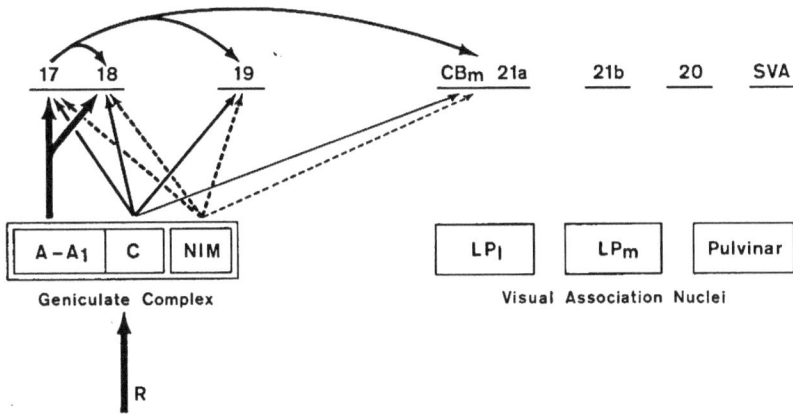

Figure 7 Schematic diagram illustrating the retino-geniculo-striate pathway in the cat. The neocortex is shown at the top with the striate cortex (area 17) and several areas in the extrastriate cortex individually represented (compare with the side view of Figure 1 illustrating these regions on outline drawings of the hemisphere). Below is the dorsal lateral geniculate complex, with laminae A and A1, the C laminae and the medial interlaminar nucleus (NIM), and the three subdivisions of the LP-pulvinar triad (LPl, the striate-recipient zone; LPm, the tectorecipient zone; and the pulvinar, the pretectorecipient zone). Indicated by the arrows are the principal retino-geniculo-cortical paths to areas 17 and 18, and the other more extended thalamocortical projections of the geniculate complex. Note that of the outlying extrastriate subdivisions shown, only the medial Clare–Bishop area (CBm) and area 21a receive direct input from the geniculate. Also shown by arrows are the transcortical projections leading out from area 17. Note that these association pathways lead to geniculorecipient cortex.

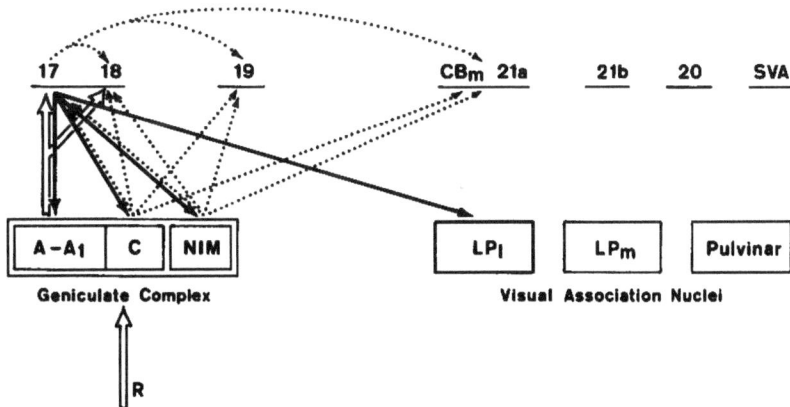

Figure 8 Schematic diagram showing the corticothalamic projections of area 17 (solid lines) against the background (dotted lines and open arrows) of the geniculocortical projections and transcortical projections of area 17 (compare with Figure 7). Note that just as area 17 projects to the medial Clare–Bishop area and area 21a in addition to areas 18 and 19, so it projects to LPl in addition to the various components of the geniculate complex. Abbreviations same as those in Figure 7.

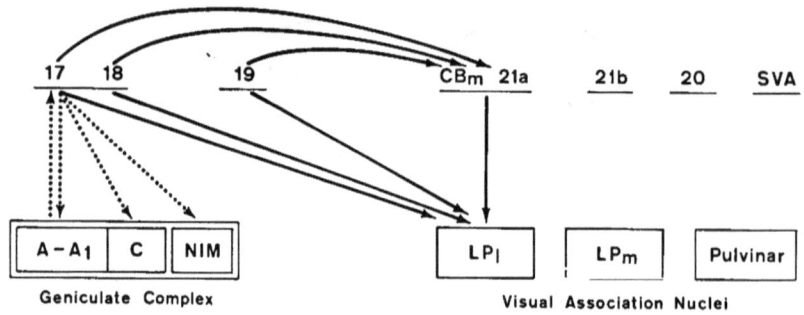

Figure 9 Continuation of the sequence of diagrams begun with Figure 7 to show the close relationship between the geniculostriate pathway, the LPl subdivision of the extrageniculate thalamus, and the medial Clare–Bishop area (CBm) and area 21a of the extrastriate cortex. Both LPl and CBm receive input from areas 17, 18, and 19. LPl also receives a direct projection from CBm. Abbreviations same as those in Figure 7.

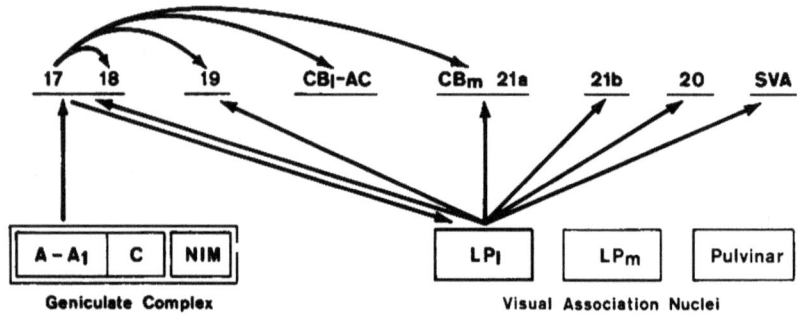

Figure 10 Schematic diagrams illustrating the striate-recipient zone of the LP-pulvinar complex (LPl) and emphasizing the large degree of overlap between the group of extrastriate areas to which LPl projects (the LPl family) and the group of areas receiving direct transcortical projections from area 17 (striate-recipient cortex). The LPl family is the only cluster of cortical areas so closely tied to the striate cortex and the retino-geniculo-cortical pathway. CBl-AC, the zone of area centralis representation in the lateral Clare–Bishop area; other abbreviations as in Figure 7.

The Geniculocortical Pathway

Figure 7 shows the complex geniculocortical pathway in the cat, which can be divided into three parts. The dorsal laminae (A and A1) receive X- and Y-cell inputs from the retina and project to areas 17 and 18, which together are the presumed equivalents of area 17 in the monkey (see Rodieck, 1979, for review). This principal conduction route of the geniculostriate system terminates massively in layer IV; it is shown by heavy arrows in Figure 7. The parvocellular C laminae of the LGd (which receive W-cell inputs from the retina) project to a wider cortical field that includes areas 17 and 18, area 19 and the adjoining area 21a (LeVay and Gilbert, 1976), and (apparently a zone of sparse projection) the strip of visually responsive cortex in the medial part of the Clare–Bishop area (AMLS and PMLS of the Philadelphia group; Berson and Graybiel, in preparation). Within areas 17 and 18, corticipetal fibers from the C laminae do not terminate principally in layer IV, but instead in layer I and in the parts of layers III and V abutting layer IV (LeVay and Gilbert, 1976).

The third component of the geniculocortical pathway originates in the medial interlaminar nucleus (NIM). This nucleus does not lie within the laminar part of the LGd and has itself no overt cellular lamination. It is nevertheless considered part of the lateral geniculate complex because it adjoins the main laminae and, like them, receives a direct projection from the retina (apparently mainly an input from Y cells). The NIM, like the C laminae, projects not only to areas 17 and 18 but also to areas 19 and 21a and to the medial Clare–Bishop area, CBm (see Rodieck, 1979).

The Extended Geniculate Family

The pathways from NIM and the geniculate C layers to the medial part of the Clare–Bishop area clearly show that this cortical region, although physically removed from the striate cortex, is a part of the geniculate family. As judged by the strength of the geniculate input, however, the link is relatively weak by comparison to that of area 19 or the members of the immediate geniculorecipient family (areas 17 and 18).

It is remarkable that the closest-relation classification made for the medial Clare–Bishop area on the basis of its geniculocortical input accurately predicts the other afferent connections of this extrastriate area. At the cortical level this holds true because CBm receives a direct transcortical projection from area 17 (Garey, Jones, and Powell, 1968) and thus is part of striate-recipient cortex. Indeed, in the cat the geniculate family and striate-recipient cortex are nearly identical (see Figure 7). As to the extrageniculate thalamic inputs to CBm, the closest-relation pattern is also striking because the only part of the LP-pulvinar triad projecting densely to CBm is the striate-recipient zone, that is, the part of the triad most closely tied in with the geniculostriate system (Berson and Graybiel, 1978b; Symonds et al., 1978).

These extended-family relationships of the medial Clare–Bishop area have a counterpart in the thalamus: in the LP-pulvinar triad there is one closest-neighbor relation of the retino-geniculo-striate pathway, the striate-recipient zone (LPl). First, this zone, as just mentioned, is the only main subdivision of the LP-pulvinar that receives a direct input from areas 17 and 18 (Figure 9). Second, like the medial Clare–Bishop area at the cortical level, LPl apparently receives input from all the cortical areas in the geniculate family (Figure 9). These afferent connections of the striate-recipient zone turn out to be predictive of its efferent thalamocortical connections: LPl is singled out among the subdivisions of the extrageniculate thalamus by projecting to cortex of the geniculorecipient family, even areas 17 and 18 (Figure 10; Berson and Graybiel, 1978a; Miller and Benevento, 1979; Symonds et al., 1978).

Rules of within-Family Connectivity

From even this brief review of the connections; it can be seen that there are systematic patterns of thalamocortical and corticocortical connection setting off some extrastriate cortical areas from others, at least as regards their relationship to the geniculostriate system. In fact, what is most obvious for the striate-recipient cortex is a rule of exclusion: the striate cortex projects hardly at all to extrastriate areas outside the extended geniculorecipient family. But it is clear that more is involved, for there is a highly lawful interlocking of the transcortical circuits with transthalamic pathways, not only with those of the principal thalamic nucleus of the geniculostriate system, the LGd, but also with those of the striate-recipient zone of the LP-pulvinar (the LPl). This further differentiation of the geniculostriate system suggests the existence of an extensive set of within-family rules that govern interconnections among family members, including highly detailed rules specifying cortical layers of origin and termination according to degree of relatedness and, apparently, density of termination as well.

As an elementary heuristic for these within-family connections, the model of a nested hierarchy recommends itself. Consider the cortical areas centered on the geniculocortical pathway and their thalamocortical connections: the "main" A and A1 laminae of the LGd project to areas 17 and 18 only (level I), and within these areas, most densely to layer IV. The "geniculate complex," including the C layers and NIM as well as the A layers, projects strongly to areas 17–19 (level II) and weakly to CBm and area 21a (level III). The differentiation between levels I and II is respected in the pattern of distribution of the C-layer pathways, because they do not terminate in layer IV in areas 17 and 18 as do the A layers. Though no comparable difference in laminar distribution is known to be correlated with the level II–III distinction, it is reflected not only in the relative strengths of the corticipetal pathways just men-

A. M. Graybiel and D. M. Berson

tioned, but also in the contrast between the dense corticofugal projection from areas 17–19·to the lateral geniculate body and the much weaker corticogeniculate projection from CBm and area 21a. All cortex of level III receives input from the single zone of the main LP-pulvinar triad known to be tightly linked to this cortical family, the striate-recipient zone (LP1). This thalamic region observes the distinction between levels I and all others in its corticipetal projection, for LP1 fibers destined for areas 17 and 18 avoid layer IV, the center of the geniculate family cluster, while elsewhere they do terminate in the middle layers (Berson and Graybiel, in preparation; Miller and Benevento, 1979).

As shown in Figure 10, nearly all of the regions receiving input from the thalamic striate-recipient zone (LP1) also receive direct transcortical projections from area 17 (and, for that matter, directly from the LGd). However, LP1 projects also to certain regions of visual cortex beyond the cluster defined as the geniculorecipient family. This wider cortical field comprises the "LP1 family." It must be reiterated that the LP1 family bears an especially close relation to the extended geniculate family. In fact, the LP1 family can be viewed as the fourth level of the nested hierarchy of the geniculate family if transthalamic conduction through the striate-recipient zone is taken into account. As will be described below, clusters of cortical areas preferentially linked to the extra-geniculate thalamic subdivisions other than the striate-recipient zone do not bear such a close association to the geniculostriate system.

Efferent Connections of the Striate Cortex and the Striate-Recipient Cortex

If one now considers these connections from the point of view of the outputs of area 17, the following routes are available:

(1) A set of apparently directly reciprocal pathways leading to the LGd. This connection observes the general principle that a corticothalamic projection directly reciprocating its principal thalamic input originates within layer VI (direct recursion; Graybiel, 1979). The corticogeniculate pathway also observes the classification by levels just defined. For example, area 19 projects to the C laminae and NIM (level II) but not to the A laminae (level I) of the LGd (Updyke, 1975).

(2) A set of transcortical pathways that are restricted, with only one unequivocal exception to be discussed below, to geniculorecipient cortical areas (that is, areas of level III). This could be considered a doubling of the direct geniculocortical inputs to these areas, but almost certainly the information is more heavily preprocessed, coming mainly (and perhaps exclusively) from the upper cortical layers. These pathways must in some way interlock the levels defined above for the cat, but are the sole direct links from the geniculostriate pathway to the extrastriate cortex in the monkey, and apparently most other species for which direct geniculocortical projections to extrastriate cortex do not exist. It is not

clear, therefore, whether one should expect to find a differentiation among striate-recipient cortical areas in the monkey comparable to that deduced in the cat from the nested geniculocortical relations of these areas.

(3) A transthalamic pathway leading from area 17 to the striate-recipient zone of the LP-pulvinar complex, and from this zone to the medial Clare–Bishop area and other members of the extended geniculate family and also to cortical regions that are apparently not part of the striate-recipient cortex (area 21b, the splenial visual area, and probably area 20). This is a key observation because it suggests that by way of the striate-recipient zone of the thalamus, area 17 has access to a greater range of cortical areas than through its direct transcortical connections. It probably also means that area 17 has access to different target neurons as well because of the different laminar distributions of the thalamocortical and corticocortical pathways. These connections may constitute partly autonomous conduction paths away from the striate cortex, for the cells of origin of the two sets of efferents are different from one another (and from the corticogeniculate pathway): the neurons projecting to LPl lie in layer V of area 17, whereas those projecting across the cortex lie in the supragranular layers. It will be interesting to follow up preliminary evidence for a sparse ascending projection to LPl (Graybiel and Berson, 1980b) because it may be possible to distinguish the LPl circuit in yet another way. More generally, it is important to emphasize that the side branches leading beyond striate-recipient cortex emerge not only by the well-recognized means of corticocortical connections stretching even farther away from area 17, but also by indirect cortico-thalamo-cortical pathways. These cortico-thalamo-cortical "escapes" from a constellation of related cortical areas may be as lawful in their organization as the original set of pathways leading from the center of the constellation to immediate and extended family members.

Each of the three classes of corticofugal connection just mentioned is present also in the monkey. It is important to make this point explicit because the striking difference between the widespread geniculocortical projections in the cat and the restricted geniculocortical projection in the monkey has tended to obscure the fact that the visual system in cats and primates has a similar organization in many other respects, as though reflecting a common mammalian plan. On this account we would suspect that there is a restricted set of cortical areas in the monkey that comprises the equivalent of the geniculorecipient cortex in the cat, namely, the set of cortical areas receiving direct transcortical projections from area 17. We would predict further that the large degree of overlap between geniculate-family and LPl-family cortex in the cat has an equivalent in the monkey in a close concordance between striate-recipient cortex and the cluster of cortical areas receiving input from the striate-recipient region of the pulvinar.

Other Affiliations of the Striate Cortex

Before leaving a consideration of the geniculate-family and striate-recipient cortex and its extensions, it remains to mention briefly efferent connections of the striate cortex not included in the thalamic and cortical circuitry discussed above. These include (a) variably massive descending fiber projections to the pontine grey matter, superior colliculus and pretectal region, and the ventral nucleus of the lateral geniculate body, and (b) fiber projections to noncortical telencephalic regions: the striatum and the claustrum.

Two details of these other efferent conduction routes are directly pertinent to the present account. First, the corticocollicular pathway from area 17 terminates in the superior colliculus in a layer just ventral to the main upper tier of contralateral retinal input except in one region of the colliculus, the rostral zone in which the area centralis is represented. In this zone, the retinotectal projection is markedly reduced in density and fibers from area 17 terminate within the tier elsewhere occupied by retinal afferents (see Graybiel, 1975; Kawamura, Sprague, and Niimi, 1974; Updyke, 1977). This exception may help account for the apparently special status of the area centralis representation in the cortical target of the tectal channel, the lateral division of the Clare–Bishop complex. This part only of the lateral Clare–Bishop area receives a direct projection from area 17 (and other members of the geniculate family), as though the transcortical connections were reflecting, at the cortical level, the domination of the area centralis part of the tectal mechanism by the descending projection from area 17 (see Berson and Graybiel, in preparation; Segraves, 1978).

The second point concerns the interconnections between area 17 and the claustrum recently described by the Duke group (Bear and Carey, 1979; Carey, Fitzpatrick, and Diamond, 1979). Their latest findings suggest that it is layer VI of the striate cortex that projects to the claustrum, and that the claustrum projects to layers IV and IIIb as well as to layers I and VI of area 17. Within the framework of the present account these layers of origin and termination suggest that the claustrum has a status otherwise reserved for the main A and A1 laminae of the lateral geniculate body (receiving input from layer VI and sending output to layer IV). The corticipetal connections of the claustrum can in this respect be sharply distinguished from those of the thalamic striate-recipient zone, which do not directly engage the IVth and VIth layers of the striate cortex. Neither the claustral nor the transthalamic loop system is closed to other inputs: other areas of extrastriate cortex project to claustrum and to LPl, and LPl receives in addition a weak ascending fiber projection. The "loop connections" linking the main A and A1 laminae with area 17 (+18) seem, by contrast, more exclusive: as mentioned above, it is the C layers, but not layers A and A1, that receive projections from areas beyond the 17–18 core. Even the main A layers, however, are open to some influence from regions other than the retina and striate cortex; they are innervated by noradrenergic fibers apparently originating in the coeruleal-subcoeruleal region (Maeda et al., 1973) and also receive a diffuse pretectal input from the nucleus of the optic tract (Graybiel and Berson, 1980a).

Families of Cortical Areas in Extrastriate Cortex

An important conclusion to be drawn from the studies just reviewed is that much of the extrastriate cortex is insulated from the direct influence of area 17. This large remainder of vision-related cortex appears itself to be divided up into family clusters analogous to the LPl family but distinguished from it (a) by being related principally to other subdivisions of the thalamic LP-pulvinar complex and (b) by lacking the direct transcortical input from area 17 characteristic of nearly all members of the LPl family. Two such groupings are shown in Figures 11 and 12, each linked to a major line of ascending extrageniculate conduction.

Cortical Areas Related to the Tectorecipient and Pretectorecipient Zones of the Thalamus

The cortical projection of the principal tectorecipient zone, LPm, defines a cluster including (1) the visually responsive areas in the lateral set of LS areas of Palmer, Rosenquist, and Tusa (1978) including the caudally located representation of the area centralis (CBl-AC), (2) an adjoining rostral part of so-called area 20, and probably (3) a zone buried in the depths of the anterior ectosylvian sulcus (Berson and Graybiel, 1978b; Symonds et al., 1978). Apparently, none of these cortical regions receives a direct fiber projection from area 17 except the area centralis zone, CBl-AC, which may, as just discussed above, be considered to be as closely affiliated with the striate as with the tectal channel when the pattern of corticotectal projection from area 17 is taken into

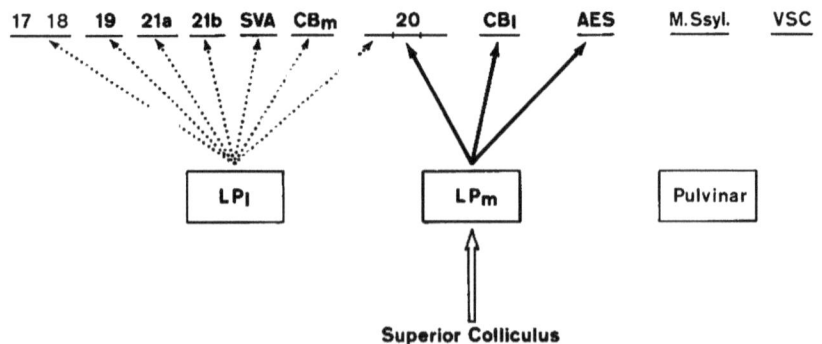

Figure 11 Schematic illustration of the tecto-thalamo-cortical channel in the cat emphasizing the restricted group of cortical areas receiving projections from the tectorecipient zone (the LPm family). Note that there is little if any overlap between the projections of the LPm (shown in solid lines) and LPl (shown in dotted lines).

A. M. Graybiel and D. M. Berson

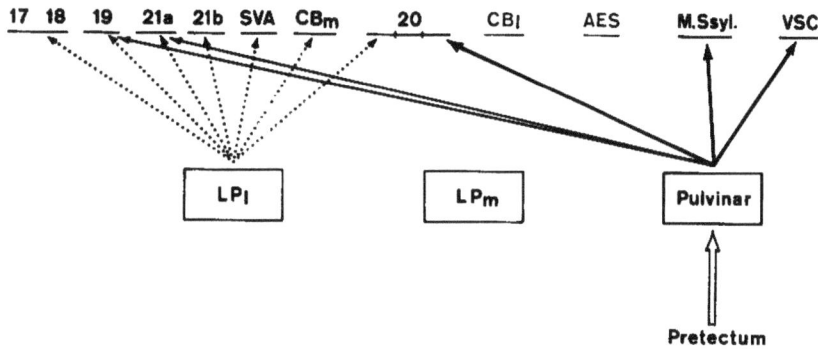

Figure 12 Schematic illustration of the pretecto-thalamo-cortical pathway in the cat. There is no overlap of "pulvinar cortex" with the LPm family (compare with Figure 11), but areas 19 and 21, both in the LPl family, receive thalamocortical projections from the pulvinar as well.

account. Nor is there any overlap with cortex of the LPl family, possible exceptions being at the border of CBm and CBl and in part of area 20.

The second extrastriate family illustrated in Figure 12 is defined by its association with the pretectorecipient zone of the pulvinar. This cluster of cortical regions includes (1) the crown of the middle suprasylvian gyrus, (2) a region in the splenial sulcus adjoining the splenial visual area (labeled "ventral splenial cortex" in Figure 1), (3) a part (probably mainly caudal and ventromedial) of "area 20," and, at least weakly, (4) area 19 and the adjoining 21a. Of these areas, all but the 19–21a complex lie outside striate-recipient cortex, and also outside the LPl family.

The corticocortical connections of these extrastriate areas are still only very incompletely known, but available information suggests that pathways linking different families are tightly restricted, whereas within-family connections are more common. For example, neither "LPm-cortex" nor "LPl-cortex" projects, as far as we know, to the crown of the middle suprasylvian gyrus ("pulvinar-cortex"). Nor, apparently, does the middle suprasylvian crown project to cortical areas of the LPl and LPm families. Connections between the LPl and LPm areas are also few. As we shall discuss in the next section, however, the three extrastriate families are by no means completely isolated from one another, for despite the generally limited number of transcortical ties linking different families, there appear to be certain nodal crossover points from one family cluster to another.

It is important to point out that for most of these areas of the extrastriate cortex, we have so far little evidence suggesting the presence of major pathways leading to the prefrontal cortex or limbic cortex of the ventral cingulate or parahippocampal gyri. An exception is the middle suprasylvian crown (area 7) which projects directly to the cingulate cortex. This supports the general distinction between *proximal association cortex*, most tightly linked to the sensory areas of the neocortex and to ancillary sensory pathways, and *distal association cortex*, representing cortical areas farther removed from the major sensory fields and projecting to prelimbic or limbic cortex (Graybiel, 1972a,c). Within the broad category of proximal association cortex further distinctions can now be made, for clearly there are sharp differences in the degree of relatedness of extrastriate cortex to the geniculostriate channel. All of LPl-cortex is related to area 17 either by direct transcortical connections or by the indirect transthalamic LPl route (or both); by contrast, nearly all areas beyond the LPl-cortex are less directly linked to area 17, but are associated with the visual modality nonetheless by way of ascending extrageniculate channels.

The cortex of the middle suprasylvian crown was classified as a distal association cortex because this cortical field has fewer transcortical ties with the sensory cortex and stronger direct ties with the limbic cingulate cortex than most of the remainder of the posterior association cortex. The pretectal channel (or at least, the pulvinar) appears to provide the suprasylvian crown its main link with the visual modality; but why the pretectal channel, in particular, should project to the distal association cortex is a puzzle. There are still many other unknowns here: for instance, the transcortical efferent connections of area 20 and of the splenial cortex (both themselves in part pulvinar-recipient cortex) have not been analyzed by modern axon-transport techniques but, because these areas lie so close to the parahippocampal and cingulate cortex, they might be expected to project directly into these limbic areas. Until we know more about such pathways it will be impossible to state whether there is a detailed hierarchy in the relation of the different extrastriate cortical families to the limbic (or, by analogy, to the premotor) mechanisms of the cerebral cortex. The same is true for the other corticofugal connections of these areas with regions in the noncortical hemisphere and brain stem. However, the crossover pathways to be described below may provide at least initial hints about how between-family connections are organized within the extrastriate cortex itself.

Crossover Pathways Linking One Extrastriate Cortical Family to Another

Bridging pathways linking different family clusters can be seen both in the transthalamic and in the transcortical connections of area 19 (Figure 13; Berson and Graybiel, in preparation). On the basis of thalamic affiliations, area 19 is clearly part of the LPl family, receiving a dense projection from LPl (and also a thalamic input from the LGd). But area 19 may also be included in the pulvinar family because it receives at least a weak projection from the pretectorecipient zone of the pulvinar and also receives, like other members of the pulvinar family, an input from LIc. A thalamocortical input to area 19 may originate in the tectorecipient zone, but this matter is not settled: injections of horseradish peroxidase in area 19 do label a small number of neurons in LPm but these are close

A. M. Graybiel and D. M. Berson

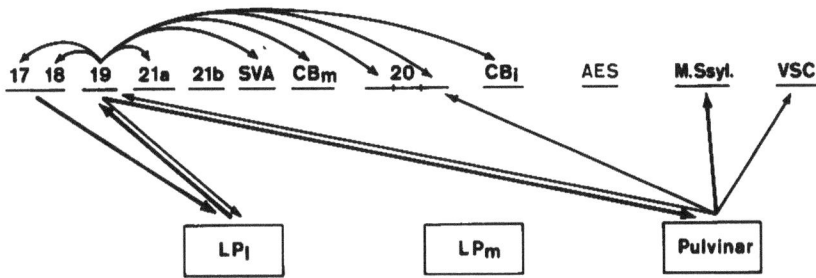

Figure 13 Schematic illustration of crossover pathways linking different family clusters in the extrastriate cortex. *Transcortical* pathways lead from area 19 to other members of the LPl (and geniculate) family but also to the LPm cortex (lateral Clare–Bishop area, CBl) and to the part of area 20 that is in the pulvinar family. *Transthalamic* crossover pathways are shown linking the LPl (and geniculate) families to the pulvinar family. Note pathway shown in heavy arrows follows the sequence: area 17 → LPl → area 19 → pulvinar → middle suprasylvian crown (M. Ssyl.). By contrast, no direct transcortical pathway links areas 17 or 19 with the cortex of the middle suprasylvian crown.

to the LPm–LPl border. In any event, at least one and possibly two of the subdivisions of the LP-pulvinar triad send pathways to area 19 supplementing the main LPl-to-19 route.

At the cortical level, the association pathways originating in area 19 clearly also cross family lines: area 19 projects both to the LPl cluster (areas 17, 18, 21a, CBm, the splenial visual area, and the part of area 20 related to LPl) and to cortex of the LPm family (CBl, probably weakly to the anterior ectosylvian cortex as well). Injections of tritiated amino acids in area 19 also appear to label the pulvinar-recipient part of area 20, but we have seen no evidence of a projection to the main pulvinar-family cortex of the middle suprasylvian crown and ventral splenial cortex. It is difficult, for technical reasons, to rule out completely the possibility that some part of this large cortical outflow originates from the cortical areas adjoining area 19. It seems more likely, however, that pathways to cortex of both the LPl and LPm families do originate in area 19 proper and that this area therefore represents a "crossover zone" of the extrastriate cortex providing access to and from cortical families that are otherwise notably insulated from one another.

The corticothalamic projections of area 19 also cross family boundaries but in a manner that reciprocates the thalamocortical connectivity and contrasts sharply with the pattern of corticocortical connections just described. Area 19 projects to the LGd complex (C laminae and NIM), densely to LPl (striate-recipient zone), densely to the lateral part of the pulvinar, and at least weakly to the rest of the pulvinar (Updyke, 1977) and to LIc (both pretectorecipient). Finally, area 19 may project to LPm, but this is questionable, as is the presence of a projection from LPm to area 19. Thus, area 19 appears to be reciprocally related to the thalamic striate-recipient and pretectorecipient zones, but to project transcortically to members of the tectorecipient and striate-recipient families and hardly at all to pretectorecipient cortex.

The implications of this pattern are at least threefold:

(1) There clearly are ties linking different families of extrastriate areas by way of transcortical pathways, but these crossover connections appear to be strictly limited. Just what the limiting rules are should be a major point for further study. For example, it is possible that the family-cluster mode of organization is embedded in a transcortical flow of information typically depicted in sequential processing models of the neocortex.

(2) Because area 19 projects both to LPl and to the pulvinar and LIc, there exists a second set of crossover pathways not evident in the pattern of transcortical projection of area 19. For example, although there is no convincing evidence for a direct corticocortical projection from area 19 to the middle suprasylvian crown (pulvinar family), there apparently are indirect, transthalamic pathways linking area 19 to this suprasylvian cortex by way of the pulvinar and LIc (see Figure 13). This observation suggests that the degree of relatedness of cortical areas should not be defined solely on the basis of their transcortical associations: cortical areas may be linked to one another by way of cortico-thalamo-cortical pathways not easily predicted from their intracortical associations.

(3) A final and related conclusion is that transthalamic crossover projections may provide a crucial means of linking lines of apparently independent ascending conduction. In the case of area 19, for example, the ascending pretectal channel is linked to the ascending tectal channel by the circuit pretectum-pulvinar-area 19-CBl. There are important similarities between these transthalamic crossover connections and the patterns of indirect recursion followed by the projections from layer V of area 17 to the tectum and pretectum (Graybiel, 1979). Both link related lines of conduction in a way that permits some measure of autonomy to be maintained. But while by indirect recursion a cortical area can influence a parallel conduction route at the prethalamic level, the crossover pathway is a device permitting a stepwise extension of the sphere of influence of one cortical family at the level of thalamus and cortex. This is the design feature stressed by the example of area 19: a systematic interlocking of parallel ascending pathways by transthalamic escape routes leading from one cortical family domain into another.

Family Clusters beyond the Visually Mapped Extrastriate Cortex

Connectional patterns suggesting a division of association cortex into families of related areas are by no means limited to visual areas proper. Figure 14 was prepared to make this point by showing the fiber connections of the most medial subdivision of the thalamic pulvinar-posterior region, the so-called LM-Sg complex (see Graybiel and Ber-

A. M. Graybiel and D. M. Berson

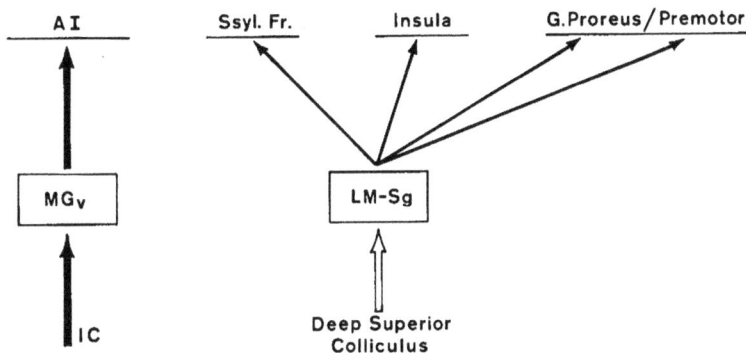

Figure 14 Schematic diagram of the thalamocortical projections of the LM-Sg complex in the cat. To the left is shown the main auditory path leading from the inferior colliculus (IC) to the ventral nucleus of the medial geniculate body (MGv) to area AI of auditory cortex. S.Syl.Fr., suprasylvian fringe.

son, 1980b). This thalamic subdivision forms part of the posterior nuclear group shown in physiological studies to contain units responsive to auditory and somatic sensory stimulation (Poggio and Mountcastle, 1960). It is not known whether cells in LM-Sg are visually responsive, but considering its afferents from the deep collicular layers (and from the insula) this would not be particularly surprising.

As shown in Figure 14, the LM-Sg complex projects to at least three cortical areas: the suprasylvian fringe; the insula; and the frontal cortex including the gyrus proreus. Experiments in progress also suggest that the LM-Sg region projects to part of the perirhinal cortex. The important point for the present argument is that if the hypothesis of family clusters is correct, then from the thalamocortical connections of these cortical areas we should be able to predict most of their corticocortical projections: there should be high within-family connectivity and restricted cross-family ties. This turns out to be the case insofar as the connections are known. The insula and gyrus proreus project to both of the other family members, and the suprasylvian fringe projects to at least one other area, the insula. In addition to corticothalamic projections reciprocating the LM-Sg projections, there are crossover pathways analogous to those discussed in connection with the extrastriate cortex. For example, the main thalamic nucleus of the gyrus proreus is the mediodorsal nucleus, which means that the LM-Sg, by way of its proreal connections, actually represents a crossover nucleus linking auditory association cortex and limbic frontal cortex. We know of only two direct links between the LM-Sg family and the families of extrastriate cortex discussed in the preceding section: a pathway from the suprasylvian fringe to the crown of the middle suprasylvian gyrus (Heath and Jones, 1971) and a weak transcortical projection to this cortical area from the insula. It is interesting that the middle suprasylvian crown is also in a line of conduction leading to another pole of the limbic cortex, the

Connections of Visual Association Cortex

cingulate gyrus: it projects there directly (Cragg, 1965) and also apparently has a weak transthalamic link by way of the nucleus lateralis dorsalis (LD) (Graybiel and Berson, 1980b).

A Modified View of Cortical Processing

The model of cortical processing that has dominated for nearly a century is that of the reflex: sensory afflux reaches the cerebral mantle by means of lemniscal line and adjunct pathways, is "processed" step by step through the association cortex, and finally is relayed to effector channels, in much modified form, by way of pathways whose archetype is the pyramidal tract. So much of cortical processing was conceived of as depending exclusively on transcortical pathways that a sizable part of the association cortex was considered to be "athalamic" (Walker, 1938), that is, without any source of ascending input and relying exclusively on association pathways epitomized in the Pavlovian notion of irradiation.

An early step toward modifying this view came when Rose and Woolsey (1949), working on the auditory cortex in the cat, introduced the notion that, aside from the so-called nonspecific intralaminar fibers, thalamocortical connections were of at least two types: if the metabolic machinery of the thalamic neurons depended on the thalamocortical connection, so that they would degenerate in its absence, the connection was called *essential;* if a restricted lesion of the cortex would not cause such retrograde damage, the thalamocortical pathway was considered to be a *sustaining connection*, probably composed of fibers widely distributed in the cortex by virtue of axon collaterals. "Athalamic cortex" was replaced by association cortex with sustaining thalamocortical connections.

A second important modification resulted from the realization, attributable to studies such as those by Pandya and Kuypers (1969) and Jones and Powell (1970), that there are reverse projections from frontal to parietal cortex as well as irradiating cortical association pathways of variable lengths leading toward the frontal lobe and limbic lobes. More recent anatomical studies have demonstrated extensive fiber projections from the cingulate gyrus to the parietal lobe (Mesulam et al., 1977) and even from the hippocampal formation to adjoining parts of the neocortex (Rosene and van Hoesen, 1977). In effect, these studies still emphasize the model of the stepwise sensory-to-limbic progression as the dominant scheme of cortical processing, but add cortical feedback and feedforward to the model.

A main purpose of the present paper is to point out the need for a third modification that would emphasize transthalamic conduction no less than the association (and commissural) pathways intrinsic to the cerebral hemisphere itself. Thalamocortical and cortico-thalamo-cortical circuits are extensive in their distribution, in the association cortex as

A. M. Graybiel and D. M. Berson

much as in the sensory and motor cortex, and these transthalamic pathways appear to be systematically interlocked with lines of transcortical conduction. To try to appreciate the function of the cerebral cortex by studying it alone would, therefore, surely be a mistake; for much of what we ordinarily think of as processing by the neocortex is actually the result of reciprocal and nonreciprocal circuiting of information between thalamus and neocortex.

In Figure 15 we have tried to schematize very simply dominant patterns of transthalamic conduction for the main thalamic nuclei, leaving aside the intralaminar and reticular nuclei. The first panel shows the model of the "relay nucleus," in which an ascending pathway is driving the thalamus and the thalamus is driving the neocortex. As Ramón y Cajal first realized, a reciprocal link from cortex to thalamus is a ubiquitous feature of thalamocortical connectivity. In the second part of the figure, the ascending pathway to the thalamus is lost, or is very small, so that the thalamus is driving the neocortex and is itself being driven by the neocortex. Note that two thalamocortical pathways have been drawn in, one part of a cortico-thalamo-cortical pathway that is not a reciprocal loop circuit but a transthalamic adjunct to direct transcortical paths. Another pattern of transthalamic conduction, in which the subcortical hemisphere influences the neocortex, is shown in the third panel by the neocortex projecting to the corpus striatum, which in turn projects to the thalamus which drives the motor cortex. This is an extrapyramidal circuit, presumably modulated by the ascending nigrostriatal pathway; but there are other transthalamic pathways originating in the subcortical hemisphere, for example, pathways from the amygdaloid complex to the mediodorsal nucleus and then on to the granular frontal cortex. The last panel shows the amygdala, but instead of the transthalamic circuitry associated with it, a direct intratelencephalic pathway from the amygdala to the orbital frontal cortex (Krettek and Price, 1977). This pattern, in which subcortical hemisphere bypasses the thalamic gate and projects directly to the cerebral cortex, is not unique to the amygdala; labeling of neurons in the putamen has been observed following large injections of the retrograde tracer horseradish peroxidase into the parietooccipital association cortex (Berson and Graybiel, unpublished).

Each of these patterns appears in the circuitry of the extrastriate cortex and its thalamic correspondents, but it is the first two that are the most familiar: the "relays" in the lateral geniculate body, tectorecipient zone, and pretectorecipient zone; and the transthalamic association paths in, for example, the line of conduction leading from area 17 to LPl and then from LPl to the medial Clare–Bishop area. Note, however, that these two patterns are actually blended together in many instances: for example, even though the input from the visual cortex is quantitatively dominant in LPl, there is a weak ascending projection to this zone from the superior colliculus. The striate-recipient zone therefore does not

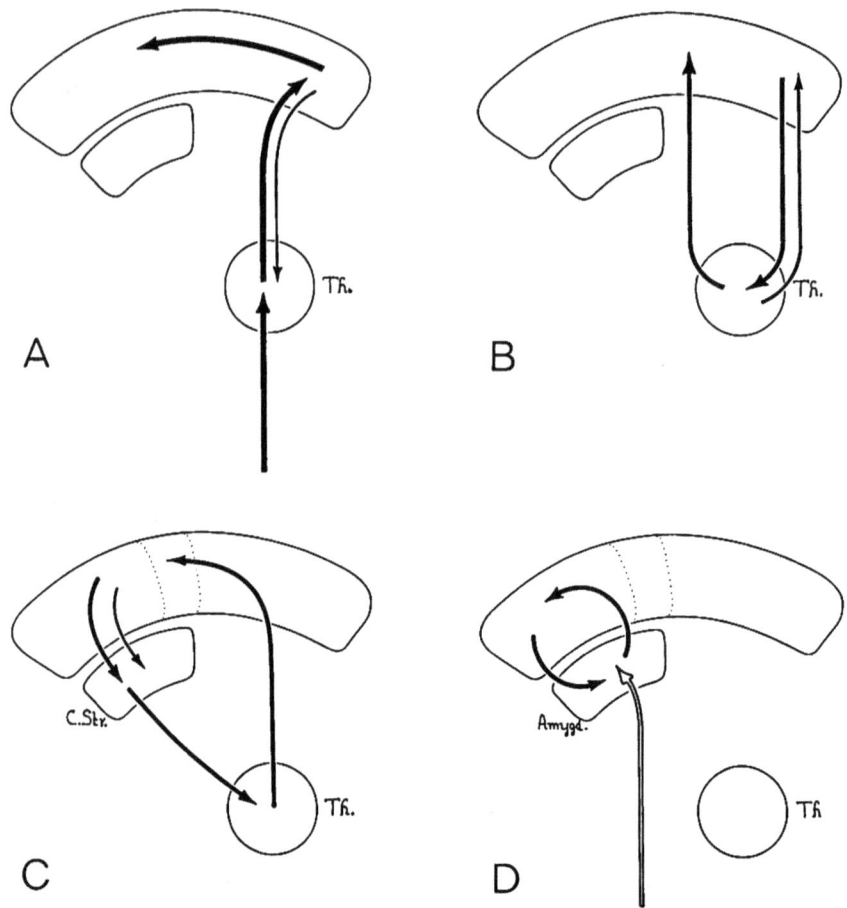

Figure 15 Schematic diagrams illustrating four patterns of access to the neocortex. (A)–(C) show transthalamic circuits, (D) a thalamic bypass. (A) The model of the relay nucleus, with a corticothalamic path reciprocating the thalamocortical connection. An extrinsic connection is shown ascending to the thalamic nucleus. (B) A cortico-thalamo-cortical circuit. Note that this can include a mode of indirect conduction from one part of the neocortex to another. (C) Forebrain circuit involving links in the subcortical hemisphere as prelude to the transthalamic pathway (C.Str., corpus striatum). (D) One of a number of forebrain circuits bypassing the thalamus. In the instance shown, the trans-amygdaloid pathway may represent a means for ascending fiber systems to influence the neocortex without synapsing in the thalamus. Not shown are biogenic amine pathways, "generalized" or "nonspecific" thalamocortical projections, and combinations of the different major classes of cortical access route.

A. M. Graybiel and D. M. Berson

fully qualify as an intrinsic thalamic nucleus, that is, a nucleus lacking ascending afferent connections altogether.

The weight of evidence suggests that it is the second transthalamic pattern that dominates in the extrageniculate visual system of primates. Most of the subdivisions of the pulvinar in advanced primates are thought to be intrinsic thalamic nuclei whose main afferents come from the neocortex. Even when ascending projections can be identified in the monkey (for example, the tectal projection to the inferior pulvinar), corticothalamic input apparently still dominates at least in the quantitative sense (Ogren and Hendrickson, 1979). It therefore may not be possible, or may be misleading, to rely in the monkey on an ascending connection as the essential or defining attribute of a particular extrageniculate thalamic subdivision and its cortical affiliates. Instead, one or more corticothalamic projections must be sought for characterization of these zones.

This does not affect the classification of cortical areas preferentially related to a particular subdivision of the extrageniculate thalamus as being part of a family cluster. There is no reason to think that groupings based upon a well-defined corticothalamic projection would be any less principled than those that can be referred to a line of ascending conduction. The difference is that the cortico-thalamo-cortical plan emphasizes a pattern of intrinsic connectivity of the forebrain rather than one of extrinsic connectivity. Even so, the lack of dense ascending projections to much of the pulvinar in the monkey may make the task of discovering family clusters in its extrastriate cortex more difficult than it has been in the cat, where the ascending inputs to the LP-pulvinar serve as reference markers. Consider the advantages of working with the ascending tectothalamic projection. Though we do not yet know the functional significance of this pathway, the thalamic tectorecipient zone is delineated by it, and in turn the LPm family can be defined in the extrastriate cortex. The advantage here is that the superior colliculus has been established as an anatomical and functional unit: it has relatively well-defined borders, a well-delineated retinotopic map, and a set of known input–output connections. For much of the posterior association cortex, especially in the monkey, comparable "units" remain difficult to define, and accordingly, it is difficult to identify thalamic subdivisions on the basis of tracing all and only all of the corticothalamic projections of a particular cortical "area." Physiological mapping studies have already begun to help in subdividing the extrastriate cortex in primates, but it will probably be necessary also to study a constellation of anatomical connections to find distinguishing markers for individual cortical zones. This will also be necessary before adequate species comparisons can be made, because it is in the patterning of a group of neural affiliations of each thalamic zone and its cortical correspondents that the notion of the family cluster rests.

In relation to studies of the extrastriate cortex, the important point to be made is that very little of the neocortex follows the simple plan of being tightly tied to the sensory or motor periphery by a single pathway. Most of the connections, instead, form parts of complex circuits that seem to represent in sum the internal processing mechanism of the forebrain itself. Accordingly, once we are a few steps out from the primary visual areas, there is no guarantee that we are even correct in analyzing the multiple representations of the visual field from the standpoint only of the visual stimulus. Part of our confusion about these maps in fact may arise from such a point of view, because they may reflect, at least in part, the organization of the equally complex and equally multiplistic effector mechanisms of the brain. Nor is it clear that we should view the pathways in the forebrain as being parceled out strictly along the lines of the behavioral categories that have been formulated so far. It may be that part of what we are seeing in them is a computational network whose logic requires a different level of analysis altogether. It is partly with this thought in mind that we have stressed the remarkable orderliness of the pathways linking thalamus and neocortex in the extrageniculate visual system. For there are hints that there may be generally applicable flow diagrams and logical sequences underlying the orderliness.

Summary and Conclusions

(1) Study of the fiber connections of the visual cortex provides little evidence for a simple hierarchical arrangement in which the striate cortex lies at the origin of a serial chain of conduction extending step by step across the visual association cortex. Instead, the extrastriate cortex is divided into clusters of cortical areas, some of these apparently quite far removed, in the connectional sense, from area 17.

(2) The cortical areas in each cluster appear to receive thalamic input primarily from one (or sometimes two) of the principal subdivisions of the LP-pulvinar complex. On this basis it has been possible to define the following family clusters: the LPl family, receiving the thalamocortical projection of the striate-recipient zone; the LPm family, receiving input from the tectorecipient zone of the thalamus; and the pulvinar family, receiving fiber projections from the pretectorecipient zone. A fourth grouping, less closely tied to the visual modality, comprises parts of auditory and frontal association cortex receiving thalamocortical projections from the LM-Sg complex.

(3) Cortical areas identified on the basis of their thalamic input as part of the same family cluster tend to be interconnected directly by transcortical pathways. The thalamocortical and corticocortical connections of individual areas of the neocortex thus appear to be related in a systematic way.

(4) In contrast to the rule of high within-family connectivity, cross-family connectivity in the extrastriate cortex appears to be restricted. Crossover pathways do exist, however, and appear to be part of an intricate and systematic interlocking of the extrastriate families that occurs both by direct transcortical pathways and by indirect transthalamic loops.

(5) The corticipetal projections of the extrageniculate thalamus are of at least two main types: those that continue a line of ascending conduction (for example, the tecto-thalamo-cortical pathway), and those that form part of a cortico-thalamo-cortical circuit (for example, the path from striate cortex to LPl to the medial Clare–Bishop area). In several instances, individual subdivisions of the LP-pulvinar complex in the cat have been shown to participate in both types of transthalamic conduction. In the monkey, pathways of the second type are probably dominant.

(6) Nonreciprocity in cortico-thalamo-cortical loop circuits appears in some instances to provide a mechanism for the stepwise extension from one family of cortical areas to another. Because these transthalamic routes interlock networks that are separate or sparsely interconnected at the cortical level, it is not sufficient to judge the relatedness of cortical areas by transcortical connectivity alone.

(7) Rules of cortical connectivity considered at the level of tracts appear to have morphological signatures in the arrangement of the layers of termination of corticipetal projections and the layers of origin of corticofugal pathways. These laminar organizations may be a defining characteristic of a particular type of connection (for example, pathways of direct recursion originate in layer VI). Laminar arrangements may also reflect hierarchical ordering of within-family connections (for example, in the contrast between the geniculocortical projections of the A layers and the parvocellular C layers of the lateral geniculate body). An important point for further study is whether the rules of circuitry also have chemical signatures indicative of a range of excitatory, inhibitory, or even metabolic and trophic influences.

(8) Structural and developmental constraints, and the need for particular sequential orderings in the connectivity, may be of crucial importance in the design of connections in the forebrain. Thus the detailed plan of organization of individual pathways may be related only partly, if at all, to particular functional classifications at the behavioral level of analysis despite the fact that these pathways make up part of biologically adaptive functional networks underlying the behaviors of the organism. A major effort should be made to distinguish among these different constraining factors and their consequences in determining the configuration of connections. It may then be possible to see exceptions to the patterns as keystones instead of points of confusion and to see

species differences in the connectivity as clues to the behavioral significance of the pathways in question.

Acknowledgments

It is a pleasure to thank Mr. Henry F. Hall and Miss Elaine Yoneoka for their assistance with some of the experimental work described here. The studies were funded by the National Institutes of Health (RO1 EY 02866-01 and 1-P30-EY02621) and the National Science Foundation (BNS75-18758 and 78-10549).

References

Allman, J. M., and J. H. Kaas, 1975. The dorsomedial cortical visual area: A third tier area in the occipital lobe of the owl monkey (*Aotus trivirgatus*). *Brain Res.* 100:473–487.

Bear, M. F., and R. G. Carey, 1979. Visual projections of the tree shrew claustrum: An anterograde and retrograde transport study. *Soc. Neurosci. Abst.* 5:777.

Berson, D. M., and A. M. Graybiel, 1978a. Parallel thalamic zones in the LP-pulvinar complex of the cat identified by their afferent and efferent connections. *Brain Res.* 147:139–148.

Berson, D. M., and A. M. Graybiel, 1978b. Thalamo-cortical projections and histochemical identification of subdivisions of the LP-pulvinar complex in the cat. *Soc. Neurosci. Abst.* 4:620.

Carey, R. G., D. Fitzpatrick, and I. T. Diamond, 1979. Layer I of striate cortex of *Tupaia glis* and *Galago senegalensis:* Projections from thalamus and claustrum revealed by retrograde transport of horseradish peroxidase. *J. Comp. Neurol.* 186:393–438.

Cragg, B. G., 1965. Afferent connexions of the allocortex. *J. Anat.* 99:339–357.

Fujii, M., and N. Yoshii, 1979. Hypothalamic projection to the pulvinar-LP complex in the cat: A study by the silver impregnation method. *Neurosci. Lett.* 12:247–252.

Garey, L. J., E. G. Jones, and T. P. S. Powell, 1968. Interrelationships of striate and extrastriate cortex with the primary relay sites of the visual pathway. *J. Neurol. Neurosurg. Psychiat.* 31:135–157.

Glendenning, K. K., J. A. Hall, I. T. Diamond, and W. C. Hall, 1975. The pulvinar nucleus of *Galago senegalensis. J. Comp. Neurol.* 161:419–458.

Graybiel, A. M., 1972a. Some ascending connections of the pulvinar and nucleus lateralis posterior of the thalamus in the cat. *Brain Res.* 44:99–125.

Graybiel, A. M., 1972b. Some extrageniculate visual pathways in the cat. *Invest. Ophthal.* 11:322–332.

Graybiel, A. M., 1972c. Some fiber pathways related to the posterior thalamic region in the cat. *Brain Behav. Evol.* 6:363–393.

Graybiel, A. M., 1974. Studies on the anatomical organization of posterior association cortex. In *The Neurosciences: Third Study Program*. F. O. Schmitt and F. G. Worden, eds. Cambridge, MA: MIT Press, pp. 205–214.

Graybiel, A. M., 1975. Anatomical organization of retinotectal afferents in the cat: An autoradiographic study. *Brain Res.* 96:1–23.

Graybiel, A. M., 1979. Some patterns of connectivity in the central nervous system: A tribute to Rafael Lorenté de Nó. In *Integration in the Nervous System: A Symposium in Honor of David P. C. Lloyd and Rafael Lorenté de Nó*. H. Asanuma and V. J. Wilson, eds. New York: Igaku-Shoin, pp. 69–96.

Graybiel, A. M., and D. M. Berson, 1980a. Autoradiographic evidence for a projection from the pretectal nucleus of the optic tract to the dorsal lateral geniculate complex in the cat. *Brain Res.* 195:1–12.

Graybiel, A. M., and D. M. Berson, 1980b. Histochemical identification and afferent connections of subdivisions in the LP-pulvinar complex and related nuclei in the cat. *Neuroscience* 5:1175–1238.

Heath, C. J., and E. G. Jones, 1971. The anatomical organization of the suprasylvian gyrus of the cat. *Ergebn. Anat. Entwicklungsgesch.* 45:1–64.

Hubel, D. H., and T. N. Wiesel, 1969. Visual area of the lateral suprasylvian gyrus (Clare-Bishop area) of the cat. *J. Physiol.* 202:251–260.

Hubel, D. H., and T. N. Wiesel, 1970. Cells sensitive to binocular depth in area 18 of the macaque monkey cortex. *Nature* 225:41–42.

Itoh, H., and N. Mizuno, 1979. A cerebello-pulvinar projection in the cat as visualized by the use of anterograde transport of horseradish peroxidase. *Brain Res.* 171:131–134.

Jones, E. G., and T. P. S. Powell, 1970. An anatomical study of converging sensory pathways within the cerebral cortex of the monkey. *Brain* 93:793–820.

Kalia, M., and D. Whitteridge, 1973. The visual areas in the splenial sulcus of the cat. *J. Physiol.* 232:275–283.

Kawamura, K., 1973. Corticocortical fiber connections of the cat cerebrum. III. The occipital region. *Brain Res.* 51:41–60.

Kawamura, S., J. M. Sprague, and K. Niimi, 1974. Corticofugal projections from the visual cortices to the thalamus, pretectum and superior colliculus in the cat. *J. Comp. Neurol.* 158:339–362.

Kinston, W. J., M. A. Vadas, and P. O. Bishop, 1969. Multiple projection of the visual field to the medial portion of the dorsal lateral geniculate nucleus and the adjacent nuclei of the thalamus of the cat. *J. Comp. Neurol.* 136:295–316.

Krettek, J. E., and J. L. Price, 1977. Projections from the amygdaloid complex to the cerebral cortex and thalamus in the rat and cat. *J. Comp. Neurol.* 172:687–722.

LeVay, S., and C. D. Gilbert, 1976. Laminar patterns of geniculocortical projection in the cat. *Brain Res.* 113:1–19.

Maeda, T., C. Pin, D. Salvert, M. Ligier, and M. Jouvet, 1973. Les neurones contenant des catecholamines du tegmentum pontique et leurs voies de projection chez le chat. *Brain Res.* 57:119–152.

Mason, R., 1978. Functional organization in the cat's pulvinar complex. *Exp. Brain Res.* 31:51–66.

Mesulam, M.-M., G. W. Van Hoesen, D. N. Pandya, and N. Geschwind, 1977. Limbic and sensory connections of the inferior parietal lobule (area PG) in the rhesus monkey: A study with a new method for horseradish peroxidase histochemistry. *Brain Res.* 136:393–414.

Miller, J. W., and L. A. Benevento, 1979. Multiple thalamic inputs to primary visual cortex in the monkey and cat. *Anat. Rec.* 193:623–624.

Ogren, M. P., and A. E. Hendrickson, 1979. The morphology and distribution of striate cortex terminals in the inferior and lateral subdivisions of the *Macaca* monkey pulvinar. *J. Comp. Neurol.* 188:179–200.

Palmer, L. A., A. C. Rosenquist, and R. J. Tusa, 1978. The retinotopic organization of lateral suprasylvian visual areas in the cat. *J. Comp. Neurol.* 177:237–256.

Pandya, D. N., and H. G. J. M. Kuypers, 1969. Cortico-cortical connections in the rhesus monkey. *Brain Res.* 13:13–36.

Poggio, G. F., and V. B. Mountcastle, 1960. A study of the functional contributions of the lemniscal and spinothalamic systems to somatic sensibility. *Bull. Johns Hopkins Hosp.* 106:266–316.

Rodieck, R. W., 1979. Visual pathways. *Ann. Rev. Neurosci.* 2:193–225.

Rose, J. E., and C. N. Woolsey, 1949. Organization of the mammalian thalamus and its relationships to the cerebral cortex. *Electroenceph. Clin. Neurophysiol.* 1:391–403.

Rosene, D. L., and G. W. Van Hoesen, 1977. Hippocampal efferents reach widespread areas of cerebral cortex and amygdala in the rhesus monkey. *Science* 198:315–317.

Segraves, M. A., 1978. Cortical afferents to two visual areas in the lateral suprasylvian sulcus of the cat. *Anat. Rec.* 190:537.

Symonds, L., A. Rosenquist, S. Edwards, and L. Palmer, 1978. Thalamic projections to electrophysiologically defined visual areas in the cat. *Soc. Neurosci. Abst.* 4:647.

Tusa, R. J., L. A. Palmer, and A. C. Rosenquist, 1975. The retinotopic organization of the visual cortex in the cat. *Soc. Neurosci. Abst.* 1:52.

Updyke, B. V., 1975. The patterns of projection of cortical areas 17, 18 and 19 onto the laminae of the dorsal lateral geniculate nucleus in the cat. *J. Comp. Neurol.* 163:377–396.

Updyke, B. V., 1977. Topographic organization of the projections from cortical areas 17, 18 and 19 onto the thalamus, pretectum, and superior colliculus in the cat. *J. Comp. Neurol.* 173:81–122.

van Essen, D. C., 1979. Visual areas of the mammalian cerebral cortex. *Ann. Rev. Neurosci.* 2:227–263.

Walker, A. E., 1938. *The Primate Thalamus.* Chicago: University of Chicago Press, pp. 190–193.

Zeki, S. M., 1978. Functional specialisation in the visual cortex of the rhesus monkey. *Nature* 274:423–428.

Chemical Signaling and Circuitry in Cerebral Cortex and Its Interconnections

Introduction

Floyd E. Bloom

Important questions concerning the intercellular operations within the cerebral cortex remain even after the experimental advances defining the details of cellular connections. In simplest terms, these remaining questions focus on the identification of the neurotransmitter systems operating within the cortex, the nature of the synaptic mechanisms executed by these specified chemical transmitters, and the possible modifications of these events by other locally active nonneuronal chemical factors. These are the questions addressed by the three chapters in this section.

Emson and Hunt focus their chapter on the active front of neurochemical mapping studies directed at the organization of the cerebral cortex. By combining micromethods for assay of neurotransmitter amino acids, monoamines, and neuropeptides with mapping strategies, a new chemical dimension is being added to the emerging details of cortical cells, especially their afferent and efferent projections. Direct neurochemical mapping is achieved through biochemical and immunochemical reagents that identify cells and fibers containing probable transmitters or their pertinent synthetic or catabolic enzymes. These details can then be verified by the aftereffects of lesions or by studying developmental processes to provide a picture of both the small number of cases for which the transmitters are already established and the still large number of cells and circuits for which the transmitters remain unknown. In this picture, certain neuropeptides such as substance P, choleocystokinin, and vasoactive intestinal peptide are revealed as probable important intercellular signals intrinsic to cortex, especially the cortex of man.

Taylor and Stone consider the functional characteristic of the monoaminergic projections to cerebral cortex as they influence the activity of pyramidal-tract neurons. Emphasizing the association between certain presumptive dopaminergic or beta-type noradrenergic synapses, on the one hand, and muscarinic cholinergic synapses, on the other hand, with their receptors coupled to activation of adenylate cyclase or guanylate cyclase, respectively, they contrast the monoaminergic systems and cyclic nucleotides with effects of amino acids or peptides. In addition, they draw attention to the possibility that noncyclic purine nucleotides, principally adenosine, could be released from sources within cortex to modify further the effectiveness of the monoaminergic systems on their target neurons. These differences in functional process attributable to monoamines and to other transmitter systems carry the chemical anatomical sketch of cortical circuitry into the functional dimension.

In the third chapter, I take the view that there are three large classes of transmitters already demonstrable for specified circuits of the cerebral cortex: amino acids, monoamines, and peptides. Although substances not yet characterized may eventually be added to each of these three lists as the chemical anatomy of cortex becomes progressively more complete, I have tried to focus attention on the distinctive properties of chemistry, cytoarchitecture, and synaptic action of these three classes of transmitter systems to attempt an integrated view of how each of these different systems of chemical neurotransmission contributes to the complex array of information-processing events which occur in cortex. Until the time when future workers can indicate any chemical or transmission properties unique to cortex, one may hold to the simplest view that the essence of the cortex resides in the enormous quantity of its cells, connections, chemicals, and synaptic mechanisms.

Floyd E. Bloom

13 Anatomical Chemistry of the Cerebral Cortex

P. C. Emson and S. P. Hunt

ABSTRACT By sensitive immunohistochemical techniques, intrinsic neurons containing cholecystokinin (CCK), vasoactive intestinal polypeptide (VIP), and glutamic acid decarboxylase (GAD) immunoreactivity have been visualized in the rat neocortex. Based on the distribution of these neurons and the known actions of these peptides (VIP and CCK) and γ-aminobutyric acid (GABA) on cortical neurons, it is suggested that the VIP and CCK neurons may be excitatory neurons, while the GAD positive neurons are possibly inhibitory. The possibility that glutamate and/or aspartate may be cortical neurotransmitters is also considered, along with evidence for monoamine and peptidergic afferents to the cortex.

Until recently our knowledge of the specific chemical circuitry of the mammalian neocortex has been limited to the study of the distribution of monoamine-containing afferents demonstrable by the fluorescent technique of Falck and Hillarp (Falck, 1962). Fortunately, significant advances have occurred in neurochemistry and immunohistochemistry which have allowed the visualization of cortical neurons containing material cross reacting with antibodies directed against glutamic acid decarboxylase (Ribak, 1978), vasoactive intestinal polypeptide, and the cholecystokinin-like peptides (Emson and Lindvall, 1979). These three antisera have been applied to the rat neo- and allocortex and have enabled the visualization of specific cortical neuronal types (see later). (In the immunohistochemical technique used here the specific antibody-antigen complex is visualized using two further antibodies, the second of which carries a peroxidase enzyme; Sternberger, 1979.) As well as considering the distribution of cortical neurons containing glutamic acid decarboxylase, vasoactive intestinal polypeptide, and cholecystokinin, the evidence in support of a neurotransmitter role for the amino acids L-glutamate and L-aspartate in the cortical projection neurons will be considered. Finally, the possible neuronal localization of several other cortical neuropeptides will be considered together with more recent data on the distribution of amine-containing afferents.

P. C. EMSON AND S. P. HUNT MRC Neurochemical Pharmacology Unit, Department of Pharmacology, Medical School, Hills Road, Cambridge, CB2 2QD, England

γ-Aminobutyric Acid (GABA)

The evidence in favor of γ-aminobutyric acid (GABA) as a cortical in-hibitory transmitter has been reviewed by Krnjević (1974) and Ribak (1978). In brief, iontophoretic application of GABA to cortical units pro-duces a strong inhibition (Dreifuss, Kelly, and Krnjević, 1969; Wal-lingford et al., 1973). Significant amounts of GABA are found through-out the cortical layers (Hirsch and Robins, 1962; Emson and Lindvall, 1976) and some 30% of cortical synaptosomes accumulate [^{3}H]-GABA under conditions favoring the high-affinity uptake system which is be-lieved to represent part of the transmitter inactivation mechanism for GABA (Iversen and Bloom, 1972). This evidence suggests that GABA is likely to be a major cortical inhibitory transmitter. In support of this suggestion, immunohistochemical localization of neurons and nerve terminals in the rat cortex which cross react with antisera raised against the specific GABA synthetic enzyme glutamic acid decarboxylase (GAD) have revealed GAD-positive nonpyramidal neurons and their nerve terminals in all cortical layers (see Figure 1 and Ribak, 1978). Parallel studies of the rat cortex using autoradiographic techniques to visualize neurons and terminals accumulating [^{3}H]-GABA have re-vealed a similar distribution of GABA-accumulating neurons and pro-cesses (Chronwall and Wolff, 1978). Comparison of the morphology of these GAD-positive neurons in the rat cortex with Golgi studies of non-pyramidal neurons in the rat cortex indicates that most of the GAD-positive neurons correspond to multipolar nonspiny stellate neuron types (Figure 2).

Examination of the type of synaptic arrangement made by the GAD-positive neurons or by the multipolar nonspiny stellate neurons indi-cates that both types of neuron make symmetrical, or "Gray type II end-ings" (Gray, 1959), with the dendritic shafts and somata of pyramidal neurons and other stellate neurons (Ribak, 1978; Peters and Fairen, 1978). This finding provides support for the idea that, in the central cortex at least, symmetrical synapses with small flattened vesicles may be inhibitory. The predominantly vertical organization of the dendrites and axons of the nonspiny multipolar stellate neurons demonstrated by Peters and Fairen (1978) is similar to the organization of the processes of the GAD-positive neurons as far as these can be visualized with the immunohistochemical technique (compare Figures 1 and 2). Finally, one extremely characteristic feature of the organization of the GAD-positive terminals is their "basket-like" localization around the somata of the cortical pyramidal neurons (Figure 4D). The presence of GABA-containing inhibitory terminals on the cell bodies of the output neurons seems to be a constant feature of cortical organization as a similar lo-calization of GAD-positive terminals has been seen in the monkey cor-tex (unpublished observations).

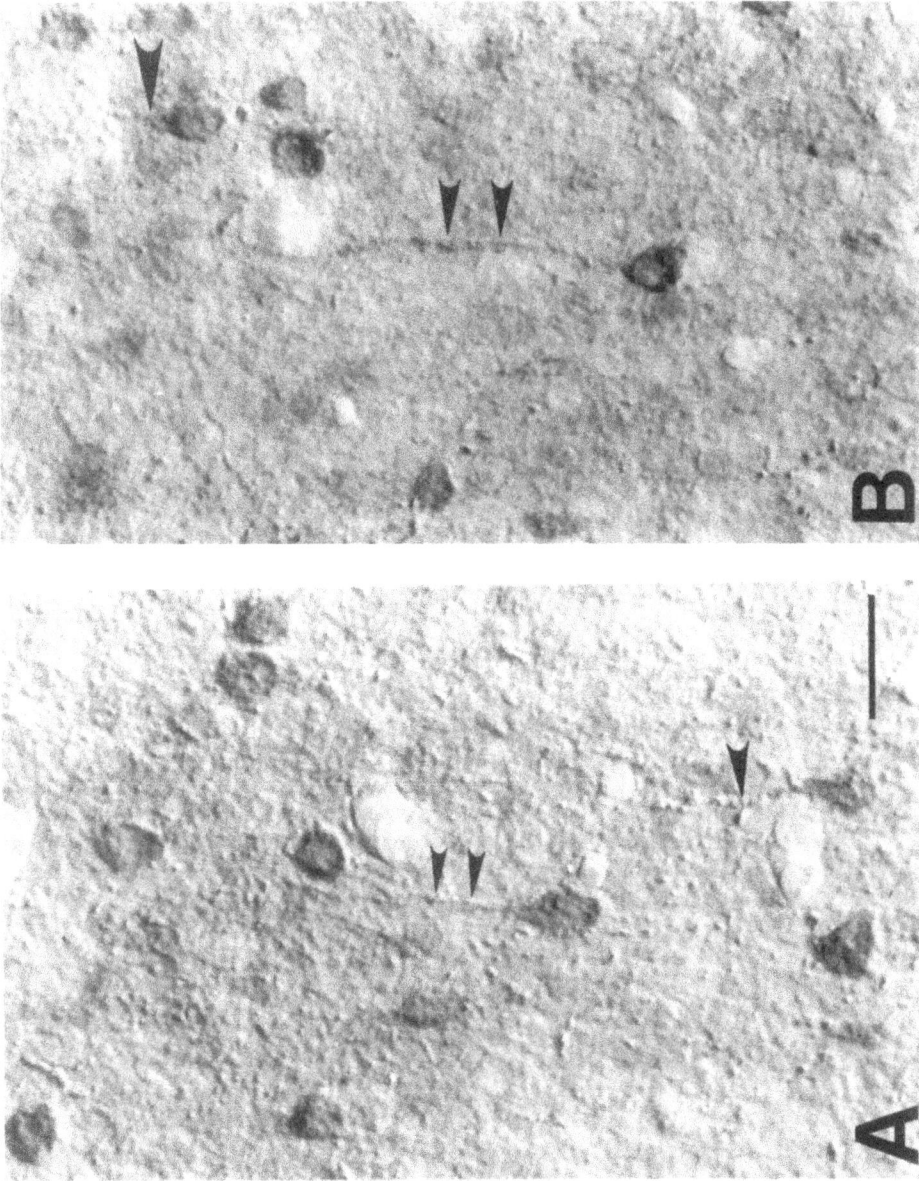

Figure 1 Immunoperoxidase-positive neurons stained for GAD immunoreactivity in the rat parietal cortex. Radially directed processes are marked (◄). Scale bar 30 μm. Bright-field interference-contrast photomicrographs.

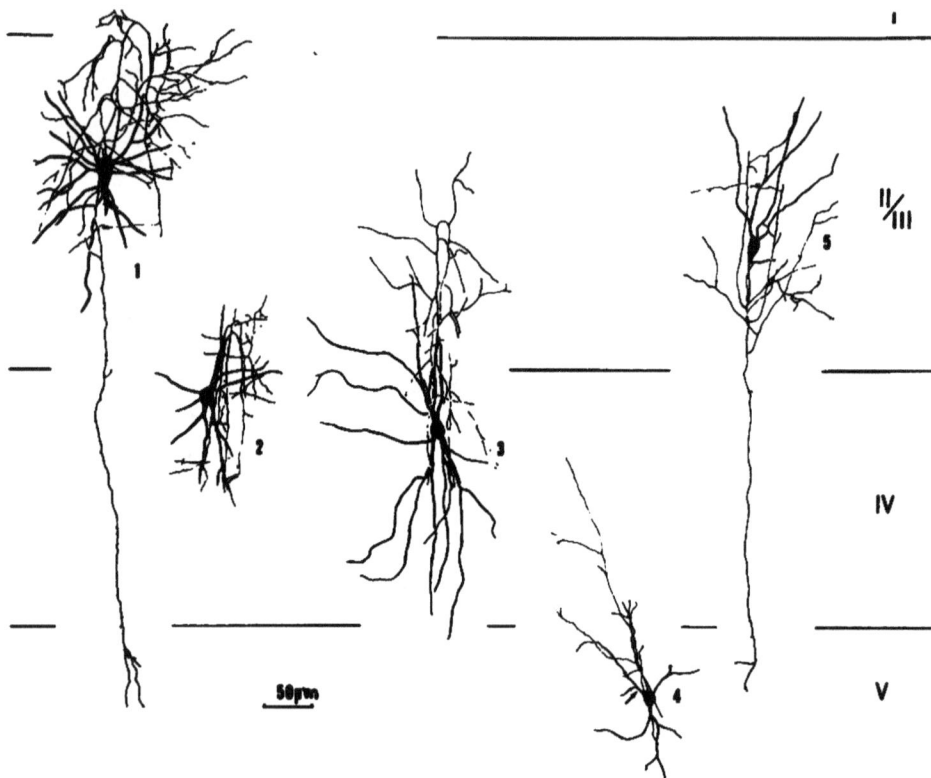

Figure 2 Camera lucida drawings of nonspiny stellate neurons in the rat visual cortex. The neurons are placed in their appropriate positions within the depth of the cerebral cortex. The horizontal lines indicate the borders between cell layers. (From Peters and Fairen, 1978, with permission.)

Excitatory Amino Acids

There is now considerable evidence that the amino acids L-glutamate and L-aspartate may be excitatory neurotransmitters in the mammalian central nervous system (CNS; Krnjević, 1974; Davidson, 1976). However, unlike GABA, both these excitatory amino acid transmitter candidates are generated by normal Krebs-cycle activity, and there is thus no possibility of purifying a specific enzyme marker, such as GAD, which could be used to selectively label neurons which may use these amino acids as transmitters. Thus the investigation of the role of glutamate and aspartate as CNS transmitters and their localization has been hindered by the lack of any suitable transmitter-specific (biochemical) marker. In 1977 several groups of workers (McGeer et al., 1977; Divac, Fonnum, and Storm-Mathisen, 1977) discovered that ablation of specific cortical areas produced a selective loss of the glutamate–aspartate high-affinity amino acid uptake system (Wofsey, Kuhar, and Snyder, 1971) in the appropriate projection area in striatum, thalamus, brain stem, or spinal cord. These observations have led to the use of this method to investigate putative glutamatergic corticocortical, transcallosal, and cortical efferent pathways. Thus, the loss of glutamate uptake sites in the corpus striatum following removal, or undercutting, of the frontoparietal cortex has been taken to indicate that glutamate or aspartate may represent the transmitter in the terminals of the layer V pyramidal neurons known to project to the striatum (Jacobson, 1964). This suggestion would be consistent with a variety of electrophysiological experiments that indicate that pyramidal-tract collaterals can monosynaptically excite layer IV interneurons with "exquisite" sensitivity, a response which can be antagonized by putative glutamate antagonists such as glutamate diethylester and 1-hydroxy-3-amino-pyrrolidone-2 (HA 966) (Stone, 1976). The best case, however, for glutamate as a cortical efferent transmitter comes from studies of the perforant pathway which carries corticofugal efferents from the cortex through the subiculum to the hippocampus proper and also to the molecular layer of the dentate gyrus. In the molecular layer, Cotman and Hamberger (1978) have shown that glutamate fulfills many of the criteria for a neurotransmitter. These are, it shows a calcium-dependent release, it is concentrated in synaptosome fractions, and it shows potent excitatory effects when iontophoretically applied on to the granule cells. In addition, Cotman and Hamberger (1978) have shown that [^{3}H]-glutamate uptake in the molecular layer is considerably reduced by perforant pathway lesions. In a parallel study, Storm-Mathisen and Iversen (1979) have shown that these characteristic perforant nerve endings, which disappear after perforant pathway lesions, accumulate [^{3}H]-glutamate (Figure 3A,B). It is to be hoped that further detailed studies of glutamate (and/or aspartate) uptake in the cerebral cortex itself will provide further evidence for glutamate (and/or aspartate) as a cortical transmitter. However, it seems likely that as the pyramidal neurons of layers III and V provide the major cortical efferents, then at least some of these neurons may use glutamate (and/or aspartate) as excitatory neurotransmitters.

Vasoactive Intestinal Polypeptide (VIP)

VIP was originally isolated from porcine intestine by Said and Mutt in 1970 (Said and Mutt, 1970a,b). VIP is a 28-amino acid peptide (Table I; Mutt and Said, 1974) with, as its name implies, potent vasodilatory activity. VIP was originally thought to be a local gastrointestinal hormone, but since the development of sensitive antibodies to porcine VIP (Fahrenkrug, 1979) its distribution has been studied in more detail. VIP is now known to be localized in neurons in both the gut and the forebrain (especially cerebral cortex; Fuxe et al., 1977; Loren et al., 1979b).

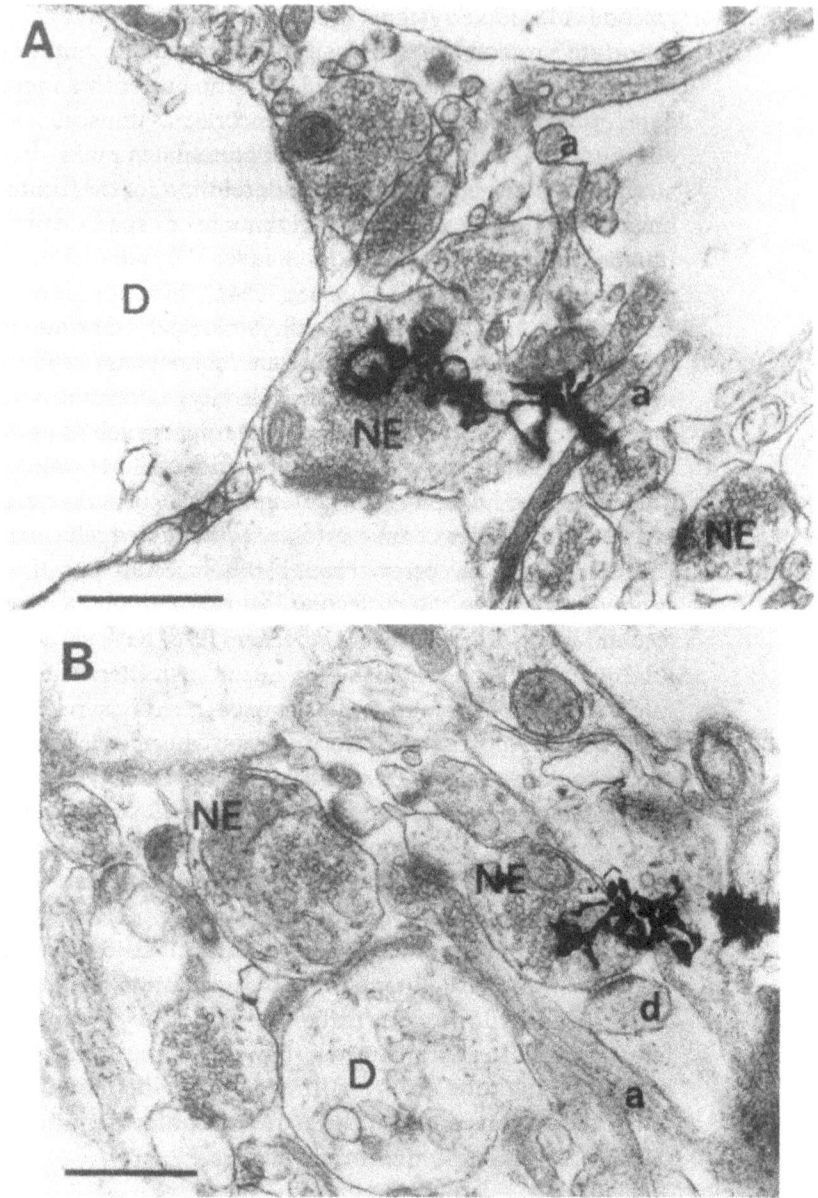

Figure 3 Electron-microscopic autoradiographs from the molecular layer of area dentata showing accumulation of [³H]-glutamate in nerve endings. (A) Several labeled nerve endings NE are seen, one of which synapses with a dendrite profile D. (B) Labeled nerve ending synapsing with asymmetrical thickening on a dendrite spine (d). This is the type of synapse typical of the perforant path terminals. (From Storm-Mathisen and Iversen, 1979, with permission.)

Table I Amino acid sequences of vasoactive intestinal polypeptide (VIP) and cholecystokinin octapeptide (CCK-8)

VIP	His-Ser-Asp-Ala-Val-Phe-Thr-Asp-Asn-Tyr-Thr-Arg-Leu-Arg Lys-Gln-Met-Ala-Val-Lys-Lys-Tyr-Leu-Asn-Ser-Ile-Leu-Asn-NH$_2$
CCK-8	Asp-Tyr-HSO$_3$-Met-Gly-Trp-Met-Asp-Phe-NH$_2$

Iontophoretic application of VIP to neurons of the cerebral cortex or hippocampus indicates that VIP is strongly excitatory (Phillis, Kirkpatrick, and Said, 1978; Dodd, Kelly, and Said, 1980). VIP is concentrated in nerve-terminal fractions isolated from the cortex, from which VIP can be released in a calcium-dependent fashion (Giachetti et al., 1977). This evidence, together with the presence of VIP binding sites in the cerebral cortex (Taylor and Pert, 1979), suggests that VIP should be seriously considered as a neurotransmitter candidate (see Emson, 1979).

In the rat neocortex, VIP immunoreactivity can be demonstrated in neurons in layers II–IV, with the highest numbers of positive neurons in layers II and III. The majority of VIP cell bodies are fusiform and bipolar, having their long processes oriented perpendicular to the pial surface (Figure 4A,B). These bipolar, fusiform cells correspond closely to the nonspiny or sparsely spiny bipolar neurons described from Golgi studies of the rat cortex (Feldman and Peters, 1978; Figure 5). Furthermore, the laminar distribution described by Feldman and Peters (1978) for nonspiny bipolars is consistent with the observed laminar distribution of these VIP neurons; that is, they are found in layers II–IV. The Golgi study of Feldman and Peters indicates that the axons of these bipolar cells originate from an apical or basal dendrite and are radially organized, overlapping the perpendicular dendritic field, but with the occasional horizontally directed axon. This finding is in good agreement with the histochemical observations that VIP terminals are concentrated in layers I–IV and are directed radially toward the pial surface. The very close correspondence between the morphology of VIP-positive neurons and the Golgi-stained nonspiny bipolar neurons makes it likely that most of the VIP neurons belong to this type of cortical nonpyramidal neuron.

Using the presence of immunoreactive VIP as a marker for this type of neuron cell body, we have studied the ontogenetic appearance of these neurons in the rat cortex (Emson et al., 1979). As our lesion studies had indicated that there were no significant VIP-containing afferent systems projecting to the rat cortex, we used the increase in VIP content of the rat cerebral cortex during development as an indication of synaptogenesis. Immunohistochemical studies showed that at the first post-

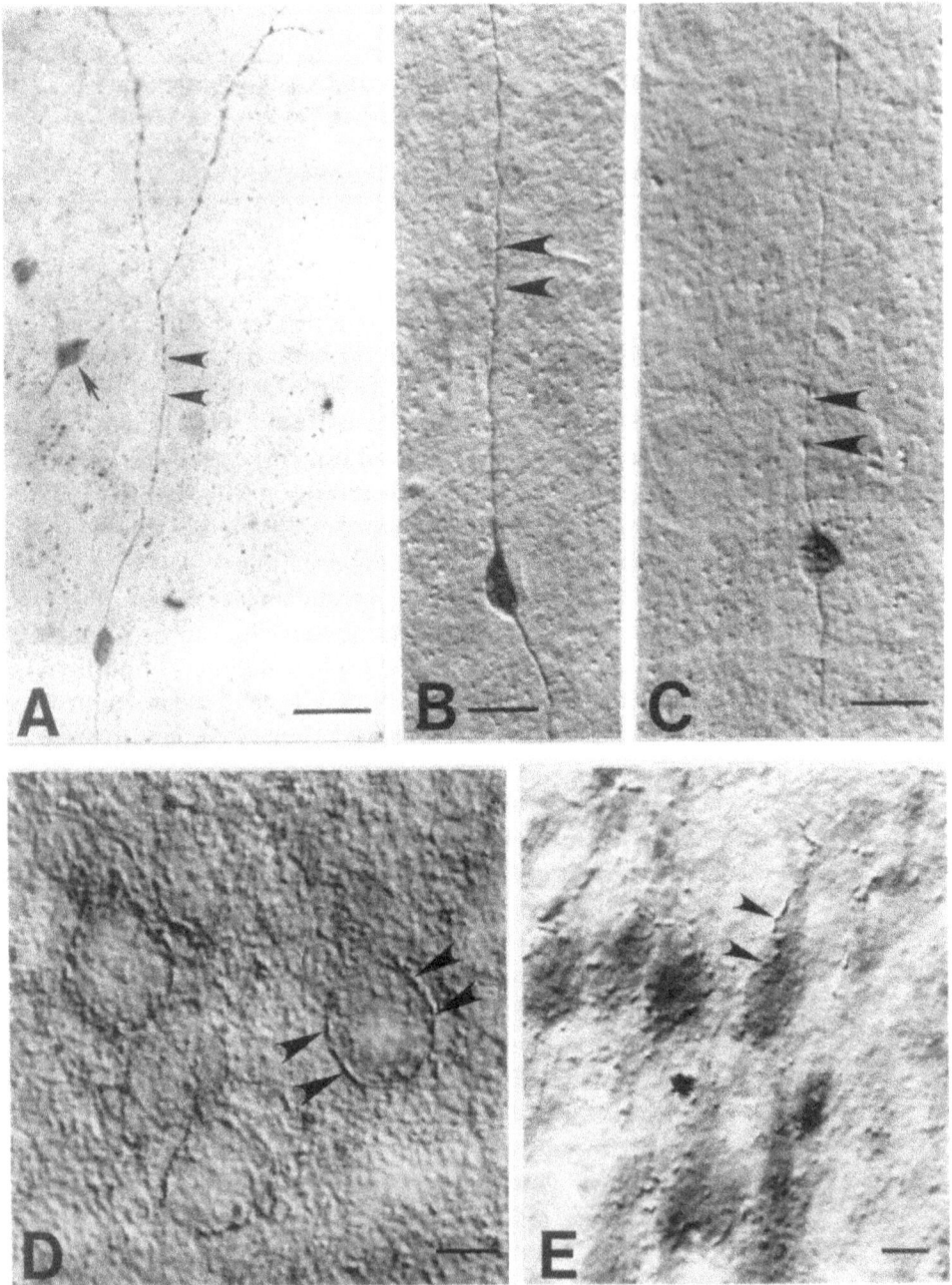

Figure 4 (A), (B) VIP-like immunoreactivity within the rat neocortical bipolar neurons. Note the long apical processes (◄) which reach up into layer I. A small positively stained multipolar neuron can also be seen (◄). Scale bars: (A) 40 μm; (B) 20 μm. (C) CCK-like immunoreactivity within a rat bipolar cortical neuron. Scale bar 20μm. (D) GAD immunoreactivity in terminals (◄) surrounding cortical pyramidal cells (layer V). Scale bar 10 μm. (E) CCK-like immunoreactivity within fibers (◄) running over CA3 hippocampal pyramidal neurons. There is also some nonspecific staining of the pyramidal cell bodies. Scale bar 10 μm.

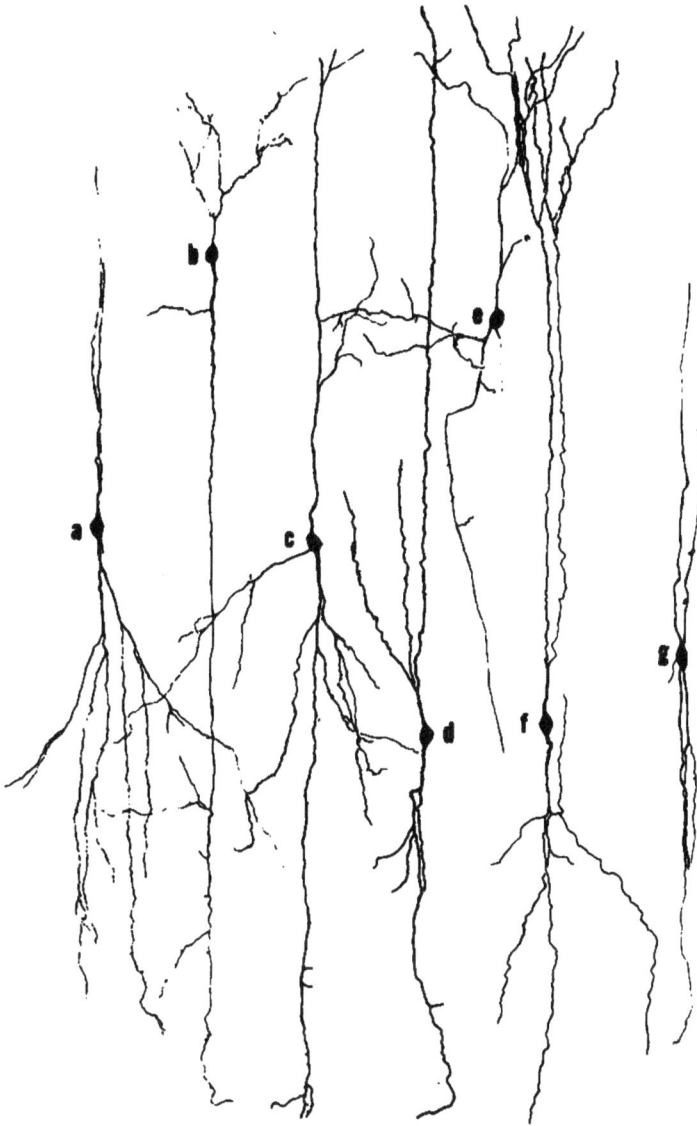

Figure 5 Examples of nonspiny bipolar neurons of the rat visual cortex (compare Figure 4A–C). (From Feldman and Peters 1978, with permission.)

natal day, no cortical neurons could be detected containing VIP. Cortical VIP neurons could be visualized, however, by the seventh postnatal day, and these were faintly staining, were grouped together, and were found in the deeper layers of the neocortex. By day 14 the neurons had reached their adult position and were demonstrable as fusiform neurons in layers II–IV of the cortex. The cell-body content of VIP, demonstrated immunohistochemically, was most noticeable at this stage in development; it resembled the content usually seen after colchicine treatment of adult rat cortex. (Colchicine stops axonal transport from the cell body and produces accumulation of immunoreactivity in the cell body. This procedure is used to increase the possibility of demonstrating cell bodies in the immunohistochemical procedure.) Between days 14 and 28 the number of cortical terminals increased substantially, and there was a drop in cell body content of VIP, making the cell bodies more difficult to demonstrate histochemically. The histochemical data correlated with radioimmunoassay data indicated a dramatic increase in cortical VIP content between days 14 and 28, presumably reflecting the development of the adult axonal tree (Table II).

Cholecystokinin

"Gastrin-like" material in extracts of cerebral cortex was first described by Vanderhaegen, Signeau, and Gepts (1975). Subsequent studies (Dockray, 1976; Muller, Straus, and Yalow, 1977; Rehfeld, 1978a,b) have shown that the gastrin-like material is in fact identical to, or closely related to, the cholecystokinin octapeptide (CCK-8; Table I), which shares the same tetrapeptide carboxy terminal amino acid sequence as gastrin. Cholecystokinin octapeptide (CCK-8), or the carboxy terminal tetrapeptide fragment of CCK-8 (CCK-4), fulfills the majority of criteria for potential neurotransmitters. Thus, CCK-8 and CCK-4 are concentrated in synaptosomes, show a calcium dependent release, and exert powerful excitatory effects when applied to hippocampal pyramidal neurons (Dodd and Kelly, 1979). Furthermore, studies of the incorporation of [^{35}S]-methionine into cortical peptides have suggested that both CCK and VIP undergo a rapid biosynthesis and turnover (Golterman, Rehfeld, and Røigaard-Petersen, 1980; Golterman, personal communication). A rapid biosynthesis and turnover might perhaps be expected if these cortical peptides were to be used as neurotransmitters, especially as there is no evidence for recapture of released peptides.

Immunohistochemical studies using CCK or gastrin-directed antisera reveal a number of CCK-positive neuron cell bodies in the rat cerebral cortex (Figure 4C). Some of these neurons, like those containing VIP, are fusiform bipolar neurons, whereas others are probably multipolar nonspiny stellates like the GAD-containing neurons (Figures 1 and 2).

Table II VIP content of developing rat brain[a]

Region	Age							
	E16	P0	P7	P14	P21	P28	P42	Adult
Anterior cortex +	0	0.7 ± 0.1 (5)	7.3 ± 2.0 (4)	27.1 ± 5.3 (4)	102.8 ± 17.7 (4)	170.5 ± 15.1 (6)	116.5 ± 27.9 (5)	100.9 ± 8.9 (5)
Posterior cortex +	0	1.3 ± 0.3 (5)	3.5 ± 0.4 (4)	20.2 ± 1.9 (4)	107.7 ± 6.5 (4)	149.1 ± 15.0 (4)	109.1 ± 9.0 (5)	112.4 ± 25.9 (5)
Spinal cord	0	0.7 ± 0.1 (5)	2.1 ± 0.1 (4)	7.3 ± 1.0 (6)	5.9 ± 0.6 (4)	5.7 ± 1.2 (4)	11.1 ± 3.9 (5)	10.0 ± 1.8 (5)
Hypothalamus	0	2.6 ± 0.5 (9)	4.4 ± 0.9 (8)	5.4 ± 1.0 (8)	12.7 ± 3.0 (9)	16.0 ± 3.4 (9)	18.6 ± 7.6 (4)	9.3 ± 2.2 (5)
Olfactory tubercle	0	0.2 ± 0.2 (4)	1.2 ± 0.5 (5)	13.7 ± 2.1 (8)	25.9 ± 3.4 (4)	48.7 ± 13.0 (4)	36.7 ± 7.3 (5)	11.55 ± 1.87 (5)

a. VIP content expressed as pM/g tissue wet weight. Values are means ± SEM for number of animals in brackets. Lower limit of accurate measurement was 0.1 pM/g tissue. (The region indicated as posterior cortex corresponds to the dorsal entorhinal cortex immediately underlying the parietal bone, and the anterior cortex represents the dorsal frontal cortex underlying the frontal bone.) E = embryo, P = postnatal.

The morphology of the fusiform CCK neurons is similar to the VIP neurons, indicating that like the VIP cells, they belong to the class of nonspiny or sparsely spiny bipolar neurons described by Feldman and Peters (1978). The numbers of CCK-containing neurons (nonspiny bipolars and multipolar stellates) are substantially greater than the number of VIP neurons, and there are many more CCK than VIP terminals in the neocortex (Figure 6A). The CCK terminals are particularly concentrated in layers II–V, and, unlike the VIP terminals, they do not spread appreciably into layer I. This type of difference in terminal pattern, together with the much greater numbers of CCK neurons, indicates that the VIP and CCK neurons belong to separate populations of cortical neurons, which include some nonspiny bipolar neurons. A similar distinction can be made in the allocortex, where the CCK neurons are located in stratum radiatum and terminate on the pyramidal-cell somata (Figure 4E), whereas the VIP neurons are found in both stratum oriens and radiatum and terminate on the dendrites of pyramidal cells (Figure 6B); Loren et al., 1979a; Larsson and Rehfeld, 1979).

Immunohistochemistry has not yet been carried out at the electron-microscope level to localize the type of synapses containing VIP and CCK, but from their distribution and presumed excitatory role we may expect them to be asymmetrical or "Gray type I" synapses. This suggestion is supported by the finding that the axons of the fusiform nonspiny bipolar neurons (among which are some of the CCK and VIP neurons) so far studied by the Golgi–electron-microscope methods make asymmetrical synapses (Peters, personal communication).

Other Peptides

In addition to the two peptides CCK and VIP which are localized to cortical neurons, preliminary immunohistochemical evidence indicates that immunoreactivity to somatostatin (growth hormone-release-inhibiting factor) may be localized in terminals and neurons in the rat allo- and neocortex (Petrusz et al., 1977; Hökfelt, personal communication). Furthermore, an antiserum directed against the amino acid sequence of avian pancreatic polypeptide (Kimmel, Hayden, and Pollock, 1975) has revealed some positive neurons in the rat neocortex (Loren et al., 1979a). The staining of these neurons cannot be abolished by adsorption of the antiserum with VIP or CCK, and on the basis of their morphology these neurons may represent an additional small population of peptide-containing nonspiny bipolar neurons. Nothing is known about the actions of avian pancreatic polypeptide (APP) on neurons in the neocortex and the identity of the material which cross reacts with these antisera remains to be established.

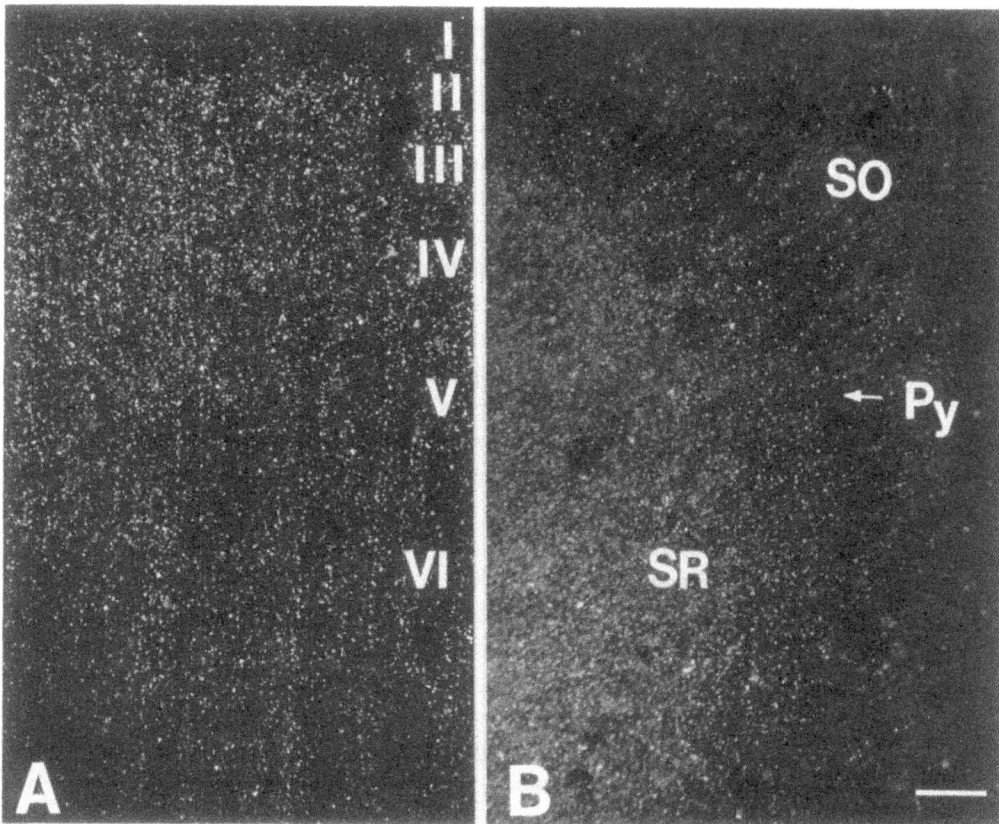

Figure 6 (A) CCK and (B) VIP-like immunoreactivity in the neocortex (A) and hippocampus (B) of the rat. Immunoperoxidase technique photographed with dark-field illumination. SO, stratum oriens; Py, pyramidal cell layer; and SR, stratum radiatum. Scale bar 40 μm.

Afferent Inputs

The bulk of our current knowledge of afferent inputs to the neocortex is based on data arising out of histochemical techniques used to demonstrate monoaminergic afferents (see Emson and Lindvall, 1979). As our histochemical techniques for amines have improved, we have realized that these afferents are more heterogeneous than originally supposed—in "limbic" cortical areas particularly. However, we still have no knowledge of the transmitters used by the main excitatory thalamic inputs. The organization of noradrenergic and dopaminergic inputs to the cortex has been extensively discussed, and it would not be appropriate to review these in detail here. However, a significant technical development in the visualization of cortical serotoninergic (5-HT) systems has been provided by the development of antibodies recognizing serotonin as an antigen (Steinbusch, Verhofstad, and Joosten, 1978).

Using the serotonin-directed antibody for immunohistochemistry reveals that serotoninergic fibers densely innervate all regions of the rat cerebral cortex with a fairly uniform density throughout all cortical layers (Steinbusch, personal communication). The serotoninergic fibers are finer than those containing norepinephrine, and, in agreement with the higher cortical serotonin content relative to norepinephrine, the number of cortical serotoninergic fibers exceeds the number of noradrenergic fibers. One area of cortex, the posterior cingulate, receives an apparently atypical innervation in that the serotonin fibers are concentrated in layers I and III (Steinbusch, personal communication). The posterior cingulate cortex also receives a specific thalamic innervation the terminals of which overlap with this serotoninergic innervation. In a similar fashion, the noradrenergic and dopaminergic innervations in the frontal and anterior cingulate cortices overlap the terminals of the particular thalamic relay nucleus to that area (Emson and Lindvall, 1979; Lewis et al., 1979; Lidov, Rice, and Molliver, 1978). In the somatosensory cortex also, the noradrenergic terminals in the cortical barrel fields in layer IV were relatively concentrated within the barrels, but additional tangential axons result in norepinephrine fibers bridging between the barrels.

The functions of the serotoninergic and noradrenergic projections to the cortex are so far unknown. However, their widespread distribution and brain-stem origin suggests that they would be particularly suited to mediate general cortical arousal or inhibition (see Bloom, this volume). The dopaminergic innervation is restricted solely to the association cortex; thus it would not be suited to a role in general arousal, and its function remains unknown. The frontal cortex is also unique in receiving a radially organized substance P input to laminae 2–4 (Ljungdahl, Hökfelt, and Nilsson, 1978).

The remaining well-established afferent input is cholinergic and originates in part from the magnocellular forebrain nuclei (see Emson and Lindvall, 1979). Examination of the acetylcholinesterase (AChE) staining pattern of the neocortex reveals a fairly uniform staining throughout all cortical layers, with a relative sparsity in layers III and an enrichment in layer IV, a pattern also reflected in the choline acetyltransferase (ChAT) distribution. Undercutting of the cortex results in a parallel loss of AChE and ChAT content, and the available data do not suggest the presence of significant numbers of intrinsic cortical cholinergic neurons. The cholinergic innervation is organized topographically; lateral and caudal magnocellular neurons project to the lateral and caudal cortex, and medial and frontal magnocellular neurons project to medial and frontal cortex.

Cortical Organization

Study of the termination of thalamic afferents in the mouse sensorimotor cortex (which has similar VIP-, CCK-, and GAD-containing neurons to those described here in the rat) indicates that both classes of interneuron to which these VIP-, CCK-, and GAD-containing neurons belong receive somatic thalamic inputs (White, 1978; Figure 7). A somatic as opposed to a dendritic innervation is likely to be more effective in modifying the activity of the neurons, so it would seem that the VIP, CCK, and GABA neurons may be among the first cortical cells activated by excitatory thalamic input. In the case of the VIP- and CCK-containing neurons, the radial and interlaminar organization of their axons, together with their potent effects on neuronal excitability, would seem to make them ideally suited to activate and synchronize neuronal activity within a vertical column of cortical cells. The ability of VIP to enhance local blood flow in the cortical area influenced by the radial processes of the VIP neurons could produce the marked regional differences in metabolic activity in the cortex revealed by the deoxyglucose technique (Sokoloff et al., 1978). Similarly the number of GABA-containing nonspiny stellates activated by thalamic stimulation (Figure 7) and the horizontal spread of their axons may provide a mechanism for limiting the outward spread of activity induced by thalamic stimulation. This type of function would allow the GABA neurons to provide temporary boundaries defining the physiological cortical columns activated by different patterns of sensory stimulation (Mountcastle, 1957).

As has been noted by several authors (Shepherd, 1974; White, 1978), the neocortex differs from phylogenetically older areas of cortex in that the excitatory input to the principal neurons is provided by the intrinsic neurons which receive the specific thalamic inputs. This is in contrast to the hippocampus, dentate gyrus, or pyriform cortex, where the main input is directly onto the principal neurons. This shift in input may be reflected in the movement of the CCK terminals from the principal neuronal somata in phylogenetically older cortical areas (hippocampus-dentate gyrus, pyriform cortex) onto the apical dendrites of the neocortical neuron. The position of VIP terminals on the principal neurons does not change in the transition from allo- to neocortex, as these terminals remain on the apical dendrites. Another feature which remains constant is the localization of GAD terminals on the somata of the principal neurons, presumably reflecting the continued importance of somatic inhibition in the neocortex. The altered position of the CCK

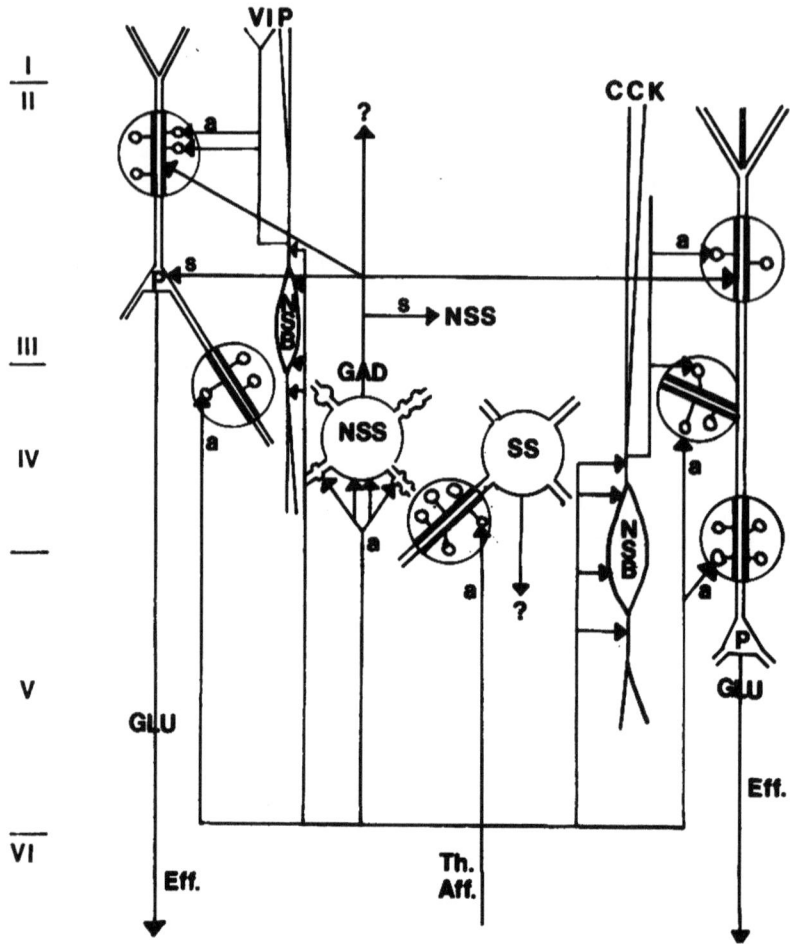

Figure 7 Diagram showing the various cell types (P, pyramidal; NSS, nonspiny stellate; SS, spiny stellate; NSB, nonspiny bipolar cells) in the rodent primary somatosensory cortex that are postsynaptic to thalamocortical afferents. (Modified from White, 1978, with permission.) The possible chemical transmitters associated with the various cell types are indicated (GLU, glutamate; GAD, γ-aminobutyric acid; VIP and CCK, vasoactive intestinal polypeptide and cholecystokinin). Note that excitatory thalamic afferents have been described as synapsing on to the somata of layer IV, nonspiny bipolars and nonspiny stellate neurons. This would provide a direct route for interlaminar excitation by VIP or CCK neurons (NSB) and, via the axons of the GABA neurons (NSS), could also limit the spread of thalamic excitation. Synaptic function types are indicated as a for asymmetrical and s for symmetrical. Ef, efferent; Th.Aff, thalamic afferent.

terminals on the neocortical neurons may reflect the altered role of the CCK neuron from providing a *parallel* excitatory input, for example to the hippocampal pyramidal neurons, to providing the *principal* excitatory input to certain neocortical neurons. Such a developmental scheme for the neocortex is illustrated in Figure 8.

It remains to be seen how much of this model for cortical organization and development can be substantiated. It is clear, however, that with the localization of several neuropeptides in the cerebral cortex, and the ability to visualize these together with neurons containing GAD by immunohistochemical techniques, powerful new tools are available with which morphologists can begin to dissect the organization of the cerebral cortex.

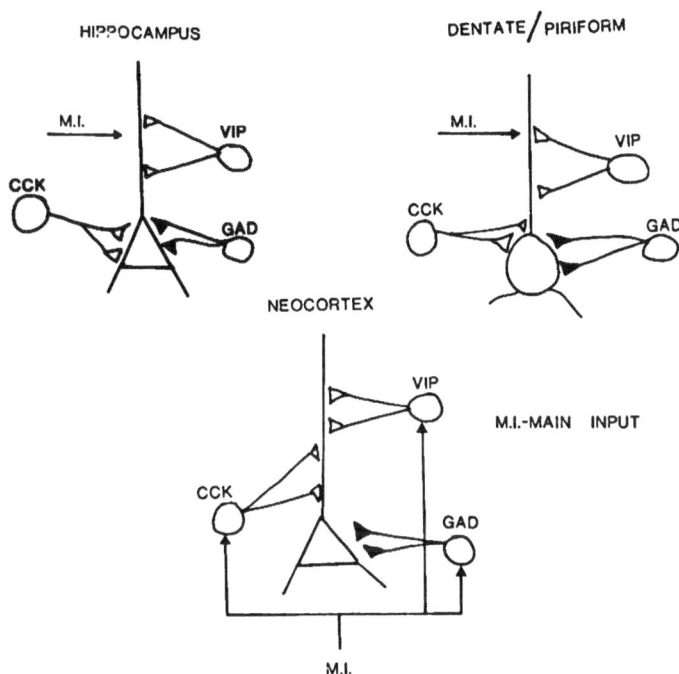

Figure 8 Speculative scheme to show the possible modifications of cortical circuitry during evolution of the neocortex. In the hippocampus and dentate and pyriform cortexes, the dendrites of the output neurons (pyramidal cells or granule cells) receive the main extrinsic excitatory afferent input. In contrast, the main input to neocortex terminates principally upon interneurons, which may include those containing the putative transmitters CCK, VIP, and GABA. M.I., main input; CCK, cholecystokinin-containing neuron; VIP, vasoactive intestinal polypeptide-containing neuron; GAD, glutamic acid decarboxylase (GABA-) containing neuron.

Acknowledgments

The authors wish to thank the Neurosciences Research Program for their invitation to attend this meeting. We are particularly grateful to Dr. Floyd Bloom and to Dr. Leslie Iversen for their suggestions, encouragement, and revision of the manuscript. Thanks are also due to Dr. Angus Mackay, who read and criticized various versions of the text, and in particular to the patience of Mr. George Marshall, who prepared the illustrations. Finally, this study would not have been possible but for the generosity of Dr. J. Y. Wu, Dr. J. Fahrenkrug, and Professor J. Rehfeld, who provided the antisera used in this study.

References

Chronwall, B. M., and J. R. Wolff, 1978. Classification and location of neurons taking up ³H-GABA in the visual cortex. In *NATO-ASI Series: Amino Acids as Neurotransmitters.* F. Fonnum, ed. New York: Plenum Press, pp. 297–303.

Cotman, C. W., and A. Hamberger, 1978. Glutamate as a CNS neurotransmitter: Properties of release, inactivation and biosynthesis. In *NATO-ASI Series: Amino Acids as Chemical Transmitters.* F. Fonnum, ed. New York: Plenum Press, pp. 379–412.

Davidson, N., 1976. *Neurotransmitter Amino Acids.* New York: Academic Press.

Divac, I., F. Fonnum, and J. Storm-Mathisen, 1977. High affinity uptake of glutamate in the terminals of corticostriatal axons. *Nature* 266:377–378.

Dockray, G. J., 1976. Immunochemical evidence of cholecystokinin-like peptide in brain. *Nature* 264:568–570.

Dodd, J., and J. S. Kelly, 1979. Excitation of CA1 pyramidal neurones of the hippocampus by the tetra- and octapeptide C-terminal fragments of cholecystokinin. *J. Physiol. (London)* 295:61–62.

Dodd, J., J. S. Kelly, and S. I. Said, 1980. Excitation of CA1 pyramidal neurones of the hippocampus by vasoactive intestinal polypeptide. *Brit. J. Pharmacol.* (in press).

Dreifuss, J. J., J. S. Kelly, and K. Krnjević, 1969. Cortical inhibition and γ-aminobutyric acid. *Exp. Brain Res.* 9:137–154.

Emson, P. C., 1979. Peptides as neurotransmitter candidates in the mammalia CNS. *Prog. Neurobiol.* 13:61–116.

Emson, P. C., and O. Lindvall, 1976. Distribution of neurotransmitter candidates in the rat neocortex. *Exp. Brain Res. Suppl.* 1:329–336.

Emson, P. C., and O. Lindvall, 1979. Distribution of putative neurotransmitters in the neocortex. *Neuroscience* 4:1–42.

Emson, P. C., R. F. T. Gilbert, I. Loren, J. Fahrenkrug, F. Sundler, and O. B. Schaffalitzky de Muckadell, 1979. Development of vasoactive intestinal polypeptide (VIP) containing neurones in the rat brain. *Brain Res.* 177:437–444.

Fahrenkrug, J., 1979. Vasoactive intestinal polypeptide: Radioimmunochemical studies on its distribution and function as a putative neurotransmitter. *Digestion* 19:149–169.

Falck, B., 1962. Observations on the possibilities of the cellular localization of monoamines by a fluorescence method. *Acta Physiol. Scand. Suppl.* 56:197.

Feldman, M. L., and A. Peters, 1978. The forms of nonpyramidal neuron in the visual cortex of the rat. *J. Comp. Neurol.* 179:761–794.

Fuxe, K., T. Hökfelt, S. Said, and V. Mutt, 1977. Vasoactive intestinal polypeptide and the nervous system: Immunohistochemical evidence for localization in central and peripheral neurons particularly intracortical neurons of the cerebral cortex. *Neurosci. Lett.* 5:241–246.

Giachetti, A., S. I. Said, C. R. Rolland, and F. C. Koniges, 1977. Vasoactive intestinal polypeptide in brain: Localization in and release from isolated nerve terminals. *Proc. Nat. Acad. Sci. USA* 74:3424–3427.

Golterman, N. R., J. F. Rehfeld, and H. Røigaard-Petersen, 1980. In vivo biosynthesis of cholecystokinin in rat cortex. *J. Biol. Chem.* (in press).

Gray, E. G., 1959. Axo-somatic and axo-dendritic synapses of the cerebral cortex: An electron-microscope study. *J. Anat.* 93:420–433.

Hirsch, H., and E. Robins, 1962. Distribution of γ-aminobutyric acid in the layers of the cerebral and cerebellar cortex. *J. Neurochem.* 9:63–70.

Iversen, L. L., and F. E. Bloom, 1972. Studies of the uptake of ^{3}H-GABA and ^{3}H-glycine in slices and homogenates of rat brain and spinal cord by electron microscopic autoradiography. *Brain Res.* 41:131–143.

Jacobson, S., 1964. Intralaminar, interlaminar, callosal and thalamocortical connections in frontal and parietal areas of the albino rat cerebral cortex. *J. Comp. Neurol.* 124:131–146.

Kimmel, J. R., L. J. Hayden, H. G. Pollock, 1975. Isolation and characterization of a new pancreatic polypeptide hormone. *J. Biol. Chem.* 250:9369–9376.

Krnjević, K., 1974. Chemical nature of synaptic transmission in vertebrates. *Physiol. Rev.* 54:418–540.

Larsson, L. I., and J. F. Rehfeld, 1979. Localization and molecular heterogeneity of cholecystokinin in central and peripheral nervous system. *Brain Res.* 165:201–218.

Lewis, M. S., M. E. Molliver, J. H. Morrison, and H. G. W. Lidov, 1979. Complementarity of dopaminergic and noradrenergic innervation in anterior cingulate cortex of the rat. *Brain Res.* 164:328–333.

Lidov, H. G. W., F. L. Rice, and M. E. Molliver, 1978. The organisation of the catecholamine innervation of somatosensory cortex. The barrel field of the mouse. *Brain Res.* 153:577–584.

Ljungdahl, A., T. Hökfelt, and G. Nilsson, 1978. Distribution of substance P-like immunoreactivity in the central nervous system of the rat. I. Cell bodies and nerve terminals. *Neuroscience* 3:861–944.

Loren, I., J. Alumets, R. Håkanson, and F. Sundler, 1979a. Immunoreactive pancreatic polypeptide (PP) occurs in the central and peripheral nervous system. Preliminary immunocytochemical observations. *Cell Tissue Res.* 200:179–186.

Loren, I., P. C. Emson, J. Fahrenkrug, A. Björklund, J. Alumets, R. Håkanson, and F. Sundler, 1979b. Distribution of vasoactive intestinal polypeptide (VIP) in the rat and mouse brain. *Neuroscience* 4:1953–1976.

McGeer, P. L., E. G. McGeer, U. Scherer, and K. Singh, 1977. A glutamergic corticostriatal pathway. *Brain Res.* 128:369–373.

Mountcastle, V. B., 1957. Modality and topographic properties of single neurones of cats' somatic sensory cortex. *J. Neurophysiol.* 20:408–434.

Muller, J. E., E. Straus, and R. S. Yalow, 1977. Cholecystokinin and its COOH-terminal octapeptide in the pig brain. *Proc. Nat. Acad. Sci. USA* 74:3035–3037.

Mutt, V., and S. I. Said, 1974. Structure of the porcine vasoactive intestinal octacosapeptide. *Eur. J. Biochem.* 42:581–589.

Peters, A., and A. Fairen, 1978. Smooth and sparsely-spined stellate cells in the visual cortex of the rat: A study using combined Golgi-electron microscope technique. *J. Comp. Neurol.* 181:129–172.

Petrusz, P., M. Sar, G. H. Grossman, and J. S. Kizer, 1977. Synaptic terminals with somatostatin-like immunoreactivity in the rat brain. *Brain Res.* 137:181–187.

Phillis, J. W., J. R. Kirkpatrick, and S. I. Said, 1978. Vasoactive intestinal polypeptide excitation of central neurons. *Canad. J. Physiol. Pharmacol.* 57:337–340.

Rehfeld, J., 1978a. Immunochemical studies in cholecystokinin II. Distribution and molecular heterogeneity in the central nervous system and small intestine of man and hog. *J. Biol. Chem.* 253:4022–4030.

Rehfeld, J. F., 1978b. Localization of gastrins to neuro and adenohypophysis. *Nature* 271:771–773.

Ribak, C. E., 1978. Aspinous and sparsely-spinous stellate neurons in the visual cortex of rats contain glutamic acid decarboxylase. *J. Neurocytol.* 7:461–478.

Said, S. I., and V. Mutt, 1970a. Polypeptide with broad biological activity. Isolation from small intestine. *Science* 169:1217–1218.

Said, S. I., and V. Mutt, 1970b. Potent peripheral and splanchnic vasodilator peptide from normal gut. *Nature* 225:863–864.

Shepherd, G. M., 1974. *The Synaptic Organisation of the Brain*. Oxford: Oxford University Press.

Sokoloff, L., M. Reivich, C. Kennedy, M. H. Des Rosiers, C. S. Portlak, K. D. Pettigrew, O. Sakurada, and M. Shinohara, 1978. The ^{14}C-deoxyglucose method for measurement of local cerebral glucose utilization: Theory, procedure and normal values in the conscious and anaesthetized albino rat. *J. Neurochem.* 28:897–916.

Steinbusch, H. W. M., A. A. J. Verhofstad, and H. W. J. Joosten, 1978. Localization of serotonin in the central nervous system by immunohistochemistry: Description of a specific and sensitive technique and some applications. *Neuroscience* 3:811–819.

Sternberger, L. A., 1979. *Immunocytochemistry*, 2nd ed. New York: John Wiley.

Stone, T. W., 1976. Is glutamic acid the pyramidal tract neurotransmitter? *Experientia* 32:581–583.

Storm-Mathisen, J., and L. L. Iversen, 1979. Selective uptake of ^{3}H-glutamic acid in excitatory nerve endings: Light and electron microscopic observations in the hippocampal formation of the rat. *Neuroscience* 4:1237–1254.

Taylor, D. P., and C. B. Pert, 1979. Vasoactive intestinal polypeptide: Specific binding to rat brain membranes. *Proc. Nat. Acad. Sci. USA* 76:660–664.

Vanderhaegen, J. J., J. C. Signeau, and W. Gepts, 1975. New peptide in the vertebrate CNS reacting with antigastrin antibodies. *Nature* 257:604–605.

Wallingford, E., R. Ostadahl, P. Zarzecki, P. Kaufman, and G. Somjen, 1973. Optical and pharmacological stimulation of visual cortical neurones. *Nature* 242:210–212.

White, E. L., 1978. Identified neurons in mouse Sm1 cortex which are post synaptic to thalamocortical axon terminals: A combined Golgi-electron microscopic and degeneration study. *J. Comp. Neurol.* 181:627–662.

Wofsey, A. R., M. J. Kuhar, and S. H. Snyder, 1971. A unique synaptosomal fraction, which accumulates glutamic and aspartic acids, in brain tissue. *Proc. Nat. Acad. Sci. USA* 68:1102–1106.

14 Neurotransmodulatory Control of Cerebral Cortical Neuron Activity

D. A. Taylor and T. W. Stone

ABSTRACT   The microiontophoretic application of norepinephrine, dopamine, and serotonin to cortical neurons in the rat has suggested that these substances may play a role as inhibitory neurotransmitters in the cerebral cortex. The localization of inhibitory responses to dopamine corresponds reasonably well with the presumed anatomical distribution of such nerve fibers within the frontal cortex. Norepinephrine and serotonin, while producing their inhibitory effects on a larger population of neurons, appear to act through different mechanisms. The very long duration, slow-onset inhibition produced by iontophoretically applied norepinephrine is mimicked closely by electrical stimulation of the nucleus locus ceruleus and could well be mediated intracellularly by cyclic adenosine monophosphate (AMP). Serotonin, however, induces a prompt, powerful inhibition of cortical neurons which is mimicked by electrical activation of the median raphe. In addition, the adenine nucleotides have provoked considerable interest recently with respect to their interaction with norepinephrine. The evidence presented here supports both a presynaptic and postsynaptic interaction between adenosine and norepinephrine and suggests that perhaps these classes of compounds may function as "neurotransmodulators" in the control of cortical-neuron activity. Thus, while these substances produce direct neurotransmitter-like effects on the neurons within the cerebral cortex, they also modulate the sensitivity of these neurons to other neurotransmitter candidates.

One of the major goals of neuroscience has been to identify and characterize those chemical elements responsible for the control of the central nervous system. However, the demonstration that a given substance is a neurotransmitter has succeeded only in isolated instances. In large part, the complexity under which the brain operates has contributed a major obstacle in the characterization of central neurotransmitters. Furthermore, the lack of identified pathways for several putative transmitters has prevented studies aimed at the physiological role which these systems might play in central function. Likewise, with increasing research regarding the mechanism of action of neuroactive drugs, it is becoming readily apparent that many compounds interact with several

D. A. TAYLOR AND T. W. STONE Merck Institute for Therapeutic Research, West Point, Pennsylvania 19486; Department of Physiology, St. George's Hospital Medical School, University of London, London SW17 ORE, England

proposed "transmitter" systems. Perhaps one of the most well-defined and intensively studied neuronal projections to the cerebral cortex, to date, is that containing monoamines.

The description by fluorescence histochemistry (Dahlström and Fuxe, 1965; Fuxe, 1965; Ungerstedt, 1971) of cortical innervation by noradrenergic nerve fibers prompted considerable investigation into the electrophysiological effects of norepinephrine. The noradrenergic innervation arises from cell bodies located in the pontine nucleus locus ceruleus (Ungerstedt, 1971), and provides a very widely distributed projection to all layers of the cerebral cortex with some predominance in the outer molecular layer (Levitt and Moore, 1978). On the other hand, dopaminergic cell bodies in the substantia nigra (Fuxe et al., 1974; Hokfelt et al., 1974) extend nerve terminals primarily to the lower layers of the cortex and appear to restrict their distribution to the frontal areas of the cortex (Thierry et al., 1973; Berger et al., 1974; and Lindvall et al., 1974). Serotonin-containing nerve fibers arising from the raphe seem to provide a norepinephrine-type innervation to all areas of the cerebral cortex (Kuhar, Aghajanian, and Roth, 1972; Descarries, Beaudet, and Watkins, 1975; Beaudet and Descarries, 1976). Thus, biochemical and histochemical evidence strongly favors the idea that monoaminergic innervation plays a role in the functioning of the cerebral cortex.

The electrophysiological analysis of the effects of the monoamines has been limited in large part to a study of the actions these compounds exert on pyramidal-tract neurons since these cells comprise not only the larger neurons in this brain region, but also the major output for information processed by the cortex (Shepherd, 1974). Norepinephrine produces predominantly inhibitory effects on virtually all cortical neurons tested (Krnjević and Phillis, 1963; Phillis, 1970; Stone, 1973) (Figure 1A). Of particular interest is the fact that while norepinephrine induces a hyperpolarization of cortical neurons, there is little, if any, change in membrane resistance (Phillis, 1977). A similar paradoxical effect on membrane potential and resistance was observed in describing the noradrenergic projection to cerebellar Purkinje neurons (Bloom, 1974, 1975). It is also noteworthy that while identification of the neuron being recorded is an important criterion for classification of the action of a putative neurotransmitter, the action of norepinephrine seems to span all types of neurons within the cortex (Lake, Jordan, and Phillis, 1973; Stone and Taylor, 1977). Pharmacological studies on the response of cortical neurons to norepinephrine have indicated that both α- and β-receptors are involved in the inhibitory response (Stone, 1973). While iontophoretic studies indicate responsivity of neurons to norepinephrine, a critical question which still remains is whether there is mimicry of these responses when the neuronal pathway providing the innervation is activated. Several laboratories have observed that electrical stimulation of the nucleus locus ceruleus lowers the frequency of firing of cortical neurons (Nakamura and Iwama, 1975; Faiers and Mogenson,

D. A. Taylor and T. W. Stone

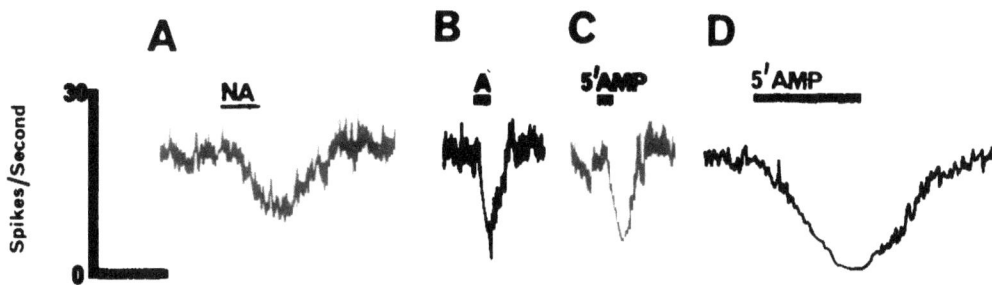

Figure 1 Ratemeter records illustrating the inhibitory effect of norepinephrine (NA), adenosine (A) and 5′-adenosine monophosphate (5′A) on pyramidal tract neurons of the rat cerebral cortex. (A), (B), (C) were obtained by microiontophoretic application of NA (80 nA), A (20 nA) and 5′-A (20 nA) to the same cortical neuron. The durations of drug ejection are indicated by the solid bars. Notice the long duration and onset of the inhibitory response to NA, particularly when compared to the rapid inhibition induced by application of either adenosine or 5′-AMP. (D) illustrates an inhibitory response obtained by allowing 5′-AMP to diffuse from the pipette tip (i.e., elimination of the holding currents indicated by solid bar). Notice that within approximately 30 sec cellular activity had ceased. Reapplication of the holding current allowed neuronal activity to return to normal.

1976; Taylor and Stone, 1980). Furthermore, data from Phillis's laboratory suggests that at least certain of these inhibitory responses to locus ceruleus activation are blocked by β-adrenergic blocking agents (Phillis, 1977; Phillis and Kostopoulos, 1977). Thus, for norepinephrine, there appears to be a strong correlation between the anatomical, biochemical, and pharmacological evidence supporting a role for this amine as an inhibitory transmitter in the cerebral cortex.

Serotonin and dopamine, though less well studied, appear to produce inhibitory responses on cerebral cortical neurons. Thus, all of the monoamines appear to act primarily as inhibitory substances in the cerebral cortex. There are some very important differences, however, which should be discussed. For example, while serotonin produces inhibition throughout a wide expanse of the cortex, the time course of the inhibitory response is markedly different than that of norepinephrine (Stone, 1973; Sastry and Phillis, 1977). Conversely, while producing an inhibitory response similar in nature to norepinephrine (i.e., long duration, slow onset) dopamine responses are more consistent and easily reproduced in the frontal areas of the cortex, and particularly in layers IV and V (Bunney and Aghajanian, 1976; Palmer et al., unpublished results). It is interesting to note that the anatomical localization of dopaminergic nerve terminals seems to be restricted to these deeper layers of the cortex (see above). Therefore, on anatomical and electrophysiological grounds, the actions of the monoamines within the cerebral cortex seem to be separate entities. Physiological activation of the serotonergic pathway has supported the inhibitory nature of this amine

349   Putative Neurotransmitter Actions and Interactions

(Frederickson, Hewes, and Norris, 1975). In this case, as with activation of the noradrenergic pathway described above, there is considerable similarity between the iontophoretic and the physiologically induced actions of these monoamines. While the evidence favoring a role for serotonin and dopamine is not as convincing, the probability is great that these amines subserve a role in the control of cortical neuronal activity. It is equally clear, however, that their functions are different from that of norepinephrine.

The characteristically long response of neurons to norepinephrine (Figure 1A) pointed the attention of several investigators toward the possible involvement of cyclic AMP in this response. Indeed, electropharmacological studies were in good agreement with biochemical investigations which supported the involvement of both α- and β-receptors in both the electrophysiological response to norepinephrine and the activation of adenylate cyclase brought by this neurotransmitter (cf. Bloom, 1975; Nathanson, 1977; Phillis, 1977). Earlier reports from our laboratory (Stone, Taylor, and Bloom, 1975; Stone and Taylor, 1977) have illustrated a strong correlation between the responses of neurons to norepinephrine and to cyclic AMP. Additional support for the idea that cyclic AMP might be involved in the response of cortical neurons to norepinephrine is obtained from studies which indicate that agents known to inhibit the catabolic enzyme of cyclic AMP, phosphodiesterase, can markedly potentiate the inhibitory response to norepinephrine. Furthermore, agents which block the postsynaptic adenosine receptor induce only a marginal reduction in the response to cyclic AMP (Taylor and Stone, 1978). It is interesting that many of the postsynaptic changes which have been ascribed to the activation of adenylate cyclase (see Figure 2) have also been suggested as possible mechanisms of action for norepinephrine (Phillis, 1977). For instance, cyclic AMP has been shown to induce alterations in calcium flux in cardiac muscle (Katz, Tada, and Kirchberger, 1975) as well as to increase the phosphorylation of a Ca^{++}-Mg^{++} ATPase in the heart (La Raia and Morkin, 1974; Tada et al., 1974; Tada, Kirchberger, and Katz, 1975; Tada et al., 1975). These two effects have also been suggested as possible mechanisms for norepinephrine's action in the central nervous system (i.e., alterations in calcium flux and/or inhibition of NA^+-K^+ ATPase). It is interesting that, as shown schematically in Figure 2, the action of norepinephrine in the central nervous system (CNS) could possibly involve all of these mechanisms. As shown diagrammatically in Figure 2, both dopamine and serotonin can also elevate cyclic AMP levels in the cerebral cortex (Bloom, 1975; Nathanson, 1977; Phillis, 1977) though the involvement of this nucleotide in the action of these neurotransmitters is yet to be defined.

In an effort to control for the inhibitory effects of cyclic AMP, the response of cortical neurons to cyclic guanosine monophosphate (GMP) was also tested. Cortical pyramidal-tract neurons exhibit a specific ex-

D. A. Taylor and T. W. Stone

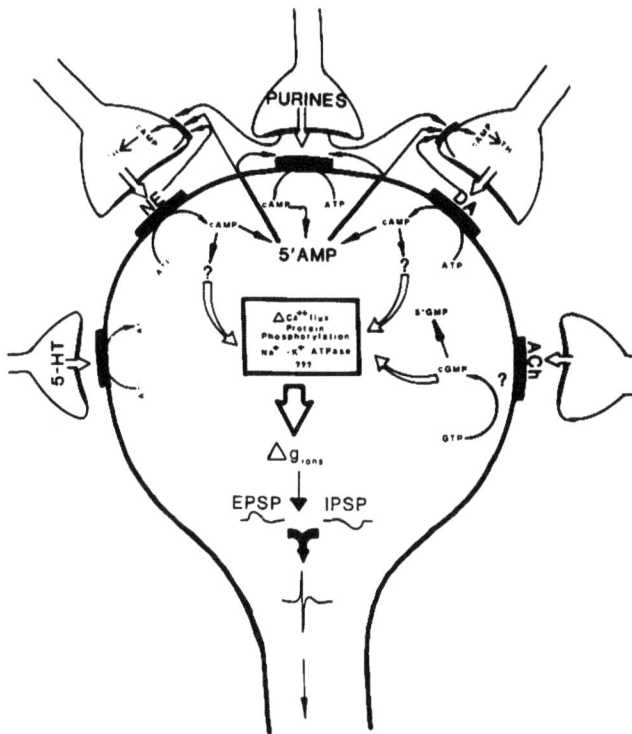

Figure 2 A schematic diagram of a few of the possible transmodulator candidates in the cerebral cortex and possible mechanisms for actions and interactions. Possible mechanisms of action for NE, DA, and purines include the elevation of cyclic AMP and/or alterations in Ca^{++} flux or interactions with NA$^+$–K$^+$ ATPase. Likewise, the purines could interact both presynaptically on both NE and DA neurons and postsynaptically via the adenosine receptor. Little conclusive evidence is available to prove or disprove the mediation of acetylcholine responses by cyclic GMP, and the mechanism of serotonin action remains obscure. It is clear that the output of a cortical neuron can be determined by a wide variety of factors acting alone or in concert with each other. Several possibilities for the role of these substances in cortical neuron control are discussed in the text and by Bloom (this volume).

citatory response to acetylcholine, while nonpyramidal-tract neurons can be inhibited by the same compound. It was noticed that the response of the neurons in the cerebral cortex to cyclic GMP was highly correlated to the response to acetylcholine (Stone and Taylor, 1977). Furthermore, when the muscarinic antagonist atropine was applied to these cells the response to cyclic GMP was maintained in spite of a total abolition of the acetylcholine response. Thus, it was suggested (Stone, Taylor, and Bloom, 1976; Stone and Taylor, 1977) that perhaps cyclic AMP and cyclic GMP might mediate the opposing responses of norepinephrine and acetylcholine. Additional evidence has recently been obtained (Schwartz and Woody, 1979) which indicates that cyclic GMP mimics the action of acetylcholine. These authors utilized intracellular recording with extracellular iontophoresis and observed a high degree of correlation between membrane potential and resistance changes induced by acetylcholine and cyclic GMP. Futhermore, while atropine antagonized the responses to acetylcholine, it exerted no effect on cyclic-GMP responses. However, a circumspect examination of the available evidence would indicate, as illustrated in Figure 2, that sufficient knowledge of the possible intracellular mediation of acetylcholine by cyclic GMP has not yet been obtained to permit a definitive conclusion regarding the interaction of these two substances.

A noteworthy sidelight to the study of the role of monoamines in the CNS has been the increasing interest in purine nucleotides other than cyclic AMP. The demonstration that a synergistic interaction exists in the cerebral cortex between adenosine and norepinephrine (Sattin and Rall, 1970) focused considerable attention on adenosine as a modulator of neuronal function. Additional studies have indicated that the ability of norepinephrine to stimulate the formation of cyclic AMP may be critically dependent upon the presence of adenosine (Daly, 1976). While no direct evidence has been forthcoming concerning the possibility that the "purinergic" nerves reported to be present in the periphery (Burnstock, 1972) are present in the CNS, considerable attention has focused on the adenine nucleotides as, at least, local regulators of neuronal function. When adenosine, AMP, or ATP (adenosine triphosphate) is applied iontophoretically to cortical neurons, a prompt, powerful depression of firing rate ensues which is very rapidly reversible (Phillis, Kostopoulos, and Limacher, 1974; Stone and Taylor, 1977). As illustrated in Figure 1, the response of cortical neurons to these nucleotides is clearly different than that produced by norepinephrine. Biochemical evidence indicated that the activation of adenylate cyclase by adenosine occurs via a postsynaptic adenosine receptor which could be blocked by theophylline and other methylxanthenes (Daly, 1976). Electrophysiological studies have shown that theophylline produces a blockade of the inhibitory effect of iontophoretically applied adenosine (Kostopoulos and Phillis, 1977; Stone and Taylor, 1977; Taylor and Stone, 1978). Based on the marked congruence between biochemical and electrophysiological studies on adenosine, a logical extension of these studies was to test whether synergistic effects could be seen between adenosine and norepinephrine. The interesting observation from these studies (Stone and Taylor, 1978; Taylor and Stone, 1980) was that while the potentiation between adenosine and norepinephrine was readily induced, there appeared to be a similar interaction between norepinephrine and gamma-aminobutyric acid (GABA), another putative inhibitory transmitter. Furthermore, no interaction could be seen between GABA and adenosine. These data raised the possibility that, as has been suggested in both the cerebellum (Freedman et al., 1976) and cortex (Reader et al., 1979), norepinephrine might function as a

D. A. Taylor and T. W. Stone

modulator of neuronal activity. To further examine the possibility, the interaction of adenosine with physiologically released norepinephrine was studied (Taylor and Stone, 1980); it was determined that, in the presence of adenosine, the inhibitory effect of activation of the nucleus locus ceruleus was reduced. Similar effects on neurotransmitter release have been observed in the peripheral nervous system (Clanachan, Johns, and Paton, 1977; Sawynok and Jhamandas, 1976; Hedqvist and Fredholm, 1976). However, when adenosine is applied simultaneously with or immediately after locus ceruleus stimulation, the exaggerated effect of the two is observed (Taylor and Stone, 1980). Thus, it is quite likely that adenosine may function at both a presynaptic site as well as postsynaptically to exert its influence on neuronal activity as shown in Figure 2.

One intriguing possibility for the interaction between putative neurotransmitters has been suggested from studies which indicate that certain nucleotides are not only released with neurotransmitters (Burnstock, 1972; Silinsky, 1975), but also from apparently postsynaptic sites (Fredholm, 1976). A wealth of evidence exists supporting both the in vitro (Pull and McIlwain, 1972; Kuroda and McIlwain, 1974) and in vivo (Schubert et al., 1977; Sulakhe and Phillis, 1975) release of adenosine from the cerebral cortex. Thus, as depicted schematically in Figure 2, the interesting possibility exists that released adenine nucleotides, either presynaptic or postsynaptic, might act as a local modulator of presynaptic neuronal function, as well as postsynaptically on pyramidal-tract neurons. In fact, the possibility exists that the role of both the monoamines and the adenine derivatives could well be that of neurotransmodulators (i.e., chemicals which act as both neurotransmitters and neuromodulators). Considerable work remains, however, in determining the role of adenine nucleotides in the cerebral cortex. The potent inhibitory effect of the noncyclic nucleotides would suggest a role greater than that of a neuromodulator or regulator.

On the basis of these data, it is tempting to speculate that norepinephrine and other monoamines might act in the CNS to modulate and regulate the activity of neurons via interactions with other putative neurotransmitters. Likewise, the effect of these compounds need not be strictly confined to electrical activity. It is quite conceivable that such an effect might be related to changes in the chemical or metabolic environment of the cell and occur over long periods of time. Furthermore, the idea that locally released substances might exert profound effects on neuronal activity provides some interesting possibilities for adaptation within the CNS (Stone, 1978). It is apparent, however, that the actions and interactions between putative neurotransmitters and neuromodulators could well lead to a reexamination and redefinition of the role of these chemicals in the regulation of cerebral cortical activity (see also the chapter by Bloom, this volume).

Acknowledgments

The authors would like to express appreciation to the Neurosciences Research Program for the kind invitation to participate in this colloquium. In addition, the helpful insights of Drs. F. E. Bloom, G. R. Siggins, B. J. Hoffer, and R. Freedman have provided invaluable assistance during many of the studies presented here. D. A. T. was supported in part while at the University of Colorado Medical Center by grants from the Pharmaceutical Manufacturers' Association Foundation and a grant from the National Heart, Lung and Blood Institute. T. W. S. was supported in part by the Medical Research Council.

References ·

Beaudet, A., and L. Descarries, 1976. Quantitative data on serotonin nerve terminals in adult rat neocortex. *Brain Res.* 111:301–309.

Berger, B., J. P. Tassin, G. Blanc, M. A. Moyne, and A. M. Thierry, 1974. Histochemical confirmation for dopaminergic innervation of the rat cerebral cortex after destruction of the noradrenergic ascending pathways. *Brain Res.* 81:332–337.

Bloom, F. E., 1974. To spritz or not to spritz: The doubtful value of aimless iontophoresis. *Life Sci.* 14:1819–1934.

Bloom, F. E., 1975. The role of cyclic nucleotides in central synaptic function. *Rev. Physiol. Biochem. Pharmacol.* 74:1–103.

Bunney, B. S., and G. K. Aghajanian, 1976. Dopamine and norepinephrine innervated cells in the rat prefrontal cortex: Pharmacological differentiation using microiontophoretic techniques. *Life Sci.* 19:1783–1792.

Burnstock, G., 1972. Purinergic nerves. *Pharmacol. Rev.* 24:509–581.

Clanachan, A. S., A. Johns, and D. M. Paton, 1977. Presynaptic inhibitory actions of adenine nucleotides and adenosine on neurotransmission in the rat vas deferens. *Neuroscience* 2:597–602.

Dahlström, A., and K. Fuxe, 1965. Evidence for the existence of monoamine-containing neurons in the central nervous system. I. Demonstration of monoamines in the cell bodies of brain stem neurons. *Acta Physiol. Scand.* 62 (Suppl. 232):1–55.

Daly, J. W., 1976. The nature of receptors regulating the formation of cyclic AMP in brain tissue. *Life Sci.* 18:1349–1358.

Descarries, L., A. Beaudet, and K. Watkins, 1975. Serotonin nerve terminals in adult rat neocortex. *Brain Res.* 100:563–588.

Faiers, A. A., and G. J. Mogenson, 1976. Electrophysiological identification of neurons in locus coeruleus. *Exp. Neurol.* 53:254–266.

Frederickson, R. C. A., C. R. Hewes, and F. H. Norris, 1975. Microiontophoresis of a selective neuronal uptake inhibitor [3-(p-trifluoromethylphenoxy)-N-methyl-3-phenyl-propylamine, Lilly 110140]: Assessing serotonin (5-HT) as a cortical neurotransmitter. *Fed. Proc.* 34:801.

Fredholm, B. D., 1976. Release of adenosine-like material from isolated perfused dog adipose-tissue following sympathetic nerve stimulation and its inhibition by adrenergic alpha-receptor blockade. *Acta Physiol. Scand.* 96:422–430.

Freedman, R., B. J. Hoffer, D. Puro, and D. J. Woodward, 1976. Noradrenaline modulation of the responses of the cerebellar Purkinje cell to afferent synaptic activity. *Brit. J. Pharmacol.* 57:603–605.

Fuxe, K., 1965. Evidence for the existence of monamine neurons in the central nervous system. IV. Distribution of monoamine nerve terminals in the central nervous system. *Acta Physiol. Scand.* 64 (Suppl. 247):37–85.

Fuxe, K., T. Hökfelt, O. Johansson, G. Jonsson, P. Lidbrink, and Å. Ljungdahl, 1974. The origin of the dopamine nerve terminals in limbic and frontal cortex. Evidence for meso-cortical dopamine neurons. *Brain Res* 82:349–355.

Hedqvist, P., and B. B. Fredholm, 1976. Effects of adenosine on adrenergic transmission; prejunctional inhibition and postjunctional enhancement. *Naunyn-Schmiedebergs Arch. Pharmacol.* 293:217–223.

Hökfelt, T., K. Fuxe, O. Johansson, and Å. Ljungdahl, 1974. Pharmacohistochemical evidence for the existence of dopamine nerve terminals in the limbic cortex. *Europ. J. Pharmacol.* 25:108–112.

Katz, A. M., M. Tada, and M. A. Kirchberger, 1975. Control of calcium transport in the myocardium by the cyclic AMP-protein kinase system. *Adv. Cyclic Nucleotide Res.* 5:453–472.

Kostopoulos, G. K., and J. W. Phillis, 1977. Purinergic depression of neurons in different areas of the rat brain. *Exp. Neurol.* 55:719–724.

Krnjević, K., and J. W. Phillis, 1963. Actions of certain amines on cerebral cortical neurones. *Brit. J. Pharmacol. Chemother.* 20:471–490.

Kuhar, M. J., G. K. Aghajanian, and R. H. Roth, 1972. Tryptophan hydroxylase activity and synaptosomal uptake of serotonin in discrete brain regions after midbrain raphe lesions: Correlations with serotonin levels and histochemical fluorescence. *Brain Res.* 44:165–176.

Kuroda, Y., and H. McIlwain, 1974. Uptake and release of C^{14}-adenine derivatives at beds of mammalian cortical synaptosomes in a superfusion system. *J. Neurochem.* 22:691–699.

Lake, N., L. M. Jordan, and J. W. Phillis, 1973. Evidence against cyclic adenosine 3',5'-monophosphate (AMP) mediation of noradrenaline depression of cerebral cortical neurones. *Brain Res.* 60:411–421.

La Raia, P. J., and E. Morkin, 1974. Adenosine 3',5'-monophosphate dependent membrane phosphorylation: A possible mechanism for the control of microsomal Ca^{++} transport in heart muscle. *Circ. Res.* 35:298–306.

Levitt, P., and R. Y. Moore, 1978. Noradrenaline neuron innervation of the neocortex in the rat. *Brain Res.* 139:219–232.

Lindvall, O., A. Björklund, R. Y. Moore, and U. Stenevi, 1974. Mesencephalic dopamine neurons projecting to neocortex. *Brain Res.* 81:325–331.

Nakamura, S., and K. Iwama, 1975. Antidromic activation of the rat locus coeruleus neurons from hippocampus, cerebral and cerebellar cortices. *Brain Res.* 99:372–376.

Nathanson, J. A., 1977. Cyclic nucleotides and nervous system function. *Physiol. Rev.* 57:157–256.

Phillis, J. W., 1970. *The Pharmacology of Synapses*. Oxford: Pergamon Press.

Phillis, J. W., 1977. The role of cyclic nucleotides in the CNS. *Canad. J. Neurol. Sci.* 4:151–195.

Phillis, J. W., and G. K. Kostopoulos, 1977. Activation of a noradrenergic pathway from the brainstem to rat cerebral cortex. *Gen. Pharmacol.* 8:207–211.

Phillis, J. W., G. K. Kostopoulos, and J. J. Limacher, 1974. Depression of corticospinal cells by various purines and pyrimidines. *Canad. J. Physiol. Pharmacol.* 52:1226–1229.

Pull, I., and H. McIlwain, 1972. Adenine derivatives as neurohumoral agents in the brain. The quantities liberated on excitation of superfused cerebral tissues. *Biochem. J.* 130:975–981.

Reader, T. A., A. Ferron, L. Descarries, and H. H. Jasper, 1979. Modulatory role for biogenic amines in the cerebral cortex. Microiontophoretic studies. *Brain Res.* 160:217–229.

Sastry, B. S. R., and J. W. Phillis, 1977. Inhibition of cerebral cortical neurones by a 5-hydroxytryptaminergic pathway from median raphe nucleus. *Canad. J. Physiol. Pharmacol.* 55:737–743.

Sattin, A., and T. W. Rall, 1970. The effect of adenosine and adenine nucleotides on the cyclic adenosine 3',5'-phosphate content of guinea pig cerebral cortex slices. *Mol. Pharmacol.* 6:13–23.

Sawynok, J., and K. H. Jhamandas, 1976. Inhibition of acetylcholine release from cholinergic nerves by adenosine, adenine nucleotides and morphine: Antagonism by theophylline. *J. Pharmacol. Exp. Ther.* 197:379–390.

Schubert, P., G. Rose, K. Lee, G. Lynch, and G. W. Kreutzberg, 1977. Axonal release and transfer of nucleoside derivatives in the entorhinalhippocampal system: An autoradiographic study. *Brain Res.* 134:347–352.

Schwartz, B. E., and C. D. Woody, 1979. Correlated effects of acetylcholine and cyclic guanosine monophosphate on membrane properties of mammalian neocortical neurons. *J. Neurobiol.* 10:465–488.

Shepherd, G. M., 1974. *The Synaptic Organization of the Brain*. Oxford: Oxford University Press.

Silinsky, E. M., 1975. On the association between transmitter secretion and the release of adenine nucleotides from mammalian motor nerve terminals. *J. Physiol.* 247:145–162.

Stone, T. W., 1973. Pharmacology of pyramidal tract cells in the cerebral cortex. Noradrenaline and related substances. *Arch. Pharmacol.* 278:333–346.

Stone, T. W., 1978. Possible roles for purine compounds in neuronal adaptation. *Biochem. Soc. Trans.* 6:858–862.

Stone, T. W., and D. A. Taylor, 1977. Microiontophoretic studies of the effects of cyclic nucleotides on excitability of neurones in the rat cerebral cortex. *J. Physiol.* 266:523–543.

Stone, T. W., and D. A. Taylor, 1978. An electrophysiological demonstration of a synergistic interaction between norepinephrine and adenosine in the cerebral cortex. *Brain Res.* 147:396–400.

Stone, T. W., D. A. Taylor, and F. E. Bloom, 1975. Cyclic AMP and cyclic GMP may mediate opposite neuronal responses in the rat cerebral cortex. *Science* 187:845–846.

Sulakhe, P. V., and J. W. Phillis, 1975. The release of ^{3}H-adenosine and its derivatives from cat sensorimotor cortex. *Life Sci.* 17:551–556.

Tada, M., M. A. Kirchberger, and A. M. Katz, 1975. Phosphorylation of a 22,000-dalton component of the cardiac sarcoplasmic reticulum by cyclic AMP-dependent protein kinase. *J. Biol. Chem.* 250:2640–2647.

Tada, M., M. A. Kirchberger, J. M. Iorio, and A. M. Katz, 1975. Control of cardiac sarcolemmal and sodium-potassium-activated ATPase activities. *Circ. Res.* 36:8–17.

Tada, M., M. A. Kirchberger, D. I. Repke, and A. M. Katz, 1974. The stimulation of calcium transport in cardiac sarcoplasmic reticulum by adenosine 3',5'-monophosphate dependent protein kinase. *J. Biol. Chem.* 249:6174–6180.

Taylor, D. A., and T. W. Stone, 1978. Neuronal responses to extracellularly applied cyclic AMP: Role of the adenosine receptor. *Experentia* 34:481–482.

Taylor, D. A., and T. W. Stone, 1980. The action of adenosine on noradrenergic neuronal inhibition induced by stimulation of locus coeruleus. *Brain Res.* 183:367–376.

Thierry, A. M., G. Blanc, A. Sobel, L. Stinus, and J. Glowinski, 1973. Dopaminergic terminals in the rat cortex. *Science* 182:499–501.

Ungerstedt, U., 1971. Stereotaxic mapping of the monoamine pathways in the rat brain. *Acta Physiol. Scand.* 82 (Suppl. 367):1–48.

15 Chemical Signaling and Cortical Circuitry: Integrative Aspects

Floyd E. Bloom

ABSTRACT In attempting to sort out the functional interrelationships between elements of the neocortex, some specific circuits that can be defined by their neurotransmitter provide a focus for an initial simplified cortical scheme. Three levels of analysis from this perspective can be developed. Amino acid-mediated transmission processes are illustrated by the presumptive excitatory glutamatergic excitatory efferent projections from motor cortex to corpus striatum and by presumptive intracortical interneurons. Inhibitory interneurons using γ-aminobutyrate (GABA) as transmitter operate on similar rapid time scales by inducing hyperpolarizations through probable increases in Cl conductance. Monoamine-mediated extrinsic projections to neocortex are generally subsumed within the so-called "nonspecific afferent" systems, but recent cytochemical studies indicate some organizational principles, within cortical layers and regions. In general, the amine afferent systems to cortex operate more slowly, in greatly decreased frequency, and act more broadly than junctions attributed to amino acids. Those amine systems thus far characterized influence membrane potentials by mechanisms in which membrane conductance is decreased.

A third class of chemically defined intracortical neurons consists of those attributed to the peptides, Substance P, cholecystokinin (CCK), and vasoactive intestinal peptide (VIP). Potential mechanisms of peptide action in cortex, presently based largely on examples of their effects in other central nervous system (CNS) regions, suggest that alternative molecular mechanisms may characterize those peptidergic elements.

Introduction

Perhaps one of the few certainties about the circuits of the cerebral cortex and the neurotransmitters which mediate the interconnections there is that most remain to be determined. Although the details of cortical connectivity are being rapidly characterized, and although—as the chapters by Emson and Hunt and by Taylor and Stone have indicated—the presence and action of some transmitters are coming under increasing scrutiny, much remains to be discovered. In trying to conceptualize the key properties which may provide the functional description of the cortical circuits, while realizing that many have not yet

F. E. BLOOM The Arthur Vining Davis Center for Behavioral Neurobiology, The Salk Institute, La Jolla, California 92037

even been recognized, I have developed this chapter around the following notion: there are three main classes of cortical neurotransmitter molecule, namely, simply amino acids, monoamines, and peptides. By focusing attention on these classes of transmitter, I highlight distinctive properties of circuits already studied in some detail as a means of comparing the different functional roles that transmitters may play in the cortex. Furthermore, I have used the known and partially known cerebral circuits to extend the spatial, temporal, and energy domains with which I recently tried to characterize the integrative aspects of chemical neurotransmission in the whole brain (Bloom, 1979).

Amino Acid Neurotransmission in Cerebral Cortex

Excitatory Amino Acid

Of all the naturally occurring amino acids with excitatory effects when tested iontophoretically, glutamate and aspartate have gained the most attention as transmitter candidates (see Giorguieff, Kemel, and Glowinski, 1977; Hosli, Andres, and Hosli, 1973; Karlsen and Fonnum, 1978; Krnjević, 1974; Roskoski, 1979; Stone, 1979). Changes in high-affinity active uptake systems, in cortex and in areas to which the neocortex projects, have strongly supported the existence of both these amino acids as highly probable synaptic mediators. Based upon the properties of synapses in other regions of the brain in which these amino acids may also be the transmitter, the properties of an excitatory amino acid-mediated synapse are rapid, on–off responses based upon a depolarization mechanism briefly and reversibly increasing transmembrane conductance for Na. Nevertheless, the available information does not distinguish between the effects of the two amino acids, although tests of analogs of glutamate and of possible antagonists of glutamate and aspartate have revealed that there may be separate receptors for glutamate and for aspartate. Therefore, while lacking direct comprehensive evidence that either of these amino acids is the transmitter for a system projecting into or out of cortex, this type of excitatory transmission would currently seem to be the most typical of classical cortical excitatory transmission.

Inhibitory Amino Acids

Evidence documenting the existence of probable GABA-mediated inhibitory synapses in cerebral cortex is considerably stronger than for excitatory amino acids because of the availability of sensitive immunohistochemical mapping studies (Emson and Lindvall, 1979; Ribak, 1978). Antisera raised against the enzyme glutamic acid decarboxylase, the synthetic enzyme which converts glutamate into γ-aminobutyrate (GABA), reveal that relatively large numbers of intracortical circuits, particularly those attributable to the large class of basket-type interneurons, exhibit the presence of this enzyme and are therefore probably GABAergic. Although another fairly potent inhibitory amino acid, taurine, is found in cerebral cortex in even higher concentration, it is not yet possible to determine whether it is present in neurons and whether it may act as a transmitter. Tests of the electrophysiological effects of GABA in cortex, and in other brain regions more easily investigated, indicate that GABA inhibits by means of a hyperpolarization due to temporary enhancement of Cl conductance. Although it has not yet been possible to examine the specific transmission properties of a definitive intracortical interneuron that has been identified cytochemically as a probable GABAergic circuit, the probable role of such systems has been partially described by Sillito (1977; also see Patel and Sillito, 1978) for the cat visual cortex. In these studies, spontaneously active neurons in area 17 of the anesthetized cat were tested for their responses to directional motion of a test slit across the visual fields and for the effects of the iontophoretic application of the GABA antagonist drug bicuculline (Curtis and Johnston, 1974; Krnjević, 1974) on these responses. The cells were initially characterized according to the scheme of Hubel and Wiesel (1962) as simple, complex, or hypercomplex units. The possible role of GABA-mediated synaptic inhibitions in the directional responses of these three types of units was then assessed by the degree to which bicuculline could alter the response. For example, all simple cells tested lost their directional selectivity during the iontophoretic application of bicuculline, suggesting that the apparent basal selectivity they exhibited was in fact due to a postsynaptic interneuron modifying an excitatory input which is not directionally specific, that is, the directional specificity for these cells arises within the cortex as a result of a GABA-mediated interneuronal element.

Cells with the response properties of complex cells were further subclassified on the basis of their responses to the drug. The type 1 complex cell behaved to bicuculline like the simple cells: during bicuculline directional selectivity was eliminated; all such cells were encountered above layer IV. The type 2 complex cell was unaffected by iontophoresis of bicuculline, even when it could be shown that sufficient antagonist was administered to antagonize simultaneous iontophoretic applications of GABA. These cells were concentrated largely in layer V, but some more superficial neurons of this type were also seen. The type 3 complex cells also showed a directional selectivity which was unaffected by bicuculline, and were also concentrated in layer V. Their distinguishing property is of added interest because it epitomizes the problem of attempting to understand cortical synaptic mechanisms. Type 3 complex cells were generally spontaneously active cells, and this spontaneous activity was powerfully suppressed when the cells were stimulated with a slit object moved in the nonpreferred direction. This strong inhibition was also not affected by bicuculline, which at the least indicates the existence of another potent intracortical synaptic transmission system. Finally, the directional selectivity of the hypercomplex cells was also unaffected by bicuculline, indicating that the complex cells of type 2 and the hypercomplex cells probably exhibit directional selectivity as a result of a directionally selective excitatory input, but that the directional selectivity of the other cortical types may result from the interposition of an inhibitory interneuron. Similar circuit properties may also characterize the velocity sensitivity of area 17 neurons to the excitatory input from X and Y directionally selective units of the lateral geniculate (Patel and Sillito, 1978).

Monoaminergic Neurotransmission to Cerebral Cortex

Taylor and Stone's chapter has already dealt in depth with many of the pharmacological interactions on cortical pyramidal neurons of the catecholamines and their possible functional interactions with the purine adenosine (also see Stone and Taylor, 1977). In general, the effects of these receptors would appear to be largely analogous to the β-adrenergic receptor of the coeruleo-Purkinje circuit and the coeruleopyramidal circuits of the hippocampus and cerebral cortex, respectively (Bloom, 1975; Dillier et al., 1978). I wish now to call attention to three aspects of monoaminergic function in cerebral cortex which were not emphasized by the previous contributors: (1) principles of anatomical organization exist; (2) monoamine receptors are distinctively different than those executing amino acid effects; (3) the spatial and temporal domains of cortex regulated by monoamine systems are considerably broader (i.e., less detailed) than those mediated by amino acids.

Principles of Cortical Organization of Monoamine Afferents

While many have focused on the apparent nonspecific nature of the monoamine projections to cerebral cortex (Moore and Bloom, 1978, 1979), it should also be recognized that the pronounced broad innervation of large numbers of target neurons in cortex by the relatively few neurons of the noradrenergic locus coeruleus, the serotonergic dorsal and median raphe, and the dopaminergic neurons of the substantia nigra and ventral-tegmental area is neither totally diffuse nor chaotic. In fact in many respects the innervation patterns exhibit obvious constraints. For example, in both their thalamic and cortical target areas of innervation, the dopaminergic afferents and the noradrenergic afferents appear to be mutually exclusive; furthermore, those areas of supragenual cingulate cortex which receive both dopaminergic and noradrenergic projections still remain in separate layers of that cortical region. While the dopaminergic system seeks mainly the frontal association areas which are concurrent targets of the mediodorsal thalamic nucleus to which the same dopamine fibers go (Bjorklund, Divac, and Lindvall, 1978; Divac et al., 1978; Lindvall et al., 1974; Freedman, Foote, and Bloom, 1975; Gatter and Powell, 1977; Thierry et al., 1973; Tassin et al., 1978; Mishra et al., 1975), the noradrenergic fibers preferentially innervate the posterior cingulate cortex and the anterior thalamic nuclei, which also innervate anterior cingulate cortex (see Vogt, Rosene, and Pandya, 1979). The noradrenergic systems also innervate the primary sensory cortices and the primary relay nuclei of the thalamus which give rise to these specific cortical projections. It is not yet clear whether the cholinergic and serotonergic projections to cerebral cortex also hold to any such broad circuitry constraints, and it remains to be determined just how detailed the constraints of convergent patterns of innervation the dopamine and norepinephrine systems exhibit. However, electrophysiological tests at the cellular level clearly demonstrate a layer-by-layer correspondence between the responsivity and the innervation pattern in the frontal association areas of the rat cortex (Bunney and Aghajanian, 1976), with noradrenergic β receptors predominating in superficial cortical layer II and dopaminergic responses predominating in deeper layer V test cells. In addition, Dillier et al. (1978) report a reserpine-sensitive poststimulus inhibition of cingulate cortex units for about 50% of cells tested with trains of locus coeruleus stimuli. Yet another suggestion of intracortical organization of the catecholaminergic innervation of cortex stems from the recent studies by Molliver and associates revealing orderly patterns of the noradrenergic innervation which is common to most cortical areas (Coyle and Molliver, 1977; Levitt and Moore, 1978; Morrison et al., 1978) in which a strong tangential orientation can be ascribed to the fibers in layers I and VI; these orderly arrays in the tangential directions appear to be well positioned to act as integrators across the vertically oriented internal organization of the cortex. This latter aspect is also borne out by the relatively more intense innervation of the "hollows" of the barrel field of the anterior frontal cortex (Lidov, Rice, and Molliver, 1978).

Monoamine Receptor Mechanisms

Reviewed in detail elsewhere (Bloom, 1975; McIlwain, 1977) are the numerous studies which deal with the association of cortical catecholamine receptor mechanisms with adenylate cyclase and—as pointed out in the chapter by Taylor and Stone—the possible association of certain cortical muscarinic cholinergic receptors with the effects similarly produced by cyclic guanosine 3'-5'-monophosphate. When tested at the intracellular level, these receptor mechanisms differ distinctively from those produced by amino acids, in that the hyperpolarizations and depolarizations produced by the cyclic adenosine monophosphate- (cAMP-) and cyclic guanosine monophosphate- (cGMP-) related receptors, respectively, appear to be associated with decreases in membrane conductance rather than with increases of ionic conductance associated with the amino acids (also see Woody and Gruen, 1978). In addition, when tested for the duration of postsynaptic action, the noradrenergic responses in cingulate cortex are one to two orders of magnitude longer than the amino acid-mediated events. While it is not yet possible to generalize the association between the cyclic nucleotide mediation of the synaptic action and the long-lasting synaptic duration, the combination of these two properties in the probable instances of the noradrenergic and dopaminergic projections would tend to emphasize their effects. Several years ago, Foote, Freedman, and Oliver (1975) reported that when iontophoretic applications of norepinephrine and GABA were tested for their ability to change the patterns of activity evoked in units of the squirrel monkey auditory cortex by vocalization stimuli, both transmitter substances altered the response in favor of the vocalization-induced activity over the spontaneous (or background) activity. Given the greater spatial domain of the noradrenergic innervation and its longer time course of action, the biasing induced by the vocalization activity could represent one function of the broad distributed adrenergic innervation. Furthermore, recent studies of the discharge patterns of locus coeruleus neurons in the awake squirrel monkey (Foote, Bloom, and Schwartz, 1978) and in the awake rat (Jones et al., 1978) reveal that these neurons tend to fire in relatively slow tonic discharge patterns during quiet waking activity, but yet are also found to exhibit sensitive responses to a variety of orienting sensory stimuli, leading to episodes of short bursts of firing until the sensory stimulus becomes habituated. This arousal effect of sensory stimuli on locus coeruleus neurons, and the possible effects of the evoked locus activity on the cortical targets of this system, could then lead to a cellular effect that is similar to that of the iontophoretic application of norepinephrine, that is, a gated change in the sensitivity of the target neuron to its primary sensory input. As a result of the possible changes in transmembrane properties, the combination of a specific sensory signal and a concurrent gate of hyperpolarization and increased membrane resistance would lead to a suppression of activity in cortical cells then being activated, and an enhancement of these cortical targets, which during the noradrenergic gate were activated. Thus the monoaminergic innervation properties of cortical units revealed from available studies of the afferent pathways, and of the neurons that give rise to these monoamine projections, strongly suggest that they differ on the spatial, temporal, and functional domains from the more common and precise amino acid-mediated systems (also see Bloom, 1979).

Peptidergic Neurotransmission in Cerebral Cortex

As Emson and Hunt have indicated in their chapter, an impressive and growing list of neuropeptides has been ascribed to the neocortex. Prominent among this list of peptides likely to play important roles in the cerebral cortex, especially the cortex of the primate brain, are such unlikely sounding candidates as vasoactive intestinal polypeptide (VIP;

Borghi et al., 1979; Fuxe et al., 1977; Phillis, Kirkpatrick, and Said, 1978); the terminal octapeptide of cholecystokinin (CCK; Innis et al., 1979; Pinget, Straus, and Yalow, 1978); and substance P (Belcher and Ryall, 1977; Gale et al., 1978; Hökfelt et al., 1976; Paxinos, Emson, and Cuello, 1978; Phillis and Limacher, 1974). Other peptides, such as enkephalin, neurotensin (Kabayashi, Brown, and Vale, 1977; Uhl, Kuhar, and Snyder, 1979), somatostatin (Finley et al., 1978), and bradykinin (Correa et al., 1979) may also participate in cortical mechanisms on a somewhat less frequent basis, judging by the density of immunocytochemically detectable fibers and of the radioimmunoassayable peptide. Even less clear than the relative cytological distribution of these peptides is the functional mechanism by which they work. Based upon their effects on spinal neurons in vivo or in vitro, some workers have suggested that a new mode of transmitter action, termed modulation, is necessary to explain the observed effects of these peptides. In this sense, modulation is defined as the altered conductance-change response to a "true" transmitter produced by a substance (i.e., peptide) when that substance itself produces neither a conductance nor membrane potential change. Such types of modulation have been reported for interactions between substance P and nicotinic cholinergic receptor responses in spinal cord and in adrenal medulla (Krnjević and Lekić, 1977; Livett et al., 1979), and for interactions between enkephalin receptors and excitations due to glutamate (Davies and Dray, 1977; Zieglgansberger and Champagnat, 1979). In one report on spinal neurons, the excitation produced by substance P was also found to modulate responses induced by iontophoresis of opiates and opiate peptides. Little testing of this type has been done in cortex with peptides known to be present in cortex, and in no case thus far described has a cortically occurring peptide been tested against a pathway in which an amino acid or amine transmitter is known. It is therefore difficult to know at this stage whether the modulatory action is typical of all peptides or only of some, and whether these interactions between some peptides and some other transmitters will be uniquely paired in specific target areas. The excitatory action described in cortex for VIP (Phillis, Kirkpatrick, and Said, 1978) shows some potent effects, provided the tests are done at well-separated intervals; if this property were a general one in cortex, one might infer that the intracortical neurons which react immunocytochemically for VIP content fire infrequently.

Conclusions

With the evidence available to us now—the current menu of cortical transmitters viewed in the light of their relative density of innervation, their discrete or general properties of innervation pattern, and their emerging physiological properties of transmitter action—the several partially defined systems can be contrasted. The most common mechanisms, probably mediated by amino acids, would generate excitatory projections into, within, and out of cortex on brief, precise, and succinct transmission, perhaps mediated by either glutamate or aspartate. Almost as frequent would appear to be intracortical inhibitory interneurons mediated in equally brief and precise terms by GABA. The monoamine systems, while considerably less specific in innervation pattern, nevertheless hold to certain broad organizational principles which need further elucidation and testing. These systems, frequently operating on density scales one to two orders of magnitude lower than the amino acid connections, also operate for considerably longer time periods. The peptide-mediated events of cortex have scarcely begun to be described, but the actions of some peptides in other regions of the central nervous system suggest that in some cases the peptides may be paired with a certain amino acid or amine transmitter to modify the sensitivity of common target cells. How these two effects (that of the amino acid or amine transmitter and of the postulated peptide modulator) are coordinated has not yet been elucidated. Taken together, the existing evidence of chemical signaling within cerebral cortex suggests that so far there are no unique transmitter arrangements that distinguish cortex. If unique arrangements of transmitters are required to generate the information process in capacity of cortex, such properties are as likely to be derived from the sheer numbers of participating cells as from any new—and as yet uncharacterized—chemical mode of information processing.

References

Belcher, G. and R. W. Ryall, 1977. Substance P and Renshaw cells: A new concept of inhibitory synaptic interactions. *J. Physiol.* 272:105–119.

Bjorklund, A., I. Divac, and O. Lindvall, 1978. Regional distribution of catecholamines in monkey cerebral cortex, evidence for dopaminergic innervation of the primate prefrontal cortex. *Neurosci. Lett.* 7:115–119.

Bloom, F. E., 1975. The role of cyclic nucleotides in central synaptic function. *Rev. Physiol. Biochem. Pharmacol.* 74:1–103.

Bloom, F. E., 1979. Chemical integrative processes in the central nervous system. In *The Neurosciences: Fourth Study Program.* F. O. Schmitt and F. G. Worden, eds. Cambridge, MA: MIT Press, pp. 51–58.

Borghi, C., S. Nicosia, A. Giachetti, and S. I. Said, 1979. Vasoactive intestinal peptide (VIP) stimulates adenylate cyclase in selected areas of rat brain. *Life Sci.* 24:65–70.

Bunney, B. S., and G. K. Aghajanian, 1976. Dopamine and norepinephrine innervated cells in the rat pre-frontal cortex: Pharmacological differentiation using microiontophoretic techniques. *Life Sci.* 19:1783–1792.

Correa, F. M. A., R. B. Innis, G. R. Uhl, and S. A. Snyder, 1979. Bradykinin-like immunoreactive neuronal systems localized histochemically in rat brain. *Proc. Nat. Acad. Sci. USA* 76:1489–1493.

Coyle, J. T., and M. E. Molliver, 1977. Major innervation of newborn rat cortex by monoaminergic neurons. *Science* 196:444–447.

Curtis, D. R., and G. A. R. Johnston, 1974. Amino acid transmitters on the mammalian central nervous system. *Ergebn. Physiol.* 69:98–188.

Davies, J., and A. Dray, 1977. Substance P and opiate receptors. *Nature* 268:351–352.

Dillier, N., J. Laszlo, B. Muller, W. P. Koella, and H.-R. Olpe, 1978. Activation of an inhibitory noradrenergic pathway projecting from the locus coeruleus to the cingulate cortex of the rat. *Brain Res.* 154:61–68.

Divac, I., O. Lindvall, A. Bjorklund, and R. E. Passinghaur, 1978. Converging projections from medio-dorsal thalamic nucleus and mesencephalic dopaminergic neurons to the neocortex in three species. *J. Comp. Neurol.* 180:59–72.

Emson, P. C., and O. Lindvall, 1979. Distribution of putative neurotransmitters in the neocortex. *Neuroscience* 4:1–30.

Finley, J. C. W., G. H. Grossman, P. Dimeo, and P. Petrusz, 1978. Somatostatin-containing neurons in the rat brain: Widespread distribution revealed by immunocytochemistry after pretreatment by pronase. *Amer. J. Anat.* 153:483–488.

Foote, S. L., F. E. Bloom, and A. Schwartz, 1978. Behavioral and electroencephalographic correlates of locus coeruleus neuronal discharge activity in the unanesthetized squirrel monkey. *Soc. Neurosci. Abst.* 4:272.

Foote, S. L., R. Freedman, and A. P. Oliver, 1975. Effects of putative neurotransmitters on neuronal activity in monkey auditory cortex. *Brain Res.* 86:229–242.

Freedman, R., S. L. Foote, and F. E. Bloom, 1975. Histochemical characterization of a neocortical projection of the nucleus locus coeruleus in the squirrel monkey. *J. Comp. Neurol.* 164:209–232.

Fuxe, K., T. Hökfelt, S. I. Said, and V. Mutt, 1977. Vasoactive intestinal polypeptide and the nervous system. Immunohistochemical evidence for localization in central and peripheral neurons, particularly intracortical neurons of the cerebral cortex. *Neurosci. Lett.* 5:241–246.

Gale, J. S., E. D. Bird, E. G. Spokes, L. L. Iversen, and T. M. Jessell, 1978. Human brain substance P: Distribution in controls and Huntington's chorea. *J. Neurochem.* 30:633–634.

Gatter, K. C., and T. P. S. Powell, 1977. The projection of the locus coeruleus upon the neocortex in the macaque monkey. *Neuroscience* 2:441–445.

Giorguieff, M. F., M. L. Kemel, and J. Glowinski, 1977. Presynaptic effect of L-glutamic acid on the release of dopamine in rat striatal slices. *Neurosci. Lett.* 6:73–78.

Hökfelt, T., B. Meyerson, G. Nilsson, B. Pernow, and C. Sachs, 1976. Immunohistochemical evidence for substance P containing nerve endings in the human cortex. *Brain Res.* 104:181–186.

Hosli, L. P., P. F. Andres, and E. Hosli, 1973. Ionic mechanisms underlying the depolarization of L-glutamate on rat and human spinal neurons in tissue culture. *Experientia* 29:1244–1246.

Hubel, D., and T. N. Wiesel, 1962. Receptive fields, binocular interactions and functional architecture in the cat's visual cortex. *J. Physiol.* 160:106–154.

Innis, R. B., F. M. A. Correa, G. R. Uhl, B. Schneider, and S. H. Snyder, 1979. Cholecystokinin octapeptide-like immunoreactivity: Histochemical localization in rat brain. *Proc. Nat. Acad. Sci. USA* 76:521–525.

Jones, G., S. L. Foote, M. Segal, and F. E. Bloom, 1978. Locus coeruleus neurons in freely behaving rats exhibit pronounced alterations of firing rate during sensory stimulation and stages of the sleep wake cycle. *Soc. Neurosci. Abst.* 4:274.

Karlsen, R. L., and F. Fonnum, 1978. Evidence for glutamate as a neurotransmitter in the corticofugal fibers to the dorsal lateral geniculate body and the superior colliculus in rats. *Brain Res.* 151:457–467.

Kobayashi, R. M., M. Brown, and W. Vale, 1977. Regional distribution of neurotensin and somatostatin in rat brain. *Brain Res.* 126:584–588.

Krnjević, K., 1974. Chemical nature of synaptic transmission in vertebrates. *Physiol. Rev.* 54:418–540.

Krnjević, K., and D. Lekić, 1977. Substance P selectively blocks excitation of Renshaw cell by acetylcholine. *Canad. J. Physiol. Pharmacol.* 55:958–961.

Levitt, P., and R. Y. Moore, 1978. Noradrenaline neuron innervation of the neocortex in the rat. *Brain Res.* 139:219–231.

Lidov, H. G. W., F. L. Rice, and M. E. Molliver, 1978. The organization of the catecholamine innervation of somatosensory cortex: The barrel field of the mouse. *Brain Res.* 153:577–584.

Lindvall, O., A. Bjorklund, A. Nobin, and V. Stenevi, 1974. The adrenergic innervation of the rat thalamus as revealed by the glyoxylic acid fluorescence method. *J. Comp. Neurol.* 154:317–348.

Livett, B. G., V. Kozousek, F. Mizobe, and D. M. Dean, 1979. Substance P inhibits nicotinic activation of chromaffin cells. *Nature* 278:256–257.

McIlwain, H., 1977. Extended roles in the brain for second messenger systems. *Neuroscience* 2:357–372.

Mishra, R. K., C. Demirjian, R. Katzaman, and M. H. Makman, 1975. A dopamine-sensitive adenylate cyclase in anterior limbic cortex and mesolimbic region of primate brain. *Brain Res.* 96:395–399.

Moore, R. Y., and F. E. Bloom, 1978. Central catecholamine neuron systems: Anatomy and physiology of the dopamine systems. *Ann. Rev. Neurosci.* 1:129–169.

Moore, R. Y., and F. E. Bloom, 1979. Central catecholamine neuron systems: Anatomy of the norepinephrine and epinephrine systems. *Ann. Rev. Neurosci.* 2:113–168.

Morrison, J. H., R. Grzanna, M. E. Molliver, and J. T. Coyle, 1978. The distribution and orientation of noradrenergic fibers in neocortex of the rat: An immunofluorescence study. *J. Comp. Neurol.* 181:17–40.

Patel, H. H., and A. M. Sillito, 1978. Inhibition and velocity tuning in the cat visual cortex. *J. Physiol.* 285:113–114P.

Paxinos, G., P. C. Emson, and A. C. Cuello, 1978. The Substance P projections to the frontal cortex and the substantia nigra. *Neurosci. Lett.* 7:127–131.

Phillis, J. W., and J. J. Limacher, 1974. Substance P excitation of cerebral cortical Betz cells. *Brain Res.* 69:158–163.

Phillis, J. W., J. R. Kirkpatrick, and S. I. Said, 1978. Vasoactive intestinal polypeptide excitation of central neurons. *Canad. J. Physiol. Pharmacol.* 56:337–340.

Pinget, M., E. Straus, and R. W. Yalow, 1978. Localization of cholecystokinin-like immunoreactivity in isolated nerve terminals. *Proc. Nat. Acad. Sci. USA* 75:6324–6326.

Ribak, C. E., 1978. Aspinous and sparsely-spinous stellate neurons in the visual cortex of the rats contain glutamic acid decarboxylase. *J. Neurocytol.* 7:461–478.

Roskoski, R., 1979. Net uptake of aspartate by a high-affinity rat cortical synaptosomal transport system. *Brain Res.* 160:85–93.

Sillito, A. M., 1977. Inhibitory processes underlying the directional specificity of simple, complex, and hypercomplex cells in the cat's visual cortex. *J. Physiol.* 271:699–720.

Stone, T. W., 1979. Selective antagonism of amino acids by a-aminoadipate on pyramidal tract neurons but not Purkinje cells. *Brain Res.* 166:217–220.

Stone, T. W., and D. A. Taylor, 1977. Microiontophoretic studies of the effects of cyclic nucleotides on excitability of neurons in the rat cerebral cortex. *J. Physiol.* 266:523–543.

Tassin, J. P., J. Bockaert, G. Blanc, L. Stinus, A. M. Thierry, S. Lavielle, J. Premont, and J. Glowinski, 1978. Topographical distribution of dopaminergic innervation and odopaminergic receptors of the anterior cerebral cortex of the rat. *Brain Res.* 154:241–251.

Thierry, A. M., G. Blanc, A. Sobel, L. Stinus, and J. Glowinski, 1973. Dopaminergic terminals in the rat cortex. *Science* 182:499–501.

Uhl, G., M. J. Kuhar, and S. H. Snyder, 1977. Neurotensin: Immunohistochemical localization in rat central nervous systems. *Proc. Nat. Acad. Sci. USA* 74:4059–4063.

Vogt, B. A., D. L. Rosene, and D. N. Pandya, 1979. Thalamic and cortical afferents differentiating anterior from posterior cingulate cortex in the monkey. *Science* 204:205–207.

Woody, C. D., and E. Gruen, 1978. Characterization of electrophysiological properties of intracellular recorded neurons in the neocortex of awake rats: A comparison of the response to injected current in spike overshoot and undershoot neurons. *Brain Res.* 158:343–357.

Zieglgansberger, W., and J. Champagnat, 1979. Cat spinal motoneurons exhibit topographic sensitivity to glutamate and glycine. *Brain Res.* 160:95–104.

The Role of Cerebral Cortex in Higher
Brain Function

Introduction

Herbert H. Jasper

The ultimate aim of research on the functional anatomy of cerebral cortex is to understand its role in higher brain functions—the neuronal mechanisms underlying perceptual awareness, discriminative learning, goal-directed intentional behavior, and abstract thought processes such as are involved in language and cognition.

Although we are now able to study certain of these complex "higher" brain functions at the single cellular or modular level, we have little detailed understanding of the interrelationships in space and time between these unit functions and conscious cognitive and purposeful patterned behavior. Possible solutions to some of these problems are presented by a number of participants in this and other sections, and especially in the more theoretical papers at the end of Edelman, Cooper, and Crick, Marr, and Poggio.

One of the most important advances in our understanding of the functional organization of cerebral cortex has been the discovery of radially oriented assemblies of cells, columns, or modules which respond selectively to significant features of a stimulus pattern (e.g., form, orientation, and location in space, or direction of movements) in somatic, visual, or auditory cortical sensory receiving areas. The features of the stimulus pattern to which such assemblies of cells are attuned become more and more complex as they are removed from primary receiving areas either in a given column in different cortical laminae, or especially at a distance from a primary cortical receiving area in "association" cortex. Mountcastle (1978) has postulated that the entire cerebral cortex may be composed of such local neuronal assemblies with highly specific though more and more complex functional organization, which might even include modules mediating "intentional behavior" in parietal cortex. In the context of "higher" brain functions, this conception poses some interesting problems. Can the melody of the mind be played on a keyboard mosaic of modules or cortical columns with rigidly determined functional characteristics? (See also Kuffler, 1973.)

This view must, of course, be coupled with the conception of much more widely distributed neuronal networks with interrelated local cortical modules in widespread areas, as well as with specific and nonspecific subcortical systems of neurons responsible for their activation and integration with highly organized neuronal activity throughout the neuraxis. In fact, microelectrode studies in behaving animals, either awake or asleep, have shown that widely distributed neuronal systems in many cortical and subcortical structures play a role in "higher" brain functions, utilizing no doubt the remarkable concatenation of information processing provided by local modules in cerebral cortex, though these retain nevertheless remarkably specific simple or highly complex functions.

Herbert Jasper begins this section by introducing the stage upon which the various specific cortical characters must perform, namely, the predetermined excitatory state, the pattern of ongoing activity and preset reactivity that forms the background for any specific stimulus–response relationship, that is, *state-dependent reactions.*

Alan Cowey discusses behavioral anatomical studies of the organization of the visual system in the monkey, with special reference to the function of multiple representations of the visual field. Giovanni Berlucchi and James Sprague will then demonstrate a somewhat different organization of the visual system in the cat, raising some interesting questions regarding the importance of the striate visual cortex in this animal and the importance of parallel processing of visual information in general.

Finally, Jean Desmedt reviews electrophysiological studies of certain higher brain functions in man as revealed by the later components of computer-averaged evoked potentials. The perfection of such techniques has added new dimensions to our knowledge of higher brain functions in man, even though their interpretation in terms of specific neuronal mechanisms remains a challenging problem.

The role of the cerebral cortex in higher brain function is, of course, an immensely complicated subject that far exceeds the scope of the present conference. We can only present selected aspects that seem to provide principles upon which a fuller, more general understanding can eventually be based. The small samples of the extensive research being carried out on this subject will, we hope, stimulate further research and interest in what is perhaps the most challenging of all endeavors by members of our scientific community and by philosophers as well. The concerted attack that has been waged on some of these problems in recent years by scientists of varied disciplines using many new and revolutionary techniques makes this conference a particularly timely one, even though we may be able only to scratch the surface of our subject.

References

Kuffler, S. W., 1973. The single-cell approach in the visual system and the study of receptive fields. *Invest. Ophthal.* 12:794–813.

Mountcastle, V. B., 1978. An organizing principle for cerebral function: The unit module and the distributed system. In G. M. Edelman and V. B. Mountcastle, *The Mindful Brain.* Cambridge, MA: MIT Press.

16 Problems of Relating Cellular or Modular Specificity to Cognitive Functions: Importance of State-Dependent Reactions

Herbert H. Jasper

ABSTRACT   The remarkable relationship which can be shown by microelectrode studies in behaving animals between cellular or modular responses and complex-feature detection or to coordinated intentional, goal-directed behavior may lead to the conception that cognitive functions may also have very specific cellular or modular localization in cerebral cortex. Can the melody of higher mental processes be played on a keyboard mosaic of modules or cortical columns with rigidly determined functional characteristics? Higher brain functions in the behaving animal or man require, in addition, that such local functional units be integrated with more widespread neuronal assemblies throughout the neuraxis. It is also necessary to understand the dynamic nature of function in both local and distributed neuronal systems, that is, state-dependent reactions. Such reactions depend upon (A) the pattern and intensity of ongoing activity in a given neuronal system and (B) the chemically determined reactive state, both general and specific.

Electrical Signs of Cortical Excitatory State

Motivated by the search for brain mechanisms of the mind, Hans Berger, Professor of Psychiatry in Jena, published the first of a series of papers entitled "Über das Elektrenkephalogram des Menschen" in 1929, just fifty years ago (Gloor, 1969). Benefiting by the availability of veterans of World War I with skull defects, he was able to prove that reliable records of rhythmic electrical activity of the human brain could be obtained from the surface of the intact scalp, and that such records were indeed sensitive to certain mental processes such as state of alertness, attention, and perceptual awareness.

These results were received with considerable skepticism both in Germany and abroad, especially since, at the same time, attention was being directed to nerve action potentials by the work of Erlanger and Gasser, who, with the help of George Bishop, introduced the cathode-ray oscilloscope, making possible for the first time an accurate measurement of nerve impulses. There seemed at first to be a certain incompatibility between these two discoveries. The gap between 1-msec

HERBERT H. JASPER   Centre de Recherche en Sciences Neurologiques, Université de Montréal, Montréal, Québec, Canada; Montreal Neurological Institute, McGill University, Montreal, Quebec, Canada

CONTROL

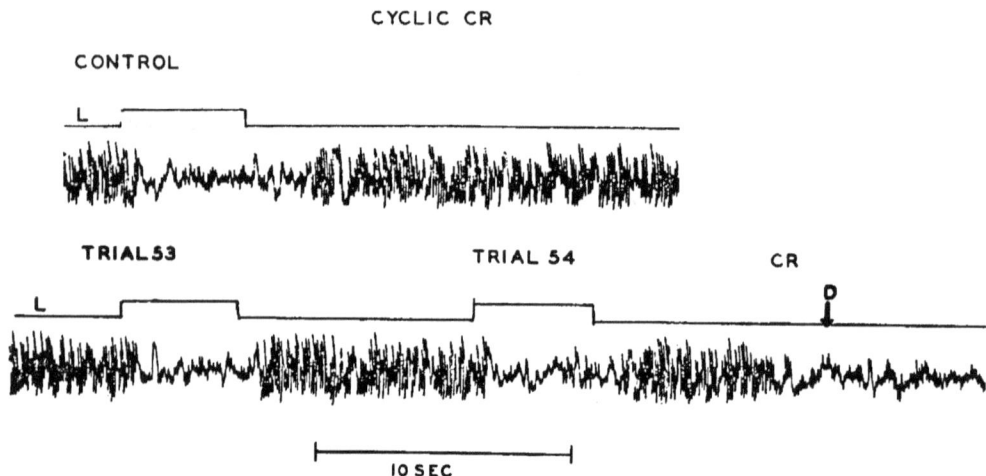

Figure 1 Cyclic conditioning of the occipital EEG in man. (From Jasper and Shagass, 1941). A light stimulus which blocked the occipital alpha waves was administered for 5 sec and regularly repeated at intervals of 10 sec. After 54 repetitions, the 55th stimulus was omitted. Note conditioned blocking of the alpha waves without a light stimulus.

spikes and 100-msec brain waves was not readily bridged before the discovery of nonpropagated synaptic potentials.

Scientific credibility was established when Adrian and Matthews were able to confirm Berger's findings and to demonstrate clear relationships to higher mental processes such as attention, imagination, and problem solving (Adrian and Matthews, 1934a,b). For example, Adrian was able to show that arrest of the occipital alpha rhythm by opening the eyes could also be produced when attempting to see in a totally darkened room. With Shagass we were able to show that a similar response could be obtained in the absence of a stimulus if, after repetition at fixed time intervals, the response occurred at the expected interval even if the stimulus was omitted (Figure 1) (Jasper and Shagass, 1941a,b).

We were then able to show that electroencephalogram (EEG) activation was accompanied by a negative dc shift in resting polarization of the cortical surface, which we described in the Cold Spring Harbor Conference of 1936 (Jasper, 1936) as a change in cortical "excitatory state," broadly defined to include inhibitory processes (chemical concomitants will be discussed later in this conference). Later, recording from the exposed sensorimotor cortex in man during neurosurgical procedures with Penfield, it was found that a similar change in electrical activity occurred during voluntary movement, and also with imagined movements in the absence of visible muscular contraction (Jasper and Penfield, 1949). The pattern of ongoing electrical activity from the cortical surface in the waking brain appeared to be sensitive not only to perceptual awareness of external stimuli but also to intrinsic "mental" processes.

The EEG, when recorded from the scalp or cortical surface, provides a sensitive sign of cortical activation during certain "higher" brain functions even though the physiological significance of these slow electrical rhythms remains obscure. The frequency and pattern of these gross electrical-field potentials ("brain waves") are also most sensitive and reliable indicators of cortical excitatory state or activation.

However, the fact that the amplitude of the EEG is inversely related to the normally integrated activation of a given cortical area, or to the "arousal" of the brain as a whole, has led to the conclusion by some investigators that these electrical rhythms may be only epiphenomena. Since they are most prominent when the cortex is relatively idle, and increase during slow-wave sleep, they may represent the synchronization of oscillating membrane potentials and reverberating synaptic circuits in relatively idle neurons which become desynchronized when they are processing afferent information or organizing patterns of motor response.

This interpretation assumes that the neuronal generators of brain waves are entirely passive and that there is no active synchronizing mechanism involved. It has been shown, however, that synchronization of cortical rhythms can be induced by electrical stimulation of certain medial forebrain structures, the septal region, the medial thalamus, and the reticular core of the brain stem. Such stimulation is also associated with arrest or impairment of behavioral responsiveness. It may be that the continuous ongoing electrical rhythms of the cortex, present during all stages of sleep and waking (the absence of which is now used as a sign of brain death), are more than epiphenomena. They may play an active role in the regulation or timing of cortical "readiness to respond" (or to not respond) to incoming afferent volleys.

When a given cortical area becomes actively engaged in integrative functions, with its finely organized asynchronous patterning of neuronal activity, the surface slow waves disappear. This has been called the "arousal," "alerting," or "orienting" response. It is this pattern of desynchronized activation which has been shown to be related to certain "higher" brain functions. On the contrary, when the surface slow waves become exaggerated, as in certain forms of epileptic discharge or in slow-wave sleep, conscious cognitive functions become abolished or severely impaired.

The most striking example of the arrest or severe impairment of cortical cognitive functions associated with hypersynchronous slow waves in the EEG is the so-called *petit mal* attack. Experimental reproduction of the characteristic spike-and-wave surface EEG pattern while recording with intracellular microelectrodes from deep-lying cortical neurons has shown that the large surface negative slow wave is associated with a

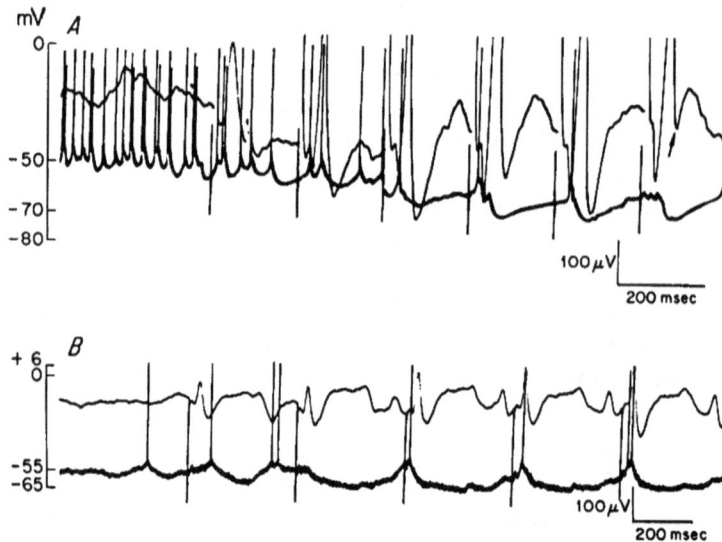

Figure 2 Surface macroelectrode (upper trace) and intracellular microelectrode records (lower trace) from the sigmoid gyrus of the cat while stimulating the intralaminar thalamus at a frequency of 3Hz. (From Pollen 1964, 1968.) In (A), a cell was firing spontaneously before thalamic stimulation; the firing was arrested during the surface negative slow wave of the experimental spike-and-wave complex. In (B), another cell was quiescent before stimulation but fired during the spike phase of the complex with an intracellular excitatory postsynaptic potential (EPSP) corresponding to the surface negative spike in the EEG. The prolonged surface negative slow wave was associated with intracellular hyperpolarization and inhibition of cell firing (calibration at right is for surface EEG only, at left for intracellular records only).

large and prolonged inhibitory hyperpolarization of cortical cells, arresting their spontaneous activity and blocking their response in incoming afferent volleys, as illustrated in Figure 2 taken from the work of Pollen (1964, 1968). This was an active process induced by thalamic stimulation under favorable states of cortical reactivity. It is not hard to understand why integrative activity is lost in cortical areas being driven by such massive excitatory and inhibitory sequences accompanying the three-per-second spike-and-wave EEG during a *petit mal* epileptic attack with sudden arrest of conscious behavior.

In minor *petit mal* attacks, frontal and parietal association cortex is principally involved bilaterally. Stereotyped sensorimotor functions may then be preserved, though there may be a loss of perceptual awareness and adaptive intentional behavior. Physiological studies of experimental models of this form of attack have shown that it involves neuronal systems of medial thalamus (intralaminar) which normally control the predominant rhythmic activity of cerebral cortex (Jasper and Droogleever-Fortuyn, 1946). In man there is a strong genetic predisposition for this unfortunate derangement of a normal control system in the brain, the nature of which is not understood. It seems to involve both

Herbert H. Jasper

cortical and subcortical interacting neuronal systems, the recruiting system of the thalamus first described by Morison and Dempsey (1942) being an important part of the mechanism generating spike-and-wave discharge as well as in controlling synchronized rhythmic activity in groups or "assemblies" of cortical neurons. This is an active process but can be shown best in the "idling" awake cortex or under light barbiturate anesthesia. The "spike-and-wave" of *petit mal* may be arrested with attention and arousing stimuli just as the normal alpha rhythm in some patients, but in others the intrinsic rhythmic activity arrests all conscious behavior and memory recording, blocking all normal response to afferent stimuli and cognitive cortical functions.

Sleep and States of Impaired Consciousness and Cognition

It has long been known that during arrest of behavioral responsiveness to external stimuli during states of sleep or light barbiturate anesthesia, primary evoked potentials from cortical sensory receiving areas are preserved or even enhanced. In the classical microelectrode studies of Hubel and Wiesel (1965) the feature selectivity of even the more complex cells in visual cortex were present even in animals immobilized by barbiturate anesthesia, presumably without perceptual awareness. Ivan Bodis-Wollner of Mount Sinai Hospital in New York has recently reported his studies with colleagues from the Department of Ophthalmology recording normal computer-averaged occipital evoked potentials in response to coarse alternating patterns of visual stimulation in a 6-year-old boy who has been completely blind since a febrile disease at the age of 2 years. Computerized tomography revealed an almost complete destruction of occipital lobes bilaterally, but with preservation of the medial striate area mainly on the left side (Bodis-Wollner et al., 1977).

Although the close relationship between EEG patterns and states of impaired consciousness or cognition is well documented, under certain conditions it is complex and seems paradoxical. Patterns similar to sleep or coma may occur with preservation of apparent vigilant reactivity (although cognitive functions are found usually to be impaired when properly tested). Conversely, normal or activation patterns may be present in states of apparent "unconsciousness," as in so-called "paradoxical sleep" or "alpha coma."

Such anomalies are more apparent than real when behavioral functions are more adequately tested, and when neurophysiological mechanisms underlying the various syndromes subsumed under the generic term "states of consciousness" are properly understood. However, the questions they raise, together with the difficulty in assigning a true functional significance to the rhythmic electrical waves of the EEG, has led some investigators to the conclusion that they are of no functional significance.

Cortical Activity during Habituation of the Arousal Response

A sleeping animal or man can be aroused repeatedly by a novel stimulus. Continued repetition of the identical stimulus without reenforcement results in extinction or habituation of the arousal response. The establishment of such an unreactive state to a specific stimulus, such as a tone of a given frequency, is fundamental to the learning process. In the cat, prepared with recording electrodes over the cortical surface and in subcortical structures, alterations in electrical activity during the habituation process can be observed. The animal was placed in a quiet box with some warm milk. It was allowed limited freedom of movement while being observed through a one-way screen. Continuous multiple-channel EEG records were begun as soon as the cat appeared to be asleep. It was awakened by a tone and then allowed to go to sleep again before the tone was repeated. Continuation of this procedure 30 to 50 times caused habituation of arousal to this frequency, while tones of a different frequency, or a stimulus of another modality (e.g., touch) were equally effective in producing an arousal response. Examples are given from experiments carried out with Seth Sharpless many years ago (Figures 3 and 4) (Sharpless and Jasper, 1956).

In some experiments a two-per-second click was used as the awakening stimulus in order that evoked potentials from auditory cortex could be recorded during sleep and awake, and following habituation.

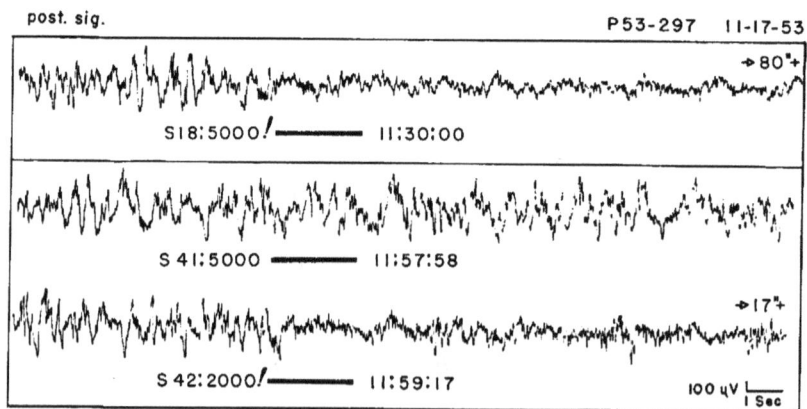

Figure 3 EEG records from chronically implanted dural surface electrodes over the suprasylvian gyrus in the cat during studies of habituation of arousal from natural sleep by different forms of repeated stimuli (tones of different frequencies). (From studies by Sharpless and Jasper, 1956.) Note desynchronized activation of the cortex for over 80 sec (with arousal from natural sleep) in response to the administration of a 5,000-Hz tone for the first time—a novel stimulus (!); 27 min later, after 21 repetitions of this tone, no activation or arousal occurred (habituation). Then, on the next trial a tone of 2,000 Hz was used which caused activation of the EEG and arousal of the animal for over 17 sec, showing frequency-specific habituation to the 5,000-Hz tone.

Herbert H. Jasper

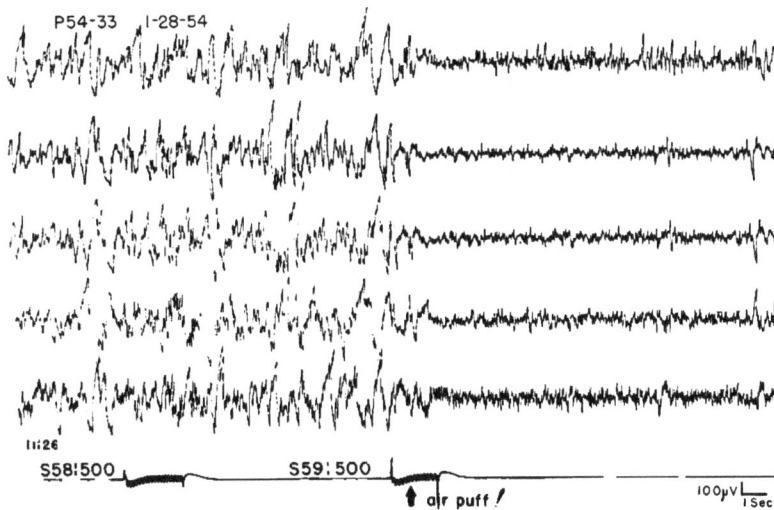

Figure 4 EEG tracings as in Figure 3 during habituation of the arousal response in naturally sleeping cats. (From studies by Sharpless and Jasper, 1956.) Records were from five different cortical areas showing generalization of the desynchronized cortical activation by arousal from slow-wave sleep. The animal was thoroughly habituated to a 500-Hz tone after the 58th repetition. Then a puff of air on the cat's nose caused immediate and prolonged arousal and activation of the EEG, demonstrating modality specificity of the arousal response.

Habituation occurred to this stimulus in 18–20 trials. Auditory evoked potentials were consistently of higher amplitude during sleep than upon awakening (Figure 5). In fact, if the arousal response was sufficiently intense, as during a second train of stimuli after the initial awakening, evoked potentials were reduced to about one half their amplitude during sleep. Following complete habituation of the arousal response to this stimulus, auditory evoked potentials were increased, as illustrated by the following example from the experiments with Sharpless. Habituation was obviously not due to blocking of sensory input to auditory cortex. This raised the question whether the auditory cortex was involved at all in this habituation process.

Habituation was then studied in animals following removal of all of auditory and adjacent cortex from both hemispheres up to and including all of somatic I and II, the suprasylvian gyrus, and the temporal lobe, leaving little more than the limbic system and motor cortex intact. Surprisingly, frequency-specific habituation to tones was still possible in these animals when tested several weeks or months following operation, as illustrated in the following example from the animal with the largest cortical removals (Figure 6). Tonal-pattern-specific habituation could not be obtained in animals after removal of auditory cortex. It was clear, however, that in the cat habituation to specific tones was not dependent upon neocortical mechanisms. This is consistent with the ob-

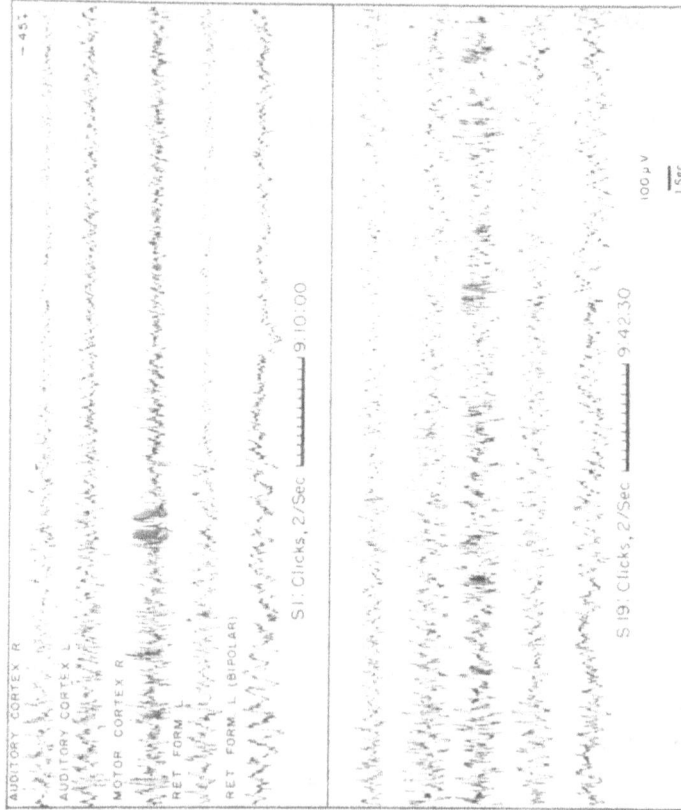

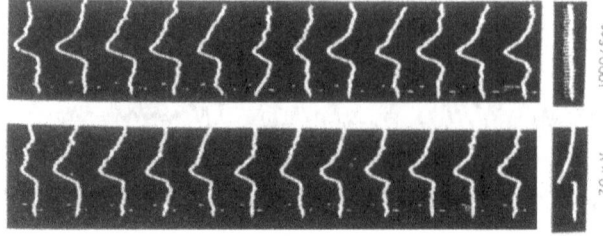

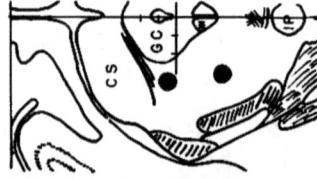

Figure 5 EEG dural surface implanted-electrode records of cortical surface electrical activity from right and left auditory cortex, right motor cortex, and midbrain reticular formation in a chronic cat preparation during studies of effect of habituation upon auditory evoked potentials in response to a 2/sec click stimulus. (From studies by Sharpless and Jasper, 1956.) Oscilloscope tracings of auditory cortical evoked potentials before (S1) and after (S19) habituation are shown at right, there being some increase in evoked potentials even though the arousal response was completely abolished as shown in EEG tracings at left.

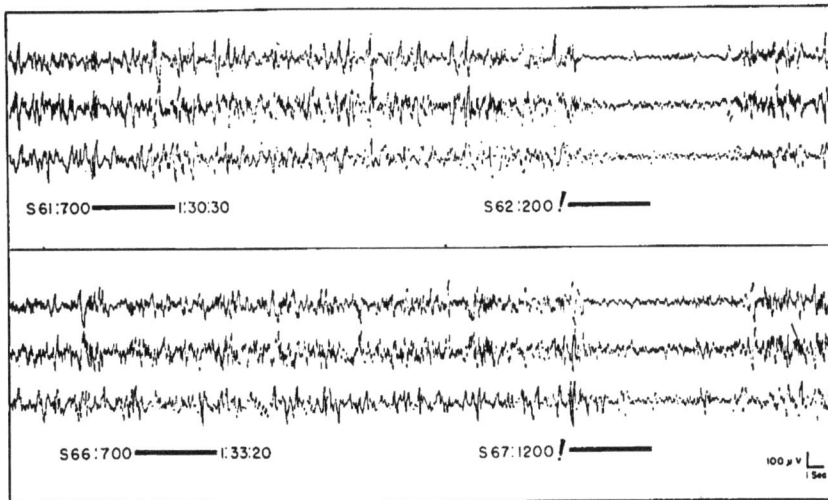

Figure 6 Cortical EEG records, as in Figures 4 and 5, from cortex surrounding a large neocortical ablation including all auditory cortex, somatic I and II, and a portion of the midsuprasylvian gyrus. (From studies by Sharpless and Jasper, 1956.) Habituation to a 700-Hz tone was complete after the 61st trial while arousal still occurred to novel 200- and 1,200-Hz tones.

servations of Diamond and Neff (1953), who found that complete ablation of auditory cortex plus somatic II did not prevent cats from acquiring differential conditioned responses to tones. Pattern discrimination
was abolished. It would appear that the auditory cortex in the cat is not
essential to the process of tonal-frequency discrimination for differential habituation or conditioning, but does play an essential role in
pattern discrimination under both of these conditions, that is, during
sleep and waking.

Relationships between Cortical Surface Rhythms and Patterns of Cellular Discharge

Microelectrode studies have shown that cortical cells are far from inactive during sleep, some being even more active in sleep than during the
waking state (Jasper, 1958; Evarts, 1964). In the visual cortex of the cat,
for example, Evarts has shown that the pattern of spontaneous firing of
cortical cells is grossly altered during different stages of normal sleep
(Evarts, 1967). Responses to photic stimulation persisted at all states of
sleep, though altered from those seen in the waking state (Jasper, 1958,
1963, 1966; Evarts, 1963).

When care is taken to record the surface slow waves from a small column of cortical cells by the use of a perspex pressure plate with a small
hole 1–2 mm in diameter in the bottom of a plastic cup filled with saline
solution through which a glass microelectrode is inserted, a close re-

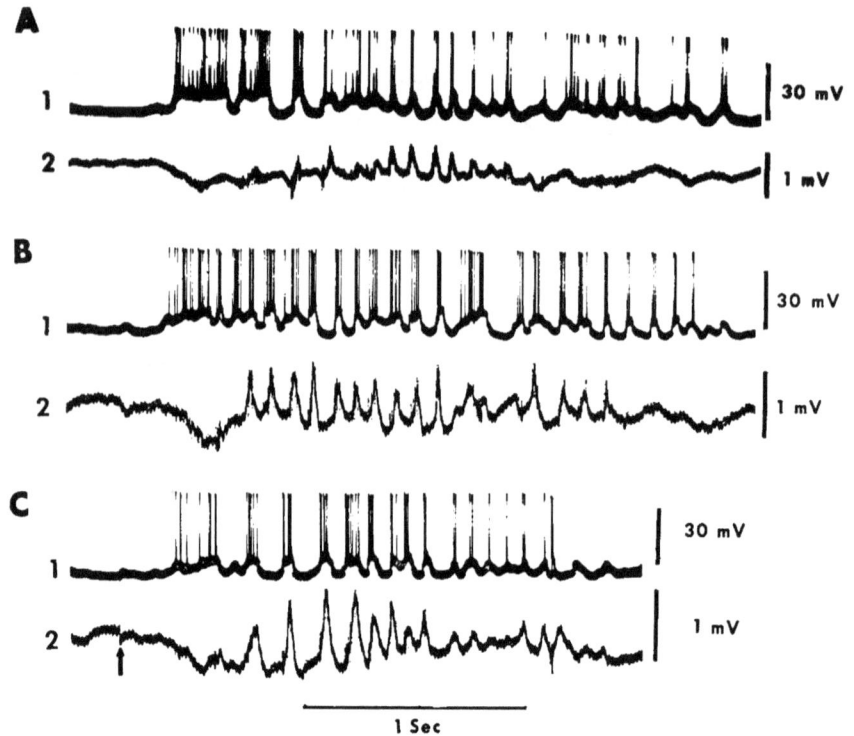

Figure 7 Intracellular (1) and cortical surface (2) tracings from motor cortex in the lightly anesthetized cat. (From studies by Jasper and Stefanis, 1965.) Two spontaneous spindles are shown in (A) and (B), each preceded by a slow surface positive wave, the spindle waves being surface negative. The initial long-lasting surface positive wave was associated with a prolonged depolarization of the cell with rapid spike discharge; then the cell firing was gated by the spindle waves firing on their surface negative phase, inhibited on their surface positive phase, showing that spindle waves contain alternating excitatory and inhibitory components and are capable of gating cell discharge.

lationship can be shown between synaptic potentials and surface potential waves. Using this technique with Costa Stefanis, by means of intracellular microelectrodes in pyramidal cells of motor cortex, there were rhythmic excitatory synaptic potentials synchronous with the surface negative phase of spindle waves, as shown in Figures 7 and 8 (Jasper and Stefanis, 1965). The intracellular synaptic potentials were 10–15 mV in amplitude, as compared to about 1–1.5 mV for the spindle waves. There were, however, other surface negative slow waves associated with large inhibitory synaptic potentials which interrupted spontaneous neuronal discharge. Larger-amplitude excitatory synaptic potentials were associated with some surface positive waves, particularly during specific evoked potentials of thalamic origin.

The surface slow waves of the EEG were shown to reflect important changes in both inhibitory and excitatory synaptic potentials, sufficient to gate the rhythmicity of spontaneous spike discharge and to modulate

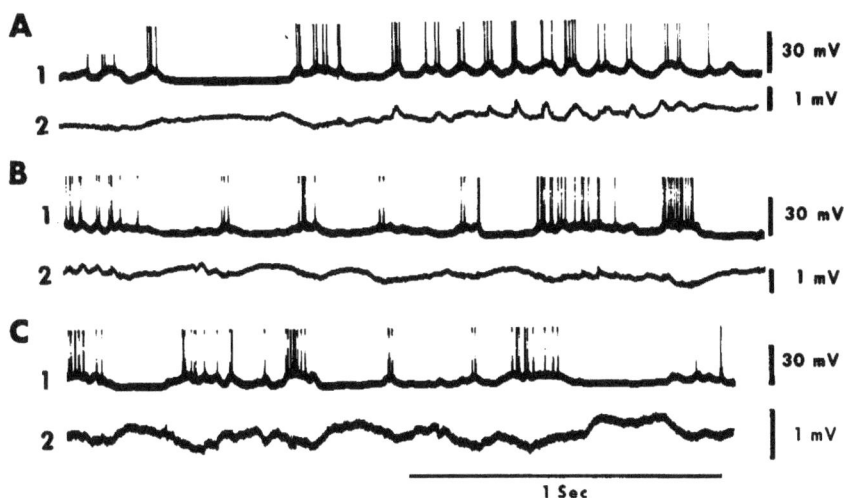

Figure 8 Intracellular (1) and surface (2) potentials from motor cortex in the cat, as in Figure 7. (From studies by Jasper and Stefanis, 1965.) Examples of spontaneous activity in a lightly barbiturated anesthetized animal are shown for three cells (A), (B), and (C), in order to show that long-lasting slow surface negative waves in the EEG may be associated with marked hyperpolarization and inhibition of cell firing, while at the same time the surface negative spindle waves are excitatory with depolarization and bursts of cell discharge. Note that a 1-mV surface wave is equal to about 10 mV of intracellular potential change, sufficient to exceed the firing threshold. Inhibitory waves are also about 10-fold larger when recorded with intracellular microelectrodes sufficient to arrest cell firing completely.

the response to incoming afferent volleys. As mentioned above, responses to afferent volleys may be almost completely blocked with greatly enhanced rhythmic slow surface negative waves characteristic of certain forms of epileptic discharge, particularly the spike-and-wave of *petit mal*, which is accompanied by a sudden brief arrest of conscious behavior or by impaired cognition. The surface negative wave of the "wave-and-spike" complex is associated with a prolonged intracellular hyperpolarization, as shown in Figure 2 (Pollen, 1964). The electrical sign of surface waves is not a reliable indication whether they are excitatory or inhibitory since deep-lying positive waves become negative on the surface, and deep-lying negative waves become surface positive, due to volume-conduction reversal of polarity.

The close relationship between surface potentials and membrane-potential changes in deep-lying nerve cells can only be demonstrated under conditions of relaxed wakefulness, drowsiness, and sleep, or with very light barbiturate anesthesia. When the animal is acutely aroused, or a given cortical area becomes actively engaged in integrative functions, with its finely organized asynchronous patterning of neuronal activity, the surface slow waves disappear. It is this pattern of *desynchronized activation* which has been shown to be related to certain "higher" brain functions. On the contrary, when the surface slow waves become exaggerated, as in certain forms of epileptic discharge or in deep slow-wave sleep, there is an increased relationship between surface waves and the firing of cells in the cortex, though this relationship may disappear under conditions which depress spike generators in cortical cells without blocking synaptic potential generation. Under these conditions, as in deep barbiturate anesthesia, the surface slow waves persist, even at increased amplitude, when spontaneous spike discharge may be almost completely absent. Steriade and coworkers have found that slow-wave sleep affects the spontaneous firing of identified cells in the cortex in different ways. Interneurons seem to fire more actively during slow-wave sleep with decreased firing in pyramidal tract cells (Steriade, 1978).

Specific Reactive States as Determinants of Unit Responses and Behavior

In most microelectrode studies of the firing of cortical cells in response to specific stimuli, or during stereotyped behavioral response, the unanesthetized animal has already been adapted to the strangeness of the experimental situation and has learned to perform certain stereotyped behavioral responses for a reward, or to avoid punishment. Microelectrode studies are then begun after states of reactivity to specific stimuli have been well established by reenforcement, and most disturbing and irrelevant responses (from the experimenter's point of view) have been abolished or attenuated by repetition without reenforcement, causing widespread habituation. This is the converse of the situation described above when habituation was produced to a specific nonreenforced stimulus.

In previous microelectrode studies of the firing of single cells in various cortical areas during the establishment of specific reactive states during delayed shock-avoidance conditioning to light flashes of different frequencies in the monkey, we found some form of response in units from all cortical areas examined before the conditioned response (CR) was well established (Jasper, Ricci, and Doane, 1958, 1960). Many of these unit responses disappeared when generalized behavioral responses also became less frequent. However, even after conditioning had been well established, there remained well-organized unit responses to the conditioning stimulus in frontal and parietal areas, as well as in sensory and motor areas, even though frequency-specific responses were observed only in occipital and parietal areas. Unit responses in frontal, motor, and sensory areas appeared to be related to the motor response since they did not contain the critical information provided by the flash frequency in the conditioning stimulus.

Parietal units responded to the reenforced flash frequency of the conditioning stimulus (CS), but not to unreenforced flash frequencies in differential conditioning. This did not occur when the animal failed to make a CR, so that cells in the parietal cortex appeared to play a critical role in the frequency discrimination involved in this form of conditioning. Most surprising was the fact that one of the earliest and most reliable electrical signs of the establishment of a CR was an anticipatory change in occipital responses to the CS during the delay period before the UCS (shock) or the CR (hand withdrawal) occurred. Even before the CR was well established, a link between the flash frequency and the delayed shock had been established, and surface visual evoked potentials were greatly reduced in amplitude, due presumably to the general alerting reaction leading up to the CR. This was associated with a marked change in occipital unit responses to the CS when the CR was established in contrast to those seen on initial trials.

It would appear that certain cells in frontal, sensory motor, parietal, and occipital cortex continued to be involved in a well-organized manner in this CR even after the more generalized irrelevant responses disappeared. Other cortical and subcortical neuronal systems were also, no doubt, involved, each with its specific contribution to make to the elaboration of this simple visuomotor CR.

One of the best examples of reactive state rather than stimulus-determined response has been provided by Evarts, who, with his colleague Tanji, observed a complete reversal in pattern of responses to the same stimulus (slight flexor movement of the hand) in cells of the motor cortex of the monkey depending upon prior instruction to "push" or "pull" signaled by red or green lights 2–4 sec before (Evarts and Tanji, 1974). This is illustrated for pyramidal-tract (PT) neurons in Figure 9 and for non-PT neurons in Figure 10, taken from their publication in *Brain Research*. The state of reactivity, push or pull, established by prior instruction with reenforcement, determined completely opposite movements and unit response from motor cortex even though the stimulus eliciting the responses was the same in both cases. The rapid reaction time of this response (20–30 msec) precluded any such thing as "voluntary control."

Another interesting example of "motor-set" determined responses to identical stimuli is provided by my colleague at the Université de Montréal, Serge Rossignol, who, following his work with Grillner in Sweden, has shown that even simple spinal reflexes can be reversed depending upon the position of the limb or upon the phase of walking movements in the spinal animal. In the following example, the crossed extensor reflex is elicited by electrical stimulation of the peroneal nerve on one side, while recording the electromyogram (EMG) from flexor and extensor muscles of both left and right hind limbs. The same stimulus elicited a crossed flexor response in the extended leg and a crossed extensor response in the flexed leg, as shown in Figure 11, soon to appear in *Brain Research* (Rossignol and Gauthier, 1979). The ipsilateral stretch reflex was not changed by alterations in limb position. This reversal in

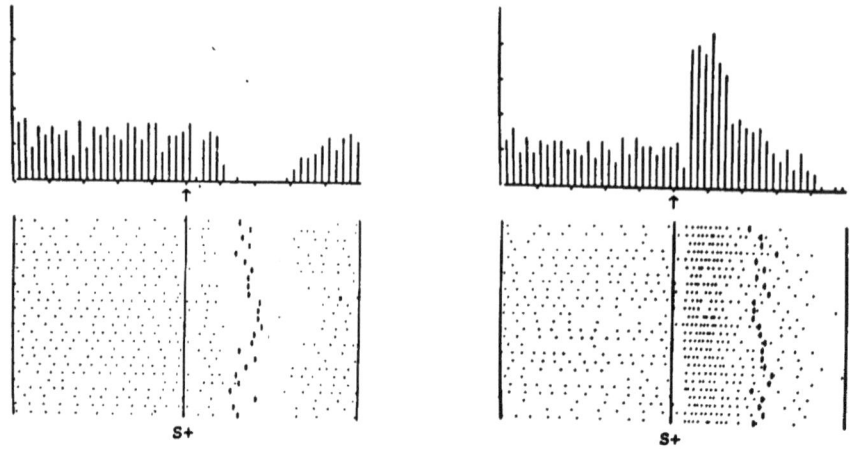

Figure 9 Records of firing of pyramidal-tract (PT) neurons in the monkey during controlled flexion and extension of the wrist. (From experiments by Evarts and Tanji, 1974.) Histograms with 20-msec bins are shown above with rasters of individual spikes shown below. The stimulus (S+) is a slight flexor perturbation of the hand in both series of records. The stimulus was preceded (2–4 sec) by a red light in records on left and by a green light for records on the right. The animal had been trained to "push" for a red light and to "pull" for a green light, although the stimulus was the same to trigger both opposite movements. The PT neuron was inhibited when instructions were to "push" and excited when prior instructions were to "pull."

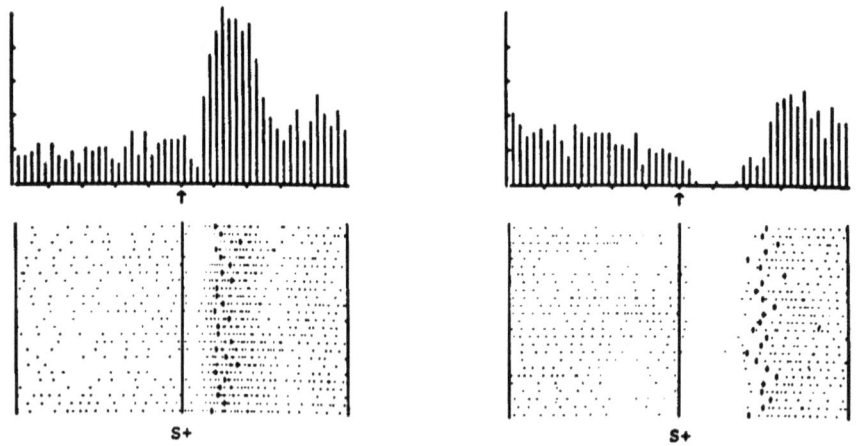

Figure 10 Record of a non-PT neuron as in Figure 9. (Recorded by Evarts and Tanji, 1974.) The same stimulus produced either excitation or inhibition depending upon prior instruction for a reactive state to be established to "push" or "pull" the bar for food reward.

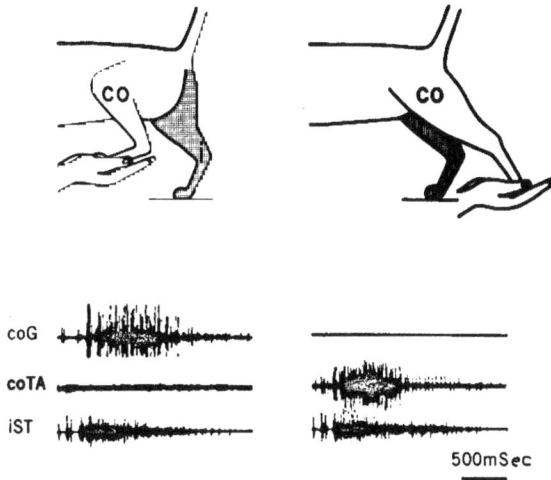

Figure 11 Electromyograms from contralateral gastrocnemius (coG), tibialis anterior (coTA), and ipsilateral semitendinosus (iST) muscles in the cat while exerting pressure on the foot pad with the leg in a flexed (left) or extended (right) position. (From experiments by Rossignol and Gauthier, 1979.) The change in position of the limb did not affect the ipsilateral stretch reflex response but it caused a complete reversal of the crossed-reflex response to the same stimulus. This was an acute spinal cat injected with Clonidine. The "reactive state" of this crossed spinal reflex was established by the position of the limb causing a reversal of the response to the same stimulus.

crossed reflexes with limb position in the spinal animal might be called "hard-wired plasticity" of synaptic connections depending upon the reactive state of spinal reflex systems.

There are many examples in the literature of modification or reversal of segmental reflexes by preprogramming of their reactive state (see also Jasper, 1975 a,b). In the studies of Evarts and Tanji cited above, they also measured the latency of the stretch reflex as seen in the EMG from flexors and extensors of the wrist. Even the shortest latency responses (12 msec) were modified by the prior instruction which had established a different reactive state for the monosynaptic stretch reflex as well as for cells of the motor cortex. They also found that motor cortical cells showed a consistent change in firing pattern within about 200 msec of the instructional stimulus (red or green light). The change in firing was sustained throughout the 1–2-sec delay period leading up to the "movement" stimulus which triggered the actual response. The nature of this response, push or pull, was determined by the anticipatory set of the system, not by the nature of the stimulus.

Lundberg and coworkers in Sweden (Lundberg, 1965; Jankowska et al., 1967a,b; Engberg, Lundberg, and Ryall, 1968a,b; Andén, Jukes, and Lundberg, 1966; Andén et al., 1966) have shown that biogenic amines (serotonin and norepinephrine) play an important role in the modulation and setting of reactive states of spinal reflexes. L-dopa administration in the spinal animal, for example, depressed short-latency spinal reflexes but caused to appear (presumably by disinhibition) a long-latency tonic multisynaptic reflex which had not been seen before. The importance of biogenic amines and other chemical substances for the establishment of reactive states in the cerebral cortex will be discussed later in this volume (see chapters by Emson and Hunt, Taylor and Stone, and Bloom). Observations that we have made in this regard will be found in the following references: Celesia and Jasper (1966); Jasper (1969); Reader, de Champlain, and Jasper (1967a,b); and Reader et al. (1979).

Conclusion

The precise nature of cortical mechanisms of higher brain function remains obscure in spite of rapid advances in our knowledge of its fine structure, interconnecting circuitry, and cell physiology during recent years. The conclusions I will draw from this brief introduction are intended to be more provocative than definitive.

1. The arrival and preliminary processing of sensory information in modality-specific cortical receiving areas may be a necessary but not a sufficient cause for perceptual awareness since such preliminary cortical processing persists during slow-wave sleep and light-barbiturate anesthesia.

2. The desynchronized activation of cortical areas is closely associated with perceptual awareness and attention to biologically significant patterns of sensory stimuli. Similar patterns of cortical electrical activity may be observed with intrinsically generated "mental" or behavioral processes such as attention, imagination, problem solving, or "voluntary" movement without concurrent sensory input.

3. Differential habituation of the generalized arousal response to a specific auditory stimulus in the cat during natural slow-wave sleep occurs without reduction of primary evoked potentials in cortical auditory receiving areas. Tonal-frequency-specific habituation persists even after removal of all auditory and somatic sensory receiving areas, including association cortex, though tonal-pattern-specific habituation was not observed following such cortical ablations. Limbic and subcortical neuronal systems, independent of primary cortical sensory systems, seem to be involved in this process, including simple modality-specific sensory discrimination during sleep.

4. The pattern of unitary responses in motor cortex, and behavioral response to a given stimulus, may be determined by preprogrammed reactive states, including alteration or reversal of segmental reflexes. There may be an important chemical component in the establishment of

these and other more complex state-dependent neuronal and behavioral reactions.

References

Adrian, E. D., and B. H. C. Matthews, 1934a. The Berger rhythm: Potential changes from the occipital lobes in man. *Brain* 57:355–384.

Adrian, E. D., and B. H. C. Matthews, 1934b. The interpretation of potential waves in the cortex. *J. Physiol.* 81: 440–471.

Andén, N.-E., M. G. M. Jukes, and A. Lundberg, 1966. The effect of DOPA on the spinal cord. 2. A pharmacological analysis. *Acta Physiol. Scand.* 67:387–397.

Andén, N.-E., M. G. M. Jukes, A. Lundberg, and L. Vyklicky, 1966. The effect of DOPA on the spinal cord. 1. Influence on transmission from primary afferents. *Acta Physiol. Scand.* 67:373–386.

Bodis-Wollner, I., A. Atkin, E. Raab, and M. Wolkstein, 1977. Visual association cortex and vision in man: Pattern-evoked occipital potentials in a blind boy. *Science* 198:629–630.

Celesia, G. G., and H. H. Jasper, 1966. Acetylcholine release from cerebral cortex in relation to state of activation. *Neurology* 16:1053–1064.

Diamond, I. T., and W. D. Neff, 1953. Role of auditory cortex in discrimination of tonal patterns. *Fed. Proc.* 12:33.

Engberg, I., A. Lundberg, and R. W. Ryall, 1968a. The effect of reserpine on transmission in the spinal cord. *Acta Physiol. Scand.* 72:115–122.

Engberg, I., A. Lundberg, and R. W. Ryall, 1968b. Is the tonic decerebrate inhibition of reflex paths mediated by monoaminergic pathways? *Acta Physiol. Scand.* 72:123–133.

Evarts, E. V., 1963. Photically evoked responses in visual cortex units during sleep and waking. *J. Neurophysiol.* 26:229–248.

Evarts, E. V., 1964. Temporal patterns of discharge in pyramidal tract neurones during sleep and waking. *J. Neurophysiol.* 27:152–171.

Evarts, E. V., 1967. Unit activity in sleep and wakefulness. In *The Neurosciences: A Study Program.* G. C. Quarton, T. Melnechuk, and F. C. Schmitt, eds. New York: The Rockefeller University Press, pp. 545–556.

Evarts, E. V., and J. Tanji, 1974. Gating of motor cortex reflexes by prior instruction. *Brain Res.* 71:479–494.

Gloor, P., (ed.), 1969. *Hans Berger on "The Electroencephalogram of Man." Supplement 28, EEG Journal.* Amsterdam: Elsevier.

Hubel, D. H., and T. N. Wiesel, 1965. Receptive fields and functional architecture in two nonstriate visual areas (18 and 19) of cat. *J. Neurophysiol.* 28:229–289.

Jankowska, E., M. G. M. Jukes, S. Lund, and A. Lundberg, 1967a. The effect of DOPA on the spinal cord. 5. Reciprocal organization of pathways transmitting excitatory action to alpha motoneurones of flexors and extensors. *Acta Physiol. Scand.* 70:369–388.

Jankowska, E., M. G. M. Jukes, S. Lund, and A. Lundberg, 1967b. The effect of DOPA on the spinal cord. 6. Half-centre organization of interneurones transmitting effects from the flexor reflex afferents. *Acta Physiol. Scand.* 70:389–402.

Jasper, H. H., 1936. Cortical excitatory state and synchronism in the control of bioelectric autonomous rhythms. *Cold Spring Harbor Symp. Quant. Biol.* 4:320–338.

Jasper, H. H., 1958. Recent advances in our understanding of ascending activities of the reticular system. In *Reticular Formation of the Brain.* International Symposium, Henry Ford Hospital, H. H. Jasper, L. D. Proctor, L. S. Knighton, W. C. Noshay, and R. T. Costello, eds. Boston: Little Brown, pp. 319–331.

Jasper, H. H., 1963. Studies of non-specific effects upon electrical responses in sensory systems. In *Progress in Brain Research, Vol. I: Brain Mechanisms.* G. Moruzzi, A. Fessard, and H. H. Jasper, eds. Amsterdam: Elsevier, pp. 272–286.

Jasper, H, H., 1966. Pathophysiological studies of brain mechanisms in different states of consciousness. In *Brain and Conscious Experience.* J. C. Eccles, ed. New York: Springer-Verlag, pp. 256–282.

Jasper, H. H., 1969. Neurochemical mediators of specific and non-specific cortical activation. In *Attention in Neurophysiology.* C. R. Evans and T. B. Mulholland, eds. London: Butterworth, pp. 377–395.

Jasper, H. H., 1975a. Structural and systems approach to central representation of motor functions: Importance of state dependent reactions. *Canad. J. Neurol. Sci.* 2:315–322.

Jasper, H. H., 1975b. Philosophy or physics—Mind or molecules. In *The Neurosciences: Paths of Discovery.* F. G. Worden, J. P. Swazey, and G. Adelman, eds. Cambridge, MA: MIT Press, pp. 403–422.

Jasper, H. H., and J. Droogleever-Fortuyn, 1946. Experimental studies on the functional anatomy of petit mal epilepsy. *Proc. Ass. Res. Nerv. Ment. Dis.* 26:272–298.

Jasper, H. H., and W. Penfield, 1949. Electrocorticograms in man: Effect of voluntary movement upon the electrical activity of the precentral gyrus. *Arch. Psychiat. Z. Neurol.* 183:163–174.

Jasper, H. H., and C. Shagass, 1941a. Conditioning the occipital alpha rhythm in man. *J. Exp. Psychol.* 28:373–388.

Jasper, H. H., and C. Shagass, 1941b. Conscious time judgments related to conditioned time intervals and voluntary control of the alpha rhythm. *J. Exp. Psychol.* 28:503–508.

Jasper, H. H., and C. Stefanis, 1965. Intracellular oscillatory rhythms in pyramidal tract neurones in the cat. *Electroenceph. Clin. Neurophysiol.* 18:541–553.

Jasper, H. H., G. F. Ricci, and B. Doane, 1958. Patterns of cortical neuronal discharge during conditioned responses in monkeys. In *The Neurological Basis of Behaviour.* Ciba Foundation Symposium, G. E. W. Wolstenholme, ed. London: Churchill, pp. 277–290.

Jasper, H. H., G. Ricci, and B. Doane, 1960. Microelectrode analysis of cortical cell discharge during avoidance conditioning in the monkey. In *Moscow Colloquium on Electroencephalography of Higher Nervous Activity. Supplement 13, EEG Journal.* H. H. Jasper and G. D. Smirnov, eds. Amsterdam: Elsevier, pp. 137–155.

Lundberg, A., 1965. Monoamines and spinal reflexes. In *Studies in Physiology.* Heidelberg: Springer-Verlag, pp. 186–190.

Morison, R. S., and E. W. Dempsey, 1942. A study of thalamo-cortical relations. *Am. J. Physiol.* 135:281–292.

Pollen, D. A., 1964. Intracellular studies of cortical neurones during thalamic induced wave and spike. *Electroenceph. Clin. Neurophysiol.* 17:398–404.

Pollen, D. A., 1968. Experimental spike and wave responses and petit mal epilepsy. *Epilepsia* 9:221–232.

Reader, T. A., J. de Champlain, and H. H. Jasper, 1979a. Interactions between biogenic amines and acetylcholine in the cerebral cortex. In *Catecholamines: Basic and Clinical Frontiers.* E. Usdin, I. J. Kopin, and J. Barchas, eds. New York: Pergamon Press, pp. 1074–1076.

Reader, T. A., J. de Champlain, and H. H. Jasper, 1979b. Participation of presynaptic and postsynaptic receptors in acetylcholine-catecholamine interactions in cerebral cortex. In *Advances in the Biosciences, Vol. 18: Presynaptic Receptors.* S. Z. Langer, K. Starke, and M. L. Dubocovich, eds. New York: Pergamon Press, pp. 363–369.

Reader, T. A., A. Ferron, L. Descarries, and H. H. Jasper, 1979. Modulatory role for biogenic amines in the cerebral cortex. Microiontophoretic studies. *Brain Res.* 160:217–229.

Rossignol, S., and L. Gauthier, 1979. An analysis of mechanisms controlling the reversal of crossed spinal reflexes. *Brain Res.* 182:31–45.

Sharpless, S., and H. H. Jasper, 1956. Habituation of the arousal reaction. *Brain* 79:655–680.

Steriade, M., 1978. Cortical long-axoned cells and putative interneurons during the sleep-waking cycle. *Behav. Brain Sci.* 3:465–514.

17 Why Are There So Many Visual Areas?

A. Cowey

ABSTRACT   It is proposed that the retina is topologically, rather than randomly, represented in the brain because it is easier to specify intracortical connections and to keep them short in a topological representation. Multiple representations, where each area is concerned mainly with one attribute of the retinal image, similarly make it possible for the excitatory and inhibitory intracortical connections involved in selective tuning to remain within a very small area of cortex concerned with a particular part of the visual field. Certain areas, farthest removed from the initial input to striate cortex, are not topologically organized, and their cells receive convergent input from other visual areas. This arrangement may minimize the number of cells and synapses involved in whatever changes underlie learned behavioral responses to visual stimuli as well as provide a possible basis for visual constancy.

In 1912 Wittenstein read a paper to the Moral Sciences Club in Cambridge. Entitled "What is Philosophy?," the talk lasted just under four minutes and showed that when the answer to a question is clear it rarely takes more than a few minutes to explain it. As this article takes substantially longer than that, the reader will correctly conclude that the answer to the question in the title is not clear. Indeed that is why it is worth discussing.

Before embarking on the answer it is necessary to state what is meant by a cortical visual area. I mean a region in which cells have visual receptive fields but do not respond, or do so unselectively, to stimuli from other modalities. This admittedly arbitrary definition therefore excludes the frontal eye fields, areas 5 and 7 of the parietal lobes, and parts of the anterior temporal lobe, where cells may have tactile or auditory as well as visual receptive fields. In many visual areas the retina is topologically represented, that is, there is a map of some portion of the visual field. However, this is not a necessary feature and one of several subsidiary questions is to ask why topological maps are sometimes present and sometimes not.

By systematically plotting the position of visual receptive fields of single neurons or clusters of neurons in the cerebral cortex, the repre-

A. COWEY Department of Experimental Psychology, University of Oxford, Oxford OX1 3UD, England

sentation of the retina has been determined in several species. There are at least 8 separate visual areas in the owl monkey (for reviews, see Allman, 1977; Kaas, 1978), and the rhesus monkey (for review, see Zeki, 1978a), 13 in the cat (Tusa, Palmer, and Rosenquist, 1975), 6 in the rat (Montero, Rojas, and Torrealba, 1973) and 4 in the mouse (Wagor and Pearlman, 1977). As only one visual area was known in monkeys in 1961 and the others have only recently been described in the more accessible parts of the occipital and temporal lobes, it will be surprising if more are not discovered. Figures 1 and 2 show the position and visuotopic arrangement of some of these areas in two species of monkey. In order to assess the significance of multiple representations of the retina it is necessary to look at the topography of each representation, at their interconnections, and at the physiological properties of their neurons, but bearing in mind that these features have yet to be fully explored in some visual areas.

The Primary Visual Area in Primates (V1)

It is known from a variety of anatomical and physiological experiments that fibers from the eye reach several terminal sites in the brain, namely: superior colliculus, suprachiasmatic nucleus, pretectal nuclei, accessory optic nuclei, nucleus of the optic tract, ventral lateral geniculate nucleus, and dorsal lateral geniculate nucleus. Only the latter projects directly to the cerebral cortex, where, in primates, the fibers terminate solely in the striate cortex (V1). In 1961 Daniel and Whitteridge electrophysiologically mapped the *entire* extent of V1 for the first time in several species of Old World monkey. The contralateral half of the visual field is represented in the striate cortex of one hemisphere but, and more important, the amount of cortex representing each degree of visual field (the magnification factor MF) declines monotonically with eccentricity from the fovea, where vision is sharpest. The latter finding is illustrated in Figure 3.

Is this very unequal cortical representation of the retina in V1 echoed in perception? Figure 3 also shows that when MF in the monkey and visual acuity in man are plotted as a function of eccentricity from the fovea, the two curves fit tolerably well, hinting that MF may be a good correlate of the perception of fine detail. Furthermore it has been shown that rhesus monkeys and squirrel monkeys, which have almost identical foveal magnification factors, have similarly close foveal acuity (Cowey and Ellis, 1967), whereas the acuity of the parafoveal retina is very different and is in accordance with the different MF for the parafovea in the two species (Cowey and Ellis, 1969). But is there more direct evidence that our brain is like this? Long ago Holmes (1918a) demonstrated that cerebral lesions of roughly comparable size produced field defects of very unequal extent depending on the location of the damage to striate cortex. For example, destruction of the occipital pole produced a small central scotoma, whereas damage in the anterior striate cortex invariably led to a much larger peripheral scotoma. However, these results were too crude to indicate MF accurately, and Cowey and Rolls (1974) therefore examined the problem in an entirely different way. The electrophysiological map is obtained in animals by stimulating the eye with light and recording the electrical activity in the brain. In a conscious human subject the reverse should be possible, that is, stimulate the brain and record the position of the illusory flash of light in the visual field. In 1968 Brindley and Lewin reported the results of implanting stimulating electrodes on the surface of the striate cortex in an attempt to recreate visual sensation in a patient blinded by glaucoma. As the patient could accurately point to the position of the apparent flash of light (phosphene) with respect to a central "fixation" point and the distance between adjacent cortical electrodes was known, Cowey and Rolls (1974) were able to calculate MF for the cortex between any given pair of electrodes by measuring the angular separation and mean eccentricity from the fovea of the corresponding phosphenes. Figure 4 shows that, as in the rhesus monkey, MF declines with eccentricity from the fovea. Moreover, the correlation between MF in this patient and normal human visual acuity at different eccentricities is impressively good (0.85). It seems safe to conclude that man has a striate cortex in which the topological representation of the retina is remarkably like that of the rhesus monkey's, and recent work shows that not only acuity but also contrast sensitivity in any part of the visual field of human subjects can be predicted from cortical MF (Rovamo, Virsu, and Näsänen, 1978; Virsu and Rovamo, 1979). The purpose of stressing this similarity in man and monkey is that it suggests that the entire visual cortex may be similarly arranged in both species and that recent discoveries with monkeys probably apply to man. One of them certainly does, as the next section shows.

Secondary Visual Areas

As in cats and rabbits, the striate cortex V1 in monkeys is adjoined by a region known as V2 in which the retina is also represented and in which the map is roughly a mirror image of that in V1 (Cowey, 1964; Allman and Kaas, 1974a). This mirror symmetry means that two points equidistant from the boundary between the two areas and lying on a line at right angles to the boundary will represent the same position on the retina. If an attempt were made to estimate MF for the cortex between two such points, the result would be absurdly high, for a large expanse of cortex would appear to represent a tiny part of the retina. Cowey and Rolls (1974) examined this possibility by selecting pairs of phosphenes corresponding to electrodes separated vertically in the human brain and which almost certainly straddled the known horizontal boundary between striate and nonstriate cortex on the medial sur-

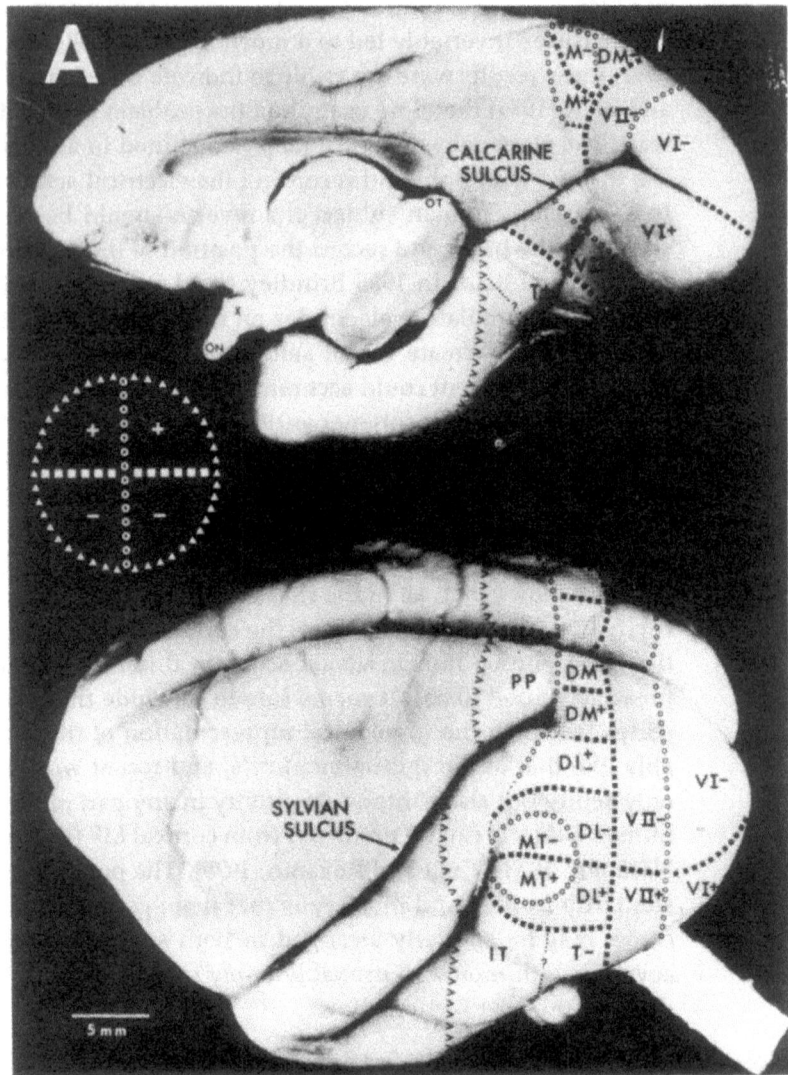

Figure 1 (A) The representation of the visual field in the cortex of the owl monkey, as seen medially (top) and dorsolaterally (bottom). The symbols from the visual field chart (center) are superimposed on the cortex. The row of V's indicates the anterior limit of known visual cortex. V1 coincides with striate cortex; D1, dorso intermediate area; DL dorsolateral crescent; IT, inferotemporal cortex; M, medial area; MT, middle temporal area; PP, posterior parietal cortex; T, tentorial area. (B) Schematic unfolding of the visual areas of the left hemisphere of the owl monkey showing the representation of the right visual field (next page). [(A) and (B) from Allman (1977), with permission.]

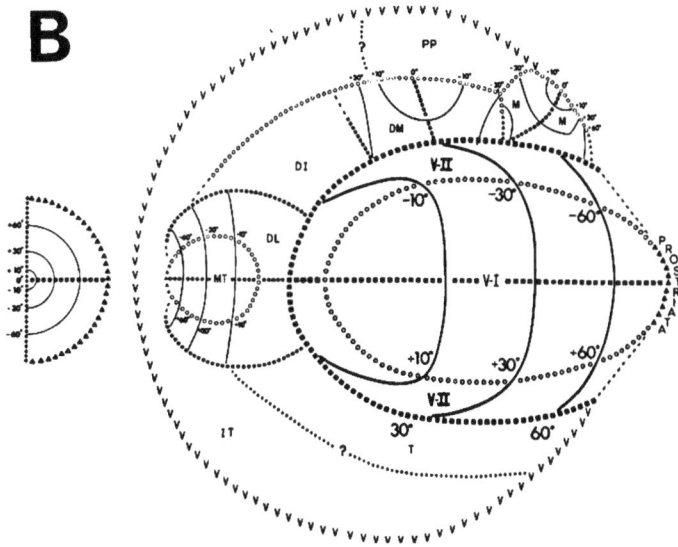

face of the occipital lobe (Figure 4). When the measurements were made in this way, the values of MF were frequently and anomalously high at all eccentricities, as would be expected if V1 and V2 are similarly arranged in the human and simian brain. Unfortunately there is no other similar evidence about the extent and arrangement of the visual cortex in man, and the remainder of the argument rests on work with monkeys.

Interconnections among Visual Areas

By making a small lesion in the cortex or injecting radioactive tracers that are transported along axons, the fibers and terminals leaving that region can be identified as they degenerate or accumulate radioactive label. For example Zeki (1978b) has shown that V1 projects to V2, V3, V4, and an area in the medial aspect of the lower bank of the superior temporal sulcus (MSTS) (Figure 2). Although the precise location of cells in V1 giving rise to all these projections is unknown, it is clear that lamina 3 projects to V2 and V3, whereas the input to MSTS arises from layer IVB and the solitary cells of Meynert in layer VI (see the chapter by Lund, this volume). So not only is there parallel processing of information from V1 to further visual areas, but different cell populations may be involved. By repeating these procedures on the secondary visual areas their interconnections and further projections have also been revealed (Zeki, 1971, 1978c,d). For example, there are two additional visual areas, V3A and LSTS, where the retina is topologically represented but whose input is not from V1. Figure 2 shows these connections and makes clear that the necessary anatomical pathways exist for both

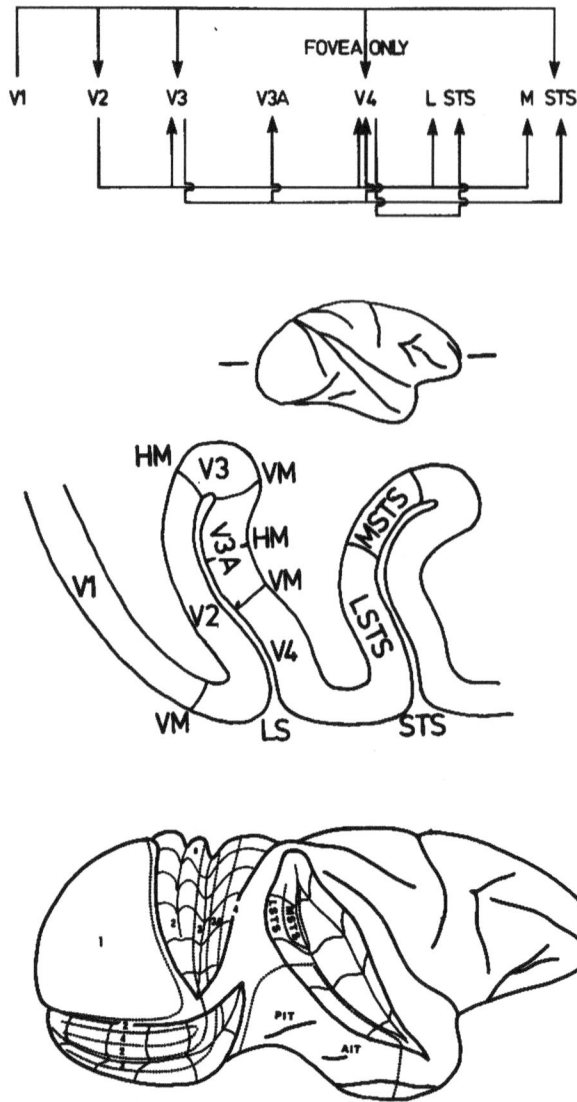

Figure 2 (Top) Demonstrated projections from visual areas described in the text. For simplicity the scheme omits subcortical projections, projections to nonvisual areas such as frontal eye fields, reciprocal connections from right to left in the diagram, and interhemispheric projections. (Middle) Horizontal section through posterior half of the right hemisphere of a rhesus monkey at the level shown in inset: LS, lunate sulcus; STS, superior temporal sulcus; LSTS and MSTS refer to lateral and medial visual areas in STS; VM, vertical meridian; HM, horizontal meridian. The precise boundary between V4 and LSTS has not been identified and may not be sharp. (Bottom) Schematic diagram of position of visual areas in occipitotemporal region of the right hemisphere of the rhesus monkey. The lunate (top) inferior occipital (lower left) and superior temporal sulci have been opened. V2 surrounds V1 but it is not clear whether V3 forms a continuous band round V2 near the foveal representation. Note that ventrally V4 is inserted like a finger into V2. This does not imply any marked discontinuity between dorsal and ventral V4, for when the sulci are closed the two ends of V4 come close together. PIT and AIT refer to posterior and anterior inferotemporal cortex. (From Cowey, 1979, with permission.)

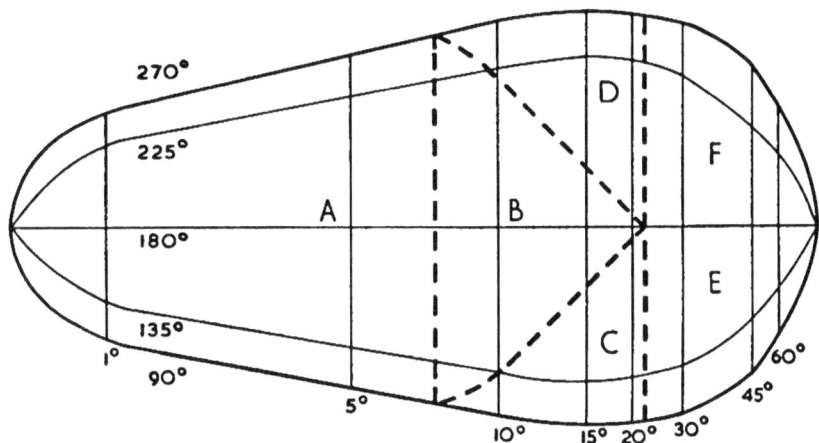

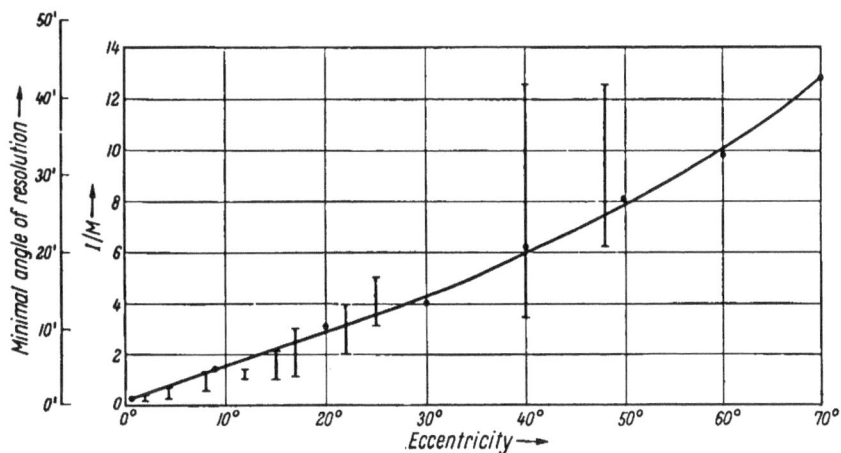

Figure 3 (Top) Flat projection of the striate cortex (V1) of the left hemisphere of the rhesus monkey to show the diminution of magnification factor with eccentricity from the foveal representation, to the left. The representation of the horizontal retinal meridian is shown at 180. The vertical meridian representation forms the periphery of the figure. Dotted lines represent the folds in the striate cortex so that F touches E, C and D touch B, and A lies on the lateral surface of the brain. (Bottom) The reciprocal of magnification factor in the rhesus monkey and minimum angle of resolution in man (solid line) in relation to eccentricity from the fovea. (Top and bottom from Whitteridge and Daniel, 1961, with permission.)

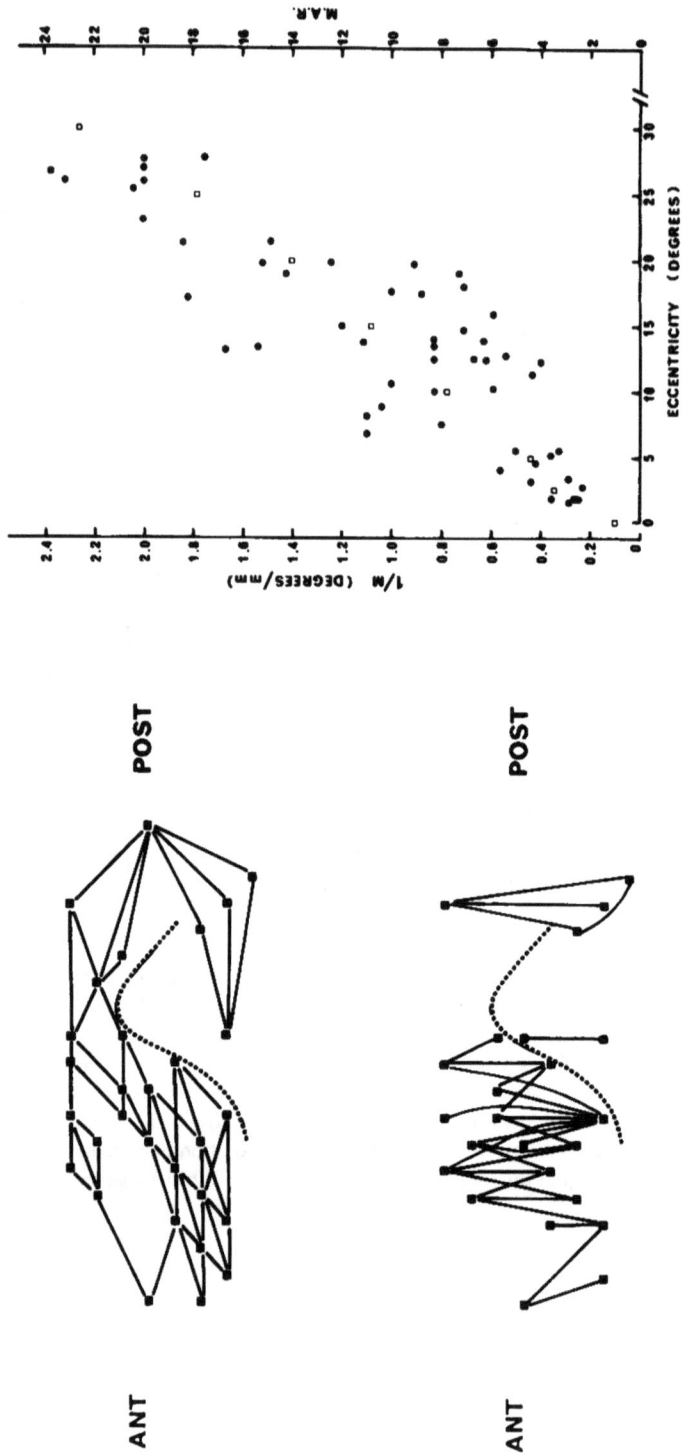

Figure 4 (Top left) Pairs of stimulating electrodes on the medial surface of the right hemisphere used to calculate magnification factor in a human subject. The dotted line shows the position of the calcarine fissure. (Right) The reciprocal of magnification factor and minimum angle of resolution as a function of eccentricity. (Bottom left) Electrode pairings used to demonstrate that adjacent to striate cortex is a second visual area in which the retinal representation is reversed. See text for details. (From Cowey and Rolls, 1974, with permission.)

parallel and serial hierarchical information processing. When lesions are made in parts of the prestriate cortex that include V3, V4, and LSTS, there is widespread terminal degeneration in the inferotemporal cortex, suggesting that information converges here from several visual areas (Kuypers et al., 1965).

Properties of Cells in the Visual Areas

The first and obvious feature of the many visual areas is their unequal size, which implies that MF probably varies widely. Although MF has rarely been precisely measured, it is known to be similar in V1 and V2 for the central parts of the retina, much smaller in MSTS, and in V3 is only one tenth its value in V1 for comparable eccentricities (Zeki, 1978c). Whatever the role of V3 and MSTS, it probably has little to do with the perception of fine detail or low contrast.

The receptive field properties of cells in V1 have been extensively investigated by Hubel and Wiesel (1968, 1977), and their classification of receptive fields into nonoriented, simple, complex, and hypercomplex is well known. There are major changes in other areas. In V2, and possibly V3, Hubel and Wiesel (1970) found that about half the cells code retinal disparity, whereas in V1 this property was absent. However, Poggio and Fischer (1977) and Fischer and Poggio (1979) have failed to confirm this sharp distinction in conscious monkeys, although it is possible that the size of the disparity tuning is much smaller in V1. According to Zeki (1978d), orientation specificity is much commoner in V2, V3, and V3A than in V4 or STS, opponent color coding is common only in V4 and LSTS, and directional selectivity is rare except in MSTS, where almost all cells show this property combined with relative indifference to exact shape and size. Finally, Gross, Rocha-Miranda, and Bender (1972) have shown that cells in the inferotemporal cortex have four properties that are not observed in other visual areas. First, their receptive fields are very large; the median size is 20° across. Second, they always include the fovea. Third, they are frequently bilateral, so that for the first time in the cortex a single cell receives information from a large part of both sides of visual space. The information from the ipsilateral field is transmitted by the forebrain commissures, for when they are severed the receptive fields become strictly contralateral again. Finally, many inferotemporal cells require a very specific but complex shape for maximum response to a 3-dimensional object, yet they show response invariance despite substantial changes in stimulus position.

Speculation

The broad picture that emerges is of a large expanse of cortex in the primate's occipital, temporal, and posterior parietal lobes, where there are multiple representations of the retina. Moreover, the various areas differ with respect to magnification factor, the precision of the retinotopic map, and the stimulus attributes that are coded by cells. Does this tell us anything about the general way in which the brain works?

A useful starting point is to consider why there is a retinotopic map at all, for it is possible to devise perceptual models which employ only random connectivity (for review, see Sutherland, 1973), and, as already mentioned, there are some visual areas where there is no map and where damage selectively and seriously impairs visual perception. The answer may be simple. One of the best-known phenomena in the retina is lateral inhibition, whereby the physiological response to luminous contrast between adjacent regions is *relatively* enhanced, that is, signals about edges are less strongly inhibited than those about other aspects of the stimulus. If lateral inhibition also occurs at the cortex and is involved in highlighting not just sharp edges but also orientation, color, disparity, spatial frequency, size, and movement, all this is most economically achieved by having a retinotopic representation so that the necessary interneurons for receptive-field tuning lie close together. If there were no map and the cells concerned with a particular part of space were scattered throughout a visual area, the average length of their interconnecting processes would have to be much longer, and the problem of specifying them during development would be enormous.

There is good evidence from a variety of sources that the vast majority of connections between cells *within* a visual area are local and that they are involved in receptive-field tuning (Cowey, 1979). For example, when a small region of V1 or V2 is damaged, degenerating excitatory and inhibitory synapses are confined to a region of only a few millimeters around the lesion (Fisken, Garey, and Powell, 1975; Colonnier and Sas, 1978). And when GABA-mediated inhibition is temporarily abolished or reduced by local application of bicuculline to the cortex, the tuning of neurons in that region to orientation, direction of movement, or ocularity is degraded (Sillito, 1977; Sillito, Patel, and Kemp, 1978). A retinotopic representation may therefore be the simplest way of organizing the local interactions that contribute to selective tuning of cells to some particular feature in a particular part of space.

A column of neurons in V1 is a thin slab of cortex wherein the initial input comes from one eye and the majority of cells are tuned to a particular orientation of a line stimulus in their receptive fields, all of which lie in the same part of the visual field. In 1974 Hubel and Wiesel introduced the idea of the hypercolumn, which is the array of columns covering either all orientations or both eyes for a particular part of space. The hypercolumn may be viewed as the basic building block of V1 and its size corresponds reasonably well with the region of degenerating terminals following very small cortical lesions. Presumably the intracortical connections between orientation columns within a hypercolumn and between adjacent hypercolumns are contributing to the orientation tuning. However, much more than orientation of a line stimulus is coded in visual cortex, and if the same anatomical substrate of numerous local intracortical connections underlies the selective tuning to contrast, spatial frequency, velocity, and direction of movement, the several forms of retinal disparity, size, and color, and if it were to take place within a single visual area, the pattern of interconnections would become immensely more complicated and their average length would grow. For example, two orientation columns concerned with adjacent parts of space might be separated by hypercolumns for several other stimulus features. The simplest solution to this problem is to have several retinotopic visual areas, each predominantly concerned with extracting information about a particular property of the retinal image, and evidence has already been given that this does occur. Although the evidence that a column of cells is concerned with a particular visual-stimulus attribute has only been systematically demonstrated for orientation in V1, there are several reports that indicate a similar columnar arrangement for distance (Hubel and Wiesel, 1970), direction (Blakemore and Pettigrew, 1970), movement (Zeki, 1974) and color (Zeki, 1973, 1977). Spatial periodicity may be an exception, for according to Maffei (1978) it changes systematically with depth in the cortex rather than with columnar shifts.

Nonretinotopic Representations

Once the visual image has been dissected and analyzed by cells in different retinotopically organized visual areas, there is no *necessity* that these cells should provide convergent input to cells in another visual area. Such an arrangement smacks of the homunculus inside the head "looking at" the combined activity of cells in a network, and, as has often been pointed out, it appears to be redundant. Yet the cells in the temporal lobe, which have enormous receptive fields and complex trigger features and which are known to receive information from several prestriate visual areas, appear to play this redundant role. There may be one reason for such an arrangement. The analysis of the visual world is only a prelude to our response to it, which includes recognition, actions, ideas, emotions, etc. And the response must vary with learning. The same stimulus may provoke different responses according to its learned significance. Whatever the structural and biochemical changes underlying learning, they would have to occur within all the visual areas in the absence of a region receiving this convergent output. The presence of such a region is therefore not surprising. This does not imply that the response properties of the cell bodies in the temporal lobe should vary according to the learned significance of a visual stimulus, and the evidence is that they do not (Rolls, Judge, and Sanghera, 1977; Ridley and Ettlinger, 1973). But at subsequent synaptic stages, for example in the substantia innominata, there is clear evidence that the response does depend on the learned significance of a complex visual stimulus (Mora, Rolls, and Burton, 1976). Of course, this is only a way of minimizing a problem in connectivity. It does not imply that any single cell can "recognize" a complex shape, and there is no physiological evidence that it can. A single cell in the temporal lobe that is maximally excited by the outline of a monkey's paw (Gross, Rocha-Miranda, and Bender, 1972) nevertheless does respond to other shapes. Its tuning is not, and cannot be, sharp enough to give an unambiguous percept, which presumably still requires the combined activity of thousands of cells.

Necessary Consequences of Having Multiple Maps

If there are several retinotopic visual areas in each of which a different aspect of the visual image is coded or emphasized, then it follows that damage restricted to one visual area ought to produce a selective disturbance of visual processing. The evidence for this is still weak, but the maps of different visual areas are so recent that the prediction has not been extensively tested. Damage to part of V1 in monkeys does produce the expected local-field defect (Cowey and Weiskrantz, 1963). Removing that part of V2 concerned with central vision seriously impairs stereoacuity without affecting global stereopsis (Cowey and Wilkinson, in preparation), whereas bilateral removal of the posterior inferotemporal region impairs global stereopsis (Cowey and Porter, 1979). Bilateral ablations anterior to V4 seriously impair pattern discrimination without affecting color discrimination (Gross, Cowey, and Manning, 1971). Fries and Zeki have shown that selective removal of V4 elevates hue discrimination thresholds but not orientation thresholds (Zeki, personal communication). Finally, the removal of the anterior inferotemporal cortex impairs visual-discrimination learning and retention for all manner of visual stimuli (Gross and Mishkin, 1977; Mishkin, 1972; Dean, 1976) as one would expect of a region receiving multiple inputs from different visual areas.

If the human brain is organized in a similar way, the same result is expected. Unfortunately accidental brain damage will rarely, if ever, be neatly confined to a single visual area, and the best one can expect is separate groups of patients with different constellations of defects (Ratcliff and Cowey, 1979). However, there is good evidence that lateroventral prestriate damage leads to achromatopsia, in which color vision is severely impaired or even abolished (Meadows, 1974; Mollon, 1979), that the position of a visual stimulus is misperceived after dorsal posterior parietal damage even though its shape and color are correctly seen (Holmes, 1918b; Cole, Schutta, and Warrington, 1962; Ratcliff and Davies-Jones, 1972), and that disturbances of stereoscopic depth perception may be selectively impaired (Rothstein and Sachs, 1972; Hamsher, 1978; Danta, Hilton, and O'Boyle, 1978). Finally, the visual impairment seen after inferotemporal damage in monkeys may be paralleled by the visual-recognition defects commonly observed after damage to the right temporal lobe in man (see reviews in Milner, 1974; Ratcliff and Cowey, 1979).

If visual perception involves the analysis of different stimulus attributes in parallel in different visual areas, the precise timing of the concurrent processes is of great importance. This is true whether or not one believes the convergent multiple input to the temporal lobe has a special significance. Any marked fluctuation in the latency and duration of responses in one area should distort what we perceive, for example by dislocating areas of different color, brightness, orientation, and movement in the visual field. Indeed, if this kind of instability were never observed, it would indicate that the general scheme outlined here is probably incorrect. However, there are many examples of such perceptual instability. Fever, toxicosis, and brain damage may all lead to what Hughlings Jackson called "positive symptoms," that is, distortion rather than attenuation of what is seen. For example, in one part of the visual field objects may seem too large or too small, contours may be doubled or further multiplied even with monocular viewing, smooth movement may appear jerky, and the position and orientation of an object may be grossly misperceived (for review, see Milner and Teuber, 1968). Gregory (1979) has also asked how the various maps maintain functional spatial registration under *normal* conditions and proposes that information about borders provided by intensity differences are of special importance. By using isoluminant figures of different color he has demonstrated highly reproducible apparent relative motion of regions of different color during systematic movement, and apparent shifts in the positions of borders when the relative luminance on either side of a border is changed across isoluminance.

Relation between Visual Areas and Anatomical Variation in Cortex

How convenient it would be if the various physiologically defined visual areas in monkeys coincided with areas distinguished from one another on purely histological criteria, for similar structural variations in the human brain would then be a good guide to our own visual areas. There is little evidence for such a neat correspondence, but the evidence against it is not nearly as strong as often supposed. Visual area 1 corresponds precisely with the striate cortex or area 17 of Brodmann. However, when the prestriate cortex was examined and divided into regions on the basis of neuronal cell-body or fiber stains, investigators disagreed about the number of different areas and the positions of the boundaries between them, and the early attempts culminated in a bleak conclusion about the uselessness of this kind of cortical geography (Lashley and Clark, 1946). Furthermore, several physiologically defined areas are known to lie within a region of apparently uniform histological appearance. For example, areas V2, V3, V3A, V4, and LSTS of Zeki (Figure 1) all lie within the region Brodmann called area 18 in the monkey. There are two rays of hope. First, where unambiguous histological boundaries do exist, they correspond to physiological boundaries (e.g., Allman and Kaas, 1971, 1974b, 1975). Second, the uniformity seen with the well-known Nissl and fiber stains may break down when more sensitive methods are used. For example, Braak (1977) has shown that the selective staining of cytoplasmic lipofuscin granules reveals that the peristriate region of the human brain is divisible into ten areas whose clear boundaries are quite invisible when using conventional stains. When this work is repeated on monkeys in which the physiologically defined areas have been mapped and marked it may be possible to say much more about the gross organization of the human occipital cortex.

Areas of Ignorance

The simplicity of the ideas presented here is deliberate and the reader will doubtless see many problems, such as the following: (1) Receptive-field properties have been extensively analyzed only for V1 in monkeys. The differences already seen in other areas may become slight on further investigation, as already described in connection with disparity tuning in V1 and V2. Furthermore, neurons in secondary visual areas that clearly respond selectively to, say, color rather than direction of movement may also prove to respond to other, as yet untested, features, like spatial frequency. (2) The functional columnar arrangement that clearly exists in V1 is not yet well demonstrated beyond V1. Nor is the local pattern of cortical interneurons known to be present, let alone concerned with, stimulus tuning. Indeed the hierarchical model of convergence on to neurons in the inferotemporal cortex suggests that a very different arrangement may exist here, and should be looked for. (3) The present description of visual areas stresses the projection from V1 onward. It is already known that some projections exist in the opposite direction to that shown in Figure 2, but their contribution to sensory analysis is unknown. We still await the results of experiments showing the effects of removing or cooling a visual area on receptive-field properties of cells in an "earlier" area. (4) Secondary visual areas receive projections from the thalamic pulvinar nucleus, but their contribution to the receptive field properties of the cells has been ignored here. As monkeys in which V1 has been totally removed can still discriminate a wide variety of patterned and colored stimuli (for review, see Butter et al., 1980), the contribution to sensory analysis of pathways other than those from V1 is presumably far from negligible. (5) The definition of a visual area as one in which the cells have only visual receptive fields may well be too divisive. Many of the arguments presented here may apply to areas containing polymodal neurons with visual receptive fields or regions containing a mixture of unimodal cells for different modalities. Furthermore, some areas that on present evidence are exclusively visual may prove to be nothing of the sort when properly analyzed with other stimuli.

Implications for Perceptual Models

It would be easy, but unjustified, to conclude that the existence of many visual areas, in which the differences in receptive field properties between areas are much greater than within any one area, is strong evidence for only that model of perceptual processing in which individual stimulus features are isolated and coded in parallel and then put together again in a hierarchical fashion to achieve a final percept. The hierarchy does seem to exist, but it may be necessary for only limited aspects of perception, for example, rapid learning or perceptual constancy or selective attention. The existence of many visual areas is not inconsistent with other schemes of information processing, for example, spatial frequency filtering. There is increasing evidence that single cells are tuned to particular spatial frequency bands (Campbell, 1978), and their other specific properties, like color or orientation preference, may be icing on the cake. Similarly the anatomical scheme outlined in this paper is compatible with the computational model of stereopsis provided by Marr and Poggio (1976) and the theory proposed by Edelman (1978) which involves dynamic interaction of neuronal groups. Such neutrality with respect to various theories of perception may seem unhelpful, if not downright weak, until it is recognized that the organization of the many visual areas tells us much more about sensory analysis than perception. Understanding the latter is still some way off.

References

Allman, J. M., 1977. Evolution of the visual system in the early primates. In *Progress in Psychobiology and Physiological Psychology*, Vol. 7. J. M. Sprague and A. N. Epstein, eds. New York: Academic Press, pp. 1–53.

Allman, J. M., and J. H. Kaas, 1971. A representation of the visual field in the caudal third of the middle temporal gyrus of the owl monkey (*Aotus trivirgatus*). *Brain Res.* 31:85–105.

Allman, J. M., and J. H. Kaas, 1974a. The organization of the second visual area (VII) in the owl monkey: A second order transformation of the visual hemifield. *Brain Res.* 76:247–265.

Allman, J. M., and J. H. Kaas, 1974b. A crescent-shaped cortical visual area surrounding the middle temporal area (MT) in the owl monkey (*Aotus trivirgatus*). *Brain Res.* 81:199–213.

Allman, J. M., and J. H. Kaas, 1975. The dorsomedial cortical visual area: A third tier area in the occipital lobe of the owl monkey (*Aotus trivirgatus*). *Brain Res.* 100:473–487.

Blakemore, C., and J. D. Pettigrew, 1970. Eye dominance in the visual cortex. *Nature* 225:426–429.

Braak, H., 1977. The pigment architecture of the human occipital lobe. *Anat. Embryol.* 150:229–250.

Brindley, G. S., and W. S. Lewin, 1968. The sensations produced by electrical stimulation of the visual cortex. *J. Physiol.* 196:479–493.

Butter, C. M., D. Kurtz, C. C. Leiby, and A. Campbell, 1980. Contrasting methods for the study of visually guided behavior in monkeys with striate cortex or superior colliculus lesions. In *Advances in the Analysis of Visual Behavior.* D. Ingle, ed. Cambridge, MA: MIT Press.

Campbell, F. W., 1978. Channels in vision: Basic aspects. In *Handbook of Sensory Physiology, Vol. VIII: Perception.* R. Held, H. W. Leibowitz, and H.-L. Teuber, eds. Berlin: Springer, pp. 3–38.

Cole, M., H. S. Schutta, and E. K. Warrington, 1962. Visual disorientation in homonymous half-fields. *Neurology* 12:257–263.

Colonnier, M., and E. Sas, 1978. An anterograde degeneration study of the tangential spread of axons in cortical areas 17 and 18 of the squirrel monkey (*Saimiri sciureus*). *J. Comp. Neurol.* 179:245–262.

Cowey, A., 1964. Projection of the retina on to striate and prestriate cortex in the squirrel monkey (*Saimiri Sciureus*). *J. Neurophysiol.* 27:366–396.

Cowey, A., 1979. Cortical maps and visual perception. The Grindley Memorial Lecture. *Quart. J. Exp. Psychol.* 31:1–17.

Cowey, A., and C. M. Ellis, 1967. Visual acuity of rhesus and squirrel monkeys. *J. Comp. Physiol. Psychol.* 64:80–84.

Cowey, A., and C. M. Ellis, 1969. The cortical representation of the retina in squirrel and rhesus monkeys and its relation to visual acuity. *Exp. Neurol.* 24:374–385.

Cowey, A., and J. Porter, 1979. Brain damage and global stereopsis. *Proc. Roy. Soc. B* 204:399–407.

Cowey, A., and E. T. Rolls, 1974. Human cortical magnification factor and its relation to visual acuity. *Exp. Brain Res.* 21:447–454.

Cowey, A., and L. Weiskrantz, 1963. A perimetric study of visual field defects in monkeys. *Quart. J. Exp. Psychol.* 15:91–115.

Daniel, P. M., and D. Whitteridge, 1961. The representation of the visual field on the cerebral cortex in monkeys. *J. Physiol.* 159:203–221.

Danta, G., R. C. Hilton, and D. J. O'Boyle, 1978. Hemisphere function and binocular depth perception. *Brain* 101:569–589.

Dean, P., 1976. Effects of inferotemporal lesions on the behavior of monkeys. *Psychol. Bull.* 83:41–71.

Edelman, G. M., 1978. Group selection and phasic reentrant signaling: A theory of higher brain function. In *The Mindful Brain*. Cambridge, MA: MIT Press, pp. 51–100.

Fischer, B. and G. F. Poggio, 1979. Depth sensitivity of binocular cortical neurons of behaving monkeys. *Proc. Roy. Soc. B* 204:409–414.

Fisken, R. A., L. J. Garey, and T. P. S. Powell, 1975. The intrinsic, association and commissural connections of area 17 of the visual cortex. *Phil. Trans. Roy. Soc. B* 272:487–536.

Gregory, R. L., 1979. Stereovision and isoluminance. *Proc. Roy. Soc. B* 204:467–476.

Gross, C. G., and M. Mishkin, 1977. The neural basis of stimulus equivalence across retinal translation. In *Lateralization in the Nervous System*. S. Harnad, R. W. Doty, L. Goldstein, J. Jaynes, and G. Krauthamer, eds. New York: Academic Press, pp. 109–122.

Gross, C. G., A. Cowey, and F. Manning, 1971. Further analysis of visual discrimination deficits following foveal prestriate and inferotemporal lesions in rhesus monkeys. *J. Comp. Physiol. Psychol.* 76:1–7.

Gross, C. G., C. E. Rocha-Miranda, and D. B. Bender, 1972. Visual properties of neurons in inferotemporal cortex of the macaque. *J. Neurophysiol.* 35:96–111.

Hamsher, K. deS., 1978. Stereopsis and unilateral brain disease. *Invest. Ophthal.* 17:336–343.

Holmes, G., 1918a. Disturbances of vision by cerebral lesions. *Brit. J. Ophthal.* 2:353–384.

Holmes, G., 1918b. Disturbance of visual orientation. *Brit. J. Ophthal.* 2:449–468, 505–516.

Hubel, D. H., and T. N. Wiesel, 1968. Receptive fields and functional architecture of monkey striate cortex. *J. Physiol.* 195:215–243.

Hubel, D. H., and T. N. Wiesel, 1970. Cells sensitive to binocular depth in area 18 of the macaque monkey cortex. *Nature* 225:41–42.

Hubel, D. H., and T. N. Wiesel, 1974. Uniformity of monkey striate cortex: A parallel relationship between field size, scatter, and magnification factor. *J. Comp. Neurol.* 158:295–306.

Hubel, D. H., and T. N. Wiesel, 1977. Functional architecture of macaque monkey visual cortex. *Proc. Roy. Soc. B* 198:1–59.

Kaas, J. H., 1978. The organization of the visual cortex in primates. In *Sensory Systems of Primates*. C. R. Noback, ed. New York: Plenum, pp. 151–179.

Kuypers, H. G. J. M., M. K. Szwarcbart, M. Mishkin, and H. Rosvold, 1965. Occipitotemporal corticocortical connections in the rhesus monkey. *Exp. Neurol.* 11:245–262.

Lashley, K. S., and G. Clark, 1946. The cytoarchitecture of the cerebral cortex of *Ateles:* A critical examination of architectonic studies. *J. Comp. Neurol.* 85:223–305.

Maffei, L., 1978. Spatial frequency channels: Neural mechanisms. In *Handbook of Sensory Physiology, Vol. VIII: Perception*. R. Held, H. W. Leibowitz, and H.-L. Teuber, eds. Berlin: Springer, pp. 39–66.

Marr, D., and T. Poggio, 1976. Cooperative computation of stereo disparity. *Science* 114:283–287.

Meadows, J. C., 1974. Disturbed perception of colours associated with localized cerebral lesions. *Brain* 97:615–632.

Milner, B., 1974. Hemispheric specialization: Scope and limits. In *The Neurosciences: Third Study Program.* F. O. Schmitt, and F. G. Worden, eds. Cambridge, MA: MIT Press, pp. 75–89.

Milner, B., and H.-L. Teuber, 1968. Alterations of perception and memory in man. In *The Analysis of Behavioral Change.* L. Weiskrantz, ed. New York: Harper and Row, pp. 268–375.

Mishkin, M., 1972. Cortical visual areas and their interactions. In *The Brain and Human Behavior.* A. G. Karczmar, and J. C. Eales, eds. Berlin: Springer, pp. 187–208.

Mollon, J. D., 1979. The theory of colour vision. In *Psychology Survey.* K. Connolly, ed. London: Allen and Unwin, pp. 128–150.

Montero, V. M., A. Rojas, and F. Torrealba, 1973. Retinotopic organization and striate peristriate visual cortex in the albino rat. *Brain Res.* 53:197–201.

Mora, F., E. T. Rolls, and M. J. Burton, 1976. Modulation during learning of the responses of neurons in the lateral hypothalamus to the sight of food. *Exp. Neurol.* 53:508–519.

Poggio, G. F., and B. Fischer, 1977. Binocular interaction and depth sensitivity in striate and prestriate cortex of behaving rhesus monkeys. *J. Neurophysiol.* 40:1392–1405.

Ratcliff, G., and A. Cowey, 1979. Disturbances of visual perception following cerebral lesions. In *Research in Psychology and Medicine*, Vol. 1. D. J. Osborne, M. M. Greeneberg, and J. R. Eiser, eds. New York: Academic Press, pp. 307–314.

Ratcliff, G., and G. A. B. Davies-Jones, 1972. Defective visual localization in focal brain wounds. *Brain* 95:49–60.

Ridley, R. M., and G. Ettlinger, 1973. Visual discrimination performance in the monkey: The activity of single cells in inferotemporal cortex. *Brain Res.* 55:179–182.

Rolls, E. T., S. J. Judge, and M. K. Sanghera, 1977. Activity of neurones in the inferotemporal cortex of the alert monkey. *Brain Res.* 130:229–238.

Rothstein, T. B., and J. G. Sacks, 1972. Defective stereopsis in lesions of the parietal lobe. *Am. J. Ophthal.* 73:281–284.

Rovamo, J., V. Virsu, and R. Näsänen, 1978. Cortical magnification factor predicts the photopic contrast sensitivity of peripheral vision. *Nature* 271:54–56.

Sillito, A. M., 1977. Inhibitory processes underlying the directional specificity of simple, complex and hypercomplex cells in the cat's visual cortex. *J. Physiol.* 271:699–720.

Sillito, A. M., H. H. Patel, and J. A. Kemp, 1978. Mechanisms influencing the ocular dominance grouping of cells in the normal visual cortex of the adult cat. *Neurosci. Lett., Suppl.* 1:383.

Sutherland, N. S., 1973. Object recognition. In *Handbook of Perception, Vol. III: Biology of Perceptual Systems*. E. C. Carterette, and M. P. Friedman, eds. New York: Academic Press, pp. 157–185.

Tusa, R. J., L. A. Palmer, and A. C. Rosenquist, 1975. The retinotopic organization of the visual cortex in the cat. *Neurosci. Abst.* 1:52.

Virsu, V., and J. Rovamo, 1979. Visual resolution, contrast sensitivity, and the cortical magnification factor. *Exp. Brain. Res.* 37:475–494.

Wagor, N. M., and A. L. Pearlman, 1977. A retinotopic map of mouse extrastriate visual cortex. *Neurosci. Abst.* 3:580.

Whitteridge, D., and P. M. Daniel, 1961: The representation of the visual field on the calcarine cortex. In *The Visual System: Neurophysiology and Psychophysics*. J. Jung and H. Kornhuber, eds. Berlin: Springer, pp. 221–227.

Zeki, S. M., 1969. Representation of central visual field in prestriate cortex of monkey. *Brain Res.* 14:271–291.

Zeki, S. M., 1971. Cortical projections from two prestriate areas in the monkey. *Brain Res.* 34:19–35.

Zeki, S. M., 1973. Colour coding in rhesus monkey prestriate cortex. *Brain Res.* 53:422–427.

Zeki, S. M., 1974. Cells responding to changing image size and disparity in the cortex of the rhesus monkey. *J. Physiol.* 242:827–841.

Zeki, S. M., 1977. Colour coding in the superior temporal sulcus of rhesus monkey visual cortex. *Proc. Roy. Soc. B* 197:195–223.

Zeki, S. M., 1978a. Functional specialization in the cortex of the rhesus monkey. *Nature* 274:423–428.

Zeki, S. M., 1978b. The cortical projections of foveal striate cortex in the rhesus monkey. *J. Physiol.* 277:227–244.

Zeki. S. M., 1978c. The third visual complex of rhesus monkey prestriate cortex. *J. Physiol.* 277:245–272.

Zeki, S. M., 1978d. Uniformity and diversity of structure and function in rhesus monkey prestriate visual cortex. *J. Physiol.* 277:273–290.

18 The Cerebral Cortex in Visual Learning and Memory, and in Interhemispheric Transfer in the Cat

Giovanni Berlucchi and James M. Sprague

ABSTRACT Understanding of the anatomical and physiological organization of the cerebral cortex is rapidly progressing, but anatomy and physiology alone cannot reveal the functional significance of cortical activity for the control of behavior. The tool of choice for this task is still the analysis of behavioral deficits following the selective removal of cortical areas. When planned and interpreted in accordance with anatomical and physiological knowledge, behavioral studies of cortical lesions are essential for constructing biologically plausible and meaningful theories of cortical and cerebral organization. In a key area of investigation, the classical visual cortex (area 17), ablation studies have failed to confirm the hypothesis that the small and exquisitely tuned receptive fields of neurons in this area are the essential substrate for contour analysis in pattern recognition. The coding of at least simple bidimensional visual patterns and shapes can and does occur outside the classical visual cortex, in other cortical areas and possibly subcortical visual centers which lack the receptive field specificity characteristic of area 17. Similarly, interhemispheric transfer of structured visual information, required for interocular transfer of pattern discriminations in split-chiasm animals, relies on callosal mechanisms independent of the classical visual cortex. Although there is little doubt that this cortex contributes significantly to visual acuity, binocular stereopsis and fusion, and probably to discrimination of textures and naturally occurring objects, we are still in need of identifying classes of visual processes that are uniquely represented in the extremely refined functional architecture of this part of the brain.

Contemporary research has gone far in providing a detailed description of the structure and function of the cerebral cortex. A cooperation of unprecedented degree between neuroanatomy, neurophysiology, and neurochemistry has resulted in the development of new methods whereby significant evidence has been marshaled on many aspects of the intrinsic organization and extrinsic connectivity of various cortical regions. Developmental studies have added information on how heredity and environment interact in the constitution of the definitive pattern of cortical organization in the individual organism, whereas comparative studies have offered evolutionary interpretations of the

GIOVANNI BERLUCCHI AND JAMES M. SPRAGUE Institute of Physiology of the University of Pisa and Laboratory of Neurophysiology, CNR, 56100 Pisa, Italy; Department of Anatomy and Institute of Neurological Sciences, University of Pennsylvania, Philadelphia, Pennsylvania 19104

cortical homologies and differences among the living mammalian species. The picture of the cerebral cortex emerging from these various analyses is one of extreme complexity, which, however, displays an extraordinary degree of order and regularity, based on general as well as local principles of structural and functional coordination.

Cytoarchitectural and myeloarchitectural subdivisions of the cortical mantle, as described by the early neuroanatomists, have been given functional meaning by the demonstration that many such anatomically identified areas have specific afferent and efferent connections, contain orderly representations of sensory receptors or motor effectors, and are made up of neurons with distinct physiological properties. Within each cortical area, in addition to the well-known segregation of cell bodies and nerve fibers into several horizontal laminae, recurrent patterns of vertical aggregations of functionally coupled neurons have been demonstrated both anatomically and physiologically. In the framework of the theory of the functional differentiation and specificity of the cortical areas, elegant models have been developed which propose that intracortical information processing and input–output operations are carried out throughout the cortex by discrete neuronal assemblies with essentially similar operating characteristics.

Considered together, all these accomplishments of modern neuroscience cannot but convey considerable aesthetic pleasure and a general sense of fulfillment; yet it is a fact that many of the most important questions about the cerebral cortex cannot be answered by purely anatomical and physiological approaches. The cortex, like the rest of the nervous system, has evolved for controlling behavior in ways appropriate to the survival of the species in its environmental niche. Since the dawn of scientific neurology, attempts at elucidating the role of the cerebral cortex in behavior have consisted chiefly in the analysis of behavioral changes following pathological or experimental lesions of the entire cortex or any of its parts. This classical method can be usefully complemented, but not supplanted, by modern electrophysiological experiments establishing correlations between behavioral responses and activities of cortical neurons in freely moving animals. When interpreted in conjunction with anatomical and physiological evidence, lesion studies of the cerebral cortex are still the tool of choice for placing our knowledge of the intrinsic cortical architecture and mechanisms in a proper context of behavioral significance.

The continuing usefulness of lesion studies for the understanding of the functional roles of the cerebral cortex is indisputable as regards man, given the limited applicability of physiological and anatomical experimentation to the human brain. But even in animals, where the techniques for direct analysis of neural activity have achieved their most significant successes, the lesion method still presents itself as a most valuable, and possibly irreplaceable, source of information on cortical functioning. As an example, one can cite the elegant anatomical and physiological demonstrations of the functional organization of the sensory and motor cortical areas into vertical arrays of neurons, along with previous lesion experiments by Sperry and coworkers. Cross-hatching lesions of the motor cortex in the monkey (Sperry, 1947), or the occipital-parietal cortex in the cat (Sperry and Miner, 1955; Sperry, Miner, and Myers, 1955), did not disrupt the capacity for skilled motor acts in the former species, nor the ability to discriminate complex visual patterns in the latter species. Since removals of those areas resulted in the loss of the corresponding behavioral abilities, the effects of the cross-hatching lesions minimized the importance of tangential connections and emphasized the role of vertical connections in the organization of these cortical areas. These results both anticipated the anatomophysiological evidence and conferred a behavioral meaning on it.

Visual Cortex and Pattern Recognition

An area of investigation in which the anatomical and physiological knowledge can be compared and contrasted with that derived from behavioral-ablation studies is that of the visual cortex. Current theories of pattern recognition rely heavily on the electrophysiological analysis of receptive fields of single neurons along the visual pathways. Concepts derived from classical psychological thinking or from information-processing theory, such as feature extraction, hierarchical organization of local analyzers, and shape coding by contour decomposition, have all been given a new status by the discovery of various classes of neuronal "detectors" of lines, edges, corners, and gratings in the visual cortex of cat, monkey, and other mammals (Hubel and Wiesel, 1959, 1962, 1965, 1968). Great popularity has been gained by the hypothesis that the identification of complex figures involves a stage in which simple, local contour constituents, such as straight-line segments, edges, or corners, are sorted out and analyzed in isolation. Other hypotheses postulate that the essential mechanism for contour processing in visual pattern perception entails a point-by-point Fourier analysis of the visual scene (Campbell, 1974; Pollen and Taylor, 1974; Maffei, 1978). The figural components selected for analysis, be they linear segments, corners, or spatial frequencies in different orientations and locations, are thought to be specifically encoded by single neurons in the classical or primary visual cortex, that is, in that part of the cortex which receives the projection of the main thalamic target of the retinofugal fibers, the dorsal lateral geniculate nucleus (LGNd). This is the region of the cortex which contains neurons that are selectively responsive to various parameters of visual stimulation such as orientation, size, direction of movement, spatial frequency, and so on.

However, if visual pattern recognition does indeed require a coding process whose primitives are uniquely represented in the primary visual cortex, pattern blindness should be the inevitable consequence of the removal of this part of the cortex. This is obviously a truism, which nonetheless is often totally ignored by the proponents of theories of vision based on the receptive-field organization of single cortical neurons.

There is now ample evidence that after total removal of primary visual cortex rats (Spear and Barbas, 1975; Hughes, 1977), squirrels (LeVey, Harris, and Jane, 1973), rabbits (Moore and Murphy, 1976), tree shrews (Killackey, Snyder, and Diamond, 1971), and cats (Spear and Braun, 1969; Doty, 1971; Sprague et al., 1977) are by no means pattern blind. Ablations or lesions of the comparable visual cortex have much more deleterious effects on pattern vision in prosimians (Atencio, Diamond, and Ward, 1975) and in primates including man (Brindley, Gautier-Smith, and Lewin, 1969; Humphrey, 1974), but even in these species discrimination of visual patterns can be successful, after visual decortication, under special conditions of training and/or testing (Atencio, Diamond, and Ward, 1975; Pasik and Pasik, 1971; Schilder, Pasik, and Pasik, 1972; Weiskrantz et al., 1974).

The surprising visual capacities of animals lacking the primary visual cortex can hardly be ascribed to subcortical mechanisms alone since the expanse of cerebral cortex receiving retinal information extends well beyond the boundaries of the classical, geniculate-recipient visual cortex. The "extrageniculate" or "extrastriate" cortical areas, which are spared by an ablation of the primary visual cortex, are reached by visual information transmitted via the midbrain (pretectum-superior colliculus) and the pulvinar nuclear complex of the thalamus (Diamond and Hall, 1969; Jones, 1974; Diamond, 1976).

There are two possibilities for reconciling these findings with the hypothesis of a unique role of the neurons in primary visual cortex for pattern recognition. The first possibility is that following ablation of the visual cortex there occurs a reorganization of the remaining visual systems, so that neurons in these systems acquire receptive-field properties similar to those of neurons in the ablated area. Where this possibility has been tested directly, no evidence has been obtained for a reorganization of visual areas or centers with either time or training. Thus, in cats with extensive visual-cortex ablations, receptive-field properties of neurons in remaining visual cortical areas become even less specific than they are in the intact brain, and no change in their organization becomes apparent with the recovery of the behavioral ability for pattern discriminations (Spear and Baumann, 1979a). Similarly, the organization of receptive fields of neurons in the superior colliculus is partially disrupted by removal of the visual cortex (Wickelgren and Sterling, 1969; Rosenquist and Palmer, 1971), and even very prolonged survival with the associated visual experience fails to bring about significant receptive-field reorganization (Stein and Magalhaes-Castro, 1975; Mize and Murphy, 1976). The second possibility is that visually decorticated animals learn to discriminate visual patterns by developing new perceptual strategies that, for example, utilize partial flux cues rather than total stimulus configuration. Although this possibility is difficult to test thoroughly, particularly in view of the fact that even intact animals may use local flux information for discriminating complex figures (see, e.g., Buchtel, 1969; Winans, 1971), substantial evidence that total configuration of visual patterns can be perceived by animals lacking the visual cortex has been obtained with tests of generalization, transposition, figural completion, figure–ground reversal, and so on (see, e.g., Doty, 1971; Schilder, Pasik, and Pasik, 1972; Ritchie, Meyer, and Meyer, 1976; Hughes, 1980).

Thus, neither receptive-field reorganization nor changes in the strategies for sampling visual information can satisfactorily account for the capacity to discriminate patterns after removal of the primary visual cortex. Therefore, it seems likely that neuronal systems lying outside the primary visual cortex must to some extent be capable of encoding visual shape. Such a capability may be partly intrinsic in extrastriate visual systems, and partly acquired after the removal of the visual cortex through a process of neural reorganization which, for reasons given above, does not affect receptive-field properties of single neurons. Following ablation of the visual cortex, the immediate retention of preoperatively learned pattern discriminations would unequivocally show the intrinsic role of the remaining visual systems in pattern recognition; whereas the loss of preoperatively learned discriminations, and their reacquisition through training, would be compatible with the hypothesis of an adaptive rearrangement of neural substrates for vision.

We have recently performed experiments (in collaboration with A. Antonini) that have produced results bearing on this point. These experiments were carried out on the cat, a species whose visual pathways differ from those of other mammals in several important respects, particularly in that the projections from LGNd are not restricted to area 17, but extend to areas 18 and 19 and to several cortical areas lying in suprasylvian gyri and sulci (see Figure 1). However, a joint ablation of areas 17 and 18 in the cat may be compared to the extirpation of the exclusive geniculate-recipient cortical area of other mammals to the extent that (1) the main laminae of LGNd (A and A1) of the cat show complete retrograde degeneration after a 17–18 removal (Doty, 1971; Sprague et al., 1977), (2) neurons in areas 17 and 18 have highly specific receptive-field properties, compatible with the hypothesis that these neurons function as simple feature analyzers in pattern recognition (Hubel and Wiesel, 1959, 1962, 1965), (3) the specificity of receptive-field properties of neurons in other visual areas or centers is to some degree dependent on the integrity of area 17 (see, e.g., Rosenquist and Palmer, 1971; Spear and Baumann, 1979b), suggesting that this area is an important node in a serial processing system, (4) the input from one functional population of ganglion cells of the retina (the X system, having the best capability to resolve high spatial frequencies) is relayed by the LGNd solely to area

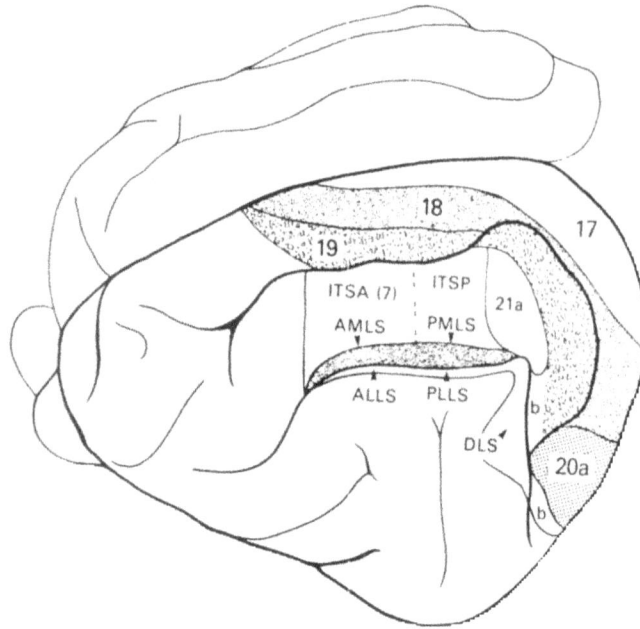

Figure 1 Visual cortical areas in the cat. From Sprague et al., 1977; based on work by Palmer, Rosenquist, and Tusa (1978); Tusa, Palmer, and Rosenquist (1978); and Tusa, Rosenquist, and Palmer (1979).

17 (see Rodieck, 1979); compared to other visual areas, area 17 has the most accurate retinotopic representation and the highest magnification factor for the area centralis of the retina (Tusa, Palmer, and Rosenquist, 1978; Tusa, Rosenquist, and Palmer, 1979; Palmer, Rosenquist, and Tusa, 1978).

The considerable capacities for spatial vision which survive ablation of areas 17 and 18 in cats have been explained on the basis of the intact projections from the nucleus interlaminaris medialis (NIM) and the C laminae of LGNd to 19 and to the lateral suprasylvian areas, as well as on the basis of the tectothalamic system relaying visual information to these same areas from the pretectum-superior colliculus via the pulvinar nuclei (see e.g., Sprague et al., 1977).

Our study, however, was planned to test whether these systems can encode visual shape independent of areas 17 and 18, so that no reorganization should be required for pattern discrimination following the removal of the latter areas.

Normal cats were trained on a simple brightness discrimination and on 7 pattern discriminations in a fixed order, as specified in Figure 2. On each discrimination each cat was trained to a criterion of two consecutive daily sessions in which 90% or more correct responses were achieved. Each daily training session consisted of 40 trials in a two-choice discrimination apparatus. Running in the apparatus was moti-

G. Berlucchi and J. M. Sprague

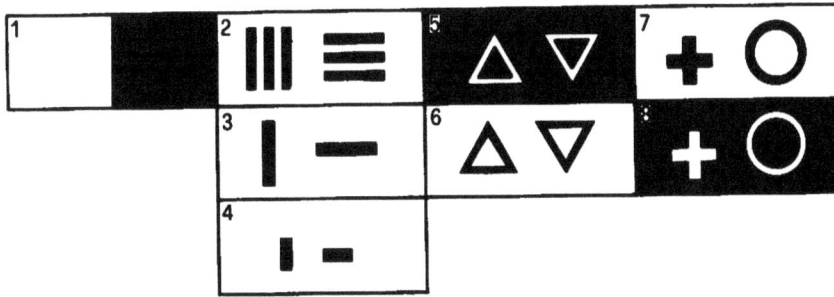

Figure 2 Pairs of stimuli used for discrimination. The 8 discriminations were learned successively from 1 to 8. In each pair, except the light–dark discrimination, the positive stimulus is on the left. In the light–dark discrimination the luminance of the light stimulus was 39 cd m^{-2}, that of the dark stimulus was 0.3 cd m^{-2}. In the pattern discrimination, the size of the stimuli is reduced to about 1/10 of the real stimuli.

vated by a 24-hr food deprivation and by food reward. Since a correction procedure was used, errors were punished by the delay in obtaining the food reinforcement and by collision against the locked, incorrect response panel. After learning the sequence of 8 discriminations, each cat underwent a preoperative retention test on each discrimination, which required the performance of a significant sequence of correct responses. A significant sequence or run is defined as a string of correct responses, including at most one error, having a chance probability of occurrence equal to or less than one in a hundred (Runnels, Thompson, and Runnels, 1968). The 8 discriminations were presented in the retention test in a random order, usually different from that used during training. After the performance of a significant run on a given discrimination, the next discrimination was immediately presented until the series was completed. Since the first significant run with a 0.01 chance probability of occurrence is 7 correct responses in the first 7 trials, a cat making no errors in the retention test could complete it in 56 trials. Following completion of the retention tests, cats were operated under Nembutal anesthesia; lesion of various areas of cortex was done by subpial suction or simply by removing the pia immediately over the areas to be destroyed. Retesting for the retention of preoperatively learned discriminations was carried out starting 14 days after the operation; during this interval the animals were housed in individual cages and were not given any further experience with the discrimination apparatus. Postoperative retesting followed the same paradigm as preoperative testing for retention; if a significant run was not performed within 200 trials, testing on that discrimination was discontinued and the next discrimination was presented to the animal. This upper limit for postoperative retention testing was adopted because during initial learning the first significant run was performed within this limit.

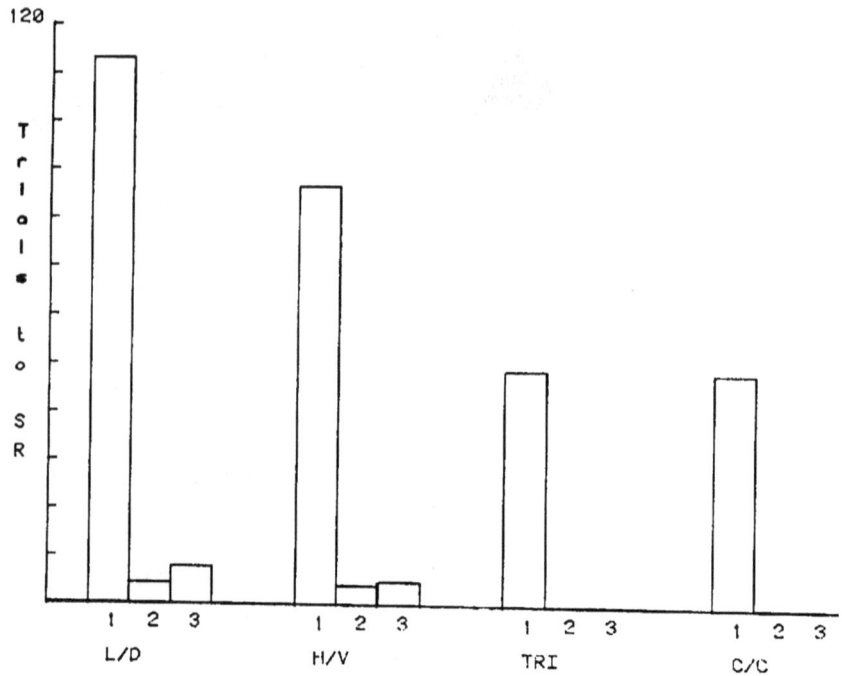

Figure 3 Mean learning, preoperative and postoperative retention scores of four cats with bilateral lesions of area 17 or areas 17 and 18. L/D = light–dark discrimination; H/V = horizontal–vertical discriminations; TRI = erect triangle–inverted triangle discriminations; C/C = cross–circle discriminations. For each discrimination or group of discriminations, each bar indicates the mean number of trials to first significant run for original learning (1), preoperative retention (2), and postoperative retention. Note perfect postoperative retention.

The 7 pattern and form discriminations (see Figure 2) were divided into three groups: (1) horizontal–vertical, including the gratings, the long bars, and the short bars; (2) upright triangle–inverted triangle, including the white triangles on a black background and the black triangles on a white background; (3) cross–circle, similarly including white stimuli on black and vice versa. This grouping was suggested both by an a priori consideration of the stimulus configurations, and by an obvious tendency of the animals to generalize from one problem to the next within each group of problems during initial learning. Each animal provided three scores for each group of discriminations, each score being the mean across problems in that group for, respectively, the number of trials to first significant run upon initial learning, number of trials to first significant run during the normal retention test, and number of trials to first significant run during the postoperative test. In addition to the scores for the pattern discriminations, similar scores for the brightness discriminations were considered.

The results are summarized in Figures 3–5. (1) The animals with a 17–18 lesion showed a perfect retention, that is, their postoperative re-

G. Berlucchi and J. M. Sprague

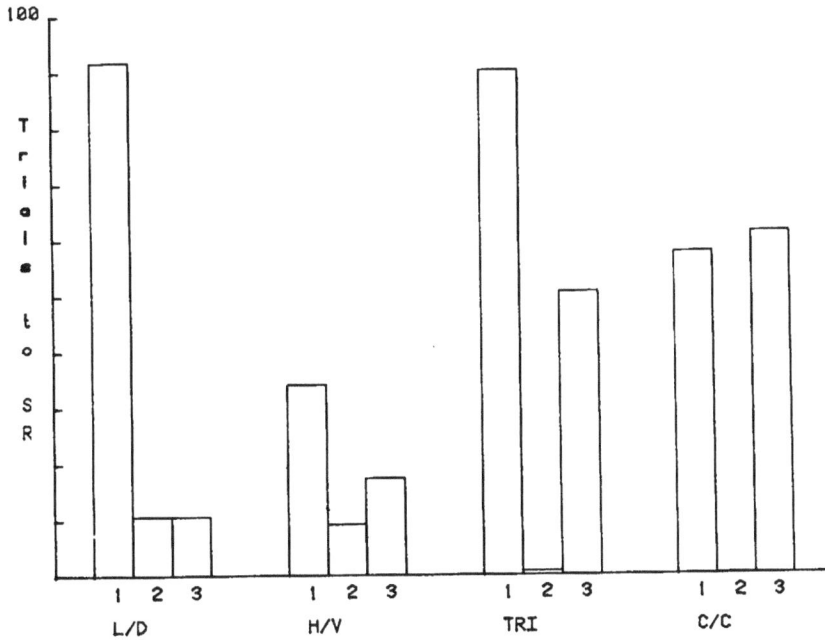

Figure 4 Mean learning, preoperative and postoperative retention scores of five cats with bilateral lesions of areas 17, 18, and 19. Conventions and indications as in Figure 3. Postoperatively these cats were generally unable to perform a significant run within 200 trials (see text).

tention scores were indistinguishable from their preoperative retention scores (Figure 3). Even on the very first postoperative discrimination, performance was usually errorless. (2) Animals with a combined lesion of areas 17, 18, and 19 were markedly deficient in retention of both brightness and pattern discriminations. Only two out of five animals could perform a significant run on the brightness problem and on the gratings within 200 trials. Otherwise, chance performances were consistently observed (Figure 4). (3) In animals with suprasylvian lesions sparing 17 and 18, postoperative retention was significantly worse than preoperative retention on both brightness and pattern discriminations. However, all cats could perform a significant run on all problems within 200 trials. On the brightness problem postoperative retention showed some savings with respect to original learning, but on the pattern problems the number of trials necessary to perform a significant run was not significantly different from the corresponding score on original learning (Figure 5). (4) Suprasylvian lesions undercutting areas 17, 18, and 19 had devastating effects on retention; no such animal was able to perform above chance in either the brightness or the pattern problems.

These results suggest a few straightforward conclusions. Specifically, perfect and immediate retention was seen only in the animals with le-

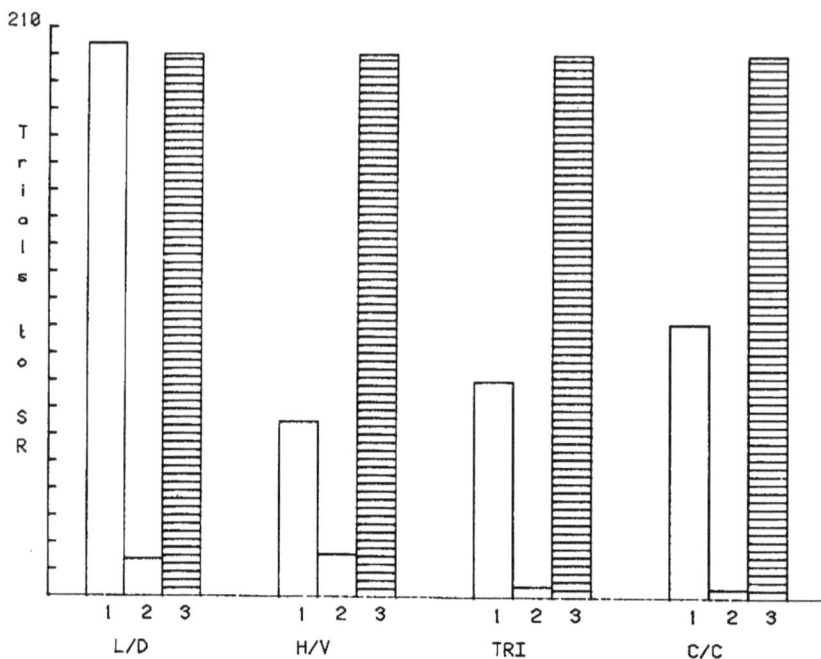

Figure 5 Mean learning, preoperative and postoperative retention scores of four cats with bilateral lesions of areas 7, 21, PMLS, and part of area 19 (see Figure 1). Conventions and indications as in Figure 3. Postoperatively these animals were able to perform a significant run within 200 trials, but on the pattern discriminations there were no significant savings with respect to initial learning.

sions limited to areas 17 and 18, a finding clearly unpredictable on the hypothesis that in the normal brain the processing of spatially patterned visual input is a unique function of neurons in these areas. The fact that cats with 17–18 lesions behaved as if they immediately recognized the discriminative stimuli can hardly be accounted for by reorganization and readaptation mechanisms, given the brevity of the time interval between the operation and the retention test, and the absence of any practice with the discriminanda during such a convalescent period. It also seems unlikely that their successful retention might have depended on the utilization of local flux cues in the pattern discriminations since this strategy would have caused considerable difficulties with the figure–ground flux reversals in the triangle and cross–circle discriminations, and yet no such difficulties were ever observed in these cats. On the other hand, retention deficits were found after suprasylvian ablations which spared areas 17–18 and much of 19. This finding is supportive of previous work and of the general concept that these parts of the brain are involved in pattern discrimination (Berlucchi et al., 1972; Hara et al., 1974; Cornwell, Warren, and Nonneman, 1976; Sprague et al., 1977; Campbell, 1978). The existence of such clear deficits after removal of a limited portion of the cortex disposes at once

G. Berlucchi and J. M. Sprague

of the frequently voiced objection that the pattern discriminations used in ablation experiments are often so crude as to be performed with subcortical centers alone. The possibility that a more prolonged retraining would have brought about a recovery of the capacity for visual discrimination in animals with retention losses (see, e.g., Spear and Baumann, 1979a) is also of no immediate concern here since the important point is the contrast between the presence of retention deficits with some cortical lesions and their absence with others.

In describing the physiological and behavioral effects of early monocular deprivation in cats, Hubel and Wiesel (1970) and Dews and Wiesel (1970) reported that occlusion of the normal eye produced some recovery of pattern vision in the initially deprived eye; this behavioral recovery, however, was not paralleled by a physiological normalization of areas 17 and 18, whose neurons remained by and large inexcitable by the initially deprived eye. These authors suggested the function of less damaged parts of the visual system as one possible physiological mechanism for the behavioral recovery. Spear and Ganz (1975) studied the effects of cortical lesions on the retention of pattern discriminations both in normal cats and in cats submitted to a monocular deprivation during the initial 14.5–17 weeks of life. The latter cats had been able to learn pattern discriminations with the deprived eye only after prolonged training. Retention of pattern discriminations was disrupted in both normal and monocularly deprived cats by a combined lesion of areas 17, 18, and 19, in agreement with our results reported above. Partial lesions of area 17 (monocular segment) or combined lesions of areas 18 and 19, plus the central visual field projection of area 17, were compatible with the retention or the reacquisition of pattern discrimination. Sprague, Levy, and DiBerardino (unpublished) removed all of area 17 and most of 18 in cats raised with a monocular deprivation for 17 and 18 months. Pattern discriminations learned with the deprived eye before the cortical ablation were perfectly retained after such ablation. These results indicate that the ability to discriminate patterns in the monocularly deprived, as in the normal cat, does not depend on areas 17 and 18. Hirsch (1972) studied visual discrimination in cats whose eyes had been exclusively exposed, during a critical postnatal period, one to vertical lines and the other to horizontal lines. This procedure results in the selective representation in separate sets of neurons in areas 17 and 18 of these two orientations alone, rather than the full complement seen in the normal cat. The capacities for discrimination of line orientations in these cats were, however, so broad that Hirsch (1972) concluded that the nervous system can encode stimulus features not corresponding to any of the available receptive fields.

While concurring with these earlier suggestions, we feel our present results justify a more extreme conclusion, namely, that the encoding of simple visual patterns and shapes in the cat's nervous system is performed outside of areas 17 and 18 even in the presence of these areas.

The X system of retinal ganglion cells with good resolution for high spatial frequencies and the exquisitely tuned receptive fields of areas 17 and 18 are probably involved in visual functions other than the analysis of contours by decomposition into spatial frequencies or sloped lines. These systems are likely to add considerable fineness and acuity to the system for **shape coding** which operates outside areas 17 and 18 (Berkley and Sprague, 1979, 1980), but their primary functions are in all likelihood still undiscovered.

Future attempts to solve this problem should take into account the discrimination of textures and 3-dimensional objects and the extraction of visual figures from a background of noise. On the other hand, computer models simulating neural systems for recognition of simple visual patterns should rely on receptive-field properties of neurons in visual centers and areas of the extrageniculate system, rather than those of areas 17 and 18. In this connection, we still lack information about the properties of receptive fields in area 19 after removal of 17 and 18. Considering the devastating effect on retention of visual discriminations by adding a 19 lesion to a 17–18 ablation in these experiments and those of others (see, e.g., Doty, 1971; Wood, Spear, and Braun, 1974; Spear and Baumann, 1979a), this information may be crucial for our understanding of the relations between receptive-field properties and pattern discrimination.

Visual Cortex and Interocular and Interhemispheric Transfer of Pattern Discriminations

Studies of interocular equivalence in the cat support the idea that neural mechanisms residing outside areas 17 and 18 can mediate pattern discriminations. After learning a pattern discrimination using one eye only, normal cats transfer the discrimination at a high level to the other eye. Granting that this capacity for interocular transfer depends on the convergence of signals from the two eyes onto one or more sets of cerebral neurons, it is only logical to look at 17 and 18, with their neurons receiving spatially matched information from both eyes (Hubel and Wiesel, 1962, 1965; Bishop, 1973), as a likely neural site for the mediation of interocular transfer. Yet in several studies, successful interocular transfer of pattern discriminations has been reported in cats with an almost complete lack of binocular neurons in areas 17 and 18 due to various forms of abnormal visual experience. More specifically, early monocular or binocular visual deprivation (Ganz, Hirsch, and Tieman, 1972; von Grünau and Singer, 1979), several types of strabismus (Sherman, 1970; Buchtel, Berlucchi, and Mascetti, 1975; Peck et al., 1979), and artificial restrictions and separations of the inputs to the two eyes (Hirsch, 1972) are all conditions that interfere with the convergence of information onto single neurons in areas 17 and 18, but not with the capacity for interocular transfer of pattern discriminations. In agreement with these findings, the removal of areas 17 and 18 does not abolish interocular transfer (Berlucchi et al., 1978). All this evidence suggests that there exist binocular neurons in areas or centers other than 17–18 mediating interocular transfer, and that the capacity of these neurons for integrating binocular information is independent of 17 and 18.

Gordon and Presson (1977) have provided evidence that alternating monocular occlusion suppresses convergence of binocular information on 17–18 neurons but not on neurons in the superior colliculus. Similarly, binocular interactions are less impaired in the superior colliculus than in areas 17 and 18 of strabismic cats (Gordon and Gummow, 1975). Although the influence of alternating monocular occlusion and strabismus on extrastriate cortical areas is not known, binocularity in these areas might be implemented by projections to the cortex from the superior colliculus via the pulvinar nuclei. Alternatively, binocularity may be built up primarily in extrastriate visual areas, and then conveyed to the superior colliculus via corticotectal projections.

The idea that binocular interactions in areas 17 and 18 may differ from binocular interactions in other centers and areas both in function and in resistance to disruptive influences is supported by experiments on Siamese cats. The retinas of Siamese cats project almost exclusively in a crossed fashion because of a genetic abnormality (see Shatz, 1977a). Binocular interactions in cortical areas can in principle be brought about by callosal connections conveying to each hemisphere the "missing" input from the ipsilateral eye. However, the callosal fibers uniting areas 17–18 on the two sides do not seem to be able to excite their target neurons in Siamese cats, possibly because they link up cortical points related to noncorresponding portions of the visual field, and their synaptic action is functionally suppressed (see Shatz, 1977b,c). As a result, 17–18 neurons in Siamese cats are almost exclusively driven from the contralateral eye. Yet these cats show good interocular transfer of pattern discriminations (Marzi, Simoni, and Di Stefano, 1976) and presumably must have binocularly driven neurons in other parts of their brain. Marzi et al. (1979) have shown that there is a high number of binocularly driven cells in the lateral suprasylvian area (medial bank of SS sulcus, PMLS of Palmer, Rosenquist, and Tusa, 1978) of Siamese cats, and that the input from the ipsilateral eye to these neurons is dependent on the integrity of the corpus callosum. The genetic abnormalities of the visual pathways that disrupt binocular interactions in areas 17 and 18 are therefore compatible with the persistence of a binocular process in other cortical areas, which presumably are involved in behavioral interocular equivalence.

Cortical and subcortical mechanisms of interocular equivalence have also been studied in split-chiasm cats, that is, in cats submitted to a restriction of the input from each eye to the ipsilateral hemisphere by a midsagittal section of the optic chiasm. Interocular transfer of pattern discriminations is still possible in these preparations (Myers, 1955;

Sperry, 1961), provided the corpus callosum, and more specifically its posterior portion, is intact (Myers, 1956; Sperry, Stamm, and Miner, 1956; Myers, 1959). Binocularly driven neurons can still be found in areas 17 and 18 of split-chiasm cats, because of the convergence onto these neurons of a direct visual input from the ipsilateral eye and an indirect visual input from the contralateral eye via the corpus callosum (Berlucchi and Rizzolatti, 1968; Berlucchi, 1972). Although it seemed reasonable that these callosum-dependent binocular interactions in areas 17 and 18 could be essential for behavioral interocular transfer, it was shown that transfer survives the removal of the sites of origin and termination of callosal fibers in areas 17 and 18 (Berlucchi et al., 1978). Interocular transfer of pattern discriminations in split-chiasm cats can be interfered with, however, by lesions of cortical areas in the middle and posterior suprasylvian gyri, leaving areas 17 and 18 intact (Berlucchi et al., 1979) (see Figure 6). A bilateral removal of areas 7, 21, and portions of area 19 and the lateral suprasylvian area (LSA) results in a deficit in interocular transfer comparable to that produced by a callosal section (Figure 7). These findings implicate the callosal connections of cortical areas other than 17 and 18 in interocular and interhemispheric transfer of pattern and form discriminations, in agreement with studies on monkeys showing a critical role of a cortical region remote from striate cortex, the inferotemporal cortex, for interhemispheric transfer (Seacord, Gross, and Mishkin, 1979). In both cat and monkey, the callosal connections mediating transfer are not limited to the representation of the vertical meridian. It has been suggested by these studies that stimulus equivalence between the two eyes of a split-chiasm cat or monkey is made possible by neurons with large receptive fields extending across the vertical meridian of the visual field. Thus the input from the contralateral eye–ipsilateral visual field is conveyed to these neurons by the corpus callosum in the cat, and by both corpus callosum and anterior commissure in the monkey (Seacord, Gross, and Mishkin, 1979). In the cat, neurons with these receptive-field characteristics are present in many extrastriate cortical areas (see review in Berlucchi et al., 1979) and at least in the lateral suprasylvian area their responsiveness to

Figure 6 (Top): Surface view of the brains of split-chiasm cats with unilateral suprasylvian lesions. (Bottom) Mean performances using the eye on the intact and on the injured side in original learning and interocular transfer for split-chiasm cats with unilateral suprasylvian lesions (upper part) and split-chiasm cats with unilateral 17–18–19 lesions. Interocular transfer is assessed on the basis of three measures: errors on first 40 trials; number of trials to final criterion (two consecutive 40-trial sessions with at least 90% correct responses); number of trials to first significant run (first sequence of correct responses, allowing for at most one error, having a chance probability of occurrence equal to or lower than 0.01). Note absence of transfer to the injured side in cats with suprasylvian lesions and presence of transfer in both directions in the cats with 17–18–19 lesions. (From Berlucchi et al., 1979.)

G. Berlucchi and J. M. Sprague

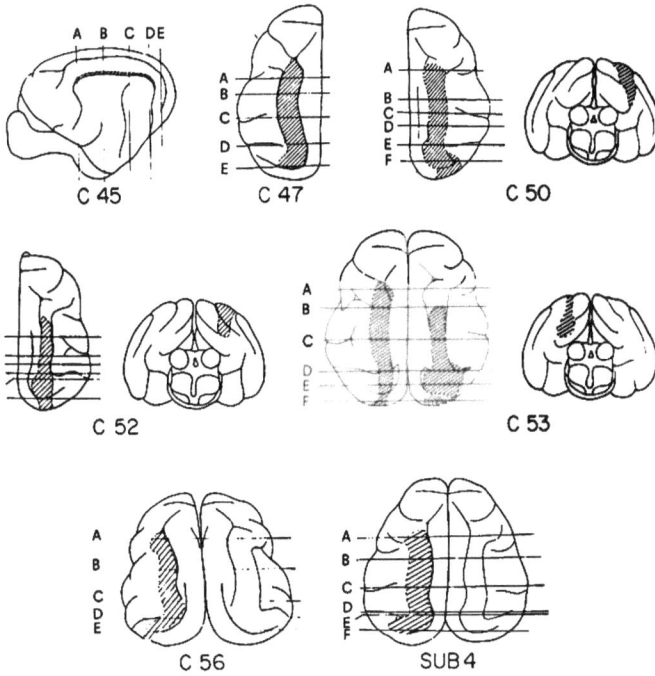

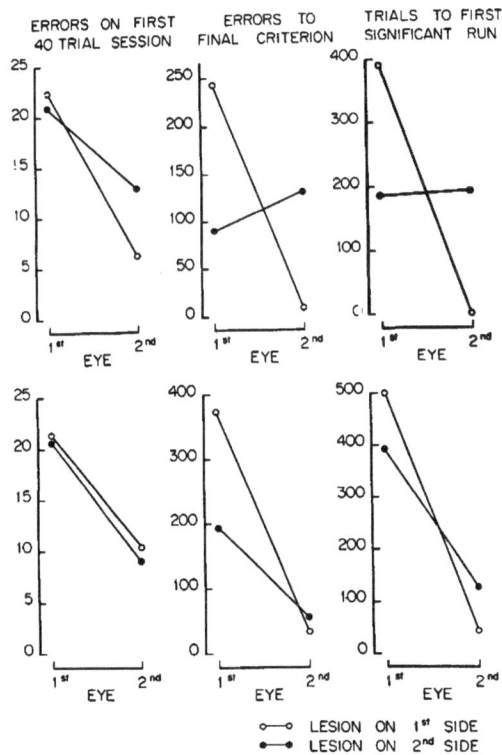

Cortical Mechanisms of Visual Learning and Transfer

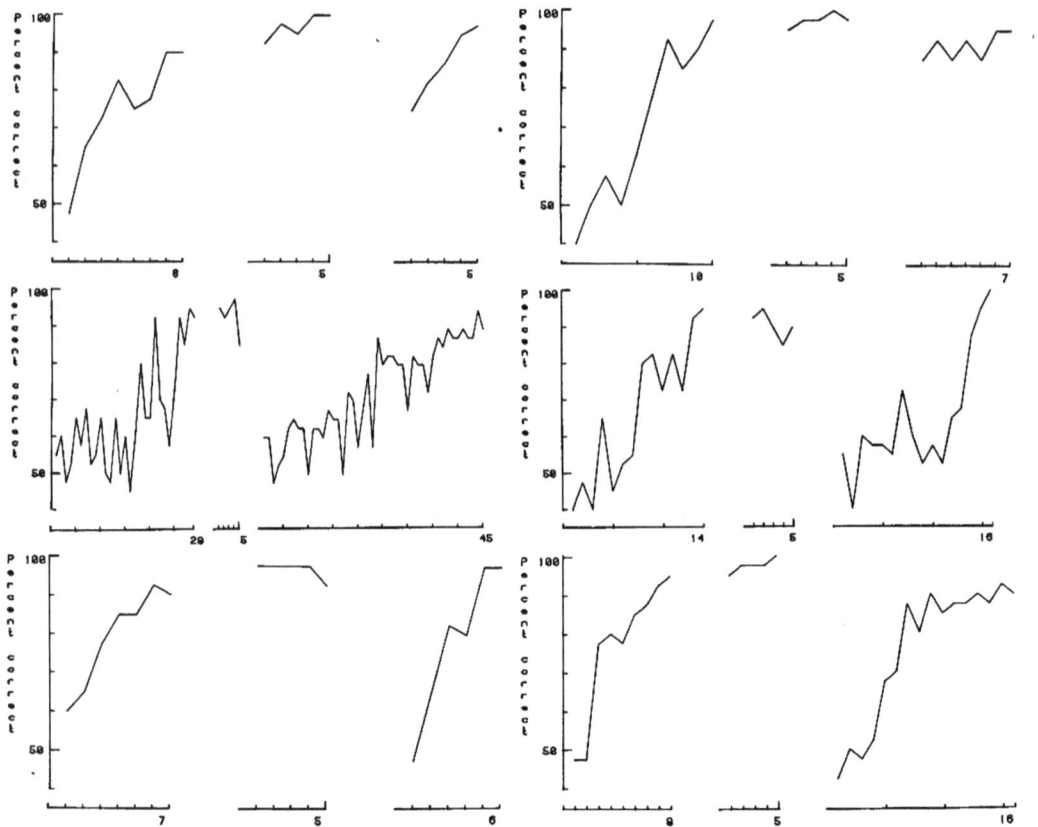

Figure 7 Interocular transfer of pattern discriminations in a split-chiasm cat (top row), a split-chiasm cat with a bilateral suprasylvian lesion (middle row), and a split-chiasm cat with a callosal section (bottom row). The left graphs refer to problem 6 of Figure 2, the right to problem 7. On the ordinates are plotted the percentages of correct responses; on the abscissae are plotted daily sessions of 40 trials each. Each graph is divided into three parts: learning with the first eye; overtraining with the same eye (five sessions); relearning with the second eye. The criterion of learning was fixed at two consecutive sessions with at least 90% correct responses. Note successful interocular transfer in the split-chiasm cat and absence of transfer in the other two cats. Note further prolonged learning in the cat with cortical lesions.

visual stimulation is not abolished by ablation of areas 17 and 18 (Spear and Baumann, 1979b).

The fact that interhemispheric transfer of pattern discriminations depends crucially on a cortical commissure such as the corpus callosum has enforced the classification of the mechanisms underlying transfer as purely cortical. Thompson (1965) first pointed out that subcortical centers as well may participate in the transfer process, since information transmitted by the corpus callosum to cortical areas subsequently can be relayed to subcortical centers for analysis and storage. We have investigated this possibility in the cat and have found that not only the visual cortical areas, but also the superior colliculus (SC), receive visual information from the opposite side of the brain via the corpus callosum. The evidence is based on the following findings.

(1) In the normal cat each SC contains not only a representation of the contralateral visual field, but also a binocular representation of a substantial portion of the ipsilateral visual field. This ipsilateral representation is largely abolished by a posterior section of the corpus callosum (Antonini, Berlucchi, and Sprague, 1978; Antonini et al., 1979a).

(2) After chiasm splitting, many binocularly driven neurons are still present in a rostral portion of the SC (see Figure 8); however, section of the corpus callosum removes the input from the contralateral eye (Antonini, Berlucchi, and Sprague, 1978; Antonini et al., 1979a) (Figure 9).

(3) After unilateral optic-tract section, neurons in the SC on the side of the section can still be activated by stimulation of either eye, but only if the corpus callosum is intact (Antonini, et al., 1979b) (Figure 10). While it cannot be excluded that cross-midline transfer of visual information to the SC by the corpus callosum is due to uninterrupted crossed corticotectal fibers (Powell, 1976), it is more likely that the transmission to the SC involved a two-stage process. Thus visual information would be transmitted first from cortical areas in one hemisphere to corresponding areas in the other hemisphere via the corpus callosum, and then from the latter areas to the SC via the uncrossed corticotectal projections. These projections originate from all visual cortical areas (Kawamura, Sprague, and Niimi, 1974) and not simply from areas 17 and 18.

These findings, along with the demonstration that section of the intertectal and posterior commissures has no effect on cross-midline transfer of visual information to the SC, either physiologically (Antonini et al., 1979a) or behaviorally (Berlucchi, Buchtel, and Lepore, 1978), indicate that sectioning the corpus callosum in split-chiasm cats deprives not only the visual cortical areas, but also the SC, of the input from the contralateral eye. Accordingly, absence of interocular transfer of pattern discriminations in split-chiasm, split-callosum cats may depend on both the cortical and subcortical visual disconnection, in agreement with the concept that the SC participates in pattern discriminations (Berlucchi et al., 1972; Sprague et al., 1977; Tunkl and Berkley, 1977) in this species.

We thus come to the conclusion that the interocular and interhemispheric equivalence of visual patterns does not require the refined circuitry for binocular interactions which is provided by neurons in areas 17 and 18. Binocular processes occurring in other cortical areas, and perhaps even in the superior colliculus, appear to be sufficient for ensuring the transfer of pattern discriminations between the eyes, or across the midvertical division of the visual field. What can then be the behavioral significance of the binocular neurons in areas 17 and 18? At least one of these functions is probably fine binocular stereopsis (see

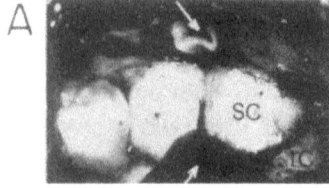

HABENULAR COMMISSURE

A

NO RESPONSE

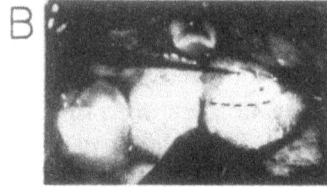

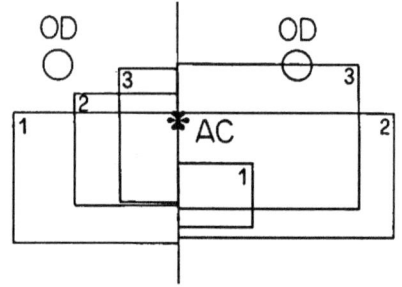

B

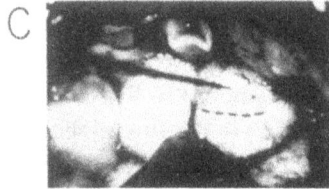

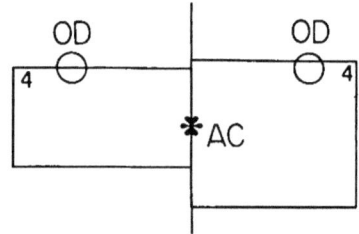

C

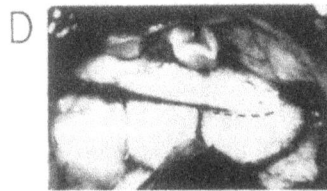

D

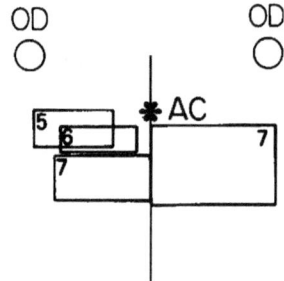

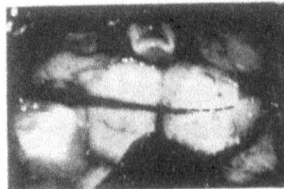

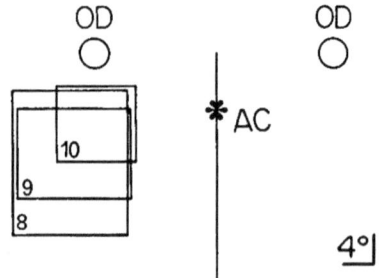

4°⌋

Figure 8 Binocularly activated portion of the superior colliculus of a split-chiasm cat as assessed by a combination of photographic and electrophysiological methods. Photographs of the superior colliculus were taken through the microscope after sacrifice and removal of the hemispheres, with the microelectrode repositioned at the beginning of tracks along which recordings were previously obtained. An illustration of the receptive fields is on the right; the vertical meridian of the two eyes is brought into register so that the receptive fields in the ipsilateral (right) eye are to the left of the midline (contralateral visual field) and the receptive fields in the contralateral (left) eye are to the right of the midline (ipsilateral visual field). In track (A) (Horsley–Clarke coordinates of the electrode: A4, L2), no units responsive to visual stimuli were found. In track (B) (A3.5, L2) and in track (C) (A3, L2), binocular units were consistently recorded. The receptive fields in the two eyes for three of these units are shown in (B) and the receptive fields in the two eyes for other units are shown in (C). Unit 1 in (B) was somewhat exceptional because of the large difference in size between the receptive fields in the two eyes. In track (D) (A2, L2), two superficial units had receptive fields only in the ipsilateral eye, and these fields were somewhat detached from the vertical meridian (units 5 and 6). Unit 7, which was encountered deeper in the track, was binocular and had receptive fields bordering on the vertical meridian in both eyes. In track (E) (A, L5, L2), all units from which recordings could be obtained had receptive fields only in the ipsilateral eye. These receptive fields were distant from the vertical meridian (see units 8–10). The interrupted line traced on the superior colliculus surface is based on similar explorations with more medial or lateral sequences of tracks. It indicates the posterior border of the binocular portion of the superior colliculus. (From Antonini, Berlucchi, and Sprague, 1978.)

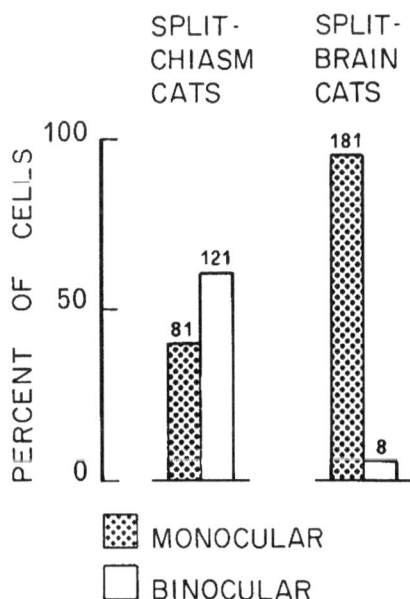

Figure 9 Most neurons in superior colliculus of split-chiasm cats can be driven from both eyes, but after an additional callosal section (split-brain cats) practically all SC neurons respond only to stimulation of the ipsilateral eye. (From Antonini et al., 1979a.)

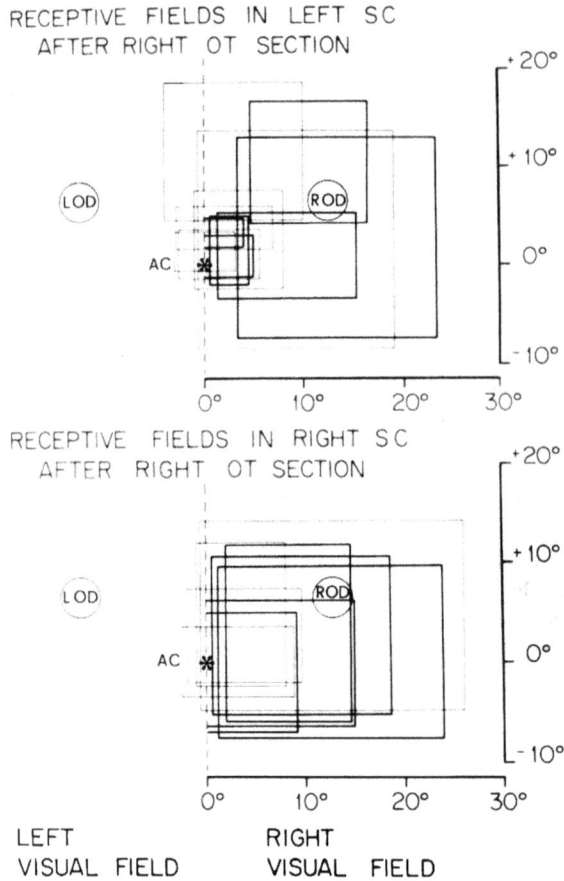

RECEPTIVE FIELDS IN LEFT SC
AFTER RIGHT OT SECTION

RECEPTIVE FIELDS IN RIGHT SC
AFTER RIGHT OT SECTION

LEFT
VISUAL FIELD

RIGHT
VISUAL FIELD

Figure 10 Examples of receptive fields in the superior colliculus contralateral (upper part) and ipsilateral (lower part) in one cat with right optic-tract section. All cells are binocular. Thin lines indicate receptive fields in the eye ipsilateral to the section and thick lines indicate receptive fields in the eye contralateral to the section. Note that fields in the eye ipsilateral to the section tend to straddle the vertical meridian. LOD, ROD = left and right optic disk; AC = area centralis. After section of corpus callosum, no responses to visual stimulation can be recorded in colliculus ipsilateral to the optic tract section. (From Antonini et al., 1979b.)

Bishop, 1973), since Siamese cats (Packwood and Gordon, 1975) and ordinary cats with alternating monocular occlusion (Blake and Hirsch, 1975), which lack binocularly driven neurons in areas 17 and 18, are stereoblind. Another function may be binocular summation in contrast-sensitivity curves, which is absent in Siamese cats and in cats raised with alternating monocular occlusion (von Grünau, 1979). It will be recalled that all these cats have excellent capacities for interocular transfer of pattern discriminations. A similar dichotomy of binocular processes is probably present also in man. Lack of interocular transfer of a variety of visual aftereffects has been reported in stereoblind subjects

G. Berlucchi and J. M. Sprague

(see, e.g., Movshon, Chambers, and Blakemore, 1972). Both stereo-blindness and absence of interocular transfer have been attributed to reduction or absence of binocular neurons in the primary visual cortex. Yet these persons must be capable of recognizing with one eye a visual pattern previously presented to the other eye, and this generalization must depend on central binocular interactions occurring in some other area of the brain. Experimental analysis of binocular interactions in stereodeficient individuals is just beginning to reveal which binocular processes, in addition to depth perception, are deficient in these subjects, and which are normal (see, e.g., Wolfe and Held, 1979). This may be the beginning of a finer classification of categories of visual perception that will lead, hopefully, to the discovery of stronger correlations between behavioral phenomena and the neuronal organization of the visual cortical areas, as it is known from anatomy and physiology.

Acknowledgment

Supported in part by United States Public Health Service Research Grant EY00577 and by Contract 77.01555.65 of the Italian National Research Council.

References

Antonini, A., G. Berlucchi, and J. M. Sprague, 1978. Indirect, across-the-midline retinotectal projections and representation of the ipsilateral visual field in superior colliculus of the cat. *J. Neurophysiol.* 41:295–304.

Antonini, A., G. Berlucchi, C. A. Marzi, and J. M. Sprague, 1979a. Importance of corpus callosum for visual receptive fields of single neurons in cat superior colliculus. *J. Neurophysiol.* 42:137–152.

Antonini, A., G. Berlucchi, C. A. Marzi, and J. M. Sprague, 1979b. Behavioral and electrophysiological effects of unilateral optic tract section in ordinary and Siamese cats. *J. Comp. Neurol.* 185:183–202.

Atencio, F. W., I. T. Diamond, and J. P. Ward, 1975. Behavioral study of the visual cortex of *Galago senegalensis. J. Comp. Physiol. Psychol.* 89:1109–1135.

Berkley, M. A., and J. M. Sprague, 1979. Striate cortex and visual acuity functions in the cat. *J. Comp. Neurol.* 187:679–702.

Berkley, M. A., and J. M. Sprague, 1980. The role of the geniculocortical system in spatial vision. In *Analysis of Visual Behavior.* D. Ingle, M. Goodale, and R. Mansfield, eds. Cambridge, MA: MIT Press (in press).

Berlucchi, G., 1972. Anatomical and physiological aspects of visual functions of corpus callosum. *Brain Res.* 37:371–392.

Berlucchi, G., and G. Rizzolatti, 1968. Binocularly driven neurons in visual cortex of split-chiasm cats. *Science* 159:308–310.

Berlucchi, G., H. A. Buchtel, and F. Lepore, 1978. Successful interocular transfer of visual pattern discriminations in split-chiasm cats with section of the intertectal and posterior commissure. *Physiol. Behav.* 20:331–338.

Berlucchi, G., J. M. Sprague, A. Antonini, and A. Simoni, 1979. Learning and interhemispheric transfer of visual pattern discriminations following unilateral suprasylvian lesions in split-chiasm cats. *Exp. Brain Res.* 34:551–574.

Berlucchi, G., J. M. Sprague, F. Lepore, and G. G. Mascetti, 1978. Effects of lesion of areas 17, 18 and 19 on interocular transfer of pattern discriminations in split-chiasm cats. *Exp. Brain Res.* 31:275–297.

Berlucchi, G., J. M. Sprague, J. Levy, and A. DiBerardino, 1972. Pretectum and superior colliculus in visually guided behavior and in flux and form discrimination in the cat. *J. Comp. Physiol. Psychol.* 78:123–172.

Bishop, P. O., 1973. Neurophysiology of binocular single vision and stereopsis. In *Handbook of Sensory Physiology*, Vol. VII/3A. Berlin: Springer, pp. 255–305.

Blake, R., and H. V. B. Hirsch, 1975. Deficits in binocular depth perception in cats after alternating monocular deprivation. *Science* 190:1114–1116.

Brindley, G. S., P. C. Gautier-Smith, and W. Lewin, 1969. Cortical blindness and the functions of the non-geniculate fibres of the optic tract. *J. Neurol. Neurosurg. Psychiat.* 32:259–264.

Buchtel, H. A., 1969. Visual form discrimination on the basis of the relative distribution of light. *Science* 164:857–858.

Buchtel, H. A., G. Berlucchi, and G. G. Mascetti, 1975. Behavioural and electrophysiological analysis of strabismus in cats. In *Plasticité nerveuse*. F. Vital and M. Jeannerod, eds. Paris: I.N.S.E.R.M., pp. 27–44.

Campbell, A., Jr., 1978. Deficits in visual learning produced by posterior temporal lesions in cats. *J. Comp. Physiol. Psychol.* 92:45–57.

Campbell, F. W., 1974. The transmission of spatial information through the visual system. In *The Neurosciences: Third Study Program*. F. O. Schmitt and F. G. Worden, eds. Cambridge, MA: MIT Press, pp. 95–103.

Cornwell, P., J. M. Warren, and A. J. Nonneman, 1976. Marginal and extramarginal cortical lesions and visual discrimination by cats. *J. Comp. Physiol. Psychol.* 90:986–995.

Dews, P. B., and T. N. Wiesel, 1970. Consequences of monocular deprivation on visual behaviour in kittens. *J. Physiol. (London)* 206:437–455.

Diamond, I. T., 1976. Organization of the visual cortex: Comparative anatomical and behavioral studies. *Fed. Proc.* 35:60–67.

Diamond, I. T., and W. C. Hall, 1969. Evolution of neocortex. *Science* 164:251–262.

Doty, R. W., 1971. Survival of pattern vision after removal of striate cortex in the adult cat. *J. Comp. Neurol.* 143:341–369.

Ganz, L., H. V. B. Hirsch, and S. B. Tieman, 1972. The nature of perceptual deficits in visually deprived cats. *Brain Res.* 44:547–568.

Gordon, B., and L. Gummow, 1975. Effects of extraocular muscle section on receptive field in cat superior colliculus. *Vision Res.* 15:1011–1019.

Gordon, B., and J. Presson, 1977. Effects of alternating occlusion on receptive fields in cat superior colliculus. *J. Neurophysiol.* 40:1046–1414.

Hara, K., P. R. Cornwell, J. M. Warren, and I. H. Webster, 1974. Posterior extramarginal cortex and visual learning by cats. *J. Comp. Physiol. Psychol.* 87:884–904.

Hirsch, H. V. B., 1972. Visual perception in cats after environmental surgery. *Exp. Brain Res.* 15:405–423.

Hubel, D. H., and T. N. Wiesel, 1959. Receptive fields of single neurons in the cat's striate cortex. *J. Physiol. (London)* 148:574–591.

Hubel, D. H., and T. N. Wiesel, 1962. Receptive fields, binocular interaction and functional architecture in the cat's visual cortex. *J. Physiol. (London)* 160:106–154.

Hubel, D. H., and T. N. Wiesel, 1965. Receptive fields and functional architecture in two nonstriate visual areas (18 and 19) of the cat. *J. Neurophysiol.* 28:229–289.

Hubel, D. H., and T. N. Wiesel, 1968. Receptive fields and functional architecture of monkey striate cortex. *J. Physiol. (London)* 195:215–243.

Hubel, D. H., and T. N. Wiesel, 1970. The period of susceptibility to the physiological effects of unilateral eye closure in kittens. *J. Physiol. (London)* 206:419–436.

Hughes, H. C., 1977. Anatomical and neurobehavioral investigations concerning the thalamo-cortical organization of the rat's visual system. *J. Comp. Neurol.* 175:311–336.

Hughes, H. C., 1980. A search for the neural mechanisms essential to basic figural synthesis in the cat. In *Analysis of Visual Behavior.* D. Ingle, M. Goodale, and R. Mansfield, eds. Cambridge, MA: MIT Press (in press)

Humphrey, N. K., 1974. Vision in a monkey without striate cortex: A case study. *Perception* 3:241–255.

Jones, E. G., 1974. The anatomy of extrageniculostriate visual mechanisms. In *The Neurosciences: Third Study Program.* F. O. Schmitt and F. G. Worden, eds. Cambridge, MA: MIT Press, pp. 215–228.

Kawamura, S., J. M. Sprague, and K. Niimi, 1974. Corticofugal projections from the visual cortices to the thalamus, pretectum and superior colliculus in the cat. *J. Comp. Neurol.* 158:339–362.

Killackey, H., M. Snyder, and I. T. Diamond, 1971. Function of striate and temporal cortex in the tree shrew. *J. Comp. Physiol. Psychol.* 74:1–29.

Levey, N. H., J. Harris, and J. A. Jane, 1973. Effects of visual cortical ablation on pattern discrimination in the ground squirrel (*Citellus tridecemlineatus*). *Exp. Neurol.* 39:270–276.

Maffei, L., 1978. Spatial frequency channels: Neural mechanisms. In *Handbook of Sensory Physiology. Vol. VIII: Perception.* R. Held, H. W. Leibowitz, and H.-L. Teuber, eds. Berlin: Springer, pp. 39–66.

Marzi, C. A., A. Simoni, and M. Di Stefano, 1976. Lack of binocularly driven neurons in the Siamese cat's visual cortex does not prevent successful interocular transfer to visual form discriminations. *Brain Res.* 105:353–357.

Marzi, C. A., M. Di Stefano, A. Antonini, and C. Legg, 1979. Binocular interactions in the Clare-Bishop area of Siamese cats which lack binocular neurones in the primary visual cortex. *Neurosci. Lett. Suppl.* 3:357.

Mize, R. R., and E. H. Murphy, 1976. Alterations in receptive field properties of superior colliculus cells produced by visual cortex ablation in infant and adult cats. *J. Comp. Neurol.* 168:393–424.

Moore, D. T., and E. H. Murphy, 1976. Differential effects of two visual cortical lesions in the rabbit. *Exp. Neurol.* 53:21–30.

Movshon, J. A., B. E. I. Chambers, and C. Blakemore, 1972. Interocular transfer in normal humans, and those who lack stereopsis. *Perception* 1:483–490.

Myers, R. E., 1955. Interocular transfer of pattern discrimination in cats following section of crossed optic fibers. *J. Comp. Physiol. Psychol.* 48:470–473.

Myers, R. E., 1956. Function of corpus callosum in interocular transfer. *Brain* 79:358–363.

Myers, R. E., 1959. Localization of function in the corpus callosum. Visual gnostic transfer. *Arch. Neurol.* 1:74–77.

Packwood, J., and B. Gordon, 1975. Stereopsis in normal domestic cat, Siamese cat, and cat raised with alternating monocular occlusion. *J. Neurophysiol.* 38:1485–1499.

Palmer, L. A., A. C. Rosenquist, and R. J. Tusa, 1978. The retinotopic organization of lateral suprasylvian visual areas in the cat. *J. Comp. Neurol.* 177:237–256.

Pasik, T., and P. Pasik, 1971. The visual world of monkeys deprived of striate cortex: effective stimulus parameters and the importance of the accessory optic system. *Vision Res. Suppl.* 3:419–435.

Peck, C. K., S. G. Crewther, G. Barber, and C. J. Johannsen, 1979. Pattern discrimination and visuomotor behavior following rotation of one or both eyes in kittens and in adult cats. *Exp. Brain Res.* 34:401–418.

Pollen, D. A., and J. H. Taylor, 1974. The striate cortex and the spatial analysis of visual space. In *The Neurosciences: Third Study Program.* F. O. Schmitt and F. G. Worden, eds. Cambridge, MA: MIT Press, pp. 239–247.

Powell, T. P. S., 1976. Bilateral cortico-tectal projection from the visual cortex in the cat. *Nature* 260:526–527.

Ritchie, D. G., P. M. Meyer, and D. R. Meyer, 1976. Residual spatial vision of cats with lesions of the visual cortex. *Exp. Neurol.* 53:227–253.

Rodieck, R. W., 1979. Visual pathways. *Ann. Rev. Neurosci.* 2:193–225.

Rosenquist, A. C., and L. A. Palmer, 1971. Visual receptive field properties of cells of the superior colliculus after cortical lesions in the cat. *Exp. Neurol.* 33:629–652.

Runnels, L. K., R. Thompson, and P. Runnels, 1968. Near-perfect runs as a learning criterion. *J. Math. Psychol.* 5:362–368.

Schilder, P., P. Pasik, and T. Pasik, 1972. Extrageniculostriate vision in the monkey. III. Circle vs. triangle and "red vs. green" discrimination. *Exp. Brain Res.* 14:436–448.

Seacord, L., C. G. Gross, and M. Mishkin, 1979. Role of inferior temporal cortex in interhemispheric transfer. *Brain Res.* 167:259–272.

Shatz, C., 1977a. A comparison of visual pathways in Boston and Midwestern Siamese cats. *J. Comp. Neurol.* 17:205–228.

Shatz, C., 1977b. Abnormal interhemispheric connections in the visual system of Boston Siamese cats: A physiological study. *J. Comp. Neurol.* 171:229–246.

Shatz, C., 1977c. Anatomy of interhemispheric connections in the visual system of Boston Siamese and ordinary cats. *J. Comp. Neurol.* 173:497–518.

Sherman, S. M., 1970. Role of the visual cortex in interocular transfer in the cat. *Exp. Neurol.* 30:34–45.

Spear, P. D., and H. Barbas, 1975. Recovery of pattern discrimination in rats receiving serial or one-stage visual cortex lesions. *Brain Res.* 94:337–346.

Spear, P. D., and T. P. Baumann, 1979a. Neurophysiological mechanisms of recovery from visual cortex damage in cats: Properties of lateral suprasylvian visual area neurons following behavioral recovery. *Exp. Brain Res.* 35:177–192.

Spear, P. D., and T. P. Baumann, 1979b. Effects of visual cortex removal on receptive field properties of neurons in the lateral suprasylvian visual area of the cat. *J. Neurophysiol.* 42:31–56.

Spear, P. D., and J. J. Braun, 1969. Pattern discrimination following removal of visual neocortex in the cat. *Exp. Neurol.* 25:331–348.

Spear, P. D., and L. Ganz, 1975. Effects of visual cortex lesions following recovery from monocular deprivation in the cat. *Exp. Brain Res.* 23:181–201.

Sperry, R. W., 1947. Cerebral regulation of motor coordination in monkeys following multiple transection of sensorimotor cortex. *J. Neurophysiol.* 10:275–294.

Sperry, R. W., 1961. Cerebral organization and behavior. *Science* 133:1749–1757.

Sperry, R. W., and N. Miner, 1955. Pattern perception following insertion of mica plates into visual cortex. *J. Comp. Physiol. Psychol.* 48:463–469.

Sperry, R. W., M. Miner, and R. E. Myers, 1955. Visual pattern perception following subpial slicing and tantalum wire implantations in the visual cortex. *J. Comp. Physiol. Psychol.* 48:50–58.

Sperry, R. W., J. Stamm, and N. Miner, 1956. Relearning tests for interocular transfer following division of optic chiasma and corpus callosum in cats. *J. Comp. Physiol. Psychol.* 49:529–533.

Sprague, J. M., J. Levy, A. DiBerardino, and G. Berlucchi, 1977. Visual cortical areas mediating form discrimination in the cat. *J. Comp. Neurol.* 172:441–488.

Stein, B. E., and B. Magalhaes-Castro, 1975. Effects of neonatal cortical lesions upon the cat superior colliculus. *Brain Res.* 83:480–485.

Thompson, R., 1965. Centrencephalic theory and interhemispheric transfer of visual habits. *Psychol. Rev.* 72:385–398.

Tunkl, J. E., and M. A. Berkley, 1977. The role of superior colliculus in vision: Visual form discrimination in cats with superior colliculus ablations. *J. Comp. Neurol.* 176:575–587.

Tusa, R. J., L. A. Palmer, and A. C. Rosenquist, 1978. The retinotopic organization of area 17 (striate cortex) in the cat. *J. Comp. Neurol.* 177:213–236.

Tusa, R. J., A. C. Rosenquist, and L. A. Palmer, 1979. Retinotopic organization of areas 18 and 19 in the cat. *J. Comp. Neurol.* 185:657–678.

Von Grünau, M. W., 1979. Binocular summation and the binocularity of cat visual cortex. *Vision Res.* 19:813–816.

Von Grünau, M. W., and W. Singer, 1979. The role of binocular neurons in the cat striate cortex in combining information from the two eyes. *Exp. Brain Res.* 34:133–142.

Weiskrantz, C., E. K. Warrington, M. D. Sanders, and J. Marshall, 1974. Visual capacity in the hemianopic field following a restricted occipital lesion. *Brain* 97:709–728.

Wickelgren, B. G., and P. Sterling, 1969. Influence of visual cortex on receptive fields in superior colliculus of the cat. *J. Neurophysiol.* 32:16–23.

Winans, S. S., 1971. Visual cues used by normal and visual decorticate cats to discriminate figures of equal luminous flux. *J. Comp. Physiol. Psychol.* 74:167–178.

Wolfe, J. M., and R. Held, 1979. Eye torsion and visual tilt are mediated by different binocular processes. *Vision Res.* 19:917–920.

Wood, C. C., P. D. Spear, and J. J. Braun, 1974. Effects of sequential lesions of suprasylvian gyri and visual cortex on pattern discrimination in the cat. *Brain Res.* 66:443–466.

19

Scalp-Recorded Cerebral Event-Related Potentials in Man as Point of Entry into the Analysis of Cognitive Processing

John E. Desmedt

ABSTRACT   Computer-averaged cerebral potentials picked up from the intact scalp disclose important features of brain function in man. Standard sensory activations elicit in primary receiving cortical areas (for example, the contralateral postcentral cortex for stimulation of fingers of the hand) electrical responses with rather stable features that relate largely to the afferent signals. When the subject is given a psychological task involving stimuli, event-related potentials (ERP) indexing various cognitive processes are added upon the hard-wired responses to the stimuli. Two classes of ERPs occurring in sequential tasks are briefly discussed. The middle-range components such as the N140 (negative component with peak latency of about 140 msec), occupying a time slot of about 70 to 250 msec after the evoking signal, are thought to index the actual processing of input signals; they become prominent in tasks with cognitive difficulties (differentiation of several types of target and nontarget signals) or in tasks that must be carried out at fast rates (overload in forced-paced conditions). The middle-range components have characteristic areal distributions on the scalp and are related to specific brain processors whose activities lead to a decision by the subject.

Another type of ERP is represented by the P300 (positive component with peak latency about 300 msec), which is bilateral and widely distributed in the brain. The P300 is not modality specific. It is interpreted here as a postdecision phenomenon that follows the identification by the subject of a task-relevant event. The neural mechanisms of ERPs appear to be different. It is proposed that P300 results from a transient reduction of the neuromodulatory pressure that is maintained in the waking performing brain by the frontal cortex acting through the mesencephalic reticular formation and neurons with widespread nonspecific distribution; the question of the respective share of cholinergic muscarinic versus catecholaminergic systems in this neuromodulation is not settled. By contrast the middle-range ERPs are also time regulated by the frontal cortex (that appears essential in serial behavior) through another more specifically distributed effector system such as the various parts of the thalamic reticular nucleus, which is known to achieve differential control over different sensory modalities.

Progress in the last decade has established the averaging of cerebral evoked potentials as one of the major methodologies for the analysis of perceptual and cognitive functions in man. The older technique of re-

JOHN E. DESMEDT   Brain Research Unit, University of Brussels, 115 boulevard de Waterloo, 1000 Brussels, Belgium

cording spontaneous brain potentials in the electroencephalogram (EEG) has largely failed to fulfill a truly useful role in this respect, although it has a number of definite uses in clinical patients. The electronic averaging of cerebral potentials related to sensory cognitive and/or motor events (event-related potentials or ERP) provide a much more versatile and powerful point of entry. ERPs are generally elicited in relation to discrete events that are separated by intervals sufficient to allow the nervous system to return to some baseline, and enough trials are added to produce clearly delineated traces from which noise and inconsistent transients have largely been averaged out. The electronic averaging is a powerful technique for extracting brain potentials as small as 0.1 μV buried in the much larger (10–100 μV) waves of the EEG; for this very reason much care must be exercised in designing the experiments and using capabilities (such as editing of raw data) so as to exclude large transient interferences from the samples (cf. Desmedt, 1977a).

A major breakthrough in 1964–1965 was the demonstration that, besides the hard-wired early potentials evoked by sensory input in the receiving areas (cf. Woolsey, Marshall, and Bard, 1942), the brain generated potentials that were related to cognitive operations at a high level of performance (Walter et al., 1964; Kornhuber and Deecke, 1965; Sutton et al., 1965; Desmedt, Debecker, and Manil, 1965). A considerable amount of research since that time has improved the methodologies and the experimental designs, thereby resolving uncertainties and putting many issues into consistent perspective (cf. Donchin and Lindsley, 1969; McCallum and Knott, 1973; Desmedt, 1977c, 1979; Begleiter, 1977; Otto, 1979). ERPs supply data that cannot be found through psychological or neuropsychological measures; unlike microphysiological recordings in acute or chronically prepared mammals, they allow noninvasive electrophysiological analysis of psychological processes in man.

Cerebral ERPs are no longer considered as unitary phenomena for which any single measure of amplitude or duration might provide meaningful data. Instead ERPs are recognized as made up of a series of different component potentials that can react differentially in various cognitive tasks and that can be specified in relation to their scalp topography and multifactorial parametric sets. These features allow genuine ERP components to be distinguished from trivial or inconsistent deflections in averaged traces. It should be realized also that any such component can vary over a certain range of amplitudes and latencies in different experiments without losing its identity or acquiring necessarily another significance. The case for identifying any ERP component that might be related to a distinct brain processor should be carefully argued on the basis of experimental parameters. In order to enhance the utility of ERP data and further narrow the division between brain neurophysiology and the study of human behavior, there is a current trend for elaborating astute paradigms that may better match the complex functional organizations underlying cognition in the performing brain (cf. Hillyard and Picton, 1979; Desmedt, Debecker, and Robertson, 1979).

Eliciting Events and Primary ERP Components

ERPs can be elicited by a variety of external or internal cues. One class of ERPs includes the readiness potential and other components that precede voluntary movements and reflect brain processor activities involved in the patterning of the central motor commands (Kornhuber and Deecke, 1965; Kornhuber, 1974; Deecke and Kornhuber, 1977; Kutas and Donchin, 1977). These motor potentials must be averaged backward from the time of beginning movement or muscle action potentials. The averaging of ERPs requires that task-relevant events occur at a definite time, so that the duty cycle of the computer can be triggered and the successive bioelectric data samples can be added consistently after analog-to-digital conversion. Certain interesting events that one may want to study with the ERP method, like sentences or complex language material, do not readily allow this to be done. On the other hand, if the sensory stimuli delivered to the subject are too simple or artificial (like flashes of light or acoustic clicks) they will of course elicit brain potentials, but may fail to engage elaborate cerebral functions. Furthermore the repetition of the same stimuli (necessary to accumulate enough samples for averaging) may result in a loss of their attention-mobilizing capacity in the course of the runs. Appropriate experimental designs must consider these conflicting requirements and control the use of cognitive resources throughout the session in order to derive pertinent and realistic ERP data.

Current problems present themselves somewhat differently for the main sensory modalities. For example, in vision the visual evoked potentials (VEP) to light flashes are disappointingly small and seem to hold little interest for brain studies. Animal experiments had indeed shown flashes to be very inefficient stimuli as compared to lines, edges, and shapes (Hubel and Wiesel, 1962). The VEP studies in man changed dramatically with the introduction of patterned visual stimulation with checkerboard or grating patterns whereby the luminance was held constant over the field while the spatial or temporal pattern varied (Spekereijse, Estevez, and Reits, 1977). This had immediate clinical relevance since patients with retrobulbar neuritis or other lesions of the visual pathways were found to present striking abnormalities in latency or shape of VEPs to patterned photic stimuli even though their VEP to flashes were within normal range (cf. Halliday, McDonald, and Mushkin, 1972; Desmedt, 1977d).

In audition, the primary cortical components are not readily identified because the receiving area in Heschl gyrus is deeply situated in the sylvian fissure (cf. Vaughan and Ritter, 1970; Peronnet and Michel, 1977). Later components of the auditory evoked potential (AEP) are poorly localized on the scalp, but readily recorded with a vertex electrode. The analysis of the first 10 msec of the vertex-recorded response to auditory clicks reveals a series of short-latency wavelets that are related to several nuclei and tracts of the brain-stem auditory pathway (Jewett, Romano, and Williston, 1970; Galambos and Hecox, 1977). The disclosure of such distant (far-field) potentials that have a consistent time relation to the sensory stimulus confirms the high sensitivity of the averaging method and has rapidly been developed into a useful clinical diagnostic test for focal brain-stem pathology (cf. Starr, 1977; Stockard and Sharbrough, 1980).

Because the parietal receiving areas are deployed on the surface of the brain, the somatosensory evoked potential (SEP) lends itself best to the study of primary cortical components elicited by sensory stimuli (e.g., to the skin). It is also possible to record and average the afferent volley directly from the peripheral nerve and over the spinal cord; furthermore, far-field components can be identified before the primary cortical response in the scalp-recorded SEP, and they reflect ascending conduction along the dorsal column and lemniscal pathways (cf. Cracco, 1973; Small, Beauchamp, and Matthews, 1980; Desmedt and Cheron, 1980a). The outstanding possibilities of the SEP approach have been exploited for clinical diagnostic tests in patients with peripheral or central neurological disorders (Desmedt, 1980). The use of somatosensory stimuli in ERP research also allows a critical evaluation of the possible role of inhibitory control of the corticipetal volleys by centrifugal pathways through monitoring the early primary SEP components (see below).

Liminal Sensation and ERP to Faint Skin Stimuli

The sensation at threshold is highly precarious; it requires on the part of the subject a decision whether a signal may or may not have occurred (Swets, Tanner, and Birdsall, 1964). The subjective threshold can be statistically defined from the S-shaped relation between the stimulus intensities and the percentage of correct conscious detections. Even when interference from other sensory stimulations is minimized (soundproofed room, etc.), and when the subject is doing his best, the relation can be shown to be influenced by the subject's own bias and by the instructions given to him (Figure 1G). Thus the subject can adopt either a more conservative criterion allowing for more secure decisions while accepting that a number of signals will be missed, or a more liberal criterion ensuring fewer such misses but with a higher incidence of false signal reports when none was in fact present (which occurs especially under forced choice conditions; Swets, Tanner, and Birdsall, 1964). In a study of ERP correlates of liminal sensation, single electric pulses of 0.1-msec duration were delivered at random intervals (2–8 sec) to one finger while averaging ERPs from the contralateral parietal scalp focus for the hand. When the highly motivated subjects detected any stimulus they pressed a light key as fast as possible with the opposite hand, which provided a measure of reaction time (Debecker, Desmedt, and Manil, 1965). In any one run, stimuli at one chosen intensity were detected with one or the other criterion. A consistent relation was observed between ERP features and the scaling of the detection curve. For example, in Figure 1E no identifiable ERP is present for faint finger stimuli that are never detected with a conservative criterion, but that elicit a "conscious sensation" in about 30% of the trials when the subject adopts a liberal criterion. False reports have been excluded, as far as possible, from these data by rejecting reaction times when they exceeded 1 sec. Finger stimuli of 1.4–1.8 mA are detected in less than 100% of trials with a conservative criterion and elicit early-component (P45) ERP that increase in amplitude and present smaller latency as the stimuli become stronger (Figure 1B–D). Figure 1F presents latencies of ERP and the corresponding reaction times. The latter increase much more than the ERP latencies when the stimuli get fainter. Reaction times also increase more when the subject is told to adopt a conservative criterion, which makes him more cautious. The larger increase of reaction times (as compared with ERP latencies) for faint stimuli points to a dissociation between stimulus evaluation processes, which are stimulus bound, and response selection and initiation processes that are elicited after the cognitive decision (cf. Kutas, McCarthy, and Donchin, 1977; Desmedt, Debecker and Robertson, 1979).

In 10 subjects tested with a conservative criterion, a contralateral ERP confined to the early primary components was clearly observed for stimuli that were detected in 10–35% of trials (6 subjects), or in 35–70% of trials (4 remaining subjects). No ERP was recorded for stimuli that were never detected when the subject used a liberal criterion. Figure 1E gives one example of no ERP for stimuli that just failed to be detected with a conservative criterion. Contrary to Libet et al. (1967), the present evidence argues against the hypothesis of subliminal exteroceptive sensation, at least under conditions when the subjects are awake, attending, and trying hard to detect the very stimuli that elicit the recorded cortical ERPs (Debecker, Desmedt, and Manil, 1965; Desmedt, Debecker, and Robertson, 1979). The common finding that early ERP components are not much changed by anesthesia or drugs affecting vigilance (cf. Saletu, 1977) is interesting, but quite unrelated to this very issue. It would indeed not be fair to say on this basis that ERPs might not bear any relation to conscious sensation. In fact when the stimuli are so faint that ERPs fail to be recorded (under adequate experimental conditions), apparently no sensation can be evoked.

On the other hand, the early SEP components to identical finger stimuli do not significantly change when the subjects switch from a conservative to a liberal criterion, the latter of which nevertheless increases

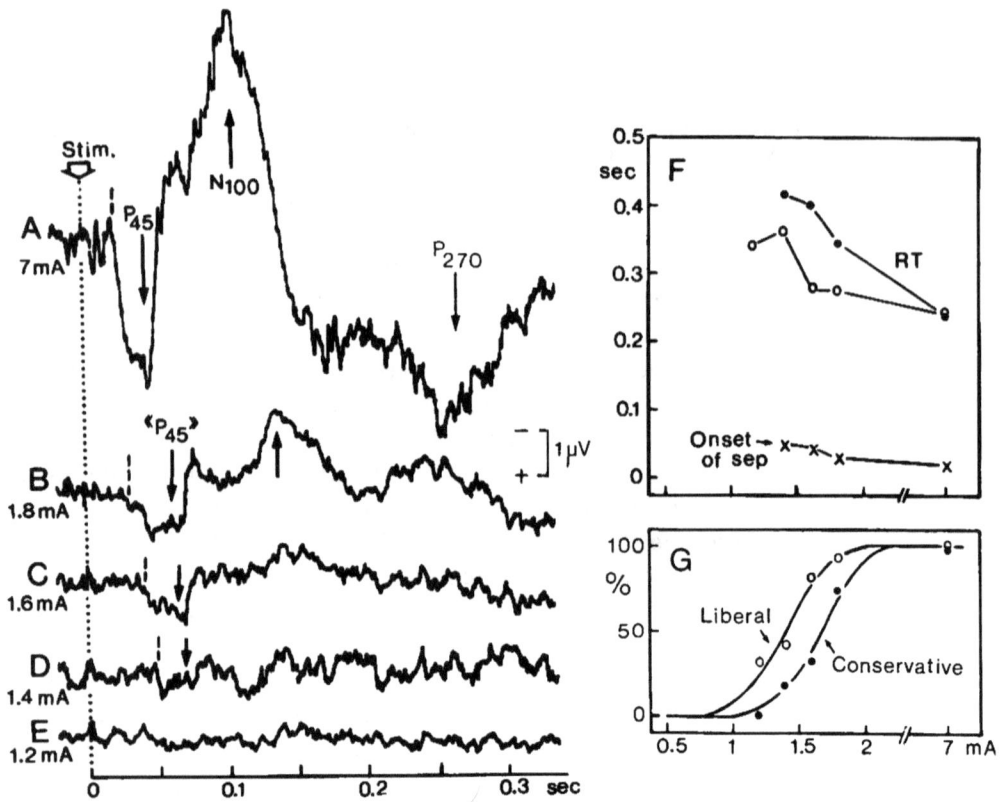

Figure 1 Subjective sensation and cortical evoked potentials for faint stimuli. Brief electrical square pulses are delivered at randomly varying intervals to the third finger of the contralateral hand. The actual intensities as measured by a current probe in milliamperes (mA) are indicated. (A)–(E) Somatosensory evoked potentials recorded from the parietal scalp focus with a front reference. The number of trials averaged for each trace is 50 (A), 200 (B), 200 (C), 200 (D), and 400 (E). The vertical row of dots indicates the time of delivery of the finger stimuli. Negativity of the active parietal electrode drives the trace upward in this and all other figures. Short vertical interrupted lines indicate the onset of the cortical SEPs, and a latency shift is apparent as the stimulus intensities are reduced from (A) to (D). No SEP can be identified for the stimuli of 1.2 mA in (E). The SEP components are indicated by arrows and labeled as P45, N100, and P270 according to recent recommendations (Donchin et al., 1977) by associating the component polarity (N for negative or P for positive) and its peak latency in milliseconds (msec). The peak latency of component "P45" increases as the stimuli become fainter. (F) Graph of the onset latency of SEP (crosses, ordinate in sec) as a function of the intensity of the finger stimuli in different runs (abscissa in milliamperes). The reaction times of the subject (RT) are also indicated for runs carried out either with a conservative (dots) or a liberal (circles) criterion of detection. (G) Number of trials correctly detected (ordinate in percentage) as a function of the stimulus intensity with either of the two criteria. (From Desmedt, Debecker, and Robertson, 1979.)

the actual detection 10–50% in the uncertain range of the detection curve (Figure 1G). This finding suggests that early SEP components elicited by the arrival of afferent signals in postcentral cortex do provide the input to the stimulus-evaluation brain processes, but apparently do not actually reflect the brain processing itself. The latter appears to be indexed by the middle-range cognitive ERP components such as N140. (Components are designated by their polarity, positive P or negative N, at the recording electrode and by their peak latency. Thus N140 is a negative component of 140-msec peak latency; see Donchin et al., 1977.) The type of criterion used by the subject does not appear to modify these components so long as he is selectively attending to the signals concerned.

The increase of SEP onset latency when the finger stimuli decrease in intensity is a common finding that is related, not to any delay in the corticopetal conduction, but rather to the longer time taken by a small input for achieving any sizable activation of the dendrites of pyramidal neurons. The cortex has integrative properties which apparently enable even small or decimated afferent signals (in clinical patients with peripheral neuropathies or with brain-stem lesions) eventually to involve enough cortical neurons so as to elicit SEPs that are delayed but of fair size (Desmedt et al., 1966; Desmedt, 1971; Noel and Desmedt, 1980). Briefly put, the early components of EPs are currently related to synaptic potentials in apical dendrites of pyramidal cells (Eccles, 1951; Purpura, Shofer, and Musgrave, 1964; Towe, 1966). Recent anatomical data show that bundles of thalamocortical axons from the ventrobasal thalamic relay terminate in discrete column-like clusters, mainly onto the spiny stellate cells or type 7 neurons of Jones (1975). The distinct vertical synaptic connectivities in cortex result in the organization of vertical modules of about 400-μm diameter in primates, and these modules appear as the essential building blocks of the cortical receiving areas (Mountcastle, 1957, 1978; Szentagothai, 1970, 1975, 1978; Jones, 1975; Eccles, 1979). The sequential activation of modules in the different cortical areas that receive connections from the postcentral receiving cortex (cf. Jones and Powell, 1970; Jones, Coulter, and Hendry, 1978; Kaas et al., this volume) probably account for a number of the SEP components that can be recorded from the human scalp (Desmedt and Cheron, 1980b).

Selective Attention, Decision, and P300

While the early SEP components are closely related to the stimuli delivered but rather unaffected by the subject's cognitive activity, the latter strongly influences the late ERP components. For example, task-relevant stimuli that allow the subject to make a definite decision elicit a P300, which is a positive component (P) with a modal peak latency of about 300–400 msec (Sutton et al., 1965; Desmedt, Debecker, and Manil,

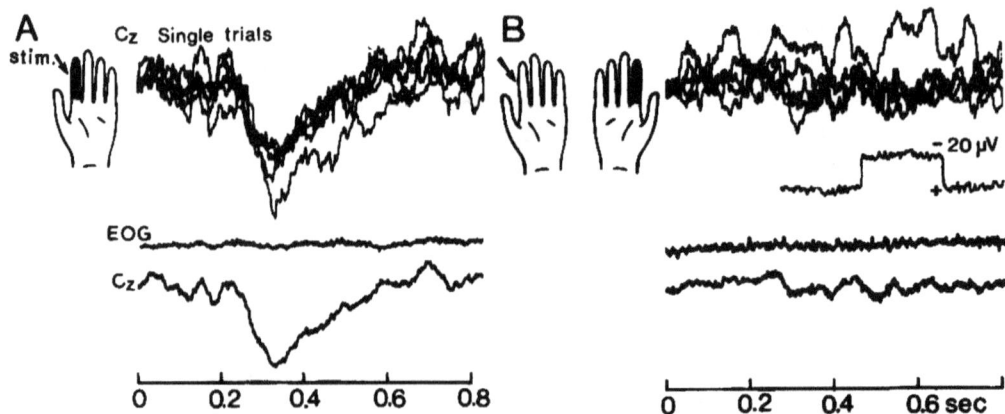

Figure 2 Single trial P300s to target-finger stimuli in selective attention within the somatosensory modality. Vertex (Cz) scalp derivation refers to linked earlobes in normal adult subject presenting very large P300 components to target stimuli. The experiment involves a four-finger paradigm with brief electrical square pulses of near-threshold intensities delivered in random sequences and at random intervals to the second and third fingers of the two hands. The mean random rate for the four fingers is 40/min. (A) Five single-trial P300s to target stimuli to the second finger of the left hand are superimposed (upper traces). The middle trace represents the control electrooculogram (EOG) and the lower trace corresponds to the average of 23 trials recorded from the vertex. (B) Same display for ERPs to identical stimuli to the second finger of the left hand in another run when the subject has to attend selectively to stimuli delivered to the second finger of the right hand. In the figures the attended finger is indicated in black, while a small arrow points to the finger whose stimulation elicits the ERP traces shown. (From Desmedt et al., 1977.)

1965; Donchin and Cohen, 1967; Ritter and Vaughan, 1969; Hillyard et al., 1971, 1973; Tueting, Sutton, and Zubin, 1971; Ford et al., 1973). Active attention directed toward the target signals of the serial cognitive task (with or without a motor response) is necessary for enhancing P300, while neglect of identical stimuli designated as task irrelevant reduces or abolishes P300 in other runs on the same subject.

In a few exceptional subjects and for unknown reasons P300 is large and easily identified in single trials (Ritter, Simson, and Vaughan, 1972; Desmedt et al., 1977). Figure 2 illustrates this in a paradigm with near-threshold stimuli delivered to four fingers of the two hands in random sequences. Large P300 are elicited when the finger stimulated for eliciting the trace is designated as target (Figure 2A), but virtually no P300 can be seen in traces evoked by identical stimuli to the same finger when this is task irrelevant because another finger of the opposite hand is now the target (Figure 2B). The near-threshold intensities of finger stimuli were carefully titrated to achieve an appropriate difficulty of decision, and this can result in a rather spectacular all-or-none manipulation of P300 that is clearly undistorted by any overlapping ERP components under such conditions.

448   John E. Desmedt

A general feature of the experimental designs in ERP studies is the delivery to the subject of random sequences of various sensory stimuli and the comparison of runs in which the verbal instructions alternatively direct the cognitive task toward different sets of stimuli. Thus the ERP components for a given set of signals designated as targets can be identified as genuinely related to the task when they are absent from control ERPs to identical stimuli that now serve as nontargets in adjacent runs. The ability to manipulate ERP components by task does not seem compatible with the view of Libet (1973), who argued that cortical activation by a signal should proceed for about 0.5 sec before a conscious sensation could be elicited, a position that appears to dissociate electrical brain events from consciousness. The position in ERP research is rather that the conscious processing of signals is actually indexed by the distinct ERP electrogeneses that are added onto the hard-wired stimulus-dependent cortical potentials (Donchin, McCarthy, and Kutas, 1977; Hillyard and Picton, 1979; Desmedt, Debecker, and Robertson, 1979).

P300 is largely independent of the characteristics and sensory modality of the evoking stimulus. Faint stimuli can elicit large P300 if task relevant. Trial-by-trial studies indicate that P300 is associated with the correctly detected stimuli (hits) and absent for the undetected stimuli (misses) in detection tasks (Hillyard et al., 1971; Paul and Sutton, 1972). Correct rejection trials, in which the subject makes the right decision that an expected stimulus was in fact absent, can be associated with an endogenously "emitted" P300 exhibiting trial-by-trial latency variability (Squires, Squires, and Hillyard, 1975a; Kerkhof, 1978; Ruchkin and Sutton, 1979). This and other evidence suggests that P300 is somehow related to a decision that allocates an event to a task-relevant category. However, it must be stressed that no P300 occurs for nontarget signals that must nevertheless be identified in order to perform the task. Therefore, P300 cannot index any brain processor involved in stimulus identification and comparison against memory, and it is proposed that P300 is rather a postdecision event elicited endogenously upon completion of certain cognitive-processing chunks (Desmedt and Debecker, 1979a,b).

It would be desirable to test this hypothesis by using an independent behavioral measure of the decision latency such as the subject's reaction time, but this is rather complicated because of the wide range of reaction-time variations in various experiments. There is indeed no fast rule for deciding how many milliseconds should be subtracted from any recorded reaction time in order to allow for initiation of voluntary response commands and muscle activation, and thus obtain the actual decision latency. When motivated subjects respond as quickly as possible with few errors the reaction times occur at about the P300 peak latency or slightly thereafter, but sometimes even before the P300 peak (Ritter, Simson, and Vaughan, 1972; Kutas, McCarthy, and Donchin, 1977; Des-

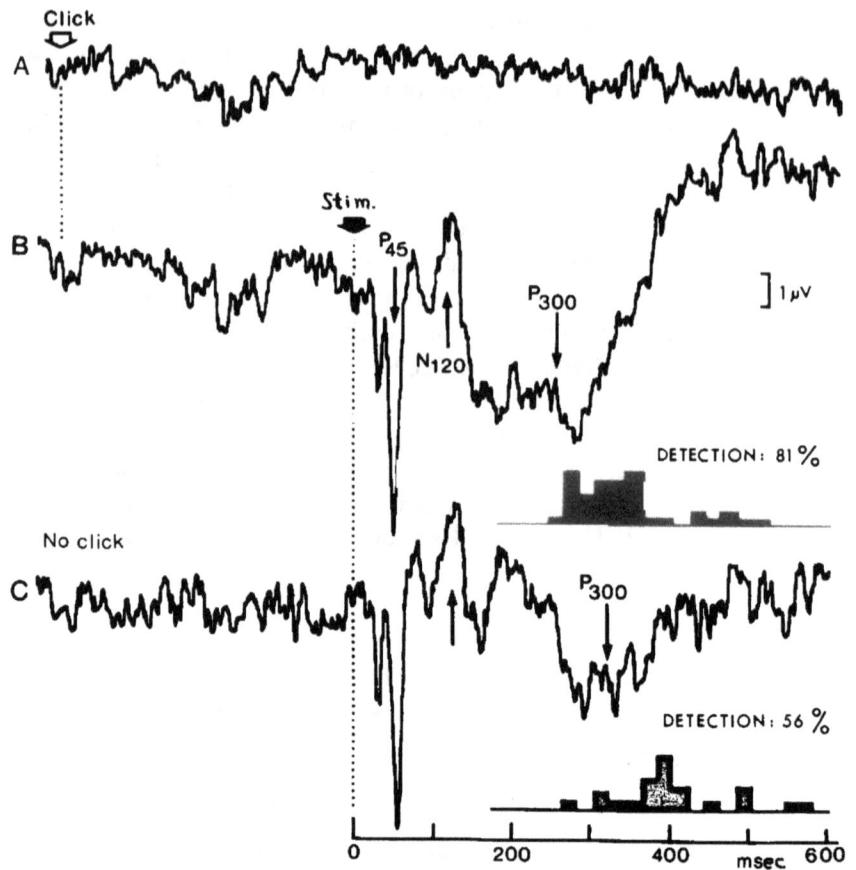

Figure 3 Influence of warning on conscious sensation, reaction time, and event-related potentials in selective-attention tasks. Averaged ERPs (*N* = 200) recorded from the parietal scalp focus for the hand. Brief square electrical pulses of near-threshold intensity are delivered at random intervals to the third finger of the contralateral hand in (B) and (C). The histogram of the subject's reaction times is presented on the same time scale. Early primary components are large and a P45 is indicated by arrows. This is followed by an N120 and a P300. The finger stimuli are delivered alone in (C). They are preceded by 350 msec by a warning click in (B), and thereby the detection percentage is improved from 56 to 81% and the peak latency of the P300 decreases along with the mean reaction times. The warning click is delivered alone, without finger stimuli, in (A) as a control. Notice that the early components are not modified when the P300 changes its features. This figure does not present ERPs to the same stimuli during runs when the subject detects other stimuli. (From Desmedt, Debecker, and Manil, 1965.)

medt, Debecker, and Robertson, 1979). The time from onset to peak of P300 is, on the average, 115 msec, and this may well roughly correspond to the time taken by response selection and initiation when the experimental conditions ensure a rather unambiguous triggering of the motor-commands package (Desmedt and Debecker, 1979a). Thus when the task is changed to decrease decision difficulty (for example by warning; Figure 3), the P300 occurs earlier and the subject's reaction

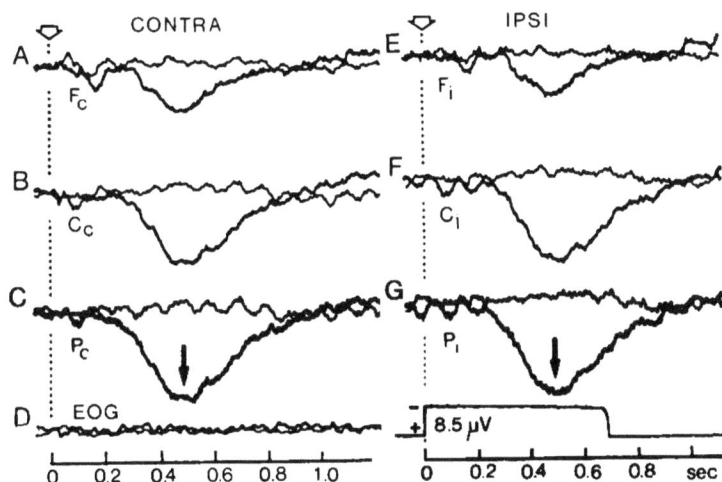

Figure 4 Scalp distribution of the P300 to target-finger stimuli. Brief square electrical pulses of 3.5 mA (1.5 mA above subjective threshold) are delivered in random sequences and at random intervals to the second and third fingers of the two hands. The four-finger paradigm is carried at the mean random rate of 2.5/min. The ERPs to target stimuli in one hand (thicker traces) are superimposed on the ERPs to identical stimuli when they are task irrelevant and the subject attends to stimuli in the opposite hand (thinner traces). The averaged traces were recorded from the contralateral [left column (A), (B), and (C)] and ipsilateral (right column) sides simultaneously at the frontal (Fc or Fi for frontal contra or frontal ipsi), central (Cc or Ci), and parietal (Pc or Pi) regions of the scalp. The horizontal distance between the frontal and central or central and parietal electrodes was 6 cm. All these active electrodes (connected to grid 1 of the amplifiers) were referred to an electrode at the earlobe (grid 2 of the amplifiers) on the same side. In this experiment the target stimuli to the designated finger had a mean probability of one fourth that of the nontarget stimuli to the three other fingers, which were task irrelevant. (D) Control oculograms (EOG). The arrows point to the P300 that had a peak latency of about 460 msec in this example. Calibration is by means of a step function of 8.5 μV. The number of trials averaged N is 130. (From Desmedt and Robertson, 1977a.)

times are also shorter. Anyway, these and other data about time relations exclude the possibility that P300 might precede (rather than follow) the point in time when the subject reaches his decision about the target stimulus and releases his motor response. Thus *P300 reflects a nonselective postdecision closure of cognitive activities,* and it should be contrasted with the middle-range ERP components (such as N140) that index predecision processing (see below).

This interpretation of P300 receives support from its diffuse bilateral scalp distribution with a maximum in the centroparietal region (Figure 4) and from the fact that P300 distribution (in contrast to that of N140) is unaffected by the sensory modality of the eliciting target (Simson, Vaughan, and Ritter, 1976, 1977; Desmedt et al., 1977; Desmedt, Debecker, and Robertson, 1979; Desmedt and Robertson, 1977a; Ritter, Simson, and Vaughan, 1979; Desmedt and Debecker, 1979a). The equal amplitude of P300 over both hemispheres is particularly striking for somatosensory target stimuli whose early components are clearly lateralized to the side opposite to the fingers stimulated (Desmedt and Robertson, 1977a,b). This statement is valid even though in tasks with motor responding, a slight asymmetry can be observed when P300 is distorted by the superimposed negativity of the readiness potential (Deecke and Kornhuber, 1977) that is larger contralateral to the responding hand (Kutas and Donchin, 1977); as a result, the positive P300 appears slightly larger ipsilaterally to that hand (Ragot and Rémond, 1979). The diffuse bilateral distribution of P300 throughout the brain is indeed in line with our proposed interpretation of P300 as reflecting a nonspecific postdecision closure (Desmedt and Debecker, 1979a,b).

It is generally believed in animal physiology that slow late components of evoked potentials have a prolonged refractoriness and habituate rapidly when the eliciting stimulus is repeated. This is only true for slow idle waves that are unrelated to a task. In contrast the P300 recorded in selective attention paradigms does not habituate in serial tasks involving even hundreds of target stimuli, and it is consistently present even when the interstimulus intervals are as short as one second or slightly less (Desmedt and Robertson, 1977a). The conditions for this lack of habituation of P300 are that the task difficulty be maintained throughout (training effects can make the task too easy in later runs of an experiment!) and that the subject be selectively attending and performing adequately. The presence of P300 thus correlates closely with the sequential cognitive activity of the subject and is not subject to any unrelated physiological habituation process.

Middle-Range ERP Components and Sensory Processing

When targets are difficult to identify in certain serial selective-attention tasks, the ERPs generally disclose a marked enhancement of N140 (a negative component with about 120–180-msec peak latency; Hillyard et al., 1973; Schwent et al., 1976; Desmedt and Robertson, 1977a,b; Desmedt and Debecker, 1979a). Several design features appear significant in these studies: (1) bisensory paradigms were used that involved a difficult decision for identifying targets of near-threshold intensity (Desmedt and Debecker, 1979a), or (2) the number of sensory events to be monitored per unit time for identifying the targets was significantly increased, thus achieving forced paced conditions (Debecker and Desmedt, 1971); or (3) more than two sets of stimuli were mixed in the series (Schwent et al., 1976). Thus the subject had to differentiate auditory inputs over either ear (Hillyard et al., 1973), or pitch and spatial location of four sets of sounds (Schwent, Hillyard, and Galambos, 1976), or electrical stimuli to four different fingers in the two hands (Desmedt and Robertson, 1977a). Both the intrinsic difficulty and the rate of signal delivery must be carefully titrated to achieve the appropriate cognitive load; for example, the middle-range ERP components can decrease or disappear when either the mean random rate of signals is reduced below a certain value (Debecker and Desmedt, 1971; Desmedt and Robertson, 1977b), or when stronger suprathreshold stimuli are delivered at the same rate (cf. Hillyard and Picton, 1979; Desmedt, Debecker, and Robertson, 1979).

When using random sequences of four different stimulus types of which one is task relevant, the mean random frequency of *targets* can be kept at 0.5–1/sec, while the total input that the subject must monitor involves a mean random rate of about 2.5/sec. This rate of 2.5/sec corresponds to the maximum rate of correct decisions that can be achieved under steady-state sequential sensory overload, regardless whether the signal delivery is changed between 3 and 5/sec (Debecker and Desmedt, 1970). This task is thus just feasible, but exacting, and it can only be achieved by motivated subjects, in the absence of fatigue. Human operators in complex control systems or high-velocity machines can normally be confronted with such forced paced conditions for short times. Figure 5 illustrates a remarkable feature of the paradigm under discussion, namely the difference in ERP to nontarget signals, which depends to some extent on whether these nontargets share neural channels with the targets (Desmedt and Robertson, 1977a). Thus the stimuli to the *third finger of the left hand* are targets to be identified in the run considered (Figure 5B,C, thicker traces) and they elicit ERPs with an enhanced N140 larger contralaterally and a bilateral P300. Virtually no N140 or P300 occurs for identical stimuli to the same finger when the subject attends in other runs to a finger on the opposite hand (faint traces in Figure 5B,C). The latter traces provide the best baseline control for the cognitive components in ERPs since everything is identical, except that a brief verbal instruction has switched the task to another target just before the run started.

Now the near-threshold stimuli to fingers of the neglected hand can easily be ignored, and indeed they are barely perceived by the subject whose perceptual resources are committed to monitoring the opposite hand. However, the stimuli to the *second finger of the left hand* are quite obtrusive (introspective data) and difficult to distinguish from the target stimuli delivered to the adjacent second finger on the same hand. In fact, it is observed that the nontarget stimuli to the second finger also elicit an N140 that is larger over the contralateral scalp (Figure 5E,F, thicker traces). This can be evaluated with respect to the baseline control (thinner traces) recorded when the task involved the opposite hand in different runs. That the targets and nontargets in the left hand are well differentiated by the subject is evidenced from the accuracy of the mental counts after each run. Furthermore the data are internally consistent since P300 is virtually lacking from the ERPs elicited by these nontargets (Figure 5E,F). This is in line with the discussion of the preceding section. One essential point had not been clarified in previous publications: Do N140 and P300 represent two successive stages of the

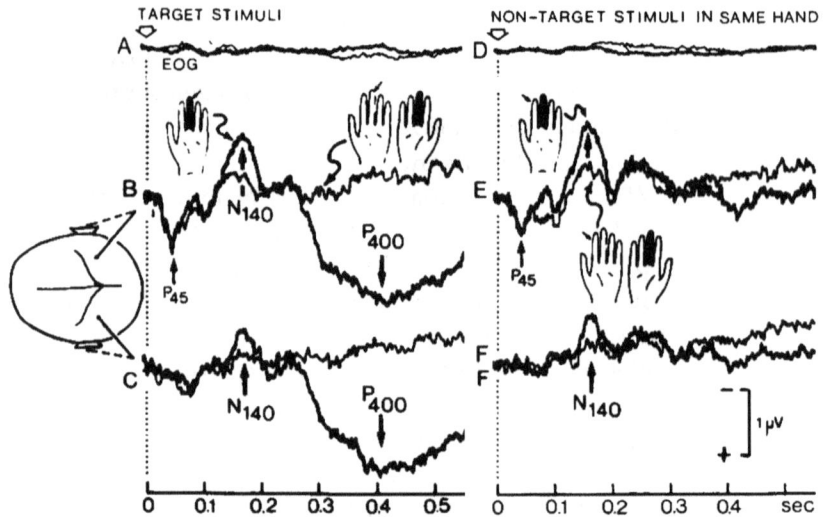

Figure 5 Dissociation of N140 and P300 ERP components in the fast four-finger random paradigm. Brief square electrical pulses of near-threshold intensity are delivered in random sequences and at random intervals to the second and third fingers of the two hands. The mean random rate for all stimuli is 150/min. The ERPs are recorded from the parietal scalp regions on either side (grid 1 of amplifiers), and the reference electrode is placed on the earlobe of the same side (grid 2 of amplifiers), indicated in the figure on the left side. (A,D) EOC controls, (B) contralateral, and (C) ipsilateral ERP to stimuli delivered to the third finger of the left hand when they are targets to be mentally counted (thicker traces), or when the subject has to neglect these stimuli in order to attend to stimuli to the third finger of the opposite hand (thinner traces). The small arrow points to the finger stimulated to evoke the trace considered. Attended fingers are in black. The early primary P45 component is present contralaterally to the finger stimulated (B) but not ipsilaterally (C), and it is not modified by task. N140 is larger contralaterally (B) when measured from the ERP baseline of thinner trace. The P300 (indicated as P400 from its peak latency in this experiment) has about the same amplitude on both sides (B,C) for the targets, and it is absent from the control baseline. (E) and (F) present ERPs to stimuli delivered to the *second* finger of the left hand in the same runs, namely, when targets to the *third* finger of the left hand are monitored and counted (thicker traces) or neglected (thinner traces). The task of differentiating stimuli to the second and third fingers of the same left hand is very difficult, but it has been carried out accurately in this experiment. N140s occur for both targets and nontargets in the attended hand, but P300s only occur to the targets. (From Desmedt and Robertson, 1977a.)

454   John E. Desmedt

processing operations whereby the subject eventually makes an appropriate decision about the signals, or are they related to brain operations of an entirely different nature? I definitely favor the latter view, which is supported by the actual experimental dissociation recorded in ERPs to nontarget stimuli delivered to the same hand as the targets. For the nontargets N140 indexes the predecision processor that must be engaged in order to achieve a difficult differentiation between signals that are anatomically close (since they arrive from the same hand and go to the same part of the contralateral postcentral primary cortex; see below).

The finding that N140 is, on the average, twice as large in the cerebral hemisphere contralateral to the hand receiving task-relevant signals (Desmedt and Robertson, 1977a) suggests that it indexes a processor in associative parietal cortex (areas 5 and 7) on that side that is closely connected to the primary postcentral cortex upon which that hand projects. The fact that the electrogenesis is not *totally* lateralized may be related to bilateral interactions, through, e.g., callosal connections known to exist between these associative areas (cf. Jones and Powell, 1969). The important points at this stage are the different parametric sets and more focal distribution of N140 as compared to P300.

The contralateral segregation of somatosensory input from the hands to the parietal area of the opposite side is documented by evoked-potential data in man (cf. Figure 5B with Figure 5C,E,F for the early ERP components; Desmedt and Robertson, 1977a; Desmedt and Cheron, 1980a,b) and is in line with anatomical data of lemniscal projections to the receiving areas 3, 1, 2 and of lack of callosal connections for the primary projections from distal limb (Jones and Powell, 1969; Pandya and Vignolo, 1969). For the present discussion of ERPs in the four-fingers paradigm, these data imply that sensory input from the neglected hand arrives to the opposite postcentral cortex and will not mix with the input from the attended hand until later stages of processing. Thus a clear situation is provided in which an *input selection mode of selective attention* (Treisman, 1969; Broadbent, 1970; cf. Hillyard and Picton, 1979) can be switched on, in conjunction with the prior instructions given to the subject, in order to prime the processors connected to the receiving cortical areas contralateral to the attended hand. Such a stimulus set is also operating in the bisensory paradigms (e.g., series of acoustic click and finger stimuli) in which, contrary to a statement by Hillyard and Picton (1979), we recorded clear enhancements of N140 even at very slow pace with large randomly varying interstimulus intervals (Desmedt and Debecker, 1979a; Desmedt, Debecker, and Robertson, 1979). Knowing in advance the places (or sensory channels) where irrelevant or relevant information is going to occur thus allows a first selection of signals to be made with relatively little perceptual analysis. Our ERP data emphasize that the early primary components of the cortical SEP response (latency range from 20 to about 70 msec; Table I) are *not* reduced in amplitude nor significantly changed for the rejected

Table I Average time features of components of event-related potentials to target-finger stimuli in serial selective-attention tasks (msec)[a]

Onset latency of primary cortical components	20
Onset latency of cognitive N140	70
Peak latency of N140	130
Onset latency of postdecision P300	250
Peak latency of P300	365
Tentative time slot for somatosensory	
Primary components	20 to 70
Middle range components	70 to 250
Postdecision components	after 250

a. Adapted from data of Desmedt and Robertson (1977a) and Desmedt and Debecker (1979a).

signals (Figure 5; Desmedt, Debecker, and Manil, 1965; Desmedt et al., 1977; Desmedt and Robertson, 1977a). Therefore the simple "filter" or channel-attenuation hypothesis of selective attention of Broadbent, or put in physiological terms, a centrifugal gating of the input (Towe, 1973; Desmedt, 1975), do not provide a ready explanation. More likely mechanisms deserving investigation could be the neuromodulation of neuron sets in association cortex or the neural synaptic control of intracortical or corticocortical transmission out of the primary receiving areas.

The analysis of ERP components tentatively can be carried out further. Under the particular conditions of serial selective-attention tasks involving simple signals, an average latency of about 250 msec appears to correspond to the decision closure after which the nonspecific P300 phenomenon is released. Predecision processing can be indexed at least in part by electrogeneses such as N140s that are associated with target signals under conditions when sufficient processing resources have been engaged by the cognitive task. In both the bisensory near-threshold detection at slow rates (Desmedt and Debecker, 1979a,b) and in the intrasensory decision sequences at fast rates (Schwent, Hillyard, and Galambos, 1976; Desmedt and Robertson, 1977a), the cognitive N140 component to somatosensory targets has been found to diverge from baseline control at latencies of 50–130 msec in different experiments, the mean value being about 70 msec (Table I, Figure 6A,B). If it is assumed that N140 would faithfully index the time course of cognitive processing of targets, this could be taken to occupy a time span of about 70–250 msec after stimulus delivery (Table I). This point is interesting for the discussion of time allocations in serial processing, even though it should not be taken to imply that no differential cortical processing can occur before 70 msec (or before the shortest delay of 50 msec seen for a cognitive N140 in some experiments; Desmedt and Robertson, 1977a).

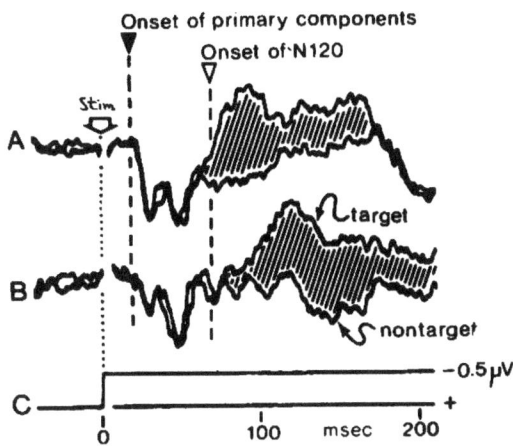

Figure 6 Early and middle-range ERP components in selective attention. The experiments involve a bisensory paradigm with random sequences of acoustic clicks and brief electrical square pulses to one finger. All stimuli are near threshold and difficult to detect. Intervals between stimuli vary at random over a range from 1 to 15 seconds. (A,B) ERPs to contralateral finger stimuli recorded from parietal scalp focus with earlobe reference. These stimuli are targets to be mentally counted in one of the superimposed traces showing a large N140. (A) and (B) correspond to two experiments on different subjects. The onset of the cortical primary components occurs at about 20 msec (first vertical interrupted line). The primary components are not changed by the task. The N140 elicited when the finger stimuli are targets diverges from control at about 70 msec (second vertical interrupted line). The divergence is slightly earlier in (A) and slightly later in (B), as indicated by the start of the hatched area. (See Desmedt and Debecker, 1979a.)

The observation that simple decisions cannot be made serially at rates exceeding about 2.5/sec (Debecker and Desmedt, 1970) is compatible because this corresponds to a time span of 400 msec that would include both the primary and middle-range ERP components as well as part of the postdecision P300 whose average peak latency is 365 msec (Table I). More relaxed conditions of serial processing are achieved in tasks at slower rates with intervals of 600–800 msec ("intervalles agréables," Fraisse, 1957) that actually correspond to the average time for completion of a standard P300 (Desmedt and Debecker, 1979a).

The proposed interpretations differ in significant respects from that of Schwent, Hillyard, and Galambos (1976) and Hillyard and Picton (1979), who associate N140 rather exclusively with stimulus-set processing and interpret P300 as reflecting a memory-dependent selection process. I do not agree with their relating P300 to a distinct signal processor, but suggest instead that P300 fulfills an entirely different postdecision closure function and is elicited when the signal processing has completed itself in a decision (Desmedt and Debecker, 1979a,b). It is also emphasized that N140 can be elicited in the absence of any forced paced conditions in conjunction with the difficult detection of near-threshold targets (Figure 6). As a matter of fact, it is not necessary to have irrelevant stimuli in the selected channel for N140 to be elicited. But if such irrelevant nontargets do occur, as with the stimuli to the finger adjacent to target in Figure 5E,F, then the N140 processor will also be engaged by these nontarget signals for the purpose of telling them apart from the targets (Desmedt and Robertson, 1977a). Obviously a simple stimulus-set condition, whatever this implies in terms of physiological mechanisms (see above), cannot cope with such non-targets whose ambiguity, and possible equivocation with targets, appears related to proximity or interaction of the respective afferent connectivities.

Neural Basis of ERP Components

While most current studies restrict their scope to the psychological correlates of ERPs, it is also necessary to consider their possible neural mechanisms, which eventually should be related as far as possible to molecular neurobiology of the brain. Besides the differences in ERP components associated with brain maturation from birth (cf. Courchesne, 1979) or pathological conditions (cf. Goodin, Squires, and Starr, 1978), a wide variety of ERP features has been described. The present discussion is restricted to the more characteristic and reproducible items that can be recorded in the sequential processing of target and nontarget stimuli when the subject consistently fulfills a definite serial cognitive task. For example, the P300 considered is a well-defined component with centroparietal scalp distribution that is elicited by task-relevant stimuli (component P3b of Squires, Squires, and Hillyard, 1975b).

The transient positivity of P300 is bilateral and diffuse throughout the brain. It does not index any modality-specific processor and can be interpreted as a postdecision closure phenomenon that has to do with the kinetics of cognitive sections in time. It is indeed possible that P300 represents a transient inhibitory process separating successive sections in serial selective attention (Desmedt and Debecker, 1979b). P300 can be discussed along with the contingent negative variation (CNV) recorded as a transient negativity in situations where a warning stimulus is followed at standard interval by an imperative stimulus calling for subject response (Walter et al., 1964; McCallum and Knott, 1973). The CNV presents a diffuse bilateral centroparietal distribution, much like P300, and is also recorded in depth (McCallum et al., 1973; Rebert, 1977). In split-brain human patients (cf. Sperry, 1974) a warning stimulus delivered to one hemisphere creates a unilateral expectancy and motor preparation, but it elicits a CNV with equal amplitude on both sides (Hillyard, 1973). The CNV or expectancy wave is best elicited when a brief period of attention is set (by the warning) against an undemanding background during which the subject can relax. The CNV is generally smaller in tense subjects or in situational anxiety (Low and

Swift, 1971) for which the cortical negativity is already quite large. P300 and CNV react differentially to experimental variables (Donchin et al., 1975; Chapman et al., 1979; Ruchkin and Sutton, 1979), and P300 occurs without any preceding CNV when warning cues are excluded through complete randomization of the serial task (Desmedt and Debecker, 1979a). Both P300 and CNV in fact represent transient changes of the level of dc negativity that develops and is maintained in conjunction with wakefulness and attention, as demonstrated in experiments on behaving mammals with implanted cortical electrodes (Caspers, 1963; Wurtz, 1966; Rowland, 1968).

Because of their diffuse distribution both these slow potential shifts (SPS), CNV and P300, must be related to one or more subcortical neural systems whereby widespread neuromodulatory controls are exerted throughout the telencephalon. Two systems closely related to the mesencephalic reticular formation (MRF) are likely candidates for this function, and their modes of operation, either separate or combined, are far from clear. On the one hand, cerebral activation and arousal have been associated with a diffuse muscarinic action (Yamamura et al., 1974) associated with a reduced resting potassium conductance in cerebral neurons (Krnjevic et al., 1971), and the widespread fibers releasing acetylcholine in the cortex (Celesia and Jasper, 1966; Szerb, 1967) have been found to originate from cholinergic neurons of the forebrain magnocellular nuclei (Divac, 1975; Mesulam and VanHoesen, 1976; Emson and Lindvall, 1979). The detailed interactions between this system of forebrain cholinergic neurons and the MRF have not yet been clarified. On the other hand, the noradrenergic neurons of the locus coeruleus have a widespread distribution on many neural systems including the neocortex (Moore and Bloom, 1979). This rather small number (about 3,000) of widely ramifying locus coeruleus neurons appears to represent a unitary capability for the regulation of synaptic transactions in widespread areas of the brain.

Both acetylcholine-muscarinic and noradrenergic effects on neurons occur with rather long latency and duration, presumably because the neurotransmitter binding to receptor initiates intracellular biochemical reactions that control the electrophysiological properties of the target neurons (Lee, Kuo, and Greengard, 1972; Bloom, 1976; Greengard, 1978). For example, the slow muscarinic effects of acetylcholine may be mediated intracellularly via the cyclic GMP system while the norepinephrine effects may involve the cyclic AMP system. In the rat both cyclic GMP and acetylcholine elicit facilitatory effects of spontaneous activities in most cortical pyramidal neurons, while norepinephrine and cyclic AMP have depressant effects on spontaneous activities (Stone, Taylor, and Bloom, 1975; Stone and Taylor, 1977). Besides these effects on spontaneous spikes, the two systems achieve important heterosynaptic interactions whereby acetylcholine- or norepinephrine-induced changes in membrane resistance of postsynaptic neurons result in an increased reactivity of the latter to other synaptic effects that may actually be either excitatory or inhibitory (Woodward et al., 1979; Moore and Bloom, 1979). The concept of neuromodulation indicates that, even though the diffusely produced membrane potential changes are apparently minimal and widespread throughout the cortex, a remarkable amplification of the phasic conventional synaptic actions may result that presumably exert specific control of transactions in cerebral processors. Recordings from cortical neurons in behaving mammals, taken in conjunction with ERP experiments, appear essential in order to elaborate pending issues. For example, Skinner et al. (1978) implanted a cryoplate over the parietal cortex of rats and found correlations between the cortical SPS to psychological stress recorded in the conscious animal and the cyclic AMP content of the rapidly (100-msec) frozen cortical tissue from which these SPSs had been recorded. The working hypothesis is proposed that the different SPS, CNV, and P300 electrogeneses reflect to some extent neuromodulation processes controlled by nonspecific subcortical systems including the MRF. These potentials, however, may only provide a rough index of these neurochemical processes, some of which might occur without producing any sizable change in membrane potentials of neurons.

The question may also be asked of the possible role of neuroglia in these potentials. Glial cells can present slow depolarizations, which do not appear to be endogenously generated, but are the passive consequence of increased extracellular concentration of potassium ions when adjacent neurons are excited (Ransom and Goldring, 1973; Somjen, 1975). Neuromodulatory changes do not by themselves elicit action potential discharges in neurons, and therefore they would not seem likely to evoke glial electrogeneses. However the neuroglia may fulfill another important function by controlling the extracellular concentration of released chemical transmitters. For example, glia is quite effective in taking up GABA and it may contribute to limiting its level in the extracellular space (Henn and Hamberger, 1971). It is also known that the level of cortical acetylcholine is controlled by the pseudocholinesterase (butyrocholinesterase) associated with glia (but not with neurons) in cortex; the selective pharmacological inhibition of the pseudocholinesterase results in an intense cortical activation, an effect that is not observed for the selective inhibition of the cortical acetocholinesterase (Desmedt, 1956; Desmedt and LaGrutta, 1957). Thus the glial regulation of acetylcholine may be significant in relation to the muscarinic neuromodulation in telencephalon.

The next question is whether the levels of activation in the MRF and subcortical systems just considered can be changed and paced in relation to selective-attention tasks. The MRF itself obviously cannot be considered the initiator of the pacing in conjunction with complex behavior, but it should not be considered unable to operate phasic shifts of attention. In fact it is proposed that MRF-mediated neuromodulations of the telencephalon are controlled by the prefrontal cortex (cf. Desmedt and Debecker, 1979a). There are substantial anatomical projections from frontal cortex to the preoptic region and hypothalamus, and to a paramedial zone of the mesencephalic tegmentum (Nauta, 1962, 1964, 1971; Millhouse, 1969), as well as physiological evidence that the basal forebrain and preoptic regions directly inhibit the MRF and reduce arousal (Clemente and Sterman, 1967; Bremer, 1977; Moruzzi, 1972).

Luria and Homskaya (1970) showed that prefrontal lesions in man disturb the control of arousal and of the orienting reflex to irrelevant stimuli. More specifically the studies of such patients indicate that the prefrontal granular cortex controls goal-oriented behavior, namely, when repeated task-relevant shifts of response are required (Milner, 1964; Luria and Homskaya, 1970). Thus the successive responses of the patient are no longer appropriate to the high-priority versus irrelevant items, respectively, of any serial task or changing environmental conditions. Fuster (1973) also observed in monkeys an increased activity of single neurons in prefrontal cortex during delayed-response paradigms. Conversely the orienting response to irrelevant stimuli was enhanced in cats with chronic lesions of prefrontal cortex or by transient reversible stereotaxic cooling of the efferent pathway from prefrontal cortex to diencephalon and midbrain (Skinner and Yingling, 1977; Yingling and Skinner, 1977).

That the prefrontal granular cortex should assume such controlling functions over behavior is not surprising since it receives important corticocortical projections from the associative cortex of all sensory modalities (Jones and Powell, 1970; Chavis and Pandya, 1976) in addition to a major projection from the limbic system through the medial dorsal thalamic nucleus (Akert, 1964; Nauta, 1971). Prefrontal areas indeed have unique capabilities for integrating information about the world outside (sensory modalities) and about the basic drives of the individual (limbic motivational system). These features make it possible to organize behavior in conjunction with current demands and expected events, for example, through inhibitory regulation of timed levels of activation of MRF that in turn sets levels of neuromodulation (reflected at least partially through the recorded SPS and CNV) throughout the telencephalon (Desmedt and Debecker, 1979a). Physiological differentiation among the prefrontal cortex processors should allow differential controls to be exerted on the MRF, such as for momentary adjustments of the cortical dc baseline (recorded as CNV or SPS) and the postdecision clearance operation of the P300.

In our model the MRF-mediated neuromodulation of telencephalon is implicated as a major effector of the prefrontal pacemaker for both CNV and P300 since these are largely coextensive bilateral diffuse potentials that are not specific for any sensory modality (cf. Desmedt and Debecker, 1979a,b). The opposite polarity of the positive P300 to the negative SPS and CNV can be ascribed to up or down variations of the tonic neuromodulatory pressure. The reason for not implicating the medial thalamic system as a primary effector for these diffuse potentials is that stimulation of medial thalamus in cats elicits SPS in rather restricted cortical areas (Brookhart et al., 1958), whereas MRF stimulation elicits diffuse SPS throughout cortex (Arduini, 1958; Moruzzi, 1972; Skinner and Yingling, 1977). The model by no means excludes the possibility that important interactions between prefrontal cortical areas, medial thalamus, reticular thalamic nucleus, and MRF could underlie these regulations (cf. Skinner and Yingling, 1977). For example, an increased arousal level is associated with inhibition of unit firing and with extracellular positive SPS in the reticular thalamic nucleus (Yingling and Skinner, 1977), these effects apparently being mediated through a cholinergic inhibitory mechanism (Ben-Ari et al., 1976).

Concluding Remarks

As research develops along these challenging lines, the actual contributions of a number of brain systems should gradually be identified and delineated. The cognitive processing of even simple sensory events in serial selective-attention tasks obviously involves complex brain mechanisms. Our working hypothesis attempts to identify a few key relationships in order to assist in the design of potentially useful research paradigms.

A major part of the model (Desmedt and Debecker, 1979a,b) proposes the following: (1) P300 is a diffuse generalized event without any sensory modality specificity that involves both cerebral hemispheres equally (Figure 5) as well as subcortical and brain-stem structures (McCallum et al., 1973); (2) P300 results from a transient reduction of the neuromodulation pressure that is maintained in the telencephalon during waking and attention through diffusely distributed connections involving either muscarinic cholinergic neurons, or norepinephrine neurons, or both (see above). These diffuse control systems adjusting general levels of neuromodulation are likely to be controlled by the mesencephalic reticular formation (MRF), whose operational features appear congruent with such functions. The MRF system itself is conceived as being biased and controlled by associative cortex, namely, by the prefrontal cortex, which has to do with the serial organization and integration of goal-oriented behavior; (3) P300 is elicited when the processing of target information has been completed by a positive decision. P300 thus indexes a postdecision closure of the cognitive activities (Desmedt and Debecker, 1979a). Considering the kinetics and amplitude variations of P300, this closure mechanism does not possess all-or-none properties, but can be adjusted in conjunction with relevant items in serial cognitive behavior. Both the subject's attitudes, situational urgency or complexity, and the nature of the current task issues may permit different types of cognitive decisions, which can either be clear and resolve a fair amount of ambiguity, or be partial and subject to revision pending further information input. It is therefore not surprising that the timing of successive cognitive epochs separated by P300 is far from fixed; for example, in language comprehension, P300 size and occurrence is influenced by syntax and sentence structure (cf. Desmedt, 1977c). Also the absence of P300 after nontarget signals, which must nevertheless be processed and identified for the purpose of task performance, suggests that the cognitive activities then remain open, closure being suspended in anticipation of subsequent target signals. The analysis of the dynamics of postdecision closure mechanisms in different tasks should no doubt clarify important issues.

In contrast to P300 thus viewed as a nonspecific closure mechanism, the cerebral electrogeneses occurring between the sensory input and the time of the cognitive decision (about 250 msec in the conditions considered; see Table I) have to do with actual signal processing and recognition. A clear differentiation must be made between two classes of components occupying the predecision time slot.

The early "primary" components corresponding to the arrival of input in the receiving cortical areas have only been consistently analyzed for the somatosensory modality. They have not disclosed any significant change in waveform or amplitude with task. Up to at least 50 msec the cortical components evoked by physically identical sensory stimuli are not influenced, irrespective of whether these stimuli serve as targets to be identified or as irrelevant nontargets in alternative runs of the same experiments (Figure 5). Thus the mechanism for target selection cannot be equated with any simplistic centrifugal "gating" of the sensory volley traveling up the specific (lemniscal) corticipetal pathway. In other words, and as far as one can tell from averaged cerebral evoked potentials, the cortex of the sensory modality is similarly involved up to 50–70 msec by a specific input, irrespective of the cognitive task to be accomplished on that input (Desmedt, Debecker, and Manil, 1965; Desmedt, Debecker, and Robertson, 1979; Desmedt and Robertson, 1977a; Desmedt and Debecker, 1979a).

On the other hand, the second class of predecision ERP components, of which N140 is an example, can be dramatically influenced by the task. N140 is not an "exogenous" component that would be evoked at all times by the stimulus. N140 is either elicited or enhanced (over and above the baseline provided by the control ERPs in the nontarget condition, see Figures 5, 6) by the target stimuli. Contrary to P300, N140 is not diffuse over the scalp. But it discloses different areal scalp distributions for targets in the different sensory modalities (cf. Ritter, Simson, and Vaughan, 1979). For somatosensory targets N140 is about twice as large over the cerebral hemisphere contralateral to the hand receiving the task-relevant stimuli (Desmedt and Robertson, 1977a,b). Therefore middle-range predecision components such as N140 must be related, not to the diffuse cholinergic or norepinephrine neural systems, but to more spatially differentiated neuron assemblies that perform definite processing operations. One likely neural basis appears to be the reticular nucleus of thalamus, whose different parts exert tonic inhibitory control over different thalamic relay nuclei, an effect that either can be reduced during MRF activation or increased and differentially adjusted by activation of prefrontal cortical areas (cf. Alexander, Newman, and Symmes, 1976; Skinner and Yingling, 1977). This thalamic system might mediate the neuromodulation of specific cortical processors in the attended sensory modality, as revealed by N140 or right hemisphere electrogenesis (Desmedt, 1977b). In view of the recorded stability of the early primary components of the evoked potential, this mechanism presumably involves the associative thalamocortical regions rather than the lemniscal path to the receiving areas.

It is interesting that N140 and P300 can be dissociated in various experimental paradigms (Hillyard and Picton, 1979; Desmedt, Debecker, and Robertson, 1979). N140 is associated with target signals when sufficient processing resources must be engaged to achieve the cognitive task. In easy tasks N140 may fail to be recorded even though P300 occurs after such targets. However N140 is also associated with a class of nontargets that cannot be rejected by mere input selection, for example, when they occur in the same hand as the target signals and therefore project to the same receiving postcentral cortical areas as the targets (Figure 5); such difficult decisions then elicit large asymmetrical N140 for the nontargets which do *not* evoke any P300, as indeed is to be expected (Figure 5).

Acknowledgments

This research has been supported by grants from the Fonds National de la Recherche Scientifique and the Fonds de la Recherche Scientifique Médicale of Belgium.

References

Akert, K., 1964. Comparative anatomy of frontal cortex and thalamofrontal connections. In *The Frontal Granular Cortex and Behavior*. J. M. Warren and K. Akert, eds. New York: McGraw-Hill, pp. 372–396.

Alexander, S. E., J. D. Newman, and D. Symmes, 1976. Convergence of prefrontal and acoustic inputs upon neurons in the superior temporal gyrus of the awake squirrel monkey. *Brain Res.* 116:334–338.

Arduini, A., 1958. Enduring potential changes evoked in the cerebral cortex by stimulation of brainstem reticular formation and thalamus. In *Reticular Formation of the Brain*. H. H. Jasper, L. D. Proctor, R. S. Knighton, W. C. Noshay, and R. T. Costello, eds. Boston: Little Brown & Co., pp. 333–354.

Begleiter, H., ed., 1976. *Evoked Brain Potentials of Behavior*. New York: Plenum Press.

Ben-Ari, Y., R. Dingledine, I. Kanazawa, and J. S. Kelly, 1976. Inhibitory effects of acetylcholine on neurones in the feline nucleus reticularis thalami. *J. Physiol. (London)* 261:647–671.

Bloom, F. E., 1976. The role of cyclic nucleotides in central synaptic functions. *Adv. Biochem. Psychopharmacol.* 15:273–282.

Bremer, F., 1977. Cerebral hypnogenic centers. *Ann. Neurol.* 2:1–6.

Broadbent, D. E., 1970. Stimulus set and response set: Two kinds of selective attention. In *Attention: Contemporary Theory and Analysis*. D. I. Mostofsky, ed. New York: Appleton Century Crofts, pp. 51–60.

Brookhart, J. M., A. Arduini, M. Mancia, and G. Moruzzi, 1958. Thalamocortical relations as revealed by induced slow potential changes. *J. Neurophysiol.* 21:499–525.

Caspers, H., 1963. Relations of steady potential shifts in the cortex to the wakefulness-sleep spectrum. In *Brain Function*, Vol. 1. M. A. B. Brazier, ed. Los Angeles: University of California Press, pp. 177–214.

Celesia, G. G., and H. H. Jasper, 1966. Acetylcholine released from cerebral cortex in relation to state of activation. *Neurol. Minneapolis* 16:1053–1063.

Chapman, R. M., J. W. McCrary, H. R. Bragdon, and J. A. Chapman, 1979. Latent components of event-related potentials functionally related to information processing. In *Cognitive Components in Cerebral Event-Related Potentials and Selective Attention. Prog. Clin. Neurophysiol.*, Vol. 6. J. E. Desmedt, ed. Basel: Karger, pp. 80–105.

Chavis, D. A., and D. N. Pandya, 1976. Further observations on corticofrontal connections in the rhesus monkey. *Brain Res.* 117:369–386.

Clemente, C. D., and M. B. Sterman, 1967. Basal forebrain mechanisms for internal inhibition and sleep. *Res. Publ. Assoc. Res. Nerv. Ment. Dis.* 45:127–145.

Courchesne, E., 1979. From infancy to adulthood: The neurophysiological correlates of cognition. In *Cognitive Components in Cerebral Event-Related Potentials and Selective Attention. Prog. Clin. Neurophysiol.*, Vol. 6. J. E. Desmedt, ed. Basel: Karger, pp. 224–242.

Cracco, R. Q., 1973. Spinal evoked response: Peripheral nerve stimulation in man. *Electroenceph. Clin. Neurophysiol.* 35:379–386.

Debecker, J., and J. E. Desmedt, 1970. Maximum capacity for sequential one-bit auditory decisions. *J. Exper. Psychol.* 83:366–372.

Debecker, J., and J. E. Desmedt, 1971. Cerebral evoked potential correlates in forced-paced tasks. *Nature New Biol.* 234:118–120.

Debecker, J., J. E. Desmedt, and J. Manil, 1965. Sur la relation entre le seuil de perception tactile et les potentiels évoqués de l'écorce cérébrale somatosensible chez l'homme. *C. R. Acad. Sci. Paris* 260:687–689.

Deecke, L., and H. H. Kornhuber, 1977. Cerebral potentials and the initiation of voluntary movements. In *Attention, Voluntary Contraction and Event-Related Cerebral Potentials. Prog. Clin. Neurophysiol.*, Vol. 1. J. E. Desmedt, ed. Basel: Karger, pp. 132–150.

Desmedt, J. E., 1956. A cholinergic "local hormone" mechanism in the cat's brain. *Electroenceph. Clin. Neurophysiol.* 8:701.

Desmedt, J. E., 1971. Somatosensory cerebral evoked potentials in man. In *Handbook of Electroencephalography and Clinical Neurophysiology*, Vol. 9. A. Rémond, ed. Amsterdam: Elsevier, pp. 55–82.

Desmedt, J. E., 1975. Physiological studies of the efferent recurrent auditory system. In *Handbook of Sensory Physiology*, Vol. 5. W. Keidel and W. D. Neff, eds. Berlin: Springer, pp. 219–246.

Desmedt, J. E., 1977a. Some observations on the methodology of cerebral evoked potentials in man. In *Attention, Voluntary Contraction and Event-Related Cerebral Potentials. Prog. Clin. Neurophysiol.*, Vol. 1. J. E. Desmedt, ed. Basel: Karger, pp. 12–29.

Desmedt, J. E., 1977b. Active touch exploration of extrapersonal space elicits specific electrogenesis in the right cerebral hemisphere of intact right-handed man. *Proc. Nat. Acad. Sci. USA* 74:4037–4040.

Desmedt, J. E., ed., 1977c. *Language and Hemispheric Specialization in Man: Cerebral Event-Related Potentials. Prog. Clin. Neurophysiol.*, Vol. 3. Basel: Karger.

Desmedt, J. E., ed., 1977d. *Visual Evoked Potentials in Man: New Developments.* Oxford: Oxford University Press.

Desmedt, J. E., ed., 1979. *Cognitive Components in Cerebral Event-Related Potentials and Selective Attention. Prog. Clin. Neurophysiol.*, Vol. 6. Basel: Karger.

Desmedt, J. E., ed., 1980. *Clinical Uses of Cerebral, Brainstem and Spinal Somatosensory Evoked Potentials. Prog. Clin. Neurophysiol*, Vol. 7. Basel: Karger.

Desmedt, J. E., and G. Cheron, 1980a. Central somatosensory conduction in man: Neural generators and interpeak latencies of the far field components recorded from neck and right or left scalp and earlobes. *Electroenceph. Clin. Neurophysiol.* 50.

Desmedt, J. E., and G. Cheron, 1980b. Somatosensory evoked potentials to finger stimulation in healthy octogenarians and in young adults: Waveform and central transit times of parietal and frontal components. *Electroenceph. Clin. Neurophysiol.* 50.

Desmedt, J. E., and J. Debecker, 1979a. Wave form and neural mechanism of the decision P350 elicited without pre-stimulus CNV or readiness potential in random sequences of near-threshold auditory clicks and finger stimuli. *Electroenceph. Clin. Neurophysiol.* 47:648–670.

Desmedt, J. E., and J. Debecker, 1979b. Slow potential shifts and decision P300 interactions in tasks with random sequences of near-threshold clicks and finger stimuli delivered at regular intervals. *Electroenceph. Clin. Neurophysiol.* 47:671–679.

Desmedt, J. E., and G. LaGrutta, 1957. The effect of selective inhibition of pseudocholinesterase on the spontaneous and evoked activity of the cat's cerebral cortex. *J. Physiol. (London)* 136:20–40.

Desmedt, J. E., J. Debecker, and J. Manil, 1965. Mise en évidence d'un signe électrique cérébral associé à la détection par le subjet d'un stimulus sensoriel tactile. *Bull. Acad. Roy. Méd. Belg.* 5:887–936.

Desmedt, J. E., and D. Robertson, 1977a. Differential enhancement of early and late components of the cerebral somatosensory evoked potentials during forced-paced cognitive tasks in man. *J. Physiol. (London)* 271:761–782.

Desmedt, J. E., and D. Robertson, 1977b. Search for right hemisphere asymmetries in event-related potentials to somatosensory cueing signals. In *Language and Hemispheric Specialization in Man: Cerebral Event-Related Potentials. Prog. Clin. Neurophysiol.*, Vol. 3. J. E. Desmedt, ed. Basel: Karger, pp. 172–187.

Desmedt, J. E., J. Debecker, and D. Robertson, 1979. Serial perceptual processing and the neural basis of changes in event-related potential components and slow potential shifts. In *Cognitive Components in Cerebral Event-Related Potentials and Selective Attention. Prog. Clin. Neurophysiol.*, Vol. 6. J. E. Desmedt, ed. Basel, Karger, pp. 53–79.

Desmedt, J. E., L. Franken, S. Borenstein, J. Debecker, C. Lambert, and J. Manil, 1966. Le diagnostic des ralentissements de la conduction afférente dans les affections des nerfs périphériques: intérêt de l'extraction du potentiel évoqué cérébral. *Rev. Neurol.* 115:255–262.

Desmedt, J. E., D. Robertson, E. Brunko, and J. Debecker, 1977. Somatosensory decision tasks in man: Early and late components of the cerebral potentials evoked by stimulation of different fingers in random sequences. *Electroenceph. Clin. Neurophysiol.* 43:404–415.

Divac, I., 1975. Magnocellular nuclei of the basal forebrain project to neocortex brainstem and olfactory bulb. Review of some functional correlates. *Brain Res.* 93:385–398.

Donchin, E., and L. Cohen, 1967. Average evoked potentials and intramodality selective attention. *Electroenceph. Clin. Neurophysiol.* 22:537–546.

Donchin, E., and D. B. Lindsley, eds., 1969. *Average Evoked Potentials.* Washington, DC: US Government Printing Office.

Donchin, E., E. Callaway, R. Cooper, J. E. Desmedt, W. R. Goff, S. A. Hillyard, and S. Sutton, 1977. Publication criteria for studies of evoked potentials in man: Report of a committee. In *Attention, Voluntary Contraction and Event-Related Cerebral Potentials in Man. Prog. Clin. Neurophysiol.*, Vol. 1. J. E. Desmedt, ed. Basel: Karger, pp. 1–11.

Donchin, E., G. McCarthy, and M. Kutas, 1977. Electroencephalographic investigations of hemispheric specialization. In *Language and Hemispheric Specialization in Man: Cerebral Event-Related Potentials. Prog. Clin. Neurophysiol.*, Vol. 3, J. E. Desmedt, ed., Basel: Karger, pp. 212–242.

Donchin, E., P. Tueting, W. Ritter, M. Kutas, and E. Heffley, 1975. On the independence of the CNV and the P300 components of the human averaged evoked potential. *Electroenceph. Clin. Neurophysiol.* 38:449–461.

Eccles, J. C., 1951. Interpretation of action potentials evoked in the cerebral cortex. *Electroenceph. Clin. Neurophysiol.* 3:449–464.

Eccles, J. C., 1979. *The Human Mystery.* Berlin: Springer.

Emson, P. C., and O. Lindvall, 1979. Distribution of putative neurotransmitters in the neocortex. *Neuroscience* 4:1–30.

Ford, J. M., W. T. Roth, S. J. Dirks, and B. S. Kopell, 1973. Evoked potential correlates signal recognition between and within modalities. *Science* 181:465–466.

Fraisse, P., 1957. *Psychologie du temps.* Paris: Presses Universitaires de France.

Fuster, J. M., 1973. Unit activity in prefrontal cortex during delayed-response performance: Neural correlates to transient memory. *J. Neurophysiol.* 36:61–78.

Galambos, R., and K. Hecox, 1977. Clinical applications of the brainstem auditory evoked potentials. In *Auditory Evoked Potentials in Man. Psychopharmacology Correlates to Evoked Potentials. Prog. Clin. Neurophysiol.,* Vol. 2. J. E. Desmedt, ed. Basel: Karger, pp. 1–19.

Goodin, D. S., K. C. Squires, and A. Starr, 1978. Long latency event-related components of the auditory evoked potential in dementia. *Brain* 101:635–648.

Greengard, P., 1978. *Cyclic Nucleotides, Phosphorylated Proteins and Neuronal Function.* New York: Raven Press.

Halliday. A. M., W. I. McDonald, and J. Mushin, 1972. Delayed visual evoked response in multiple sclerosis. *Lancet* 1:982–985.

Henn, F. A., and A. Hamberger, 1971. Glial cell function: Uptake of transmitter substances. *Proc. Nat. Acad. Sci USA* 68:2686–2690.

Hillyard, S. A., 1973. The CNV and human behavior. *Electroenceph. Clin. Neurophysiol.* (Supplement 33):161–171.

Hillyard, S. A., and T. W. Picton, 1979. Event-related potentials and selective information processing in man. In *Cognitive Components in Cerebral Event-Related Potentials and Selective Attention. Prog. Clin. Neurophysiol.,* Vol. 6. J. E. Desmedt, ed. Basel: Karger, pp. 1–52.

Hillyard, S. A., R. F. Hink, V. L. Schwent, and T. W. Picton, 1973. Electrical signs of selective attention in the human brain. *Science* 182:177–180.

Hillyard, S. A., K. C. Squires, J. W. Bauer, and P. H. Lindsay, 1971. Evoked potential correlates of auditory signal detection. *Science* 172:1357–1360.

Hubel, D. H., and T. N. Wiesel, 1962. Receptive fields, binocular interaction and functional architecture in the cat's visual cortex. *J. Physiol. (London)* 160:106–154.

Jewett, D. L., N. N. Romano, and J. S. Williston, 1970. Human auditory evoked potentials: Possible brain stem components detected on the scalp. *Science* 167:1517–1518.

Jones, E. G., 1975. Varieties and distribution of non-pyramidal cells in the somatic sensory cortex of the squirrel monkey. *J. Comp. Neurol.* 160:205–267.

Jones, E. G., and T. P. S. Powell, 1969. Connexions of the somatic sensory cortex of the Rhesus monkey: Contralateral cortical connexions. *Brain* 92:717–730.

Jones, E. G., and T. P. S. Powell, 1970. An anatomical study of converging sensory pathways within the cerebral cortex of the monkey. *Brain* 93:793–820.

Jones, E. G., J. D. Coulter, and S. H. C. Hendry, 1978. Intracortical connectivity of architectonic fields in the somatic sensory, motor and parietal cortex of monkeys. *J. Comp. Neurol.* 181:291–348.

Kerkhof, G. A., 1978. Decision latency: The P3 component in auditory signal detection. *Neurosci. Lett.* 8:289–294.

Kornhuber, H. H., 1974. Cerebral cortex, cerebellum and basal ganglia: An introduction to their motor function. In *The Neurosciences: Third Study Program.* F. O. Schmitt, and F. G. Worden, eds. Cambridge, MA: MIT Press, pp. 267–280.

Kornhuber, H. H., and L. Deecke, 1965. Hirnpotentialänderungen bei Willkürbewegungen des Menschen: Bereitschaftspotential und reafferente Potentiale. *Arch. Gesch. Physiol.* 284:1–17.

Krnjevic, K., R. Pumain, and L. Renaud, 1971. The mechanism of excitation by acetylcholine in the cerebral cortex. *J. Physiol. (London)* 215:247–268.

Kutas, M., and E. Donchin, 1977. The effect of handedness, of responding hand, and of response force on the contralateral dominance of the readiness potential. In *Attention, Voluntary Contraction and Event-Related Cerebral Potentials. Prog. Clin. Neurophysiol.,* Vol. 1. J. E. Desmedt, ed. Basel: Karger, pp. 189–210.

Kutas, M., G. McCarthy, and E. Donchin, 1977. Augmenting mental chronometry: The P300 as a measure of stimulus evaluation time. *Science* 197:792–795.

Lee, T. P., J. F. Kuo, and P. Greengard, 1972. Role of muscarinic cholinergic receptors in regulation of guanosine 3':5'-cyclic monophosphate content in mammalian brain, heart muscle, and intestinal smooth muscle. *Proc. Nat. Acad. Sci. USA* 69:3287–3291.

Libet, B., 1973. Electrical stimulation of cortex in human subjects and conscious sensory aspects. In *Handbook of Sensory Physiology,* Vol. 2. A. Iggo, ed. Berlin: Springer, pp. 743–790.

Libet, B., W. W. Alberts, E. W. Wright, and B. Feinstein, 1967. Responses of human somatosensory cortex to stimuli below threshold for conscious sensation. *Science* 158:1597–1600.

Low, M. D., and S. J. Swift, 1971. The contingent negative variation and the resting DC potential of the human brain: Effects of situational anxiety. *Neuropsychologia* 9:203–208.

Luria, A. R., and E. D. Homskaya, 1970. Frontal lobes and the regulation of arousal processes. In *Attention: Contemporary Theory and Analysis.* D. I. Mostofsky, ed. New York: Appleton Century Crofts, pp. 303–330.

McCallum, W. C., and J. R. Knott, eds., 1973. *Event-Related Slow Potentials of the Brain. Electroenceph. Clin. Neurophysiol.* (Supplement 33). Amsterdam: Elsevier.

McCallum W. C., D. Papakostopoulos, R. Gombi, A. L. Winter, R. Cooper, and H. B. Griffith, 1973. Event related slow potential changes in human brainstem. *Nature* 242:465–467.

Mesulam, M. M., and G. W. VanHoesen, 1976. Acetylcholinesterase-rich projections from the basal forebrain of the rhesus monkey to neocortex. *Brain Res.* 109:152–157.

Millhouse, O. E., 1969. A Golgi study of the descending medial forebrain bundle. *Brain Res.* 15:341–363.

Milner, B., 1964. Some effects of frontal lobectomy in man. In *The Frontal Granular Cortex and Behavior.* J. M. Warren and K. Akert, eds. New York: McGraw-Hill, pp. 313–334.

Moore, R. Y., and F. E. Bloom, 1979. Central catecholamine neuron systems: Anatomy and physiology of the norepinephrine and epinephrine systems. *Ann. Rev. Neurosci.* 2:113–168.

Moruzzi, G., 1972. The sleep waking cycle. *Ergebn. Physiol.* 64:1–165.

Mountcastle, V. B., 1957. Modality and topographic properties of single neurons of cat's somatic sensory cortex. *J. Neurophysiol.* 20:408–434.

Mountcastle, V. B., 1978. An organizing principle for cerebral function: The unit module and the distribution system. In *The Mindful Brain.* G. M. Edelman and V. B. Mountcastle, eds. Cambridge, MA: MIT Press, pp. 7–50.

Nauta, W. J. H., 1962. Neural associations of the frontal cortex. *Acta Neurobiol. Exp.* 32:125–140.

Nauta, W. J. H., 1964. Some efferent connections of the prefrontal cortex in the monkey. In *The Frontal Granular Cortex and Behavior.* J. M. Warren and K. Akert, eds. New York: McGraw-Hill, pp. 397–409.

Nauta, W. J. H., 1971. The problem of the frontal lobe: A reinterpretation. *J. Psychiat. Res.* 8:167–187.

Noël, P., and J. E. Desmedt, 1980. Cerebral and far-field somatosensory evoked potentials in neurological disorders involving the cervical spinal cord, brainstem, thalamus and cortex. In *Clinical Uses of Cerebral, Brainstem and Spinal Somatosensory Evoked Potentials. Prog. Clin. Neurophysiol.,* Vol. 7. J. E. Desmedt, ed. Basel: Karger, pp. 205–230.

Otto, D. A., ed., 1979. *Multidisciplinary Perspectives in Event-Related Brain Potential Research.* Washington, DC: US Environmental Protection Agency.

Pandya, D. N., and L. A. Vignolo, 1969. Interhemispheric projections of the parietal lobe in the rhesus monkey. *Brain Res.* 15:49–65.

Paul, D. D., and S. Sutton, 1972. Evoked potential correlates of response criterion in auditory signal detection. *Science* 177:362–364.

Peronnet, F., and F. Michel, 1977. The asymmetry of the auditory evoked potentials in normal man and in patients with brain lesions. In *Auditory Evoked Potentials in Man. Prog. Clin. Neurophysiol.,* Vol. 2. J. E. Desmedt, ed. Basel: Karger, pp. 130–141.

Purpura, D. P., R. J. Shofer, and F. S. Musgrave, 1964. Cortical intracellular potentials during augmenting and recruiting responses. *J. Neurophysiol.* 27:133–151.

Ragot, R., and A. Rémond, 1979. Event-related scalp potentials during a bimanual choice RT task: Topography and interhemispheric relations. In *Human Evoked Potentials.* D. Lehmann and E. Callaway, eds. New York: Plenum Press, pp. 303–316.

Ransom, B. R., and S. Goldring, 1973. Slow depolarization in cells presumed to be glia in cerebral cortex of cat. *J. Neurophysiol.* 36:869–878.

Rebert, C. S., 1977. Intracerebral slow potential changes in monkeys during the foreperiod of reaction time. In *Attention, Voluntary Contraction and Event-Related Cerebral Potentials. Prog. Clin. Neurophysiol.*, Vol. 1. J. E. Desmedt, ed. Basel: Karger, pp. 242–253.

Ritter, W., and H. G. Vaughan, 1969. Averaged evoked responses in vigilance and discrimination: A reassessment. *Science* 164:326–328.

Ritter, W., R. Simson, and H. G. Vaughan, 1972. Association cortex potentials and reaction time in auditory discrimination. *Electroenceph. Clin. Neurophysiol.* 33:547–555.

Ritter, W., R. Simson, and H. G. Vaughan, 1979. Topographic analysis of task-related cerebral potentials. In *Cognitive Components in Cerebral Event-Related Potentials and Selective Attention. Prog. Clin. Neurophysiol.*, J. E. Desmedt, ed. Vol. 6. Basel: Karger, pp. 132–139.

Rowland, V., 1968. Cortical steady potential in reinforcement and learning. *Prog. Physiol. Psychol.* 2:1–77.

Ruchkin, D. S., and S. Sutton, 1979. CNV and P300 relationships for emitted and for evoked cerebral potentials. In *Cognitive Component in Cerebral Event-Related Potentials and Selective Attention. Prog. Clin. Neurophysiol.*, Vol. 6. J. E. Desmedt, ed. Basel: Karger, pp. 119–131.

Saletu, B., 1977. Cerebral evoked potentials in psychopharmacology. In *Psychopharmacology Correlates of Evoked Potentials. Prog. Clin. Neurophysiol.*, Vol. 2. J. E. Desmedt, ed. Basel: Karger, pp. 175–207.

Schwent, V. L., S. A. Hillyard, and R. Galambos, 1976. Selective attention and the auditory vertex potential. Effects of stimulus delivery rate. *Electroenceph. Clin. Neurophysiol.* 40:604–614.

Simson, R., H. G. Vaughan, and W. Ritter, 1976. The scalp topography of potentials associated with missing visual and auditory stimuli. *Electroenceph. Clin. Neurophysiol.* 40:33–42.

Simson, R., H. G. Vaughan, and W. Ritter, 1977. The scalp topography of potentials in auditory and visual Go-Nogo tasks. *Electroenceph. Clin. Neurophysiol.* 43:864–875.

Skinner, J. E., and C. D. Yingling, 1977. Central gating mechanisms that regulate event-related potentials and behavior. A neural model for attention. In *Attention, Voluntary Contraction and Event-Related Cerebral Potentials. Prog. Clin. Neurophysiol.*, Vol. 1. J. E. Desmedt, ed. Basel: Karger, pp. 28–68.

Skinner, J. E., J. C. Reed, K. M. A. Welch, and J. H. Nell, 1978. Cutaneous shock produces correlated shifts in slow potential amplitude and cyclic 3-5 adenosine monophosphate level in parietal cortex of the conscious rat. *J. Neurochem.* 30:399–704.

Small, D. G., M. Beauchamp, and W. B. Mathews, 1980. Subcortical somatosensory evoked potentials in normal man and in patients with central nervous system lesions. In *Clinical Uses of Cerebral, Brainstem and Spinal Somatosensory Evoked Potentials. Prog. Clin. Neurophysiol.*, Vol. 7. J. E. Desmedt, ed. Basel: Karger, pp. 190–204.

Somjen, G. G., 1975. Electrophysiology of neuroglia. *Ann. Rev. Physiol.* 37:163–190.

Spekereijse, H., O. Estevez, and D. Reits, 1977. Visual evoked potentials, and the physiological analysis of visual process in man. In *Visual Evoked Potentials in Man: New Developments*. J. E. Desmedt, ed. Oxford: Oxford University Press, pp. 16–89.

Sperry, R. W., 1974. Lateral specialization in the surgically separated hemispheres. In *The Neurosciences: Third Study Program*. F. O. Schmitt and F. G. Worden, eds. Cambridge, MA: MIT Press, pp. 5–19.

Squires, K. C., N. A. Squires, and S. A. Hillyard, 1975a. Decision related cortical potentials during an auditory signal detection task with cued observation intervals. *J. Exp. Psychol. Human Percept.* 1:268–279.

Squires, N. K., K. C. Squires, and S. A. Hillyard, 1975b. Two varieties of long-latency positive waves evoked by unpredictable auditory stimuli in man. *Electroenceph. Clin. Neurophysiol.* 38:387–401.

Starr, A., 1977. Clinical relevance of brain stem auditory evoked potentials in brain stem disorders in man. In *Auditory Evoked Potentials in Man. Psychopharmacology Correlates of Evoked Potentials. Prog. Clin. Neurophysiol.*, Vol. 2. J. E. Desmedt, ed. Basel: Karger, pp. 45–47.

Stockard, J. J., and F. W. Sharbrough, 1980. Unique contributions of short-latency auditory and somatosensory evoked potentials to neurologic diagnosis. In *Clinical Uses of Cerebral, Brainstem, and Spinal Somatosensory Evoked Potentials. Electroenceph. Clin. Neurophysiol.*, Vol. 7. J. E. Desmedt, ed. Basel: Karger, pp. 231–263.

Stone, T. W., and D. A. Taylor, 1977. Microiontophoretic studies of the effects of cyclic nucleotides on excitability of neurones in the rat cerebral cortex. *J. Physiol. (London)* 266:523–543.

Stone, T. W., D. A. Taylor, and F. E. Bloom, 1975. Cyclic AMP and cyclic GMP may mediate opposite neuronal responses in the rat cerebral cortex. *Science* 187:845–847.

Sutton, S., M. Braren, J. Zubin, and E. R. John, 1965. Evoked-potential correlates of stimulus uncertainty. *Science* 150:1187–1188.

Swets, J. A., W. P. Tanner, and T. G. Birdsall, 1964. Decision process in perception. In *Signal Detection and Recognition by Human Observers*. J. A. Swets, ed. New York: Wiley, pp. 3–57.

Szentagothai, J., 1970. Les circuits neuronaux de l'écorce cérébrale. *Bull. Acad. Roy. Méd. Belg.* 10:475–492.

Szentagothai, J., 1975. The module concept in cerebral cortex architecture. *Brain Res.* 95:475–596.

Szentagothai, J., 1978. The neuron network of the cerebral cortex: A functional interpretation (Ferrier lecture). *Proc. Roy. Soc. London B* 201:219–248.

Szerb, J. C., 1967. Cortical acetylcholine release and electroencephalographic arousal. *J. Physiol. (London)* 192:329–343.

Towe, A. L., 1966. On the nature of the primary evoked response. *Exp. Neurol.* 15:113–139.

Towe, A. L., 1973. Somatosensory cortex: Descending influences on ascending systems. In *Handbook of Sensory Physiology*, Vol. 2. A. Iggo, ed. Berlin: Springer, pp. 701–718.

Treisman, A., 1969. Strategies and models of selective attention. *Psychol. Rev.* 76:282–299.

Tueting, P., S. Sutton, and J. Zubin, 1971. Quantitative evoked potential correlates of the probability of events. *Psychophysiology* 7:385–394.

Vaughan, H. G., and W. Ritter, 1970. The sources of auditory evoked responses recorded from the human scalp. *Electroenceph. Clin. Neurophysiol.* 28:360–367.

Walter, W. G., R. Cooper, V. J. Aldridge, W. C. McCallum, and A. L. Winter, 1964. Contingent negative variation: An electric sign of sensorimotor association and expectancy in the human brain. *Nature* 203:380–384.

Woodward, D. J., H. C. Moises, B. D. Waterhouse, B. J. Hoffer, and R. Freedman, 1979. Modulatory actions of epinephrine in the central nervous system. *Fed. Proc.* 38:2109–2126.

Woolsey, C. N., W. H. Marshall, and P. Bard, 1942. Representation of cutaneous tactile sensibility in the cerebral cortex of the monkey as indicated by evoked potentials. *Bull. Johns Hopkins Hosp.* 70:399–441.

Wurtz, R. H., 1966. Steady potential correlates of intracranial reinforcement. *Electroenceph. Clin. Neurophysiol.* 20:59–67.

Yamamura, H. I., M. J. Huhar, D. Greenberg, and S. H. Snyder, 1974. Muscarinic cholinergic receptor binding: Regional distribution in monkey brain. *Brain Res.* 66:541–546.

Yingling, C. D., and J. E. Skinner, 1977. Gating of thalamic input to cerebral cortex by nucleus reticularis thalami. In *Attention, Voluntary Contraction and Event-Related Cerebral Potentials. Prog. Clin. Neurophysiol.*, Vol. 1. J. E. Desmedt, ed. Basel: Karger, pp. 69–92.

Impact of Theoretical Constructs and Modeling of Cortical Function

Introduction

Gerald M. Edelman

One of the embarrassments facing theorists in the neurosciences is that there are many levels of description of both behavior and brain function. This is an embarrassment of riches; it calls for restraint and critical choices, particularly in relation to the size of the system being tackled by the theorist. The cortex and its functions are a poignant example—at least 10^{10} neurons with at least 10^{15} connections functionally linked in a distributed fashion to themselves and other neuronal systems of the brain. Moreover, there is no way that such a system can be functionally analyzed without constantly reminding oneself that the brain appears to have evolved for action and survival, not for pure thought or calculation. At least in this respect, it sharply differs from all automata so far constructed. For a theory to be useful under these circumstances, it must either enunciate a general principle based on global behavior or organization, or limit itself to a very defined problem or subsystem.

The three chapters presented in this part illustrate several such choices. Crick, Marr, and Poggio, for example, have limited their concern to very specific aspects of psychophysical observations related to visual acuity. They offer a novel view of how the early stages of vision may operate, but are modest about its linkage to detailed neurophysiology and neuroanatomy. Aside from the new interpretation of psychophysics discussed by these authors, it is an additional strength of their chapter that it clearly reflects the need to connect psychophysical constructions with the neuroanatomical and physiological facts.

Cooper has attacked a different subject, the nature of memory and recognition. In his paper, he considers both the self-consistency of a theory of associative networks and its consistency with the observed properties of recognition and distributed memory. While this theory has not yet been proved to be sharply predictive of the neuronal functions of the cortex, it too is written in awareness of the actual phenomenology of memory as well as of neuronal properties in the visual cortex. It is a contribution that points to ways of formulating questions about memory that are new and provocative. Above all, the theory of associative nets actually performs in a computer model, and whether it is verified for the visual cortex or not, it is demonstrably functional in an abstract system; therefore, there are no doubts about its self-consistency.

The last chapter, by myself, is related to Cooper's in the sense that it too is concerned with principles of organization of brain function. It takes the position that the brain and particularly the cortex is a Darwinian system in both function and ontogeny. Its major point is that individual variations of connectivity at the finest ramifications of the cortex are not just adventitious but are essential for group selection to operate during higher brain function. The chapter considers the available evidence for both ontogenetic and functional variability working along with group selection as a basis of cortical function. Much of the discussion relates to the evidence for cortical modules and their development described in earlier parts of this book. In an appendix with G. N. Reeke, an example of a group-selective system is provided in a computer model.

None of these papers pretends to be complete or very sharply predictive. But all point in new directions. Perhaps at an early stage of a science, this is the greatest value of a theory—not its falsifiability (important as that is), but its suggestive and heuristic value. Such theories can temporarily exclude searches down fruitless paths; at least, they can stimulate the experimentalist to look at his data in a new way.

Explicit theory making about the brain has not yet been a central concern of neurobiologists. If we exclude psychological dogma and pre-scientific philosophical thought, this is as it should be, for there is much still to be done of a descriptive nature before a powerful theory can be constructed. Theory making nevertheless, should be encouraged among those who can be discreet about its aims and its uses. This is the main point of the following part, and it is fair to say that all three chapters have novel and provocative viewpoints that will be of use to the experimentalist.

20 Distributed Memory in the Central Nervous System: Possible Test of Assumptions in Visual Cortex

Leon N Cooper

ABSTRACT Progress has been recently made in constructing neural networks that can organize themselves to produce distributed memories. These networks, as well as the proposed procedures by which they modify themselves with experience, are consistent with known neurophysiology as well as with what information may be available at synaptic junctions. The modification assumptions on which these ideas are based have consequences that may be testable in visual cortex. Applied to visual cortex, we assume that between lateral-geniculate and visual cortical cells there exist labile synapses that modify themselves in a fashion consistent with the assumptions above, and in addition, nonlabile synapses that contain permanent information. In the theory which results there is an increase in the specificity of response of a cortical cell when it is exposed to stimuli that are the result of normal patterned visual experience. Nonpatterned input, such as might be expected when an animal is dark reared or raised with eyelids sutured, results in a loss of specificity, with details depending on whether noise to labile and nonlabile junctions is correlated. Specificity can sometimes be regained, however, with a return of input due to patterned vision. It is proposed that this provides a possible explanation of some recent experimental results. We are presently working to extend this theory to situations in which there is binocular interaction.

Introduction

Although the properties of individual neurons are relatively well understood, the manner in which large interacting networks of these nerve cells produce mental activity remains almost a complete mystery. The many excellent papers presented at this conference have emphasized once more how complicated the situation is. We have heard that, in general, sensory input has very complex projections in cortex, that input from the visual field has an extremely elaborate representation in posterior association cortex, and that single cells or regions of cortex receive input from many areas. In addition, we know that it has not been possible to localize any region of the nervous system in which memory is stored, nor to isolate activity of single cells corresponding to higher cortical function. All of this reinforces the belief that central-

LEON N COOPER Center for Neural Science and Department of Physics, Brown University, Providence, Rhode Island 02912

nervous-system properties such as storage and retrieval of memory are of unusual subtlety, involving small changes in the activities of large numbers of neurons. It is this point of view that I would like to develop here.

For several years my colleagues and I have been analyzing a class of neural models for the acquisition and storage of distributed memories that display, on a primitive level, features such as recognition, association, and generalization, and which suggest some of the mental behavior associated with animal memory and learning (Cooper, 1973; Anderson and Cooper, 1978). The mechanisms we employ seem to be plausible biologically and are not inconsistent with known neurophysiology. In addition the networks that result seem to be a reasonable outcome of evolutionary development under the pressure of survival. Some of our ideas are related to, or are generalizations of, earlier concepts such as Perceptrons or similar models (Block, 1962; Block, Knight, and Rosenblatt, 1962; Minsky and Papert, 1969). In addition holographic or nonlocal memories have been explored previously (Longuet-Higgins, 1968a,b).

Many ways to store and retrieve information exist: filing cabinets, libraries, and computers. But the fact that an animal's memory is held in a living structure and is successfully utilized, even though the animal may have no idea of where his memories are stored or how they are ordered, places special requirements on theory. Current computer memories, for example, are made of elements in which yes–no information is recorded and which can be recalled by addressing the location of an element. These computers perform sequences of elementary operations with incredible speed and accuracy, completely beyond the capability of living cells. A basic problem in understanding the organization of memory in a biological system is to understand how a vast quantity of information can be stored and recalled by a system composed of vulnerable and relatively unreliable elements and with no knowledge of how or where the information has been filed.

The evolution of neocortex has been extremely rapid—an explosive growth of this area of the brain having occurred in only a few million years. This suggests that it may be that a simple method of organization is repeated over and over, that, as more cells were added, the cortical surface folded to create more area so that the entire structure could be fitted into a skull of reasonable volume. In addition, outside of a few well-defined regions, the results of damage to cortex are often diffuse and difficult to describe; they have been observed to depend more on the size of the lesion than on its exact location.

Such considerations led Karl Lashley to his proposal that nervous system memory is distributed: "It is not possible to demonstrate the isolated localization of a memory trace anywhere within the nervous system. . . . The same neurons which retain the memory traces of one experience must also participate in countless other activities. . . . Recall involves the synergic action or some sort of resonance among a very large number of neurons" (Lashley, 1950). From this point of view there are no privileged sites in the brain for the storage of memory items in isolation from each other. This seems, at first, very unpromising since individual memories would interfere with each other; but, as we shall see, the problem has a solution and memories so constructed can function as well as local memories.

Although the concept of distributed mappings and memory storage is less familiar than those of local storage, distributed mappings have been discussed (Anderson, 1970, 1972; Kohonen, 1972, 1977) and probably have already been observed. An example is the superior colliculus. Although the retinal efferents that project to the colliculus form a very precise, fine-grained map, cells that are just a few millimeters below the very precise cells respond to stimuli over a wide area of visual space. Thus we have the apparently paradoxical situation—which seems to be true of other parts of the brain as well—that great precision of response is generated by systems composed of cells which progressively show less and less selectivity as the motor output of the system is approached (McIlwain, 1976).

It is now commonly believed that much of the learning and resulting organization of the central nervous system occurs due to some kind of modification of the efficacy or strength of at least some of the synaptic junctions between neurons, thus altering the relation between presynaptic and postsynaptic potentials. It is also known that small but coherent modifications of large numbers of synaptic junctions can result in distributed memories.

Whether and how such synaptic modification occurs, what precise forms it takes, and what the physiological basis of this modification is, is not known. There is direct experimental evidence that at least some modification of synaptic strength occurs in invertebrates (Kandel, 1976), and there are various indications that synaptic modification is a rather general phenomenon. In recent years many conjectures have been made concerning the kind of modification that might occur at synaptic junctions. It has been suggested that the existence of a fundamental biological mechanism could lead to an entire class of interesting modifications, among which are those that could produce distributed memories with very attractive properties.

It seems to me that the central issue has become to confront the various theoretical ideas with hard experimental results. I believe that this is possible at present and indeed may have already proceeded further than is generally realized. In what follows, I present an outline of recent experimental and theoretical results relating to the development and modification of neurons in mammal visual cortex that, I feel, provides just such a meeting of experiment and theory.

Distributed Memory Mappings

For a distributed memory it is the simultaneous or near-simultaneous activities of many different neurons (the result of external or internal stimuli) that are of interest. Thus a large spatially distributed pattern of neuron discharges, each of which might not be very far from spontaneous activity, could contain important, if hard to detect, information. Let us consider the behavior of an idealized neural network (that might be regarded as a model component of a nervous system) to illustrate some of the important features of distributed mappings.

Consider N neurons $1, 2, \ldots , N$, each of which has some spontaneous firing rate r_{j0}. (This need not be the same for all of the neurons, nor need it be constant in time.) We can then define an N-tuple whose components are the difference between the actual firing rate r_j of the jth neuron and the spontaneous firing rate r_{j0}:

$$f_j \equiv r_j - r_{j0}. \tag{1}$$

By constructing two such banks of neurons connected to one another (or even by the use of a single bank which feeds signals back to itself), we arrive at a simplified model as illustrated in Figure 1.

The actual synaptic connections between one neuron and another are generally complex and redundant; we have idealized the network by replacing this multiplicity of synapses between axons and dendrites by a single ideal junction which summarizes logically the effect of all of the synaptic contacts between the incoming axon branches from neuron j in the F bank and the dendrites of the outgoing neuron i in the G bank (Figure 2). Each of the N incoming neurons, in F, is connected to each of the N outgoing neurons, in G, by a single ideal junction.

Although the firing rate of a neuron depends in a complex and nonlinear fashion on the presynaptic potentials, there is usually a reasonably well-defined linear region. We focus our attention on the region above threshold and below saturation for which the firing rate g_i of neuron i in G is mapped from the firing rates of all of the neurons f_j in F by

$$g_i = \sum_{j=1}^{N} A_{ij} f_j. \tag{2}$$

In doing this we are regarding as important average firing rates, and time averages of the instantaneous signals in a neuron (or perhaps a small population of neurons). Further, we are using the known integrative properties of neurons.

We may then regard $[A_{ij}]$ (the synaptic strengths of the N^2 ideal junctions) as a matrix or a mapping which takes us from a vector in the F space to one in the G space. This maps the neural activities $f = (f_1, f_2 \ldots$

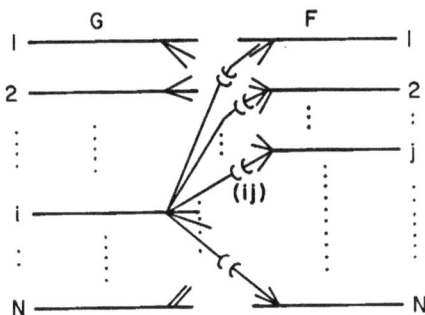

Figure 1 An ideal distributed mapping. Each of the N incoming neurons in F is connected to each of the N outgoing neurons in G by a single ideal junction. (Only the connections to i are drawn.) (From Cooper, 1973.)

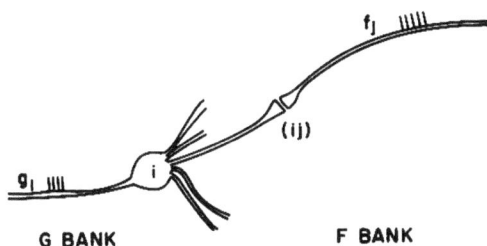

Figure 2 An ideal junction. (From Cooper, 1973.)

f_N) in the F space into the neural activities $g = (g_1, \ldots, g_N)$ in the G space and can be written in the compact form

$$g = Af. \tag{3}$$

I propose that it is in modifiable mappings of the type A that the experience and memory of the system are stored. In contrast with machine memory, which is (at present) local (an event stored in a specific place) and addressable by locality (requiring some equivalent of indices and files), animal memory is likely to be distributed and addressable by content or by association. In addition for animals there need be no clear separation between memory and "logic."

It is convenient to write the mapping A in the basis of vectors the system has experienced:

$$A = \sum_{\mu\nu} c_{\mu\nu} g^\mu \times f^\nu. \tag{4}$$

Here g^μ and f^ν are output and input patterns of neural activity, while the $c_{\mu\nu}$ are coefficients reflecting the degree of connection between various inputs and outputs. The symbol $\times$ represents the "outer" product between the input and output vectors. Although (4) is a well-known mathematical form, its meaning as a mapping among neurons deserves some discussion. The ijth element of A gives the strength of the ideal junction between the incoming neuron j in the F bank and the outgoing neuron i in the G bank (Figure 2).

Thus, if only f_j is nonzero, g_i, the firing rate of the ith output neuron, is

$$g_i = A_{ij}f_j. \tag{5}$$

Since

$$A_{ij} = \sum_{\mu\nu} c_{\mu\nu}g_i^\mu f_j^\nu, \tag{6}$$

the ijth junction strength is composed of a sum of the entire experience of the system as reflected in firing rates of the neurons connected to this junction. Each experience or association ($\mu\nu$), however, is stored over the entire array of $N \times N$ junctions. This is the essential meaning of a distributed memory: each event is stored over a large portion of the system, while at any particular local point many events are superimposed.

We show below that the nonlocal mapping A can serve in a highly precise fashion as a memory that is content addressable and in which "logic" is a result of association and an outcome of the nature of the memory itself.

Recognition and Recollection

The fundamental problem posed by a distributed memory is the address and accuracy of recall of the stored patterns. Consider first the "diagonal" portion of A,

$$(A)_{\text{diagonal}} \equiv \mathcal{R} \equiv \sum_{\nu} c_{\nu\nu}g^\nu \times f^\nu \tag{7}$$

An arbitrary event e in the external world mapped by the sensory apparatus into the pattern of neural activity f will generate the response in G

$$g = Af \tag{8}$$

[The pattern f might also be the result of some other internal pattern of neural activity.] If we equate recognition with the strength of this response, say the inner product

$$(g, g), \tag{9}$$

then the mapping A will distinguish between those events it contains, the f^ν, $\nu = 1, 2, \dots, K$, and other events separated from these.

The word "separated" in the above context requires definition. Suppose the vectors f^ν are thought to be independent of each other, and to satisfy the requirements that, on the average,

$$\sum_{i=1}^{N} f_i^\nu = 0, \qquad \sum_{i=1}^{N} (f_i^\nu)^2 = 1. \tag{10}$$

Any two such vectors have components which are random with respect to one another so that a new vector f presented in the F bank as above gives a noise-like response in the G bank since, on the average, (f^ν, f) is small. The presentation of a vector f^λ seen previously, however, gives the response in the G bank

$$f^\lambda = c_{\lambda\lambda}g^\lambda + \text{noise}. \tag{11}$$

It can be shown that if the number of imprinted events K is small compared to the dimensionality N, the signal-to-noise ratios are reasonable.

If we define separated events as those which map into orthogonal vectors, then clearly a recognition matrix composed of K orthogonal vectors $f^1, f^2, \ldots f^K$,

$$\mathcal{R} = \sum_{\nu=1}^{k} c_{\nu\nu}g^\nu \times f^\nu, \tag{12}$$

will distinguish between those vectors contained and all vectors separated from (perpendicular to) these. Further, the response of the system to a vector previously recorded is unique and completely accurate:

$$\mathcal{R}f^\lambda = c_{\lambda\lambda}g^\lambda. \tag{13}$$

In this special situation, the distributed memory is as precise as a localized memory.

In addition, **this type of memory has the interesting property of recalling an entire associated vector g^λ even if only part of f^λ is presented.** Let

$$f^\lambda = f_1^\lambda + f_2^\lambda. \tag{14}$$

If only part of f^λ, say f_1^λ, is presented, we obtain

$$\mathcal{R}f_1^\lambda = c_{\lambda\lambda}(f_1^\lambda, f_1^\lambda)g^\lambda + \text{noise}. \tag{15}$$

The result is the entire response to the full f^λ with a reduced coefficient plus noise.

Association
If we now take the point of view that presentation of the event e^ν which generates the vector f^ν is recollected if

$$\mathcal{R}f^\nu = (\text{const.})g^\nu + \text{noise}, \tag{16}$$

then the off-diagonal terms

$$\mathcal{A} \equiv \sum_{\mu \neq \nu} c_{\mu\nu}g^\mu \times f^\nu \tag{17}$$

may be interpreted as containing associations between events initially separated from one another:

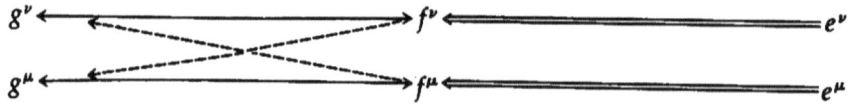

where $(f^\nu, f^\mu) = 0$.

For such terms the presentation of event e^ν will generate not only g^ν (which is equivalent to the recollection of e^ν) but also, and perhaps more weakly, g^μ, which should result with the presentation of e^μ. Thus, for example, if g^μ initiates some response, originally a response to e^μ, the presentation of e^ν when $c_{\mu\nu} \neq 0$ will also initiate this response.

We can thus divide the association matrix A into two parts:

$$A = \sum_{\mu\nu} c_{\mu\nu} g^\mu \times f^\nu = \mathscr{R} + \mathscr{A} \tag{18}$$

where

$$\mathscr{R} = (A)_{\text{diagonal}}$$

$$\equiv \sum_\nu c_{\nu\nu} g^\nu \times f^\nu \quad \text{(recognition and recollection)} \tag{19}$$

and

$$\mathscr{A} = (A)_{\text{off-diagonal}}$$

$$\equiv \sum_{\mu \neq \nu} c_{\mu\nu} g^\mu \times f^\nu \quad \text{(association).} \tag{20}$$

The $c_{\mu\nu}$ are then the direct recollection and association coefficients.

"Logic"

In actual experience, the events to which the system is exposed are not in general highly separated, nor are they independent in a statistical sense. There is no reason, therefore, to expect that all vectors f^ν printed into A would be orthogonal or even very far from one another. Rather it seems likely that large numbers of these vectors often would lie close to one another. Under these circumstances, a distributed memory might be "confused" in the sense that it will respond to new events as if they were old, if the new event is close to an old one. It will "recognize" and "associate" events never, in fact, seen or associated before.

The memory will tend to categorize stimuli on the basis of the past history of the system. For example, suppose a number of vectors in the memory are of the form

$$f^\nu = f^0 + n^\nu \tag{21}$$

where n^ν varies randomly; f^0 eventually will be recognized more strongly than any particular f^ν actually presented. This, of course, is reminiscent of psychological properties called "generalization" or "abstraction." From such a point of view, generalization grows from the loss of detail of individual instances, a trade-off that seems characteristic of distributed systems. Something like this seems to occur in a few psychological contexts where it can be checked (Anderson, 1977).

We have here an explicit realization of what might loosely be called "animal logic"—which, of course, is not logic at all. Rather what occurs might be described as the result of a built-in directive to "jump to conclusions." The associative memory by its nature takes the step

$$f^0 + n^1, f^0 + n^2, \ldots, f^0 + n^k, \ldots \rightarrow f^0, \tag{22}$$

which one perhaps attempts to describe in language as passing from particulars: cat^1, cat^2, cat^3, . . . to the general: cat.

How fast this step is taken depends on the parameters of the system. By altering these parameters, it is possible to construct mappings which vary from those which retain all particulars to which they are exposed, to those which lose the particulars and retain only common elements—the central vector of any class.

In addition to "errors" of recognition, the associative memory also makes "errors" of association. If, for example, all (or many) of the vectors of the class $\{f^\alpha\}$, defined as a class of vectors not very separated from one another, associate some particular g^β, so that the mapping contains terms of the form

$$\sum_{\nu=1}^{k} c_{\beta\nu} g^\beta \times f^\nu \qquad f^\nu \in \{f^\alpha\}, \tag{23}$$

with $c_{\beta\nu} \neq 0$ over much of $\nu = 1, 2, \ldots, k$, then the new event e^{k+1} which maps into f^{k+1} also in the class $\{f^\alpha\}$ will not only be recognized, the inner product $(\mathcal{R}f^{k+1}, \mathcal{R}f^{k+1})$ being large, but will also associate g^β $\mathcal{A}f^{k+1} = cg^\beta + \cdot\cdot$ as strongly as any of the vectors $f^1, \ldots, f^k$ explicitly contained in (23).

If errors of recognition lead to the process described in language as going from particulars to the general, errors of association might be described as going from particulars to a universal: cat^1 meows, cat^2 meows, . . . $\rightarrow$ all cats meow.

There is, of course, no "justification" for this process. Whatever efficacy it has will depend on the order of the world in which the animal system finds itself. If the world is properly ordered, an animal system that "jumps to conclusions" in the sense above may be better able to adapt and react to the hazards of its environment and thus survive. The animal philosopher sophisticated enough to argue "the tiger ate my friend but that does not allow me to conclude that he might want to eat me" could then be a recent development whose survival depends on other less sophisticated animals who jump to conclusions.

By a sequence of mappings of the form above (or by feeding the out-

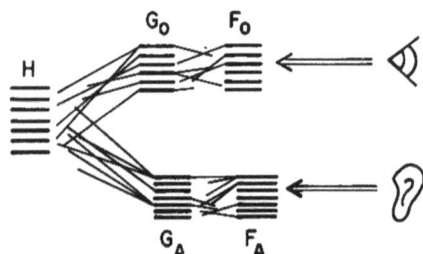

Figure 3 A model optical-auditory system. (From Cooper, 1973.)

put of A back to itself) one obtains a fabric of events and connections that is rich as well as suggestive. One easily sees the possibility of a flow of electrical activity influenced both by internal distributed mappings and the external input. This flow is governed not only by direct association coefficients $c_{\mu\nu}$ (which can be explicitly learned) but also by indirect associations due to the overlapping of the mapped events. One can imagine situations arising in which direct access to an event, or a class of events, has been lost, while the existence of this event or class of events in A influences the flow of electrical activity.

One problem in making the identifications suggested above is that such systems tend to form very large all-encompassing classes that include too much. But means have been devised to limit the extent of class formation. In fact such mappings can be made to separate classes as well as to unite them (Kohonen, 1977).

Another problem is a direct consequence of the assumption of the linearity of the system. Any state is generally a superposition of various vectors. Thus one has to find a means by which events—or the entities into which they are mapped—are distinguished from one another.

There are various possibilities; neurons are so nonlinear that it is not at all difficult to imagine nonlinear or threshold devices that would separate one vector from another. But the occurrence of a vector in a distributed memory is a set of signals over a large number of neurons each of which is far from threshold. A basic problem, therefore, is how to associate the threshold of a single cell or a group of cells with such a distributed signal. How this might come about has been shown by Nass and Cooper (1975). Further progress in separating regions that are not linearly separable has also been made.

In addition to the appearance of "pontifical" cells or groups of cells, there will be a certain separation of mapped signals due to actual localization of the areas in which these signals occur. For example, optical and auditory signals are subjected to much processing before they actually meet in cortex. It is possible to imagine that identification of optical or auditory signals (as optical or auditory) occurs first from where they appear and their immediate cluster of associations. Connections between an optical and an auditory event might occur as suggested in Figure 3.

I need hardly mention that even assuming that the physiological assumptions that underlie these constructions are possible (or even correct), there is a distance to be traveled before it is shown that such mappings or combinations of such mappings working together could produce even a portion of animal mental behavior.

Network Modification, Learning

We now ask how a mapping of the type A might be put into the network. The ijth element of A,

$$A_{ij} = \sum_{\mu\nu} c_{\mu\nu} g_i^\mu f_j^\nu, \tag{24}$$

is a weighted sum over the j components of all mapped signals f^ν and the i components of the responses g^μ appropriate for recollection or association. Such a form could be obtained by additions with each input f and output g to the element A_{ij}:

$$\delta A_{ij} \sim g_i f_j. \tag{25}$$

This δA_{ij} is proportional to the product of the differences between the actual and the spontaneous firing rates in the pre- and postsynaptic neurons i and j. [This is one realization of Hebb's form of synaptic modification (Hebb, 1949).] The addition of such changes to A for all associations $g^\mu \times f^\nu$ results finally in a mapping with the properties discussed in the previous section.

Synaptic modification dependent on inputs alone, of the type already directly observed in *Aplysia* (Kandel, 1976), is sufficient to construct a simple memory—one that distinguishes what has been seen from what has not, but does not easily separate one input from another. To construct a mapping of the form above, however, requires synaptic modification dependent on information that exists at different places on the neuron membrane—what I call two- (or higher-) point modification.

In order that this take place, information must be communicated from, for example, the axon hillock to the synaptic junction to be modified. This implies the existence of a means of internal communication of information within a neuron—in the above example, in a direction opposite to the flow of electrical signals (Cooper, 1973). The junction ij, for example, must have information of the firing rate f_j (which is locally available) as well as the firing rate g_i, which is somewhat removed (Figure 4). One possibility could be that the integrated electrical signals from the dendrites produce a chemical or electrical response in the cell body which controls the spiking rate of the axon and at the same time communicates (by backward spiking, for example) to the dendrite ends the information of the integrated slow potential.

One might guess that once the physiological mechanism for such

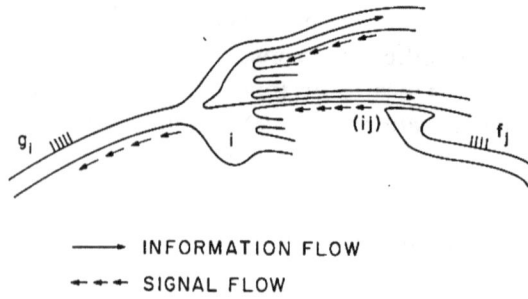

INFORMATION FLOW

SIGNAL FLOW

Figure 4 In order that the junction (*ij*) be modified in proportion to $g_i f_j$, a means is needed for communicating the firing rate g_i, which is the result of signals incoming from all the dendrites $g_i = \Sigma_j A_{ij} f_j$, back to the junction (*ij*). (From Cooper, 1973.)

communication was available, different types of two- (or higher-) point modification evolved in various ways. It is tempting to conjecture that a liberating evolutionary step was just the development of this means of internal communication that, coupled with the ability of synapses to modify, created the possibility for a new organizational principle.

There are a variety of means by which the coefficient A_{ij} might be modified, given that the necessary information is available at the *ij*th junction. Among these might be growth of additional dendritic spines, addition of new synaptic junctions, activation of synaptic junctions previously inactive, changes in membrane resistivity, and/or changes in the amount of transmitter in a synapse. Although some structural changes have been observed, there is little evidence yet to choose among the possibilities mentioned above or, in fact, to conclude that such processes take place at all in the cortex of an adult animal.

Passive Modification

To make the modification

$$\delta A \sim g^\mu \times f^\nu \tag{26}$$

by any of the mechanisms suggested above, the system must have the signal distribution f^ν in its F bank and g^μ in its G bank. It is easy to obtain f^ν since this is mapped from either an external event or is some internal pattern. But to get g^μ in the G bank is more difficult since this in effect is what the system is trying to learn.

In what we denote as active learning, the system is presented with some f^λ, searches for a response, and is given some indication of when it is coming closer. When by some procedure or another it finds the "right" response, say g^ω, it is "rewarded" and responds to the reward by printing into A the information

$$\delta A_{ij} = \eta g_i^\omega f_j^\lambda. \tag{27}$$

(The information is available at the time of the reward since at that time the system is mapping f^{λ}, responding g^{ω}, and thus has just the desired spiking frequencies in the F and G banks of neurons.) Active learning probably describes a type of learning in which a system response to an input is matched against an expected or desired response and judged correct or incorrect.

However, there is a type of animal learning that does not seem from visible external indications to require this type of a search procedure. It is the type of learning in which, as far as can be seen, an animal is placed in an environment and seems to learn to recognize and to recollect in a far more passive manner.

To arrive at an algorithm which produces what we call passive learning, we utilize a distinction between forming an internal representation of events in the external world as opposed to producing a response to these events that is matched against what is expected or desired in the external world.

The simple but important idea is that *the internal electrical activity that in one mind signals the presence of an external event is not necessarily (or likely to be) the same electrical activity that signals the presence of that same event for another mind.* There is nothing that requires that the same external event be mapped into the same neural patterns by different animals. The event e^{ν} which for one animal is mapped into the signal distributions f^{ν} and g^{ν}, in another animal is mapped into f'^{ν} and g'^{ν}. What is required for eventual agreement between animals in their description of the external world is not that electrical signals mapped be identical, but rather that the relation of the signals to each other and to events in the external world be the same (Figure 5).

If we now allow the output of a cell to be determined by the input to that cell and the already existing synaptic junction strengths, as well as by possible noise-like fluctuations (making no prior requirement on what the output should be), we arrive at a mathematical formulation of what we call passive modification (Cooper, 1973):

$$\delta A_{ij} \sim g_i f_j \sim \sum_{k=1}^{N} A_{ik} f_k f_j. \tag{28}$$

It has been shown in the above reference that with a simple form of passive modification, a system generates its own response to incoming patterns in such a way as to construct distributed mappings that can function as memories capable of recognition and association. To a limited extent these mappings can be regarded as internal representations of what has arrived from the outside world. It has further been shown (Nass and Cooper, 1975) that a form of passive modification can result in the formation of feature detectors or threshold-response units which learn to respond to repeated patterns even in the absence of any initial

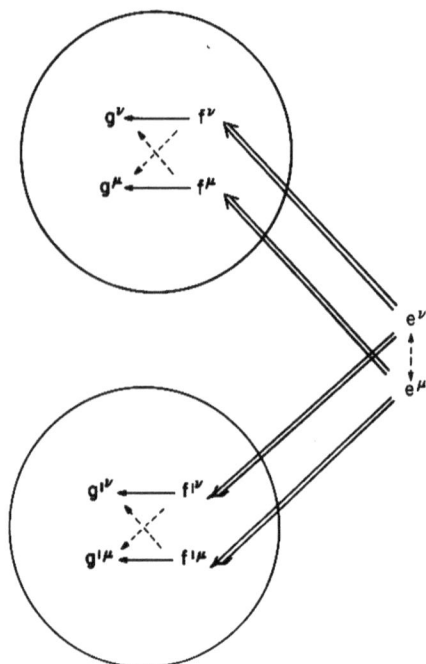

Figure 5 Representations in two different systems of the same external fabric of events. The two representations are not identical, but they each stand in a one-to-one relation to the external fabric and to each other. (From Cooper, 1973.)

bias. Such units can serve to perform some nonlinear separations mentioned in the previous section.

More detailed discussion of the consequences of these modification procedures and the properties of some of the mappings that result is contained in the references cited above. I would now like to turn to the situation in visual cortex where some of the assumptions made above may be tested.

Experimental Tests in Visual Cortex

Experimental work of the last generation, beginning with the pathbreaking work of Hubel and Wiesel (1959, 1962), has shown that there exist cells in visual cortex (areas 17, 18, and 19) of the adult cat that respond in a precise and highly tuned fashion to external patterns—in particular, to bars or edges of given orientation and moving in a given direction. Much additional work (Blakemore and Cooper, 1970; Blakemore and Mitchell, 1973; Hirsch and Spinelli, 1971; Pettigrew and Freeman, 1973) has indicated that the number and response characteristics of such cortical cells can be modified. It has been observed in particular (Imbert and Buisseret, 1975; Blakemore and Van Sluyters, 1975; Buisseret and Imbert, 1976; Frégnac and Imbert, 1977, 1978) that

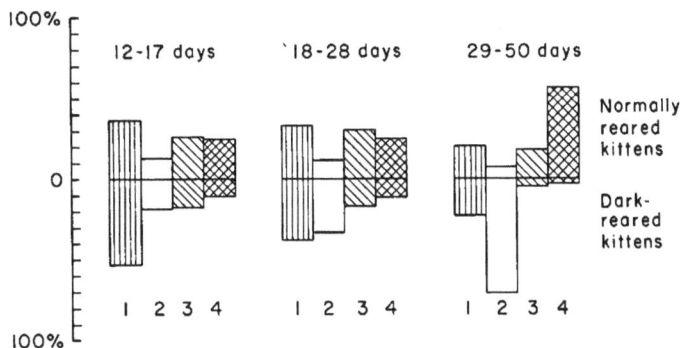

Figure 6 Distribution of the different types of cells in three age groups in normally reared kittens (upper part) and in dark-reared kittens (lower part). The ordinate is normalized so that the heights are the percentages of cells in the various functions groups. Type 1, nonactivatable (▥);¡2, nonspecific (□); 3, immature (▧); 4, specific (▨).(From Frégnac and Imbert, 1977, 1978.)

the relative number of cortical cells that are highly specific in their response to visual patterns varies in a very striking way with the visual experience of the animal during the critical period.

Imbert and Buisseret have classified cortical cells that respond to visual stimuli into three groups—aspecific, immature, and specific. They and Frégnac and Imbert have measured the relative proportions of these groups depending on the visual experience of the animal. The distribution of the different cell types in three age groups is shown in Figure 6.

Examination of these results, which were obtained from the study of 1,050 cells, shows that cells having some of the highly specific response properties of adult visual cortical neurons, especially concerning orientation selectivity, are present in the earliest stages of postnatal development independent of visual experience (Frégnac and Imbert, 1977, 1978). However, visual experience between 17 and 70 days is critical in determining the evolution of these cells. Animals reared normally showed a marked increase in the number of specific cells as compared with aspecific. (The period between 17 and 28 days is usually sufficient to reach the normal adult level of specificity). The reverse is true for animals reared in the dark. A statistical analysis of this evolution, performed by Frégnac (1978), shows clearly the striking dependence of the ratio of sharply tuned to broadly tuned cells depending on the experience of the animal.

In addition, as shown by Imbert and Buisseret (1975), Buisseret and Imbert (1976), and Buisseret, Gary-Bobo, and Imbert (1978), as little as 6 hours of normal visual experience at about 42 days of age can alter in a striking fashion the ratio of specific or immature to aspecific cells (Figure 7). That such a short visual experience can change the tuning ratios so markedly is clear evidence of the great plasticity of these cortical cells at the height of the critical period.

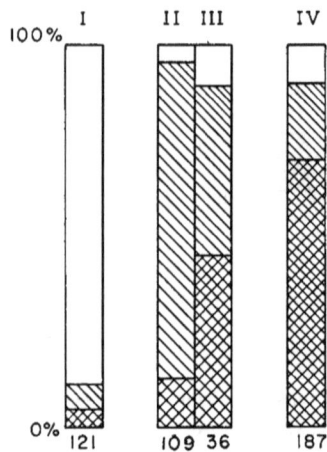

Figure 7 Distribution, in percentage, of the three types of visual cortical units (area 17) recorded after 6 hours of visual exposure for 6-week-old dark-reared kittens. Columns: I, dark-reared kittens; IV, normally reared kittens. During 6 hours of exposure, conditions were: in II and III, freely moving; in III, 12 hours in the dark followed by 6 hours of exposure. Numbers of visual cells recorded are given under each column. Specific cells (▨) are activated by oriented stimuli within a sharp angle (<60°). Immature cells (▨) are activated by oriented stimuli within a larger angle (<150°). Nonspecific cells (□) are activated by nonoriented stimuli moving in any direction. A statistical analysis reveals no significant difference in the percentages of immature and specific units between columns III and IV. Therefore it may be that for a 6-week-old dark-reared kitten, a 6-hour exposure to visual input followed by 12 hours in the dark is sufficient to produce a distribution of cortical cells similar to that of normally reared animals. (From Buisseret, Gary-Bobo, and Imbert, 1978.)

These results seem to us to provide direct evidence for the modifiability of the response of single cells in the cortex of a higher mammal according to its visual experience. Depending on whether or not patterned visual information is part of the animal's experience, the specificity of the response of cortical neurons varies widely. With normal patterned experience, specificity, developing normally, increases. Deprived of normal patterned information (dark reared or lid sutured at birth, for example), specificity decreases. Further, even a short exposure to patterned information after 6 weeks of dark rearing can reverse the loss of specificity and produce an almost normal distribution of cells.

We do not claim, and it is not necessary, that all neurons in visual cortex be so modifiable. Nor is it necessary that modifiable neurons be especially important in producing the architecture of visual cortex. It is our hope that the general form of modifiability we require to construct distributed mappings manifests itself for at least some cells of visual cortex that are accessible to experiment. We thus make the conservative assumption that the biological mechanisms, once established, will manifest themselves in more or less similar forms in different regions. If this is the case, modifiable individual neurons in visual cortex can

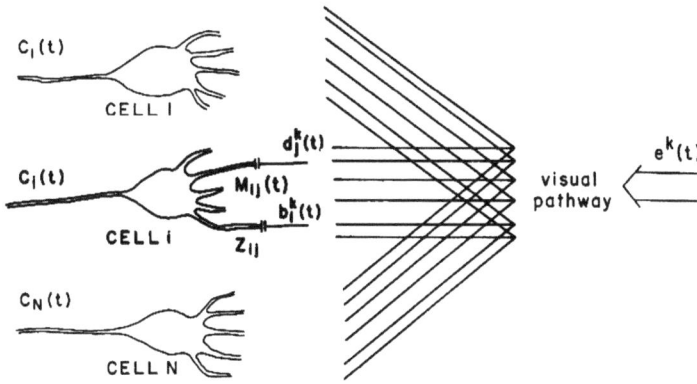

Figure 8 A visual pattern $e^k(t)$ (e.g., a bar or an edge of a given orientation and moving in a given direction) falls on the retina at time t. This pattern evokes a set of parallel responses in the axons of the cells of lateral geniculate nucleus (LGN), and these result in presynaptic inputs to a layer of modifiable neurons in visual cortex. The inputs are divided into two parts: inputs $d_j^k(t)$ that fall on modifiable junctions; and inputs $b_i^k(t)$ that fall on nonmodifiable junctions. The strengths at time t of the modifiable junctions $M_{ij}(t)$ comprise a matrix $M(t)$, while the strengths of the nonmodifiable junctions Z_{ij} comprise a matrix Z. The responses of the cortical neurons depend on the inputs and the junction strengths $M_{ij}(t)$ and Z_{ij}. (From Cooper, Liberman, and Oja, 1979.)

provide evidence for such modification more generally. In what follows, I will present some of the results of a recently developed theory (Cooper, Liberman, and Oja, 1979) which attempts to account for the experimental data mentioned above.

In this theory CLO (Cooper, Liberman, and Oja) it is assumed that between lateral-geniculate and visual cortical cells there exist labile synapses M_{ij} that are modified according to a form of passive modification, called threshold passive modification, as well as nonlabile synapses Z_{ij} that contain permanent information (Figure 8). These latter give the cortical cells a weak initial tendency to fire more strongly and readily to some orientations in the visual field than to others. Threshold passive modification is a variation of the two-point modification for which a cell can learn to respond or increases its response to a repeated external pattern while at the same time changing its response so that it responds to no more than one pattern. In this way, the tuning curve sharpens and the mapping from input to output becomes optimal.

Referring to the ijth ideal synaptic junction (Figure 8) in the CLO theory, the modifiable part of the junction changes according to

$$\delta M_{ij} = F(c_i)c_i d_j \tag{29}$$

where c_i is the output of the ith cell, d_j the input to the ijth modifiable junction M_{ij}, and $F(c_i)$ some function of the output. (Note again that in passive modification the output of a cell is determined by the input and the already existing synaptic strengths as well as by noise-like fluctuations.)

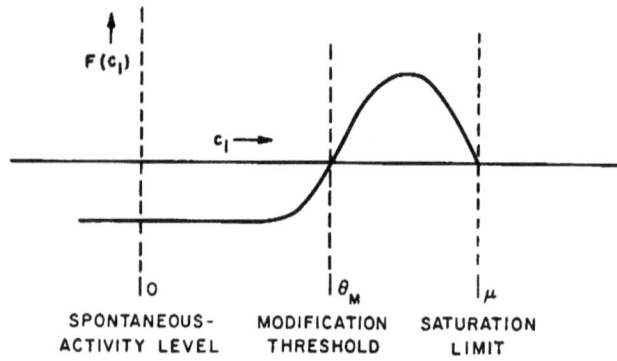

Figure 9

The precise form of $F(c_i)$ is not critical as long as it has certain general characteristics (Figure 9). What CLO have shown is that if the function F goes through zero (ideally the position of this zero is determined by some mean activity of the cell), then the sharpness of the tuning curve is altered by the visual experience of the animal, as described below. This modification might be called "Hebbian" when the output is above the modification threshold and "anti-Hebbian" when the output is below this threshold.

CLO thus assume that the modifiability of a synaptic junction is dependent on events that occur at different parts of the same cell and on the rate at which the cell responds: below θ_M, above θ_M but below the maximum rate μ, and above μ. They have proved several theorems which show that with this form of passive modification there is an increase in the specificity of the response of a cortical cell to visual input (sharpening of its tuning curve) when that cell is exposed to stimuli that are the result of normal patterned visual experience, and there is a loss of specificity when that cell is exposed to noise-like input, such as might be expected when an animal is dark reared or raised with eyelids sutured. Specificity can be regained, however, with a return of input due to patterned vision.

In addition to this basic behavior, simulations and mathematical results on the asymptotic states of the neural network show some more subtle phenomena that depend upon values of system parameters, notably, the amount decay (forgetting per-unit time), the strength of selective modification of synaptic junctions, and the different statistical properties of noise factors. In the following discussion, some of these effects are illuminated by computer simulations and simplifying approximations.

Sharpening of Tuning with Learning
With stimuli corresponding to normal visual input, the tuning curve of a cell sharpens, going from broadly tuned to sharply tuned. The neuron

Leon N Cooper

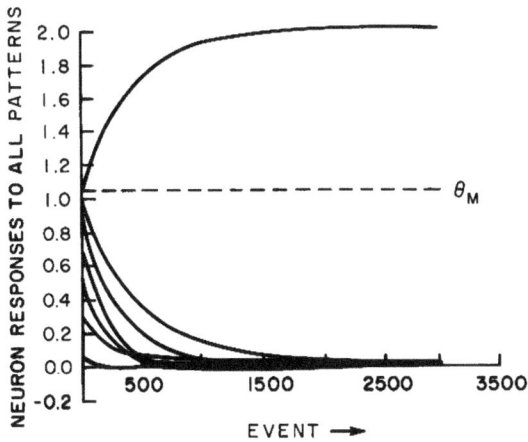

Figure 10 The responses of a neuron modified by the input of seven different noiseless patterns as a function of time. (A detailed discussion of the conditions under which the simulations, whose results are shown here, were run is given in Cooper, Liberman, and Oja, 1979.) Upper curve: the response to the leading pattern to which the initial response was higher than θ_M. Lower curve: responses to the other six patterns. (From Cooper, Liberman, and Oja, 1979.)

changes from a nonspecific unit, showing some response to all input patterns, to an immature one, for which some orientations have already lost the ability to elicit any kind of response above the spontaneous activity of the cell. Then the range of orientations for which the neuron is sensitive diminishes further until only a high and narrow peak, centered at the leading pattern for that cell, is visible in the tuning curve: the neuron has become a specific unit (Figures 10, 11, 12, and 13). This is in good agreement with experimental observation of the progression from aspecific to immature to specific as reported by Frégnac and Imbert (1977, 1978). In addition, this suggests that the classifications (Imbert and Buisseret, 1975; Buisseret and Imbert, 1976) aspecific, immature, and specific are relatively arbitrary divisions in what is really a continuum of response.

In learning with patterned stimuli, the outcome is not very sensitive to system parameters; the gross behavior of sharpening of tuning close to the optimum was achieved in simulations under a considerable range of parameter values. It is especially notable that even with relatively high noise levels, with signal-to-noise ratios considerably smaller than one, we still obtain qualitatively very similar behavior to the noiseless learning cases (Figure 13).

Loss of Specificity
With noise-like stimuli, corresponding to nonpatterned visual input, widening of the cortical-cell tuning curve takes place, practically independent of how sharp the tuning was originally. The main effect is a

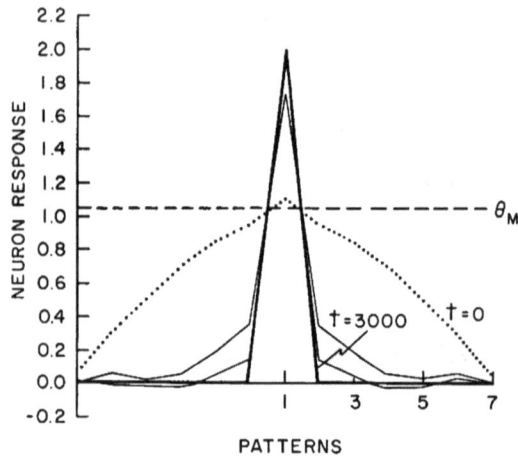

Figure 11 The responses of a neuron to seven different noiseless patterns at intervals from $t = 0$ to $t = 3,000$. (This is the same simulation as that shown in Figure 10.) (From Cooper, Liberman, and Oja, 1979.)

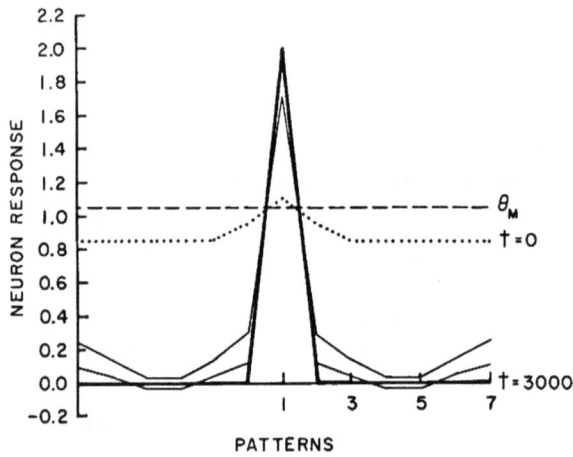

Figure 12 The responses of a neuron to seven different noiseless patterns. This simulation is identical to that of Figure 7 except that initial values are chosen to make the initial responses of the neuron relatively flat (as is the case for some aspecific cells). (From Cooper, Liberman, and Oja, 1979.)

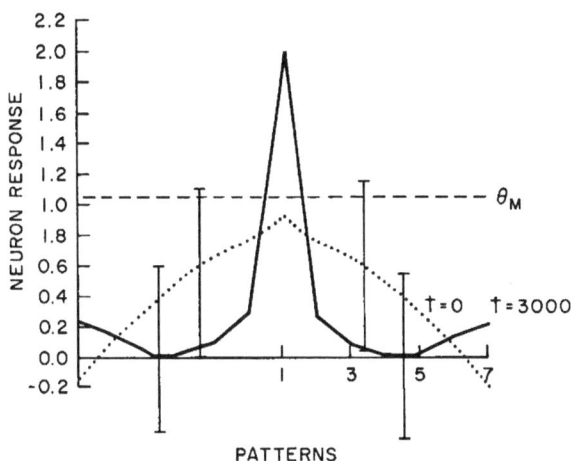

Figure 13 The responses of a neuron to the seven patterns at times $t = 0$ and $t = 3,000$. In this simulation, the input vectors were the patterns with noise. Channel noise was also present. All elements of noise vectors were uncorrelated and uniformly distributed. Channel noise was uncorrelated with signal noise. Dotted curve: responses at time $t = 0$. Solid curve: responses at time $t = 3,000$. The vertical bars represent regions inside which the responses would occur when channel noise is added. Therefore each individual realization of a "tuning curve" would be inside these regions, with the curves giving the average tuning at the respective times $t = 0$ or $t = 3,000$. (From Cooper, Liberman, and Oja, 1979.)

rapid decay of the central peak of the tuning curve; the change in response for nonoptimal patterns is smaller. The overall time constant for loss of specificity is larger than that for gain of specificity. This seems to be in agreement with experimental results indicating that exposing dark-reared animals to patterned stimuli produces remarkably fast gains of specificity (Figure 7); loss of specificity is a more gradual process.

For this situation the effect of parameters is important. In the absence of the overwhelming influence of strong patterned stimuli, some rather subtle phenomena, due to correlation properties among different noise components, become visible. Strong correlation between the noise inputs to modifiable and nonmodifiable junctions leads to a limit such that the *total* response of the cell is close to zero (Figure 14A). Weak correlation drives the modifiable part of the mapping close to zero, leaving the nonmodifiable part alone to determine the tuning of the cell (Figure 14B). A return of patterned stimuli (after noisy stimuli have broadened the response of a cell) can then restore the sharp tuning (Figure 15).

We see that if there is strong correlation between the noise inputs to labile and nonlabile junctions, the initial bias of the cell can be entirely lost. A return of specificity would then not necessarily be to the same orientation as that preferred originally. If excitation is assumed between cells in an orientation column, other cells that retained their

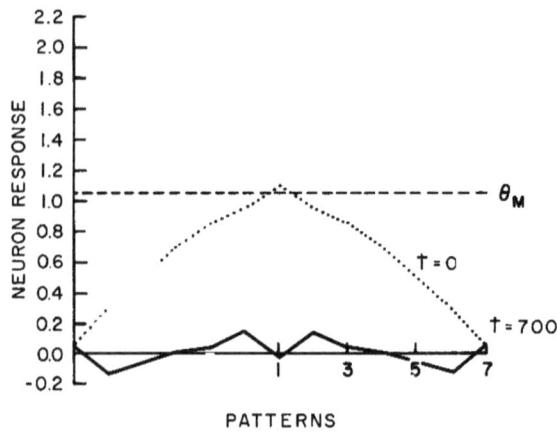

A

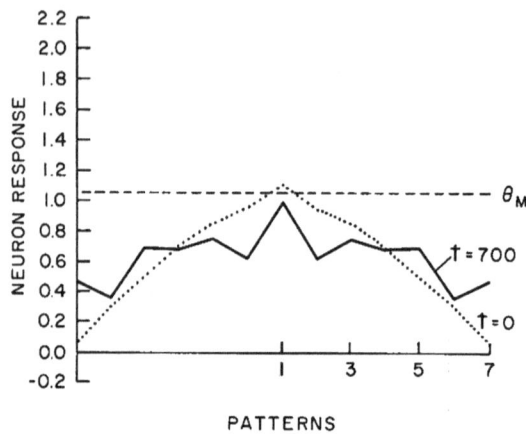

B

Figure 14 The response of a neuron to signal and channel noise. The channel noise was uncorrelated with a signal noise. Both were uniformly distributed. (A) The signal noise inputs to modifiable and nonmodifiable junctions were completely correlated. (B) The signal noise inputs were uncorrelated. In these simulations the parameters have been changed to decrease simulation time. Dotted upper curve: responses at time $t = 0$. Solid curve: responses at time $t = 700$. (From Cooper, Liberman, and Oja, 1979.)

original bias might still guide a cell that had lost its bias to its original orientation preference. However, an entire column could shift its orientation preference (Blakemore and Van Sluyters, 1974; Movshon, 1976).

These results seem to me to be, at least qualitatively, in agreement with the experimental data cited above. An extension of the CLO theory to include effects of binocular interactions is presently being pursued with E. Bienenstock and P. Munro. Initial results seem promising. When this extension is completed, we expect to have a fairly explicit theory, applicable to a wide variety of situations in visual cortex, in

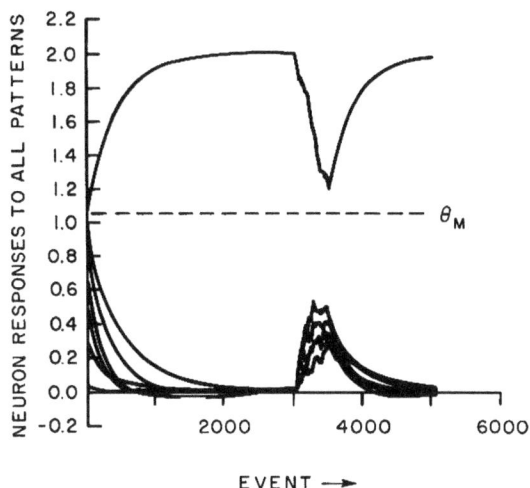

Figure 15 Loss and retrieval of specificity. This figure is plotted in a manner similar to Figure 10. From $t = 0$ to $t = 3,000$ noiseless patterns were presented and the neuron acquired a sharp tuning. Uncorrelated noise was presented to the neuron from $t = 3,001$ to $t = 3,500$, and a broadening (i.e., loss of specificity) occurred. Noiseless patterns were presented from $t = 3,501$ to $t = 6,000$ and the neuron regained its former sharp tuning —retrieval of specificity. (The parameters were changed in the course of the simulation to decrease simulation time. For the same parameters loss of specificity is slower than increase of specificity.) (From Cooper, Liberman, and Oja, 1979.)

agreement with present observation and hopefully, with a number of new and testable consequences.

Acknowledgments

The work on which this article is based was supported in part by a grant from the Ittleson Foundation, Inc.

References

Anderson, J. A., 1970. Two models for memory organization using interacting traces. *Math. Biosci.* 8:137–160.

Anderson, J. A., 1972. A simple neural network generating an interactive memory. *Math. Biosci.* 14:197–220.

Anderson, J. A., 1977. Neural models with cognitive implications. In *Basic Processes in Reading: Perception and Comprehension.* D. La Berge and S. J. Samuels, eds. Hillsdale, NJ: Erlbaum Associates, pp. 27–90.

Anderson, J., and L. N Cooper, 1978. Biological organization of memory. In *Pluriscience.* Paris: Encyclopaedia Universalis France S.A., pp. 168–175.

Distributed Memory: Experimental Tests

Blakemore, C., and G. F. Cooper, 1970. Development of the brain depends on the visual environment. *Nature* 228:477–478.

Blakemore, C., and D. E. Mitchell, 1973. Environmental modification of the visual cortex and the neural basis of learning and memory. *Nature* 241:467–468.

Blakemore, C., and R. C. Van Sluyters, 1974. Reversal of the physiological effects of monocular deprivation in kittens. Further evidence for a sensitive period. *J. Physiol. (London)* 237:195–216.

Blakemore, C., and R. C. Van Sluyters, 1975. Innate and environmental factors in the development of the kitten's visual cortex. *J. Physiol. (London)* 248:663–716.

Block, H. D., 1962. The perceptron: A model for brain functioning. I. *Rev. Mod. Phys.* 34:123–135.

Block, H. D., B. W. Knight Jr., and F. Rosenblatt, 1962. Analysis of a four-layer series coupled perceptron. II. *Rev. Mod. Phys.* 34:135–142.

Buisseret, P., and M. Imbert, 1976. Visual cortical cells. Their developmental properties in normal and dark reared kittens. *J. Physiol. (London)* 255:511–525.

Buisseret, P., E. Gary-Bobo, and M. Imbert, 1978. Ocular motility and recovery of orientational properties of visual cortical neurons in dark-reared kittens. *Nature* 272:816–817.

Cooper, L. N, 1973. A possible organization of animal memory and learning. In *Proceedings of the Nobel Symposium on Collective Properties of Physical Systems*. B. Lundquist and S. Lundquist, eds. New York: Academic Press, pp. 252–264.

Cooper, L. N, F. Liberman, and E. Oja, 1979. A theory for the acquisition and loss of neuron specificity in visual cortex. *Biol. Cybern.* 33:9–28.

Frégnac, Y., 1978. Cinétique de development du cortex visuel primaire chez lè chat. Effects de la privation visuelle binoculaire et modèle de maturation de la sélectivité à l'orientation. Doctoral Thesis: Université René Descartes.

Frégnac, Y., and M. Imbert, 1977. Cinétique de development des cellules du cortex visuel. *J. Physiol. (Paris)* 6:73.

Frégnac, Y., and M. Imbert, 1978. Early development of visual cortical cells in normal and dark-reared kittens. Relationship between orientation selectivity and ocular dominance. *J. Physiol. (London)* 278:27–44.

Hebb, D. O., 1949. *The Organization of Behavior*. New York: Wiley, p. 62.

Hirsch, H. V. B., and D. N. Spinelli, 1971. Modification of the distribution of receptive field orientation in cats by selective visual exposure during development. *Exp. Brain Res.* 12:509–527.

Hubel, D. H., and T. N. Wiesel, 1959. Receptive fields of single neurons in the cat striate cortex. *J. Physiol. (London)* 148:574–591.

Hubel, D. H., and T. N. Wiesel, 1962. Receptive fields, binocular interaction and functional architecture in the cat's visual cortex. *J. Physiol. (London)* 160:106–154.

Imbert, M., and Y. Buisseret, 1975. Receptive field characteristics and plastic properties of visual cortical cells in kittens reared with or without visual experience. *Exp. Brain Res.* 22:2–36.

Kandel, E. R., 1976. *Cellular Basis of Behavior: An Introduction to Behavioral Neurobiology.* San Francisco: W. H. Freeman.

Kohonen, T., 1972. Correlation matrix memories. *IEEE Trans. Computers C* 21:353–359.

Kohonen, T., 1977. *Associative Memory: A System Theoretic Approach.* Berlin: Springer-Verlag.

Lashley, K. S., 1950. In search of the engram. In *Symposia of the Society of Experimental Biologists, No. 4: Physiological Mechanisms in Animal Behavior.* New York: Academic Press, pp. 478–480.

Longuet-Higgins, H. C., 1968a. Holographic model of temporal recall. *Nature* 217:104.

Longuet-Higgins, H. C., 1968b. The non-local storage of temporal information. *Proc. Roy. Soc. B* 171:327–334.

McIlwain, J. T., 1976. Large receptive fields and spatial transformations in the visual system. In *International Review of Physiology: Neurophysiology II, Vol. 10.* R. Porter, ed. Baltimore: University Park Press.

Minsky, M., and S. Papert, 1969. *An Introduction to Computational Geometry.* Cambridge, MA: MIT Press.

Movshon, J. A., 1976. Reversal of the physiological effects of monocular deprivation in visual cortex. *J. Physiol. (London)* 261:125–174.

Nass, M. M., and L. N Cooper, 1975. A theory for the development of feature detecting cells in visual cortex. *Biol. Cybern.* 19:1–18.

Pettigrew, J. D., and R. D. Freeman, 1973. Visual experience without lines. Effects on developing cortical neurons. *Science* 182:599–601.

21 An Information-Processing Approach to Understanding the Visual Cortex

Francis H. C. Crick, David C. Marr, and Tomaso Poggio

ABSTRACT An outline description is given of the experimental work on the visual acuity and hyperacuity of human beings. The very high resolution achieved in hyperacuity corresponds to a fraction of the spacing between adjacent cones in the fovea. We briefly outline a computational theory of early vision, according to which (a) the retinal image is filtered through a set of approximately band-pass spatial filters and (b) zero-crossings are detected independently in the outputs of these channels. Zero-crossings may contain sufficient information for much of the subsequent processing. Consideration of the optimal filter leads to one which is equivalent to a cell with a particular center–surround type of response. An "edge" in the visual field then corresponds to a line of zero-crossings in the filtered image. The mathematics of sampling and of Logan's zero-crossing theorem are briefly explained.

In this framework we suggest, similarly to Barlow (1979), that the fine grid of small cells in layer $IVC\beta$ of the striate cortex perform an approximate reconstruction of the filtered image with the goal of representing the position of zero-crossings with a very high accuracy (around a few seconds of arc). How this might be achieved is discussed in outline. Finally it is mentioned that this picture is probably too static, as hyperacuity can be achieved with moving targets.

To make for easier comprehension much of the mathematics is set out in an appendix.

Introduction

That we see the world as well as we do is something of a miracle. What seems so direct and effortless turns out, on close consideration, to involve many rapid and complex processes the details of which we are only beginning to glimpse. In a series of papers Marr and his collaborators have outlined a general strategy for approaching some of these problems (Marr, 1976, 1977; Marr and Nishihara, 1978b; Marr and Poggio, 1977; Ullman, 1979). Two useful introductions are the general account by Marr and Nishihara (1978a) and a sympathetic review in *Nature* by Sutherland (1979). Other papers by Marr and his coworkers

F. H. C. CRICK, D. C. MARR, and T. POGGIO The Salk Institute for Biological Studies, P. O. Box 1809, San Diego, California 92112; M.I.T. Psychology Department, 79 Amherst Street, Cambridge, Massachusetts 02139; Max-Planck-Institut fuer biologische Kybernetik, 74 Tuebingen 1, Spemannstrasse 38, Germany

have made detailed suggestions about the computations the brain carries out in special cases (Marr and Poggio, 1976; Marr, 1977; Ullman, 1979). In particular, a recent paper by Marr and Poggio (1979) has proposed an algorithm for human stereopsis which has been successfully implemented in a computer program (Grimson and Marr, 1979). Computational theories of this kind based on old and new results of information theory can establish what needs to be computed and how, while psychophysical experiments can tell us, for instance, the precision of the computation. Additional constraints are determined by the biophysics of nerve cells and their recorded physiological properties as well as by the anatomical and physiological diagrams of the circuitry.

In this chapter we shall deal only with the very early stages in the main visual pathway, specifically the retina, the lateral geniculate nucleus (LGN), and the striate cortex (also called area 17 or V1). The visual system is attractive not only because it can be supplied with a well-controlled and detailed input (unlike the cerebellum), but also because it has a fairly simple and direct path from the sensory receptors to the cortex (unlike the auditory system). Moreover, a large amount of detailed experimental work has been done on it, using a variety of methods, including such different approaches as neurophysiology, neuroanatomy, and psychophysics.

To our regret we are not yet able to make detailed and explicit suggestions as to what all the neurons in this region are doing. Instead we shall try to explain the general way in which we are approaching these problems from a computational point of view. In particular, we shall apply it to the phenomenon of hyperacuity since, as Barlow (1979) has pointed out, this raises special problems, both static and dynamic.

Acuity and Hyperacuity

The main experiments (which we summarize here only very briefly) have been carried out on human beings, especially in recent years, by Westheimer and his collaborators (Westheimer, 1976, Westheimer and McKee, 1975, 1977a,b,c). If two points of light lie side by side, they can be seen to be double. If they are put closer together, they may appear to us as a single point. It is found that, with practice, an angular separation of about 1' of arc can be distinguished with 75% success (see, for instance, Westheimer, 1977). This is the classical test for two-point acuity (see Figure 1A).

Much closer angular intervals can be detected in special situations. A typical example of this is the acuity found in reading a vernier. The objects used need not be straight lines. A pattern of three points also gives good results (see Figure 1B, where the task involves determining whether the middle point lies to the right or to the left of the imaginary line connecting the outer two points (Beck and Schwartz, 1979). In such tasks 75% success can be obtained, with practice, using an angular mis-

F. H. C. Crick, D. C. Marr, and T. Poggio

A   B

Figure 1 (A) Pattern configuration for two-point acuity tests. (B) One of several patterns yielding hyperacuity. Lateral displacements of the middle point to the right or to the left of the imaginary lines connecting the outer two points can be detected down to about 5″ accuracy. A typical separation for the dots is 10′.

alignment of only 2″ to 5″ of arc, that is, of a few seconds of arc rather than the minute of arc found for two-point acuity. Acuity of this type is often called hyperacuity, though "positional accuracy" might be a better name. To achieve it the three points should not be too far apart—a few minutes of arc separation give the best performance.

What is at the root of this large difference between hyperacuity and simple two-point acuity? For such high resolution the points must be adjacent but they must not overlap. This has been clearly pointed out by Westheimer and McKee (1977b).

Hyperacuity, that is, positional accuracy, is found in a variety of situations. In particular, the acuity observed in stereopsis is hyperacuity (Westheimer and McKee, 1978). This and other data (possibly Julesz, 1971, Figures 3.6.1–3.6.3) show that hyperacuity can be binocular. For this reason it is likely to be implemented no earlier in the visual pathway than the striate cortex, since this is the first place where the inputs from the two separate eyes interact strongly. The image need not be prolonged in time. A flash of 1.5 msec is quite adequate, and in fact the different parts of the pattern need not be flashed simultaneously, provided they are not separated in time by more than 20 msec (Westheimer and McKee, 1977a). Furthermore, the random line stereogram of Julesz (1971, Figure 3.6.1) would seem to imply that vernier acuity is not restricted to forced choice tests.

Most remarkable of all, as Barlow (1979) has emphasized in a recent note, performance in a hyperacuity task is not appreciably degraded even if the target is moving at rates up to 2° to 4° per second (Westheimer and McKee, 1975). This is not due to eye movements. Westheimer has used the technique of presenting the signal for only 200 msec, with the direction of motion randomized. This is too short a time for eye movements to be initiated correctly.

The astonishing nature of this performance (which even without practice is fairly striking) can be seen when the properties of the retina are considered. The spacing of the receptors, the cones, even in the fovea where they are closest, is about 25″. In addition, the optical spread of the system has a half-width of about 30″. The spacing of the retinal ganglion cells, which connect the eye to the brain, is no finer. How then can we achieve such a high performance with such a blunt optical instrument?

Theory

To approach this problem we need to use a computational approach. The underlying idea is that the nervous system is a very complex information-processing machine. While we cannot always say exactly how visual information is handled, we can be sure that once information is lost in a pathway it cannot be recovered. But to assess whether information is lost or only concealed we need some theoretical results, and to this we must now turn.

Viewed in this way, the retina is a device for sampling the visual image at intervals which, from the point of view of hyperacuity, might appear somewhat coarse. Is it possible to sample a continuous distribution and yet not lose any information? The mathematical answer to this is well known. Provided that the pattern does not change too abruptly in space the reconstruction can, in theory, be perfect.

To make this more precise consider first the 1-dimensional (1-D) case. The condition imposed is that, if the pattern is analyzed into its Fourier components, they must be zero above a certain limiting spatial frequency. For any general spatial pattern we can achieve this by passing it through a perfect low-pass filter (see Figure 2). This allows all spatial frequencies below the cutoff frequency of the filter to pass unaltered while reducing to zero all frequencies above this limit. The sampling theorem then says that for such a pattern we need only sample it at the (regular) intervals shown in Figure 3. That is, the sampling points must

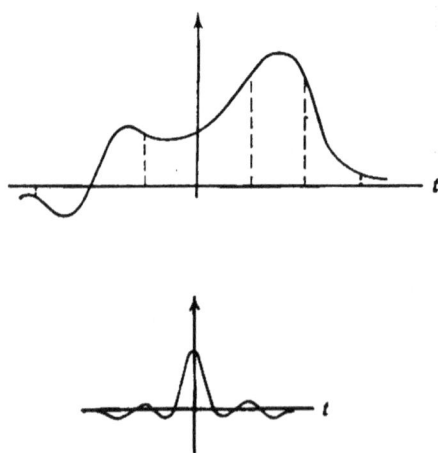

Figure 2 A perfect low-pass filter is shown on the left. Frequencies above $f = \frac{1}{2}$ are blocked, whereas frequencies below are passed undistorted. The inverse Fourier transform sinc x is outlined on the right. The function sinc has an infinite number of side lobes, not shown here, but indicated in Figure 3. Convolution of a 1-D pattern with the "receptive field" sinc x is equivalent to filtering it with $\pi(f)$.

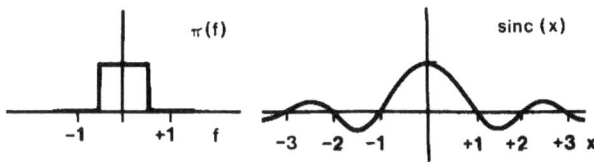

Figure 3 An illustration of the sampling theorem. The time function shown above is sampled at the Shannon rate. Convolution of the series of sampled values with the function sinc x shown below reconstructs the original function exactly.

be spaced no further apart than the zeros of the higher-frequency spatial component, as shown in the figure. The proof is elementary (see the appendix).

Moreover, there is a relatively simple method of reconstructing the continuous distribution from the samples. This involves convolving the amplitudes of the sampled points with the mathematical function sinc x = $\sin(\pi x)/\pi x$. This function is shown in Figure 3.

The operation of convolution is described in the appendix. In very rough terms, if one function is convolved with a second one, the resulting function would be considered as the first function spread everywhere by the second one (or vice versa). Thus, if the second function is Gaussian, the effect of convolving it with a more extended function is to average the latter locally on every point and thus make it everywhere smoother.

We shall need one other useful result. This is Logan's zero-crossing theorem (Logan, 1977). Again we consider the 1-D case. This time we impose not just an upper frequency limit to the filter but also a lower limit as well, to give a band-pass filter just one octave wide (see Figure 4). That is, we remove both the high frequencies and the low frequencies. This necessarily means that the filtered distribution must cross the zero-line fairly often since there are no low-frequency components to keep it on one side of zero for any considerable distance. Logan's theorem states that it is almost always possible to reconstruct the entire (filtered) distribution, given only the positions and signs of the zero-crossings, subject to a constant multiplication factor. The exact conditions under which this can be done are set out in the appendix. A similar theorem applies to the zero-crossings of a 2-dimensional (2-D) distribution (see the appendix).

However, in this case the proof is an existence proof. There appears to be no very simple way to reconstruct the distribution from the zero-crossings. Nevertheless, the theorem shows quite clearly that, provided the filter is band-pass, the zero-crossings alone are a very rich source of information. It would therefore not be surprising if the brain used them as an important way to transmit and further process visual information, especially since the positions of the zero-crossings of a function are

509   Information Processing in Vision

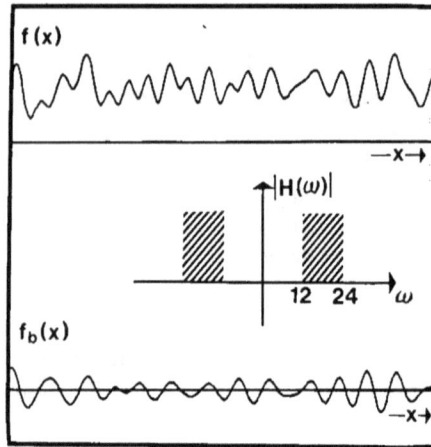

Figure 4 The meaning of Logan's theorem. A band-limited signal $f(x)$ is filtered through an ideal one-octave filter (inset) providing $f_b(x)$. Since $f_b(x)$ has a bandwidth of one octave and it has no complex zeros in common with its Hilbert transform and no multiple real zeros, Logan's theorem implies that f_b is determined, up to a multiplicative constant, by its zero-crossings alone.

unaltered if the amplitude scale is altered, that is, if the function is multiplied by a constant factor. This feature of the zero-crossings is an important aspect of Marr and Poggio's theory of stereopsis (1979).

The Optimal Filter

We must next consider what mathematical operations, in a very general sense, are likely to be performed on the intensity distribution of the retinal image as it proceeds along the visual pathway. It is well known that the ganglion cells of the retina hardly respond to an increase in general level of uniform intensity but rather to inequalities in it, in a center–surround manner. This is even more true for cells of the lateral geniculate and for cells in layer IVC of the striate cortex of the monkey, which are the main recipient of the input from the LGN (the cat's cortical cells may be somewhat different).

A useful way to approach this problem from a computational point of view is to ask what operation it would be best to perform on the visual input to the retina. Simply on computational grounds an important preliminary operation in the processing of visual information is the localization of sharp changes in image intensity, for the reason that these usually correspond to physically important items like edges in the image. A major difficulty with natural images is that changes can and do occur over a wide range of scales. It follows that one should seek a way of dealing separately with the changes occurring at different scales, since no single filter can be optimal at all scales. The appropriate filter,

F. H. C. Crick, D. C. Marr, and T. Poggio

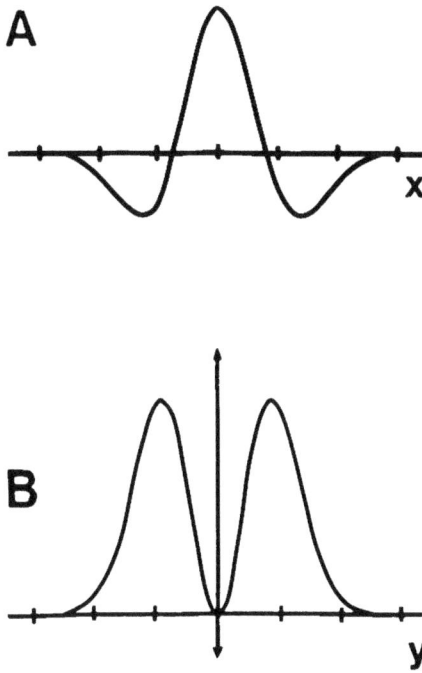

Figure 5 The 1-D $\nabla^2 G$. The corresponding 2-D receptive field is circularly symmetric with a Mexican-hat shape. (B) is the Fourier transform of (A).

at each scale, should be approximately band-pass, so that we reduce the range of scales over which intensity changes take place. The fact that there appear to be band-pass channels in vision would in any case point in this direction. In addition, since the "high" frequencies in the spatial pattern are filtered out, we can use sampling techniques. As explained in Marr and Hildreth (1979), it is sensible to choose a function which is compact both in space (because the visual world is largely made up of compact features) as well as in frequency. The function which does this best is the Gaussian, since its Fourier transform is also a Gaussian.

The first (spatial) differential of an edge has a maximum, but the second differential has a zero-crossing at the point where the edge is located. In fact, an intensity change corresponds to a zero-crossing in the second spatial derivative. Thus we need to take the second differential of the image filtered through a Gaussian. This is equivalent to convolving the image with the second differential of a Gaussian. As shown in Figure 5, this is indeed a function which gives a center–surround type of visual field. A related function (indicated as $\nabla^2 G$) can conveniently be used for a 2-D spatial pattern. A similar function, the difference of two Gaussians, has been suggested by Wilson and Giese (1977). The details are given in the appendix.

The Fourier transform of Figure 5 is shown in the same figure. As can be seen, this is not exactly a band-pass filter of width one octave, but it

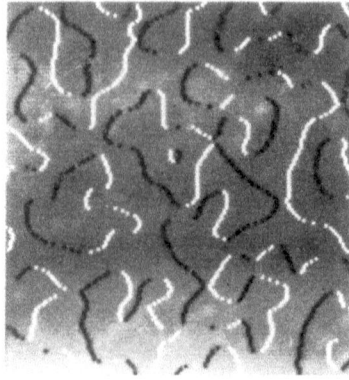

A

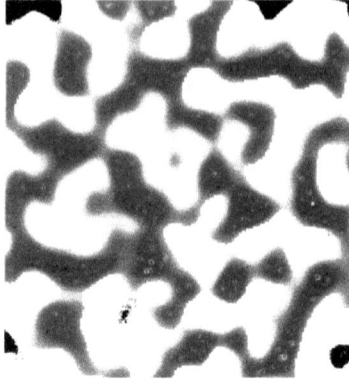

B

C

Figure 6 A pattern (A) is filtered (B) through a medium size $\nabla^2 G$ receptive field. Black areas represent negative values, white positive. Figure 6C shows the zero-crossings of (B).

F. H. C. Crick, D. C. Marr, and T. Poggio

approximates to it in that both low and high frequencies are much diminished. The "effective band width" might be considered to be about an octave and a half. Thus it is unlikely that the whole (filtered) distribution could be recaptured from the zero-crossings (see appendix) alone; nevertheless, the position of the signed zero-crossings probably contains a good fraction of the information in the continuous distribution. An example at one scale of the signed zero-crossings of a filtered 2-D image is given in Figure 6.

In summary our thesis is that the set of zero-crossings of the image filtered through independent $\nabla^2 G$ filters of three or four sizes (in order to cover the range of scales characteristic of natural images) represents the main "symbols" on which later visual processes, like stereopsis, are likely to operate.

Finally, observe that the physiological detection of zero-crossings need not depend on the detection of cells with zero-response. For instance, near an intensity edge the zero-crossings in the band-pass signal are flanked by two peaks of opposite sign. Detection of zero-crossings can thus be performed on the basis of peaks rather than zero-response. Marr and Hildreth (1979) and Marr and Ullman (1979) have proposed physiological schemes of how simple cells in area 17 may detect and represent oriented zero-crossing segments.

The Striate Cortex

The main input to the striate cortex is to layer IVC. To be more precise, in the monkey the major ganglion cell type of the retina, the X cells, which project to the parvocellular layers of the LGN, project from there mainly to IVCβ of the striate cortex. The Y cells, though larger in size, are much fewer in number. They connect to the magnocellular layers of the LGN and from there project mainly to layer IVCα. Y cells respond more transiently than X cells. X cells give a fairly sustained response and are more linear in their behavior. Here we shall mainly be considering X cells and cortical layer IVCβ. For this reason our theory will be a linear one, even though linearity may be only a first approximation to the truth.

What immediately strikes one in examining layer IVCβ is the very large number of very small cells in this layer. Thus, as Barlow (1979) has already suggested, it makes sense to consider that the visual image, or to be more precise a filtered version of it, is reconstructed there explicitly from the sampled input passed to it, via the LGN, from the ganglion cells of the retina. Barlow speaks loosely of "reconstructing" the visual image. Because of our computational theory of early visual information processing, we would prefer to express this as a more precise hypothesis: the cells of layer IVCβ represent the reconstruction on a very fine grid of the visual image passed through a $\nabla^2 G$ filter in such a way that its zero-crossings are especially well preserved.

The different sizes of the $\nabla^2 G$ operator, required by our previous scheme, may correspond to various receptive field sizes of the X cells (at any given eccentricity) in the LGN. If this is so, it seems likely that the interpolation in layer IVCβ mainly operates on the smallest of the X channels with a foveal central width of around 1.5' and a sampling density between 1' and 30" (Marr and Hildreth, 1979; Marr, and Hildreth, and Poggio, 1980).

Exactly how the reconstruction might be done in layer IVCβ is not clear at the present time. A major problem is how to represent the negative parts of a function. If all the cells of IVCβ had a steady background firing rate, then a positive value could be represented by an increase in firing rate and a negative value (relative to the mean) by a decrease—or vice versa. Alternatively, if the resting firing rate were very low, then one distribution of cells could map the positive part of the function (being silent for the negative parts) and another, somewhat separate, one would map the negative parts. That is, in this latter set of cells a high rate of firing would represent a large negative value of the function.

Even if it were known which of these two alternatives is correct, there would still remain the problem of how to interpolate from the relatively sparse input. How would the reconstruction function be implemented? It may not be necessary to do more than provide the central positive peak of this function (ideally $J_1(\rho)/\rho$; see appendix) and a surrounding, rather shallow, negative peak. The very small oscillation in amplitude beyond that could probably be ignored (see the appendix). It is known that the axonal trees of the geniculate input spread out somewhat. Could the synapses in the inner part of the axonal tree excite, whereas those of the outer portions inhibit? This would do the job very nicely, but we know of no precedent for such behavior.

A more plausible way to implement the reconstruction function would be by the sum of two Gaussians of opposite sign, a narrow positive one plus a lower, wider negative one, the total integral of one being equal and opposite to that of the other. Exactly how this would be done depends upon how the negative is represented, as discussed above.

More elaborate schemes are possible but are not without their difficulties. An alternative way, if there are indeed two "maps," one for the positive values of the function and the other for the negative ones, is to have a rather sharply localized inhibition of one map by the other. This would have the effect of sharpening up the smearing produced by axonal spread and imprecision of wiring. Though we have yet to do computer simulation of this, it seems probable that in most cases this would leave the position of the zero-crossing almost unaltered, though the nonzero parts of the function might be distorted somewhat. It is even possible that, in this case, it might only be necessary to implement the central positive part of the reconstruction function. Preliminary computer studies show that the location of the zero-crossings can be reconstructed with Vernier precision for 1-D functions via a much simpler receptive field than the ideal sinc x (Hildreth, personal communication).

Experimental Evidence

Some of the experimental evidence has already been outlined by Barlow (1979). It should be remembered that most of the psychophysical data is obtained from human beings, whereas the greater part of the detailed neurophysiological and neuroanatomical data is from the macaque monkey. As it is believed that the visual systems of man and the macaque, at least in their earlier stages, are not very different (by a factor of 2, starting from the angular separation between photoreceptors), no great harm is likely to be done by combining data from these two sources. We hope to give a detailed account of the numbers involved elsewhere. Here we merely sketch the broad features.

For the macaque the number of ganglion cells in one retina is about 1.5×10^6, and it is believed that the number of cells projecting to the striate cortex from the LGN is about the same (S. LeVay, personal communication, and Le Gros Clark, 1941). Since the area of the striate cortex in one hemisphere is about 1,400 mm^2 (Le Gros Clark, 1941, 1942; Cowey, 1964), there are, in all, about 300–500 incoming axons of each type (on and off) from the LGN per square millimeter of cortex.

The total number of cells per square millimeter of striate cortex has been estimated at 3.5×10^5 (calculated from Rockel et al., 1974). The exact fraction of these in layer IVCβ does not appear to have been reported. A reasonable estimate is 16%, giving 5.5×10^4/mm^2 (Powell, personal communication). Thus there are about 50 times more cells in Layer IVCβ than incoming LGN axons. Barlow (1979) arrived at a similar ratio (using Garey's data). These figures can only be regarded as very approximate, but they make the general point. There are many cells in IVCβ and this does indeed suggest that they might be used to make a fine-grained reconstruction of the sampled input provided by the incoming optic radiation.

If there are indeed about 5.5×10^4/mm^2, then, lumping them all together, we see that their mean spacing is about 4 μm when projected onto the surface of the cortex. To translate this into a visual angle we need the so-called magnification factor. This is of course different in different parts of the visual field. Near the fovea it is about 0.25°/mm for the macaque (Daniel and Whitteridge, 1961). Ignoring possible complications produced by ocular-dominance columns, this implies that a spacing of 4 μm corresponds to a visual spacing, near the fovea, of roughly 3" of arc. This is indeed fairly close to the observed hyperacuity limit for humans.

The above calculation can only be regarded as approximate, both because some of the numbers need to be determined more accurately and because the argument has been oversimplified. For example, we have ignored the fact that not all ganglion cells are X cells, that there might be two distinct maps (possibly more), and so forth. A similar calculation also needs to be done for the simple cells of the striate cortex, but even a rough estimate suggests that, for any one orientation, there are far fewer of them than the nonoriented cells of layer IVCβ.

If there is a rather precise reconstruction of the filtered visual input in layer IVCβ, then this should show up in single-electrode experiments. We are informed by Dr. David Hubel (personal communication) that preliminary results suggest that the mapping of the visual field in this layer is indeed rather precise. It would be useful to have an estimate of just how accurate it really is. The anatomical mapping between LGN and layer IVCβ has in fact to be quite precise. Preliminary calculations show that the ordering of the LGN inputs has to be preserved, that is, the jitter in the LGN inputs must be less than 30" (in the fovea) in order to ensure a reconstruction at vernier accuracy. Our hypothesis would furthermore require that the cells in layer IVCβ should have the same receptive field as the corresponding LGN cells, and again this seems to be supported by known physiological data. In addition, any detailed theory must take into account neuroanatomical factors such as the spread of the incoming axonal trees. For axons from the parvocellular cells of the LGN this is believed to be around 500 μm (S. LeVay, personal communication). However, it should be remembered that this is the total spread. The parameter used in the mathematics, which assumes that the axon terminals have an approximately Gaussian distribution, is σ, the "half-width" of the Gaussian (see the appendix). This may well be less than 100 μm, corresponding, in the foveal representation, to about 1'. Whether this degree of smearing at the input can be satisfactorily sharpened, and by what means, remains to be seen.

As more becomes known about the neuroanatomical details of the visual cortex (see the chapters by Lund and by Gilbert and Wiesel in this volume), it may be possible to suggest more precisely how an exact reconstruction could be implemented. More quantitative data would be especially welcomed, especially that which could be obtained fairly exactly. We know no theory yet which justifies our asking for cell counts, etc., to be as accurate as 10% or even 20%, but in some cases the relevant numbers are not known to a factor of 10 (for example, how many cells in the striate cortex project back to the LGN?). A rough estimate, to within a factor of 2, is always better than no estimate at all. A factor of about $\sqrt{2}$ might be the sort of precision to aim for at this stage.

Conclusion

Our hypothesis is that hyperacuity depends on a fairly accurate reconstruction of the filtered visual input, with well-preserved zero-crossings, in layer IVCβ of the striate cortex. As Barlow has already argued (1979), this seems plausible enough as a working hypothesis, but, as he has pointed out with especial force, it may seem to suffer from one major disadvantage: it is too static. Recent psychophysical results, especially those of Burr (Burr and Ross, 1979; Burr, 1979) have emphasized what was known before: it is not possible to understand hyperacuity without considering the response to moving objects. Whether this involves the Y cells of the retina, which project to the cortex mainly to layer IVCα; whether the effect of movement depends also on the W ganglion cells of the retina, projecting to the superior colliculus and from there to the striate cortex via the pulvinar; whether other cortical areas, such as V2 or Zeki's movement area on the posterior bank of the superior temporal sulcus (Zeki, 1974), are especially involved—all these questions remain for the future. It is pointed out in the appendix that, from the point of view of communication theory, psychophysical experiments of the Burr type may not present a problem for our proposal. They may be satisfactorily explained by a scheme in which the zero-crossings of the filtered image—but not necessarily the filtered image itself—are precisely reconstructed on the fine grid of layer IVC. This issue can be resolved only by additional psychophysical experiments. How such computations might be implemented in the brain is not immediately obvious.

Though some clues may come from neuroanatomy, we cannot help feeling that little progress will be made until the response to stationary and moving spots of light, of the type now being studied in man by Burr, is also measured in the alert monkey with electrodes in various regions of the brain; for instance, do cells in layer IVC reconstruct the pattern of activity at moments intermediate between the flashes and at locations intermediate between the stations at which the line segments are flashed?

Appendix

Mathematical Tools and Definitions

The convolution of two functions $f(x,y)$ and $g(x,y)$ is defined as the function $h(x,y)$, where

$$h(x,y) = f(x,y) * g(x,y)$$

$$= \iint_{-\infty}^{\infty} f(u,v)g(x-u,y-v)\,du\,dv. \tag{1}$$

Figure 7 illustrates graphically the meaning of this operation for 1-D functions. The importance of convolution stems from the fact that the output of a linear time-invariant system on an input function is given by the convolution of the input with the impulse response characteristic of the system. Thus, the operation of linear filtering (in space as well as in time) is equivalent to convolution.

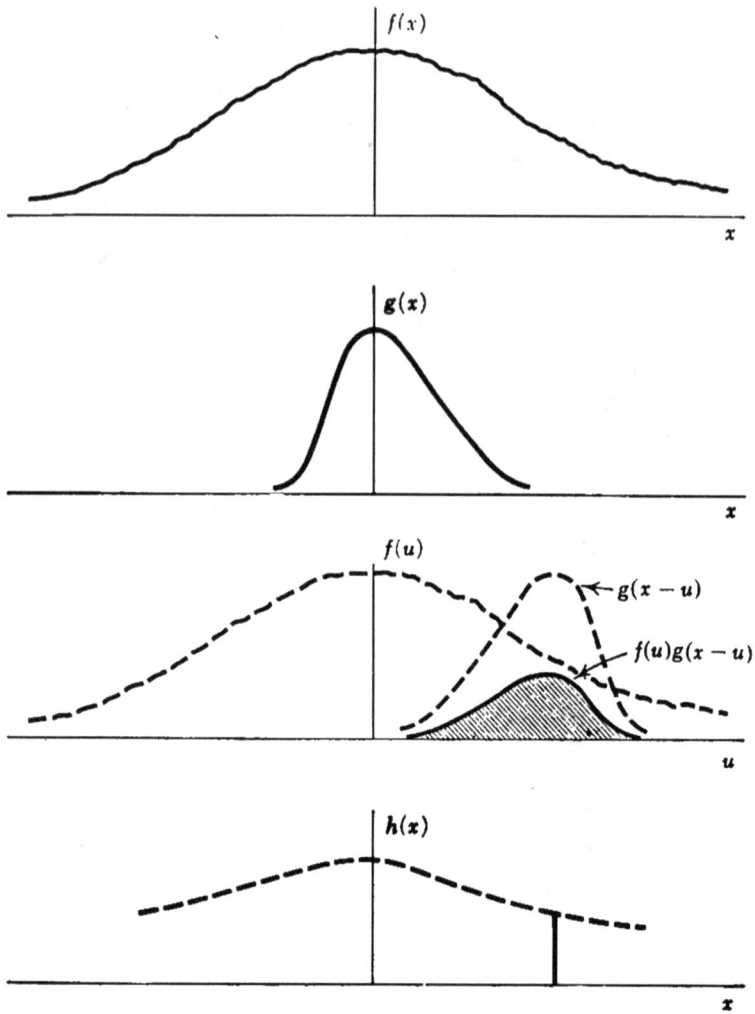

Figure 7 A pictorial illustration of the convolution operation. The function $f(x)$ is convolved with $g(x)$ according to $h(x) = \int_{-\infty}^{\infty} f(u)g(x-u)\,du$. The value $h(x)$, represented by the height of the segment in the bottom diagram, equals the shaded area above.

The Fourier transform $g(f_x, f_y)$ of the function $g(x,y)$ is defined here as

$$\tilde{g}(f_x, f_y) = \mathscr{F}\{g(x,y)\}$$

$$= \iint_{-\infty}^{\infty} g(x,y) \exp\left(-i\pi(f_x x + f_y y)\right) dx\, dy. \tag{2}$$

The transform is itself a complex-valued function of two independent variables f_x and f_y, which we generally refer to as frequencies.

The Sampling Theorem

The retinal image is sampled at a set of discrete points by the photo-receptors and it is represented by a still smaller number of nerve fibers

F. H. C. Crick, D. C. Marr, and T. Poggio

in the optic radiation. Intuitively, it is clear that if these samples are taken sufficiently close to each other, the sampled data provide an accurate representation of the original 2-D function, in the sense that the pattern can be reconstructed with considerable accuracy by simple interpolation. For band-limited functions the reconstruction can be accomplished exactly, provided only that the interval between samples is not greater than a certain limit. The retinal image is effectively band limited by diffraction at the pupil to about 60 cpd (cycles per degree) in man.

We derive here (following Goodman, 1968) a simple version of the sampling theorem for 2-D functions (possibly time dependent). We will also show how the conditions of the classical sampling theorem can be relaxed, if the pattern to be sampled is known to move at constant (known) speed. Sampling in time will not be considered; it is easy to extend the proofs to this case.

Let us consider a rectangular lattice of sampling points as shown in Figure 8. With the continuous function $g(x,y)$ we associate its sampled version

$$g_s(x,y) = g(x,y) \operatorname{comb}(x/X) \operatorname{comb}(y/Y) \frac{1}{XY}, \tag{3}$$

where $\operatorname{comb}(x) = \Sigma_n \delta(x - n)$. The sampling function $\operatorname{comb}(x/X) \operatorname{comb}(y/Y)$ consists of an array of δ functions, spaced at intervals of width X in the x direction and width Y in the y direction. The Fourier transform of $\operatorname{comb}(x/X)$ is

$$\mathcal{F}\{\operatorname{comb}(x/X)\} = \sum_n \delta(f - n/X)$$

$$= X \operatorname{comb}(Xf), \tag{4}$$

as shown in Figure 9.

The Fourier transform of g_s is

$$\tilde{g}_s(f_x, f_y) = \operatorname{comb}(f_x X) \operatorname{comb}(f_y Y) * \tilde{g}(f_x, f_y). \tag{5}$$

Thus, the spectrum of g_s can be found simply by replicating the spectrum of g about each point in the (f_x, f_y) plane corresponding to the lattice defined by $\operatorname{comb}(f_x X) \operatorname{comb}(f_y Y)$, as shown in Figure 10.

The function g is assumed to be band limited, and thus its spectrum $\tilde{g}$ is nonzero over only a finite region of the frequency space, called its support. If the sampling points are sufficiently close together (i.e., X and Y are sufficiently small), then the separations $1/X$ and $1/Y$ of the various "lobes" in Figure 10 will be great enough to ensure that adjacent regions do not overlap. We can reconstruct $g(x,y)$ from g_s if we can recover $\tilde{g}$ from $\tilde{g}_s$, and this can be accomplished exactly by passing $\tilde{g}_s$ through a linear filter that excludes all side lobes in $\tilde{g}_s$ but includes the central one. In the limiting case, adjacent regions in the spectrum $\tilde{g}_s$ just touch. This happens (see Figure 10) when $X = 1/2B_x$, $Y = 1/2B_y$, where

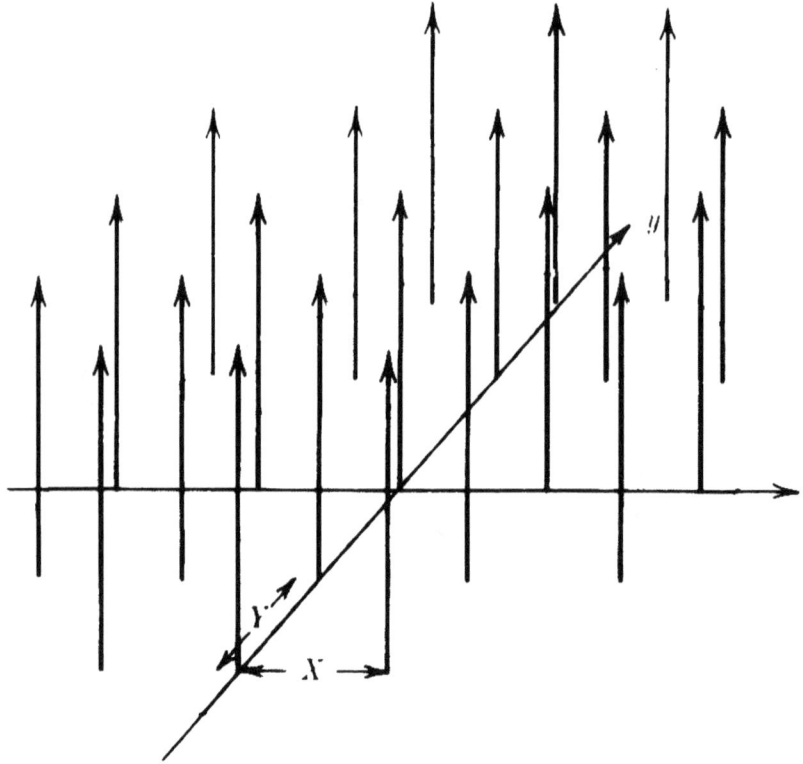

Figure 8 The "sampling function" comb(x/X) comb(y/Y). By multiplying a continuous function $g(x,y)$ with this array of delta functions, one obtains the sampled function g_s, which essentially consists of the values of the original function at the positions of the arrows.

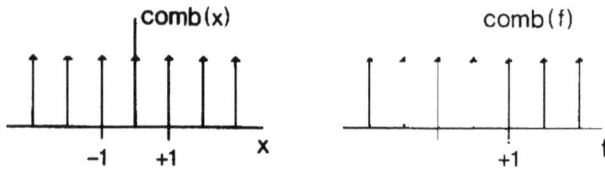

Figure 9 The function comb $x = \Sigma_n\, \delta(x - n)$ and its Fourier transform comb$(f) = \Sigma_n\, \delta(f - n)$. The comb function is thus its own Fourier transform. The small ticks show where the variable has a value of unity.

A

B

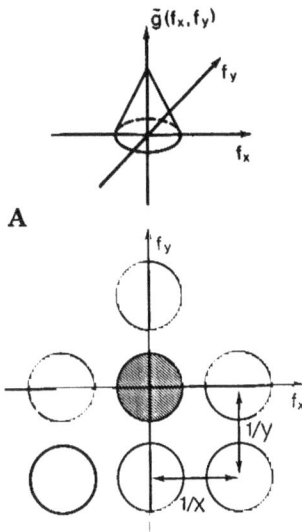

Figure 10 (A) The Fourier transform $\tilde{g}$ of a band-limited pattern $g(x,y)$, chosen as an example to be a cone. (B) The support of the Fourier transform $\tilde{g}_s$ of the sampled function
$g_s(x,y) = g(x,y)[\text{comb}(x/X)\,\text{comb}(y/Y)]$,
where the expression within brackets is the sampling function shown in Figure 8. The spectrum $\tilde{g}$ is repeated at distances $1/X$ and $1/Y$. If the sampling distances X and Y are small enough compared with the bandwidth of g, there is no overlap of the side lobes in the spectrum of g_s. Only some of the side lobes are shown here: they repeat over the whole Fourier plane.

$2B_x$ and $2B_y$ represent the width in the f_x and f_y directions, respectively, of the smallest rectangle that completely encloses the support of $\tilde{g}$ (support centered on the origin). It is as if we have tiled the Fourier plane with an infinite number of rectangular tiles, on each of which we have a replica of $\tilde{g}(f_x,f_y)$. In this case the form of the filter must be

$$H(f_x,f_y) = \pi(f_x/2B_x)\pi(f_y/2B_y), \tag{6}$$

where

$$\pi(x) = \begin{cases} 1, & x \leq 1/2 \\ 0, & \text{otherwise.} \end{cases}$$

Filtering $\tilde{g}_s$ through H one gets

$$g(x,y) = \sum_{n m} g_s\,(nX,mY) \tag{7}$$

which corresponds, as it can be seen by Fourier inversion, to the following (classical) interpolation scheme:

$$g(x,y) = \sum_{n m} g_s\,(nX,mY)$$
$$\times \text{sinc}[2B_x(x - nX)]\,\text{sinc}[2B_y(y - mY)], \tag{8}$$

where $\text{sinc}(x) = \sin(\pi x)/\pi x$.

A

B

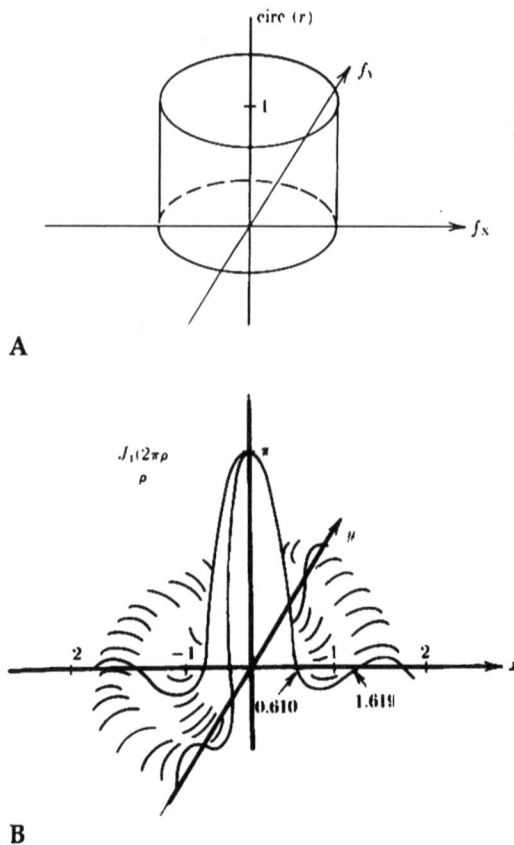

Figure 11 (A) The ideal low-pass filter circ(r) in the Fourier plane and (B) its inverse Fourier transform, i.e., the corresponding receptive field.

There are, of course, especially in 2-D, a variety of filters that could perform a correct interpolation. For instance, another choice for H may be, when g is band limited over a circular region of the Fourier plane,

$$H(f_x, f_y) = \text{circ}(B_x), \tag{9}$$

where

$$\text{circ}(r) = \begin{cases} 1, & r \leq 1 \\ 0, & \text{otherwise,} \end{cases} \tag{10}$$

as shown in Figure 11, with an inverse Fourier transform

$$\mathscr{F}^{-1}\{\text{circ}(r)\} = \frac{J_1(2\pi\rho)}{\rho}; \tag{11}$$

J_1 is the Bessel function of the first kind, order one. Figure 11 illustrates the circle function and its transform. Filtering $\bar{g}_s$ through circ(B_x) corresponds to convolving g_s with a "receptive field" of the type shown in Figure 11B. It can be easily shown that for such signals, the optimal sampling scheme involves hexagonal sampling instead of rectangular

F. H. C. Crick, D. C. Marr, and T. Poggio

sampling. In the case of hexagonal sampling the Fourier plane is tiled with an infinite number of hexagonal tiles.

We have derived in this way sufficient conditions for exact reconstruction of a 2-D function:

Theorem 1 (Whittaker, Shannon). A band-limited function $g(x,y)$, that is, $\tilde{g}(f_x,f_y) = 0$ for $|f_x| > B_x|f_y| > B_y$, can be recovered exactly from a rectangular array of its sampled values through suitable filtering. The sampling distance in the x (y) direction can be as large as $1/2B_x$ ($1/2B_y$). In this case the reconstruction can be performed according to (8). Hexagonal sampling is more efficient if the support of $\tilde{g}$ is circular. Since the retinal image is radially band limited to about 60 cpd, Theorem 1 for an hexagonal lattice implies that the maximum distance between photoreceptors should be $\Delta\phi = (1/60)°\sqrt{3} = 27$ sec, which is about right for the human fovea. The finite diameter of the photoreceptors worsens only slightly the overall transfer function of the system. The proof clearly shows that the classical interpolation function sinc does not have an exclusive role. Many other interpolation functions would do as well or almost as well, especially if the sampling density is higher than the minimum. In such a case, the side lobes in the spectrum $\tilde{g}_s$ do not touch; thus the requirement of the sharp cutoff in the filter H is removed. A variety of filter functions would exclude the side lobes while transmitting the central lobe without significant distortions.

With a suitably higher sampling density, it is clear that simple receptive fields (see, for instance, Figure 5) could interpolate almost as well as $J_1(2\pi\rho)/\rho$, especially with respect to the location of the zero-crossings (Figure 6). Recent computer experiments show indeed that very simple interpolation schemes (linear interpolation, filtering through a Gaussian, filtering through $\nabla^2 G$) can localize zero-crossings in the output of a channel having $w = 1'30''$ with vernier precision (E. Hildreth, personal communication).

As one would expect, the classical sampling scheme is stable in the sense that a small change in the amplitude of sample values leads to small changes in the reconstructed function. It can be proved that stable sampling cannot be performed at a lower rate than the Nyquist rate.

The sampling theorem can be extended (and relaxed) in various directions. For instance, if the sampling points are not equally spaced (in a known way), it is still possible to recover the original signal, under relatively weak conditions. Sampling with derivatives increases the sample spacing required, or in other words, it allows the reconstruction of the band-limited signal with a sampling rate less than the Nyquist rate.

Stronger results than Theorem 1 also hold if the band-limited function is also band-pass. For instance, a 1-D band-pass function with one octave bandwidth can be sampled at half the rate set by the classical sampling theorem. This can be easily seen in Figure 12A. In 2-D, sam-

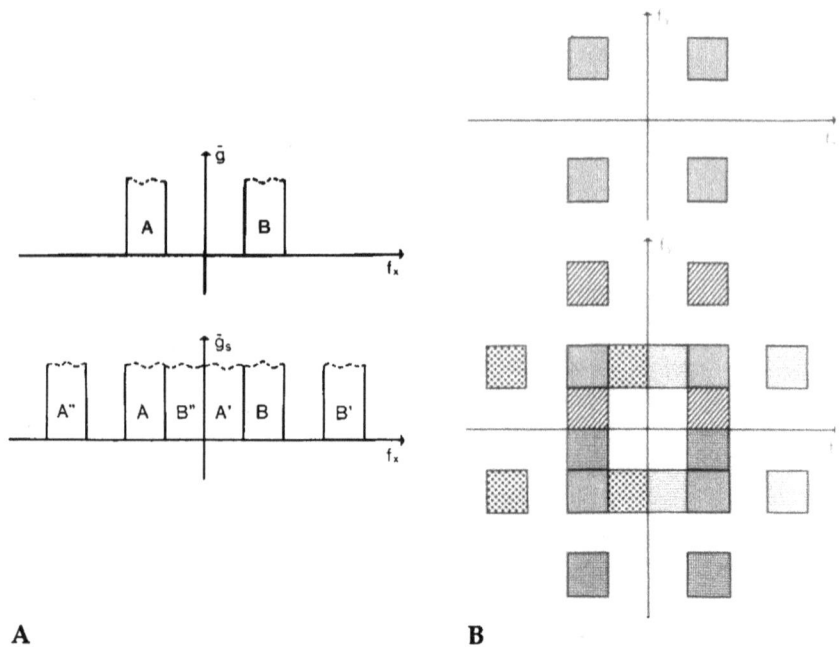

Figure 12 (A) $\tilde{g}$ is the (modulus of the) Fourier transform of a one-octave band-pass signal. If the signal is sampled at half the Shannon rate, interleaving of side lobes but no overlapping occurs in the spectrum $\tilde{g}_s$. $\tilde{g}_s$ is obtained by shifting g by all integral multiples of B_x, B_x being the bandwidth of g. Only two of the side lobes are shown in the bottom of (A). Same hatching identifies parts of the same side lobes. (B) The same situation for a 2-D pattern, assumed to be band-pass (one-octave) on f_x and f_y. Again sampling at half the classical rate corresponds to interleaving but no overlapping of the side lobes. Only some of the side lobes are shown in the lower half of (B). They are created by shifting the original spectrum (shown in the upper half) by all multiples of $1/X$ and $1/Y$, X and Y being the sampling distances. Side lobes thus fill the whole Fourier plane. Notice that if the support of $\tilde{g}$ were a ring in the Fourier plane, overlap of the side lobes in $\tilde{g}_s$ would occur for any sampling rates lower than Shannon's rate.

pling below the classic limit corresponds to interlacing of the lobes in the Fourier spectrum of the sampled function. Depending on the geometry of the band-pass support, interlacing can take place without overlapping of the side lobes. Suitable filtering can again recover exactly the original function (Figure 12B). Whereas in the band-limited case it is possible to sample at any sufficiently high rate, exploitation of the band-pass property requires in this scheme sampling at exactly the correct intervals, in order to obtain the correct interlacing effect. Notice that this scheme cannot be applied to a 2-D band-pass function with a circularly symmetric, ring-like support in the Fourier plane. However, the (sufficient) conditions given by this overlap argument are not strictly necessary in the band-pass case. It turns out that despite eventual overlap it is still possible to reconstruct exactly the band-pass function with two interlaced sampling sequences, each one having a

F. H. C. Crick, D. C. Marr, and T. Poggio

sampling interval of $1/B$, where B is the width of the band (for $f > 0$). The average sampling interval is thus $1/2B$.

The following theorem extends Theorem 1:

Theorem 2. For a band-pass function in 1-D [$\tilde{g}(f) = 0$ for $|f| > f_0$, $|f| < (1 - \alpha)f_0$] exact reconstruction can be obtained with a sampling distance as large as $1/(2\alpha f_0)$. This also holds for 2-D functions band-pass in x and y separately.

The Sampling Theorem for Moving Patterns

For simplicity we consider a 1-D pattern $f(x)$, band limited in spatial frequency, sampled at a regular 1-D array of points. Movement of the pattern $f(x)$ produces a function $f(x,t)$ whose sampling in space obeys the usual restrictions set by the sampling theorem. If we assume, however, that $f(x)$ moves at a constant (known) velocity v, it is rather clear that the sampling rate may become very low, without losing information (in fact, one "photoreceptor" clearly suffices). We analyze this problem with the same methods as in the previous part. The proof (again providing only sufficient conditions) is quite instructive, especially for situations in which the velocity is not exactly known.

Since $g(x)$ moves at constant speed v, the pattern of excitation on the "retina" is $g(x,t) = g(x + vt)$. The Fourier transform is

$$\tilde{g}(f_t,f_t) = \tilde{g}(f_x)\delta(f_t - vf_x), \tag{12}$$

where $\tilde{g}(f_x)$ is the Fourier transform of $g(x)$. Since $g(x)$ is band limited, $g(x,t)$ is band limited in both space and time if v is finite. The array of "photoreceptors" spaced by X provides a sampled version $g_s(x + vt)$ whose spectral support is shown in Figure 13. The slope of the line is v. The classical sampling theorem requires a sampling distance $X = 1/2B$. In this case a filter function like $\pi(f/2B)$ can separate the central region from the side lobes and thus retrieve $g(x + vt)$. Figure 14 shows clearly, however, that the sampling distance X can be increased much above the classical limit irrespective of the velocity v, provided that v is different from zero: in the Fourier plane the distance between the side lobes can be made arbitrarily small (corresponding to X arbitrarily large in x space) without overlapping.

The original spectrum can be retrieved by the filter depicted in the Figure 14A. The retrieval scheme in the limit of very large X would require convolution of $g_s(x,t)$ with the (noncausal) receptive field $\delta(x + vt)$.

Uncertainty in the velocity forces a finite sampling distance. The minimum allowed sampling rate depends on the geometry of the support of the Fourier transform. It can be derived easily from graphs like Figure 14.

For instance, assume that only the direction of motion is known, that

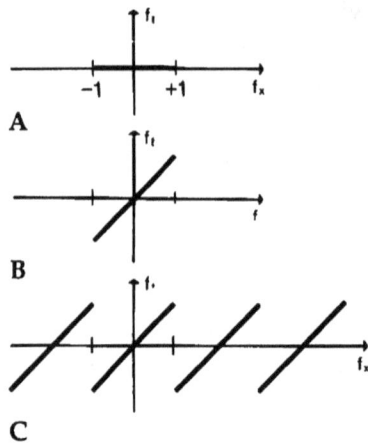

Figure 13 (A) The support (a "delta" segment) of the spectrum $\tilde{g}$ of a band-limited 1-D pattern $g(x)$ at rest ($v = 0$) in the Fourier plane of spatial (f_x) and temporal (f_t) frequencies. $\tilde{g}(f_x,f_t)$ equals $g(f_x)$ on that segment. (B) The spectral support of the same pattern moving at constant speed v. The Fourier transform of $g(x + vt)$ takes nonzero values only on the "delta" segment, whose slope is v. (C) Spectral support of $g_s(x,t)$. The pattern $g(x + vt)$ is sampled in space at the Shannon rate.

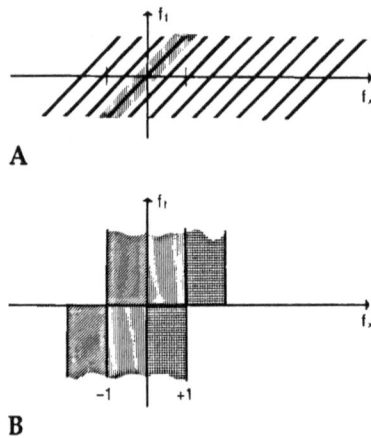

Figure 14 (A) The support of $g_s(x + vt)$, when sampling rate is lower than Shannon's rate. The original function $\tilde{g}$ (Figure 13B) can be retrieved by filtering the sampled data, for instance, with the filter indicated by hatching. The filter is arbitrary, provided it transmits without distortion the central lobe, eliminating at the same time all side lobes. (B) If it is only known that the sign of the velocity is positive, the support of $\tilde{g}$ may lie anywhere in the region shown by vertical hatching. Sampling spatially at half the Shannon rate still ensures that the side lobes do not overlap in the spectrum $\tilde{g}_s$. Compare Figure 13C.

is, the sign of v. Figure 14B shows that if only the sign of v is known, the minimum distance on the (f_x, f_t) plane to ensure no overlapping is half the classical distance. Thus, the maximum distance between the samples can be twice the limit set by the classical sampling theorem. Again from the figure it is easy to derive the required filter and the corresponding "spatiotemporal receptive field." We have proved the following:

Theorem 3. Assume that a band-limited spatial pattern $g(x)$ with a bandwidth $2B$ moves at constant velocity v. Then, if the velocity v is known with arbitrarily high precision, the distance between sampling points can be made arbitrarily large. Uncertainty in v requires, in this scheme, a well-defined maximum sampling distance, higher, however, than the classical limit ($v = 0$). As a corollary, if only the sign of the velocity is known, the maximum sampling distance X is twice the classical limit for stationary patterns (thus $X = 1/B_x$).

The Sampling Theorem and Burr's Experiment

This result can help in discussing the demonstration published very recently by Burr (1979). In his experiment, vernier line segments are displayed stroboscopically at a sequence of stations. Spatial offsets were detected with an accuracy in the 5-sec range in spite of the movement (compare Westheimer and McKee, 1975); in addition an illusory displacement occurs if the line segments are accurately aligned in space, but are displayed with a slight delay in one sequence relative to the other. The accuracy of detecting the equivalent displacement is again in the hyperacuity range. As Barlow (1979) pointed out, this suggests that the spatial pattern of activity at moments intermediate between the stroboscopic flashes is actually reconstructed. Clearly, temporal interpolation (i.e., temporal filtering) followed by the "static" spatial interpolation can reconstruct a pattern of activity $g(x,t)$ on an arbitrarily fine spatial grid from the sampled functions provided by the LGN fibers. This amounts to saying, as pointed out by S. Ullman, that almost nothing needs to be done in order to obtain the right kind of temporal filling-in. Temporal low-pass properties of the LGN pathway provide temporal blurring: spatial interpolation, for instance in layer IVCβ, would then reconstruct activity between the LGN fibers at all times. Notice that the blurring due to temporal integration can be corrected by spatial high-pass operations (for a pattern moving at constant speed, temporal and spatial variables are interchangeable). Thus, there is no problem in reconstructing the correct pattern of activity in IVCβ for a real movement of the retinal image. Difficulties may appear, however, when motion of the object is simulated by presenting the image at discrete positions at separate instants, as in the experiments by Westheimer and by Burr. If the positions at which the vernier segments are flashed correspond to the sampling grid of the LGN cells, the simulated motion is in fact completely equivalent (from the LGN point of view) to real motion. If, however, neighboring positions are much farther apart than neighboring LGN sampling points and larger than LGN receptive fields, there may be too few samples (in terms of the classical sampling theorem) to reconstruct the equivalent spatiotemporal pattern of activity between positions. It is important to stress, on the other hand, that our hypothesis requires a precise reconstruction in space and time of the zero-crossings of the filtered image, but not necessarily of the filtered image itself. Thus the necessary conditions are probably weaker. From this point of view the bounds on the sampling intervals given by the theorems of this appendix are too strong, since they refer to a correct reconstruction of a whole function and not only of its zero-crossings.

Although more psychophysical experiments are essential to determine how the vernier acuity measured by Burr actually degrades with increased separations between the positions at which the segments are flashed, it is conceivable that separations larger than the maximum allowed by the sampling theorem may not dramatically reduce performance. Clearly, these estimates depend on which channel is actually reconstructed in layer IVC: if larger receptive fields are involved, the maximum separation allowed would be correspondingly larger. For instance, for the smallest channel (w = 1' 30") the maximum distance should be not much larger than about 1'. This estimate could become up to about 16 times larger for the biggest (and transient) channel (in IVCα?). It is also conceivable that the effective receptive field size of the channel reconstructed in layer IVC may be transiently larger at the onset of a stimulus, either because of Y influences or via a mechanism similar to the one postulated by Detwiler, Hodgkin, and McNaughton (1978) for the rod network in the retina. This would provide a lower cutoff in spatial frequencies for moving stimuli, allowing a larger sampling interval (see Theorem 1). The corresponding spatiotemporal "receptive field" would have a support on the (f_x, f_t) plane with negative slope on the upper right quadrant (from low f_t and high f_x to low f_x and high f_t).

In any case, Theorem 3 shows that for an object moving at constant speed, the maximum (spatial) sampling interval could be increased. Thus, rough, and even implicit, use of velocity information may account, at least from the point of view of information theory, for eventual quite large separations in Burr's type of experiments. For instance, it is conceivable that the interpolation scheme may be based on the a priori assumption of a movement of the retinal image within a well-defined range of velocities. This idea can be easily extended, within the framework of the hypothesis of independent $\nabla^2 G$ channels tuned to different spatial sizes. Probably the simplest (but not the only!) system which can perform spatiotemporal interpolation and avoid motion smear is the following: There exist several independent channels, each

F. H. C. Crick, D. C. Marr, and T. Poggio

tuned to a different range of velocities and resembling the filter indicated by hatching in Figure 14A); these channels might correspond to different direction-selective neurons; for the channels to be "independent" there should be a "hole" around $f_x = f_t = 0$; therefore, high velocity channels have a low f_x and a high f_t cutoff and are band-pass in f_t and low-pass in f_x; low velocity channels have a low f_t and a high f_x cutoff and are band-pass in f_x and low-pass in f_t. Similar sets of channels should also exist for $v < 0$ and for "each" direction of motion. Full spatial acuity could be expected from the channels tuned at velocities below $v = f_t^c/f_x^c$, where f_t^c and f_x^c are the upper temporal and spatial frequency limits of the visual system. Approximations of this ideal situation may have similar properties. Notice that the high-velocity, low-spatial-frequency channel would be bandpass in the time domain, yielding a temporal impulse response with a positive peak followed by a negative phase. In conclusion, independent spatiotemporal channels tuned to different velocities can avoid motion smear if a pattern moves at constant speed. (If it changes velocity then the broadened spectrum may "spill over" into other channels.) At the same time, spatiotemporal interpolation could be achieved simply by spatial interpolation of the output of each independent channel. Since the spatial density of the different channels should be inversely proportional to their upper-frequency cutoff (see theorem 1), the "fast" channels (steep slope in Figure 14) are expected to be much sparser than the "slow" channels. The sparse fast channels may thus achieve a correct spatiotemporal interpolation even for quite large separations between the stations, although the corresponding vernier-type accuracy would probably be lower.

The sampling theorems outlined here do not, of course, say which neural mechanisms may be involved. But even if an explicit reconstruction on a finer grid of neurons is not done in our brain, these results characterize the conditions under which information of the vernier type can be preserved in the visual pathway.

Logan's Theorem. If a 1-D band-limited function (belonging to B_∞, i.e., the restriction to the real line of entire functions of exponential type; see Logan, 1977)

(a) has no free zeros (i.e., complex roots in common with its Hilbert transform) and no multiple real zeros, and

(b) is band-pass with enough real zeros in proportion to its bandwidth, then the function is uniquely determined, up to an overall multiplicative constant, by its (real) zero crossings.

Condition (a) is almost always satisfied. Condition (b) is critical: it is always ensured if the bandwidth of the signal is less than one octave. For particular classes of bandpass signals (b) may be satisfied even for larger bandwidths: for instance, ergodic Gaussian band-pass signals satisfy condition (b) if their bandwidth is less than 1.67 octaves (H. K.

Nishihara, personal communication). On the other hand, Logan's result is valid for ideal band-pass functions, and it cannot be extrapolated with abandon to "almost band-pass" functions.

An Extension of Logan's Theorem to 2-D Functions

It is impossible to use directly Logan's technique for proving some 2-D version of its theorem. There is, however, a simple way of translating the 2-D problem into a 1-D problem in order to use Logan's result. In this way it can be shown that zero-crossings in a suitably band-pass 2-D function (in principle) determine the function to within a multiplicative constant. The conditions under which this result is valid are likely to be too restrictive: they are sufficient but almost certainly not necessary. The argument runs as follows. The image $f(x,y)$ is filtered through one-octave bandwidth vertical masks: zero crossings are then measured along horizontal scan lines at intervals appropriate to recover all the information. Since the 1-D functions associated with each scan line are then band-pass with less than one-octave bandwidth, they satisfy Logan's theorem. The same operation can be carried out with horizontal masks and vertical scans. It can be shown that it is thus possible to reconstruct the filtered image (through horizontal and vertical marks) modulus a single scaling factor (Marr, Poggio, and Ullman, 1979; Nishihara, personal communication; Poggio, 1980). This reconstruction scheme cannot be applied to images filtered through nonoriented band-pass filters, like the circularly symmetric receptive fields of the ganglion cells.

$\nabla^2 G$

This way of locating zero-crossings in a filtered image is not the only, nor necessarily the best, method. It has been shown (Marr and Hildreth, 1979) that under certain rather weak conditions the zeros in an image filtered through a concentric-type receptive field provide an equivalent way of locating edges, whose orientation must then be represented. This suggests that zero-crossings in an image filtered through concentric receptive fields may also contain the whole information of the image. As we mentioned, however, the extension of Logan's theorem to this case is not yet available.

In a similarly negative vein, we do not have yet any formal result on the information content of the zero-crossings in a nonideal band-pass signal, although recent computer experiments (K. Nishihara, personal communication) indicate that they still contain almost full information, under rather loose conditions.

In summary, Logan's theorem cannot strictly be used in a theory of early visual processing; the important point is that it shows that zero-crossings of a band-pass signal are very rich in information. In this sense, it supports a set of computational arguments (Marr, 1976; Marr and Poggio, 1977, 1979; Marr and Hildreth, 1979) suggesting that the detection of zero-crossings in the output of independent (spatial) roughly band-pass channels is one of the first steps in the processing of visual information. Marr and Hildreth (1979) argue that intensity changes in the image at one scale may be detected by filtering (i.e., convolving) the image with the Laplacian of a 2-D Gaussian at that particular scale and then locating zero-crossings. Since the Gaussian is given (in 1-D) as

$$G(x) = \frac{1}{\sqrt{2\pi}\sigma} \exp\left(\frac{-x^2}{2\sigma^2}\right)$$

its 1-D Laplacian,

$$G''(x) = \frac{-1}{\sigma^3} \sqrt{2\pi} \left(1 - \frac{x^2}{2\sigma^3}\right) \exp\left(\frac{-x^2}{2\sigma^3}\right),$$

looks like a Mexican-hat operator (*see* Figure 5); it is approximately a band-pass operator with a half-power bandwidth of about 1.25 octaves and is very closely approximated by Wilson and Giese's (1977) difference of two Gaussians (with a ratio for their σ of about 1.6). By using a range of $\nabla^2 G$ mask sizes, one can deal with the wide range of scales over which intensity changes take place in a natural image.

These ideas may begin to account, on purely information-processing grounds, for the presence of spatial-frequency-tuned channels in early human vision (Campbell and Robson, 1968; Wilson and Giese, 1977) and for the properties of simple cells in the cortex, which are usually described as detectors of edges and bars of various widths and orientations (Hubel and Wiesel, 1962).

Acknowledgments

We are grateful to H. B. Barlow and S. Ullman for discussions, to I. Geiss for typing the manuscript, and to L. Heimburger for drawing the figures. F. H. C. Crick was supported by the Eugene and Estelle Ferkhanf Foundation, J. W. Kieckhefer Foundation, and Samuel Roberts Noble Foundation, Inc. D. Marr and T. Poggio thank the Salk Institute for their kind hospitality.

References

Barlow, H. B., 1979. Reconstructing the visual image in space and time. *Nature* 279:189–190.

Beck, J., and T. Schwartz, 1979. Vernier acuity with dot test objects. *Vision Res.* 19:313–319.

Burr, D. C., 1979. Research Note. Acuity for apparent Vernier offset. *Vision Res.* 9:835–837.

Burr, D. C., and J. Ross, 1979. How does binocular delay give information about depth? *Vision Res.* 19:523–532.

Campbell, F. W., and J. Robson, 1968. Application of Fourier analysis to the visibility of gratings. *J. Physiol. (London)* 197:551–566.

Cowey, A., 1964. Projection of the retina on to striate and prestriate cortex in the squirrel monkey, *Saimiri Sciureus*. *J. Neurophysiol.* 27:366–393.

Daniel, P. M., and D. Whitteridge, 1961. The representation of the visual field on the cerebral cortex in monkeys. *J. Physiol. (London)* 159:203–221.

Detwiler, P. B., A. L. Hodgkin, and P. A. McNaughton, 1978. A surprising property of electrical spread in the network of rods in the turtle's retina. *Nature* 274:562–565.

Goodman, J. W., 1962. *Introduction to Fourier Optics*. New York: McGraw-Hill.

Grimson, E., and D. Marr, 1979. A computer implementation of a theory of human stereo vision. *Proc. Image Understanding Workshop*.

Hubel, D., and T. Wiesel, 1962. Receptive fields, binocular interaction and functional architecture of monkey striate cortex. *J. Physiol. (London)* 195:215–243.

Julesz, B., 1971. *Foundations of Cyclopean Perception*. Chicago: University of Chicago Press.

Le Gros Clark, W. E., 1941. The laminar organization and cell content of the lateral geniculate body in the monkey. *J. Anat.* 75:419–433.

Le Gros Clark, W. E., 1942. The cells of Maynert in the visual cortex of the monkey. *J. Anat.* 76:369–377.

Logan, B. F., Jr., 1977. Information in the zero crossings of bandpass signals. *Bell System Tech. J.* 56:487–510.

Marr, D., 1976. Early processing of visual information. *Phil. Trans. Roy. Soc. B* 275:483–524.

Marr, D., 1977. Representing visual information. *AAAS 143rd Annual Meeting*.

Marr, D., and E. Hildreth, 1980. Theory of edge detection. *Proc. Roy Soc. B* 207:187–217. [Also available as MIT AI: Memo 518.]

Marr, D., and H. K. Nishihara, 1978a. Visual information processing: Artificial intelligence and the sensorium of sight. *Tech. Rev.* 81:1–23.

Marr, D., and H. K. Nishihara, 1978b. Representation and recognition of the spatial organization of three-dimensional shapes. *Proc. Roy. Soc. B* 200:269–294.

Marr, D., and T. Poggio, 1976. Cooperative computation of stereo disparity. *Science* 194:283–287.

Marr, D., and T. Poggio, 1977. From understanding computation to understanding neural circuitry. *Neurosci. Res. Prog. Bull.* 15:470–488.

Marr, D., and T. Poggio, 1979. A computational theory of human stereo vision. *Proc. Roy. Soc. B* 204:301–328.

Marr, D., and S. Ullman, 1979. Directional selectivity and its use in early visual processing MIT AI: Memo 524.

Marr, D., T. Poggio, and E. Hildreth, 1980. The smallest channel in early human vision. *J. Opt. Soc. Amer.* (in press).

Marr, D., T. Poggio, and S. Ullman, 1979. Bandpass channels, zero-crossings, and early visual information processing. *J. Opt. Soc. Amer.* 69:914–916.

Poggio, T., 1980. Trigger features for Fourier analysis in early vision: A new point of view. In *The Role of Feature Detectors*. Gough and Peters, eds. (in press).

Rockel, A. J., R. W. Hiorns, and T. P. S. Powell, 1974. Numbers of neurons through full depth of neocortex. *J. Anat.* 118:371.

Sutherland, N. S., 1979. The representation of three-dimensional objects. *Nature* 278:395–398.

Ullman, S., 1979. The interpretation of structure from motion. *Proc. Roy. Soc. B* 203:405–426.

Westheimer, G., 1976. Diffraction theory and visual hyperacuity. *Amer. J. Opt. Physiol. Optics* 53:362–364.

Westheimer, G., 1977. Spatial frequency and light-spread descriptions of visual acuity and hyperacuity. *J. Opt. Soc. Amer.* 67:207–212.

Westheimer, G., and S. P. McKee, 1975. Visual acuity in the presence of retinal-image motion. *J. Opt. Soc. Amer.* 65:847–850.

Westheimer, G., and S. P. McKee, 1977a. Integration regions for visual hyperacuity. *Vision Res.* 17:89–93.

Westheimer, G., and S. P. McKee, 1977b. Spatial configurations for visual hyperacuity. *Vision Res.* 17:941–947.

Westheimer, G., and S. P. McKee, 1977c. Perception of temporal order in adjacent visual stimuli. *Vision Res.* 17:887–893.

Westheimer, G., and S. P. McKee, 1978. Stereoscopic acuity for moving retinal images. *J. Opt. Soc. Amer.* 68:450–455.

Wilson. H., and S. C. Giese, 1977. Threshold visibility of frequency gradient patterns. *Vision Res.* 17:1177–1190.

Zeki, S. M., 1974. Cells responding to changing image size and disparity in the cortex of the rhesus monkey. *J. Physiol.* 242:827–841.

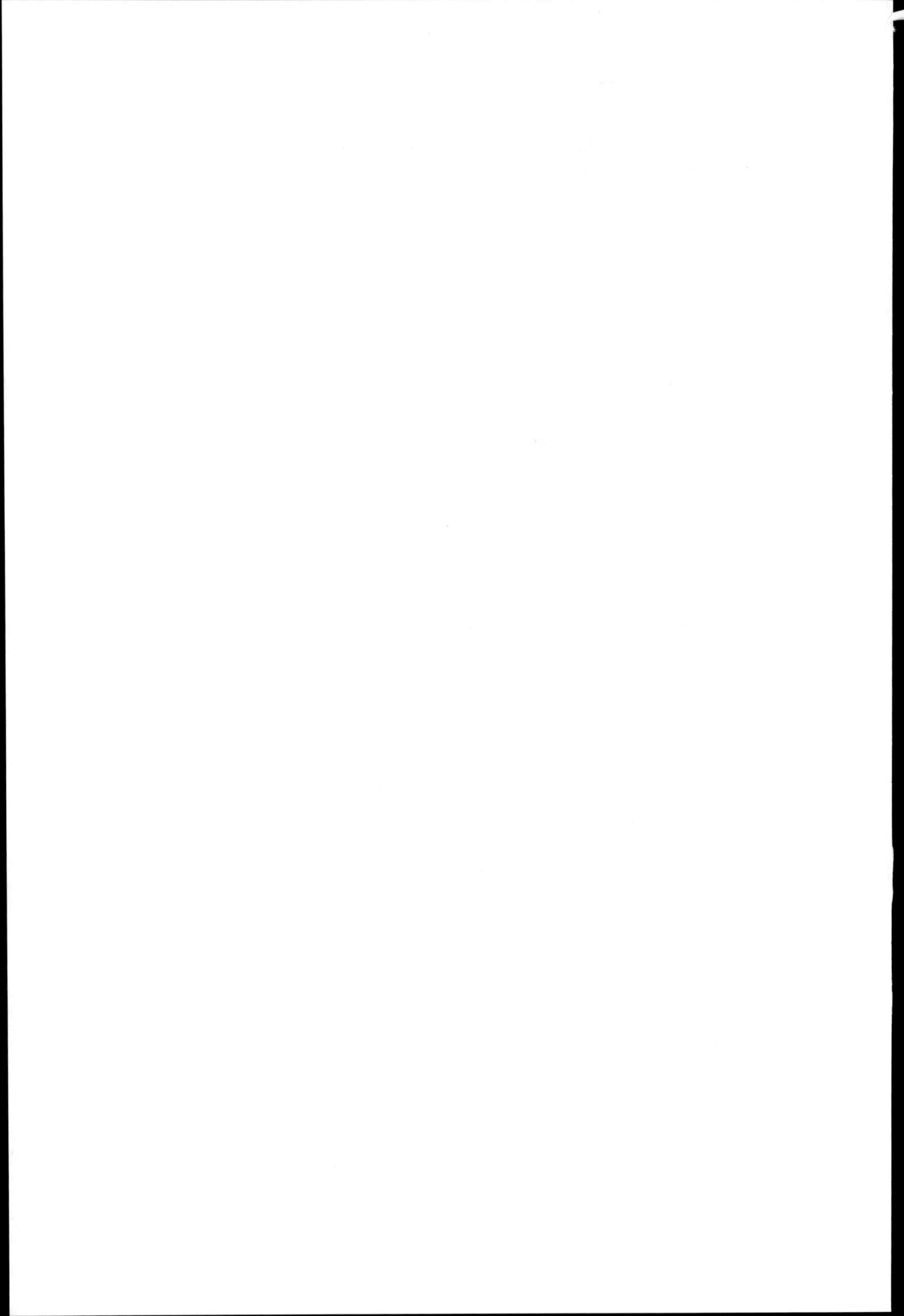

22 Group Selection as the Basis for Higher Brain Function

Gerald M. Edelman

ABSTRACT The purpose of this chapter is to consider and extend several aspects of the group-selection theory (Edelman, 1978) of higher brain function. This theory is Darwinian in outlook: its basic premise is that preexisting structural variations in multiply connected and distributed cellular groups of the brain provide a basis for selection of those groups whose function proves to be sufficient for adaptive behavior. It is meant to apply to backboned animals, mainly mammals, and specifically to man. At present, it has no direct reference to other nervous systems such as those of insects.

This theory is posed in phenomenological terms; although it does not depend upon the exact details of localization, neural coding, or synaptic plasticity, it nonetheless must directly confront these major unsolved problems of neurobiology. The assumptions that are made concerning these problems are as follows:

1. Localization. The cells of the cerebral cortex and associated structures are arranged in functioning groups or modules. Some, but not necessarily all, are arranged in a columnar fashion. These groups have intrinsic connectivities that can be sufficiently variable to form repertoires of groups with similar or identical functions. The existence of such isofunctional but nonisomorphic groups in various repertoires reflects a fundamental degeneracy which is necessary for selection to operate in a somatic system (Edelman, 1978). The extrinsic connectivities of the groups form a distributed system (Mountcastle, 1978) which in some places is hierarchically arranged, but in most others is not. This distributed arrangement is entirely consistent with the idea of a series of interconnected degenerate repertoires, each repertoire carrying out a different major function.

2. Neural Representation or Coding. Beyond the level of initial sensory processing in the primary sensory areas of the cerebral cortex, the exact nature of neural representation is unknown (Bullock, 1961). The theory therefore assumes that neuronal groups recognize, "read," or respond characteristically to specific patterns of activity of other neuronal groups, but it does not specify the nature of these spatiotemporal patterns of neural activity. On the other hand, the theory is quite unambiguous concerning certain global aspects of the mapping of external features of objects in the world. It assumes that primary receiving areas of the cortex provide a topologically ordered or topographic map of significant features of objects. In contrast, however, intrinsic ("association") or homotypical cortex is assumed to be arranged to carry out a recognition or association procedure upon features of this map leading to abstraction; in general, it does not itself contain an isomorphic representation of the maps in the primary

G. M. EDELMAN The Rockefeller University, New York, New York 10021

cortex. Despite the absence of higher-order maps, this arrangement is consistent with schemes for early preprocessing of sensory information that have been suggested for human stereoscopic vision (Marr and Poggio, 1979).

3. Synaptic Plasticity. The theory does not specify any particular molecular mechanism for synaptic alteration. But it makes the crucial assumption that selection through repeated function of particular groups in a repertoire alters their synaptic responses and increases the probability that these groups will be selected again in preference to alternative isofunctional groups in that repertoire. It has been pointed out (Edelman, 1978) that such an arrangement can lead to associative interactions consistent with a content-addressable memory.

Because neuronal groups are specified to be arranged in degenerate repertoires connected in a distributed fashion to carry out a variety of functions that are specified *prior to* adult experience, it is necessary to consider the development or ontogeny of such an arrangement. It is central to the theory that, during development, neural connections and various cellular arrangements arise largely by epigenetic selection among a large collection of possibilities; in some areas, such as homotypical cortex, this leads to degeneracy, particularly in the intrinsic connectivity of groups at the level of their finest axonal and dendritic interactions. Any more rigidly specified and strictly preprogrammed intrinsic connectivity within groups would be inconsistent with the premises of the theory, and proof of such an arrangement would disprove the theory.

A major feature of the theory is concerned with the dynamic interaction of the neuronal groups. Because the groups form a distributed and degenerate system, a means must be provided to allow for temporal and spatial coordination of immediate multimodal input so that signals are not lost, that is, so that they can be correlated in terms of the properties of the original signal object. A particular dynamic mode called phasic reenty (Edelman, 1978) is suggested as a means for this correlation. In one form of reentry, immediately previous signals that have been relayed to the cortex and processed are matched with succeeding less highly processed signals such as those reaching the thalamus. These temporally matched clusters of signals are then read again by groups in the cortex. It should be stressed that this is not the only form of reentry; reentrant signaling is assumed to occur at a variety of levels in the nervous system. Reentry provides a cyclical temporal basis consistent with the reading of related signals by groups in a distributed system. It guarantees that the spatiotemporal continuity of objects is maintained in the neural construct despite the lack of isomorphic representation or mapping in the homotypical or multimodal areas of the cortex.

The ensuing discussion will emphasize successively those aspects of the theory related to the connectivity of cell groups, the representation of objects, and the problem of correlating representations in a distributed system. In addition, some experimental evidence consistent with the theory will be discussed. A detailed discussion of the structural requirements of selective systems has been presented previously (Edelman, 1978). An appendix to the present paper will consider the requirements of selective recognition systems in terms of a minimal computer model. This model most closely resembles the immune selective system, but it contains features in common with those of the group selection theory proposed for the nervous system.

Connectivity

According to the present theory, the major basis for the preexisting diversity in repertoires of neural groups is the anatomical variation in their intrinsic circuitry that is established during development. The preexisting diversity of connections is considered to provide a basis for selection among groups of cells. Selection is not considered, however, to rely upon extensive preexistent repertoires of macromolecules on either single cells or synapses. The basic units of the cerebral cortex subject to selection are supposed to be groups of cells ranging in number from a few hundred to tens of thousands connected via intrinsic connections (local to a group) and extrinsic connections (from group to group or to target organs). The theory therefore makes an assumption about the size and nature of the unit of selection that is exactly contrary to the assumption made by Barlow (1972). He assumes that individual high-level neurons each "correspond to a pattern of external events of the order of complexity of the events symbolized by a single word." The reasons for rejecting this view are numerous; the main ones are (1) it seems inconsistent with the evidence for selection during development (see the section on experimental evidence, below), (2) it is difficult to understand how a content-addressable memory (see Cooper, this volume) could be constructed from such a collection, and (3) it requires *extensive* modifiability of individual neurons, which is tantamount to adopting an instructive theory. The objections to such a theory have been discussed previously (Edelman, 1978), and it has also been pointed out that the identification of a simple correspondence between the elements of perception and unit activity of neurons in homotypical cortex would invalidate the present theory.

In certain instances, the neuronal groups that serve as units of selection may be identified with cortical columns; other types of cell groups are not excluded, however. The groups respond to, recognize, and transform the output patterns of other groups in terms of the spatiotemporal pattern of this output. As mentioned above, the representation or code for most of these outputs is unknown.

The intrinsic and extrinsic connectivity of neuronal groups is established during development by means of a series of processes culminating in selection for circuitry. These processes are (Cowan, 1978) cell proliferation, migration, adhesion and aggregation, differentiation, cell death, process extension, synaptic connection, and selective validation or elimination of synapses. According to the theory, the selective nature of these developmental processes results in the formation of large degenerate repertoires of neuronal groups. Both the major functions and potential range of the groups in these repertoires are established before encounter with the sensory input and motor tasks that will be encountered by the adult animal. To emphasize this point, these repertoires have been called primary repertoires (Edelman, 1978).

The main point is that *two* kinds of selection are necessary for the expression of higher brain function: that which occurs during ontogeny to establish connectivity (particularly via cell death and synaptic elimination), and that which ensues as a result of alteration of synaptic function during behavior. Such an alteration results in the formation of functioning secondary repertoires. To some extent, the processes of primary and secondary repertoire formation may overlap during development.

Within the primary repertoire (the overall function of which is determined by its connectivity) are variant groups of cells that can carry out the same group functions. These variants can carry out these functions (or have similar output patterns) despite the fact that they are not isomorphic in their intrinsic connectivity. Subrepertoires of such cell groups may have similar but not completely identical extrinsic (input and output) connections (Mountcastle, 1978). The major behavioral function of such subrepertoires is also largely defined by these connections (Mountcastle, 1978). Collections of such primary repertoires can thus form a distributed system containing degenerate (i.e., *more* or *less* isofunctional but nonisomorphic) cell groups. Degeneracy can serve in the same manner as redundancy (Wilson and Cowan, 1973) to offset the potential problem of unreliability in a distributed system.

According to the theory, secondary repertoires are formed from cell groups that have already been selected by the synaptic alteration that occurs as a result of encounter of an animal with the world. Early sensorimotor experience serves particularly to select certain cell groups from the population of a subrepertoire. This selection occurs by altering their synaptic responses in such a way that, after a second encounter with a particular input, such groups are more likely to respond than previously unselected groups. Within a secondary repertoire, cell groups can have either an enhanced or diminished probability of response. Nevertheless, the primary repertoire may still contain functionally equivalent or even potentially more effective cell groups than those in the secondary repertoire. Thus, after selection, there still exists a multiplicity of possible responses to a given situation, although the likelihood of occurrence of the various responses is altered by experience.

Sharpening or tuning of the responses of such cell groups may occur by filtering processes or changes in the thresholds that define recognition events among these cell groups. Cell groups with higher repetition rates of response could, for example, be stabilized more effectively if, at the same time, inhibitory processes suppressed those cell groups having less response to the original input. Cell groups are therefore subject to competitive exclusion. This process would effectively sharpen the specificity of an overall response (Edelman, 1978). An algorithm for a similar tuning process has been recently developed and extensively modeled for networks of single cells by Cooper (this volume). With some modification, this algorithm may also be applicable to groups of cells and thus may have application to the present theory. It has not been shown, however, whether a limitation in the size of the cell populations making up a correlation matrix of the type proposed by Cooper would severely compromise its function. Moreover, the need for accuracy in the physical realization of the vectors and matrix coefficients of such a theory (corresponding to rates of firing of neurons and efficiencies of synapses) may exceed that achievable by groups of neurons of the size (up to 10,000 neurons) postulated in the present theory. Aside from these difficulties, however, there is no inconsistency between Cooper's proposal of associative networks and the present notion of group selection, provided that instruction is not allowed. However, the earlier proposal of Nass and Cooper (1975) is not consistent with the present theory; for, if correct, it would exclude group selection.

Representation and Mapping

Because the repertoires of neuronal groups constitute a degenerate and distributed system, the problems of storage and recall, representation, timing of signals, and signal correlation become particularly critical. Associative storage and recall have been discussed previously in some detail (Edelman, 1978). It has been argued that a group degenerate system is capable of associative interactions that are consistent with the operation of a content-addressable memory. The property of association results from the overlapping of the functions of different degenerate groups as well as from the sharing of similar extrinsic connectivities (Edelman, 1978). This form of association differs from that proposed by Cooper (this volume); a detailed comparison of the two notions must await the formulation of a quantitative model that can be tested by a computer (see appendix).

I have pointed out that the group-selection theory makes no detailed or explicit assumptions about neural representations or coding. It is important to stress, however, that there are a variety of related problems that the theory must consider directly even if a choice of a particular neural code from a list of candidate codes (Bullock, 1961; Uttal, 1978) cannot be made.

The first problem has to do with the representation necessary for perception. Whatever the code used, it must correlate various temporal and spatial aspects of a neural representation with the features of a real-world object. A number of questions may be asked to point up the issue. Is there a need at all in the brain for a topological and topographic representation or isomorphic map of the geometrical or physical properties of real-world objects? If so, is the brain so constructed that it makes a series of maps, for example, maps of maps? If motion occurs, how (in the neural representation that is critical to perception) are features "saved" or correlated with a second presentation of the same scene?

It seems necessary that there be at least one level of representation of encoded sensory information in the brain which has the features of a topological or topographic map of a real-world object. If there were not some topological invariance at some early stage of neural processing, it would be difficult to establish or maintain correspondences to the spatiotemporal locus or the continuity of an object in any *subsequent* neural representation. It is sufficient, however, that some early map maintain only basic features relating to the spatiotemporal continuity of an object; a complete point-to-point mapping may not be required. So far no "point-to-point" map has been shown to exist; instead, all mappings studied have been "point to area" and "area to point." Indeed, the partially shifted overlap that has been observed in primary sensory cortex (Mountcastle, 1978) appears to represent a special case of degeneracy and can be taken as some real indication that degeneracy exists at the level of function. Of course, the point-to-area relationship of afferent input to initial cerebral representation is sharpened by both lateral inhibition and by a number of dynamic properties of the system. An obvious example is the movement of the receptor sheet over the external scene. Even in audition, where this is not strictly true, head movements greatly sharpen the capacity to localize sound.

Cerebral columns not only serve to map multidimensional properties of a given modality onto a 2-dimensional sheet (Mountcastle, 1978), but they also "translate" certain physical properties of the real-world object (such as orientation, pitch, etc.) into neural properties at defined locations. Viewed in this way, a cerebral map may be considered to be a translation which makes it possible to preserve the gross order of the external scene. This appears to be a major function of cerebral columns in primary receiving areas (Hubel and Wiesel, 1977). Such an arrangement need not map all features densely, and apparently it does not (Mountcastle, 1978). By the same token, however, such a map does not appear to be sufficient for perception (Uttal, 1978).

In a selective, distributed system, this first translation and lower-level abstraction is of particular importance because it allows higher-order groups to refer without ambiguity to specific groups that already respond to particular features and properties of an object. As will be shown in the next section, the higher-order groups are freed by this arrangement from maintaining the strict correspondences required in a map.

There is some evidence to support this suggestion. For example, in rerepresentation within the parietal cortex, there is always an increase in receptive-field size. This is frequently a very large increase, and in the parietal lobe it can extend to as much as half of the region (Mountcastle, personal communication). In such regions, the property of place is no longer encoded in the same way as in the primary representation. Thus, in the theory, we specify that the topological and topographic requirement is met solely in the primary receiving areas of the cortex by recognizer groups (R). These are identified mainly with the columns of Mountcastle (1978) or the hypercolumns of Hubel and Wiesel (1977). Such R neurons or groups still have a sensory "signature," that is, they are associated with the input from sensory transducers through labeled lines and a few synapses in a most definite way. The distinction between R groups and higher-order groups would not be critically blurred, however, if in certain cases there were a gradient in the amount of topographic mapping found in primary receiving areas and that found in higher areas. Several such areas exist for the visual system (as pointed out by Cowey in this volume).

For the reasons mentioned, and despite the fact that intrinsic or homotypical cortex is also arranged in columns, it does not seem likely that it is tied as tightly to strict mapping as the primary cortex. Such a restriction would only result in a succession of maps with no new principle for carrying out abstract representations or "computations" in perception. The main need for homotypical cortex is for abstract correlation of multiple modalities and for the reflection in various actions of the resolution of potential command that must occur in effectively executing output functions. To fulfill this need, the system would require a set of neuronal groups capable of carrying out routines, procedures, or computations on the translated and mapped information from R groups. This set must meet the requirement for abstraction, that is, degradation of some of the information in the input with invariant representation of the remainder. Groups that carry out this set of routines are called R-of-R groups (recognizers of recognizers; Edelman, 1978).

R-of-R groups are supposed to be located mainly but not exclusively in homotypical cortex. They are assumed to be richly and associatively linked to each other by their degenerate responses and also by their extrinsic connectivities to the same R input as well as to each other through commissural, collateral, and local linkages. Such an arrangement defines the primitive sequence

$$S \rightarrow R \rightarrow R\text{-of-}R,$$

where S is the input.

But this sequence is neither linear, sequential, nor serial and could more properly be represented by

$$S \rightarrow R \rightarrow \overset{\frown}{R}\text{-of-}R.$$

The fundamental distinction between R groups and R-of-R groups is that collections of R groups are much less degenerate and are topographically related to some features of S within any given modality. It is postulated that R-of-R groups are highly degenerate, receive multimodal input, and are in general not topographically related to S. R-of-R groups can interact with other R-of-R groups, with R groups of different modalities, or with various outputs to motor control for action.

Correlation and Reentry

The view sketched above considers that higher brain centers abstract from a map by means of processes in which mapping, if present at all, is

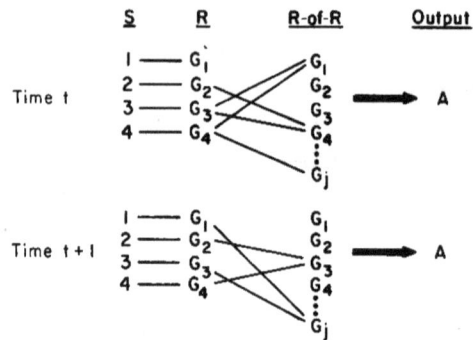

Figure 1 Diagram illustrating the same output (A) from different groups in response to a stimulus object (with characteristics labeled 1,2,3,4) and having no variation or dynamic change in the time period t to $t + 1$. Despite the identity of the output response, a dynamic change has occurred in the *representation* within R-of-R. This could occur because of changes in level set (or "arousal state"), because of alterations in command functions, or because of competitive interactions of incoming excitatory or inhibitory signals (S, stimulus; G_1, . . . , G_j, various neuronal groups in R repertoires or in R-of-R repertoires).

not a predominant feature. Such centers send outputs to action which once again possess maps, but of a different kind. The abandonment of a picture of the brain which favors "maps of maps" for a picture of procedures or computations (abstracting from a map with output to action) leads, however, to a fundamental difficulty related to the properties of a distributed system. In a dynamic situation within a distributed system, a consistent representation of the spatiotemporal continuity and correlated features of a stimulus or goal object can only be maintained in one of two ways. Either there must be a complete temporal ordering and an information exchange on correlated features of the representation within the distributed system, or the ordering must occur by sequential references back to the ordered arrangement in the stimulus object itself. A diagram (Figure 1) may sharpen this problem by underlining the fact that in a distributed system, completely *different* degenerate R-of-R groups may yield what amounts to an equivalent output at two successive moments of time.

If different but equivalent R-of-R states or successive R-of-R states corresponding to features of an object are to be related to the same object *solely* within the brain, then a real-time correlation must occur between the states. This requirement becomes even more stringent in the case of representations of multiple objects in motion that stimulate various sensory modalities. Because of the distributed nature of the system, however, the correlation of temporal sequences of signals from multimodal inputs becomes a formidable problem. In general, even a partial ordering of such sequences requires considerable housekeeping—time or date stamps, stacks, and a complex set of informational tags (Lamport, 1978). While schemes have been devised to route information in networks to the site of a "request" without specific information on the location of that site, they require precise restrictions on the local directivity of input and output (Sahin, 1973). This severe requirement, and the parallel arrangement and complexity of nervous systems, makes it unlikely that such schemes would be applicable. Thus, any distributed degenerate system that does not refer back to the stimulus object but only to the representations of that object must maintain (1) multiple representations, as well as tags corresponding to these representations and correlating any single feature with all other features of the object, and (2) a complex system of real-time clocks cross-correlating the inputs from the very recent past. If one adds to these requirements the need to cross-correlate various *degenerate* neural representations of the object (Figure 1), the informational burden becomes immense.

One solution to this problem is reentry at a particular place of the higher order of more abstract signals, so that they may be correlated in time with the next input signals (Edelman, 1978). Reentry, which must occur in several locations, could occur, for example, at various levels of R groups or between R groups and R-of-R groups or even at the level of thalamocortical input. A possible anatomical basis for this last possibility exists in the corticothalamic radiation. Such a reentered signal could be correlated with the mapped features of the next signal in a temporal sequence. This temporal correlation could then be read by R-of-R neurons responsive to the paired reentrant signals (Edelman, 1978). This mode of correlation would guarantee a continuous spatiotemporal representation of the object. In particular, it would obviate the need for elaborate cross-correlation of R-of-R tags and relieve the requirement for a complete ordering by multiple real-time clocks of various signals in the distributed system. Because of the distributed and degenerate nature of the system, the requirement for reentry is a strong one—if reentry can be shown not to occur, the group-selection theory is likely to be invalid.

In accord with the associative properties (Edelman, 1978) of such a distributed degenerate system, each cycle of reentry would call upon a very large number of associable neuronal groups. The associations would continually shift in response to small variations in the sensory input, to motor demand, or to changes in the arousal system. Whatever other functions the arousal system carries out, the theory postulates (Edelman, 1978) that it helps to coordinate the temporal simultaneities of cellular response required both for reentry and for resolution of redundancies of potential command.

Reentry in itself, however, is not sufficient for adequate functioning of a group-selective system. The brain functions for action and the output to motor systems is required for two essential tasks. The first task is to aid in selecting appropriate inputs by altering the relationship of sensory systems to the surroundings. This further focuses or reinforces the selective features of the system. The second task is to verify and corroborate the instantaneous and dynamic picture as well as the stored routines that result from the action of groups in both primary and secondary repertoires. Both of these tasks serve to update (MacKay, 1970) the instantaneous and the stored information in these repertoires. While the process of reentry is itself one of continuous updating, this process is reinforced by motor activity, and therefore a number of errors of correlation that might arise are canceled by motor responses. In this sense, the informational picture in both R and R-of-R groups is subject to continual verification or to checks for internal consistency by means of motor activity.

It has been pointed out (Edelman, 1978) that long-term storage of abstract patterns of R-of-R repertoires, combined with multiple reentry, updating, and verification through action, can lead to a system consistent with states of awareness.

Experimental Evidence and Some Suggested Lines of Experimentation

The group-selection theory is a global theory concerned with the principles according to which the cortex and associated structures develop and function. It does not (and at present, cannot) deal in any sufficiently detailed manner with the mechanisms and function of particular neuronal subassemblies. Nevertheless, it provides a scheme that directly addresses several fundamental problems of neural development, the nature of the functional unit of the cortex, the associative and distributive nature of cerebral groups, the global organization of representation and mapping, and the dynamics of access in associative groups by means of reentry. When coupled to the associative potential of degenerate repertoires and mechanisms of secondary repertoire formation, the idea of phasic reentry suggests an approach to an understanding of the problem how, by means of association, immediate sensory representations can interact with a content-addressable store.

It is important to identify those parts of such an ambitious and abstract description that might be subject to experimental test and also to note certain experimental observations that already seem consistent with the theory. Some of the latter task has been carried out previously (Edelman, 1978); here, some additional examples may be worthy of note.

Before mentioning these examples, however, it may be useful to list some essential features of the theory, disproof of which would effectively invalidate it. Some of these areas can be examined by means of presently available methods; others are not presently accessible to experimental checks because of the unavailability of adequate techniques.

Feature 1. Extensive degeneracy and selective processes characterize the embryonic development of cortical assemblies. Invalidating counter-examples would include the following:

a. The finding of a molecular repertoire expressed on single cells as a result of gene programming and accounting for specific and predetermined neuron-neuron interaction and assembly.

b. The finding of completely precise specification of neural connections at the level of the finest ramifications of dendrites, with no evidence of great variability. Neuroanatomical evidence already suggests that this is unlikely. Alternatively, the finding of variability with no functional significance, as a simple by-product of development.

Feature 2. The postulation of degeneracy of neuronal repertoires containing isofunctional but nonisomorphic groups. Invalidating counter-examples:

a. Redundancy but no degeneracy in groups of homotypical cortex.

b. An insufficient number of groups from which to select for a given function (Edelman, 1978; also see the appendix).

Feature 3. Synaptic alteration with formation of secondary repertoires. Invalidating counterexample:

a. Evidence for lack of distinctive synaptic alterations *of a group* or a column of cells after experience and behavior.

Feature 4. Reentrant signaling directly correlated with thalamic nuclear function, with activity of primary cortex, or with portions of the cortex immediately associated with primary cortex. Invalidating counter-example:

a. Failure to find phasic correlations of cellular activities between any two of the above-named areas or the finding only of phasic correlations that are very much longer than 100–200 msec (Edelman, 1978).

I shall take up in turn some experimental evidence related to these four features.

Feature 1. A body of experiments is now accumulating to provide support for the selective aspects of development. Notable are the evidence for selective elimination of neurites or synapses (Cowan, 1979; Changeux and Danchin, 1976; Sohal and Weidman, 1978; Landmesser and Pilar, 1976; Landmesser and Pilar, 1978; O'Brien, Östberg, and Vrbová, 1978), the evidence that the adhesion of neurites is mediated by a single type of molecule which is found in cells of the retina and brain at early and late stages of differentiation (Brackenbury et al., 1977; Thiery et al., 1977; Rutishauser et al., 1978; Rutishauser, Gall, and Edelman, 1978), and the accumulating evidence that connections maintaining a specific order, such as retinotectal connections, are specified mainly by the organization of neurites in bundles rather than by specific chemoaffinity (Scholes, 1979; Chung and Cooke, 1975).

Feature 2. At present, it is difficult to perform a stringent test of the notion of degeneracy in the cortex. From the anatomical point of view, a stereological reconstruction of a cerebral column would be required as a reference for comparing variation within other columns; clearly, this is a realizable but still formidable task. At the functional level, the essential operational requirement would be having at hand a direct means of measuring and correlating the simultaneous activity of several hundreds or thousands of cortical neurons. Obviously, this is beyond the capability of single-cell electrode techniques that are currently available. Were a multielectrode procedure or possibly an adequate optical technique at hand, a systematic search could be made for degenerate and distributed repertoires of cells. Both changes in response (that could be distinguished from simple level setting) and, more important, changes in selectivity could provide evidence consistent with degeneracy.

A recent study of lability in the responses of auditory-cortex neurons of squirrel monkeys (Glass and Wollberg, 1979) provides evidence of this type, but because of technical limitations of extracellular recording, only 28 neurons in AII could be tested. During the recording of the responses to 7 different species-specific vocalizations, 22 cells revealed a change in pattern or strength of their response to at least one vocalization over a 6-hour period of recording. Twenty-one cells changed selectively, that is, changed in such a fashion that they responded to a different type or number of the vocalizations which were presented. These alterations in the response pattern were not exclusive of each other. The authors have suggested that their results may be accounted for by a system consisting of an ensemble of cells in which the response of individual cells is labile, but the overall response of a particular ensemble or cell assembly is stable. They were clearly aware of the need for analyzing a larger sample of cells in order to substantiate their suggestion. The main point to be stressed here is that the lability of selectivity of cells cannot be explained simply in terms of level of arousal. The evidence is consistent with the existence of degeneracy in AII but, of course, does not provide definite proof.

I have previously mentioned partially shifted overlap (Mountcastle, 1978) as a special case of degeneracy. Another special case may be represented by the experiments of Wall and Eggars (1971) indicating that partial lesions in the course of the somatosensory pathway lead to unexpected responses in parts of the body map adjacent to the deafferented region. Related studies (Millar, Busbaum, and Wall, 1976; Dostrovsky, Millar, and Wall, 1976) suggest that each dorsal root segment projects more broadly in the nucleus gracilis and nucleus cuneatus than the area from which one may elicit a *physiological* deafferentiation response. In addition to surgical deafferentiation, cold blocks were effective, suggesting that axon sprouting is not the cause of the broader connectivity. Thus, even this far in the periphery, absolute precision of connections is less likely than degeneracy with functionally filtered inhibition as an explanation for the transmission of a precise map through the various higher brain areas.

Feature 3. The question of lability of synapses is being studied actively. Until the existence of degeneracy is established, however, it will be difficult to search directly for the formation of secondary repertoires. But it is conceivable that learning situations could be set up to test the labile behavior of neurons in the parietal cortex of young monkeys in the fashion being carried out by Mountcastle (1980, in press). The search would be for correlations and contrast between the behavior of striate cortical neurons and parietal cortical neurons in a very young animal subjected to a stringent learning situation. The finding of functionally equivalent groups, of similar groups that abstract differently from the same input signals, and of groups with altered probabilities of responses after learning would tend to corroborate the theory. Such a study would have to be a statistical one, however; present technology rules out simultaneous neuronal recording from large numbers of single cells. The main goal in any case is to look for *different* cortical representations in R-of-R of the properties of the *same* R neuron. At the same time, the expectation would be for diffuse R-of-R responses in the early behavior of the inexperienced animal as contrasted with specific or selected R-of-R responses in the older trained animal.

Feature 4. An important test of the group-selection theory is whether or not reentry occurs. Here, the difficulty appears to be twofold: the locus of reentry must be established, and then dynamic correlations must be made. There may be a number of loci of reentry in the cortex or in various tracts. One of the most promising candidates is the corticothalamic radiation because of its anatomy, its obvious relationship to early signals, and its accessibility. Its main interest would be its correlation and possible functional registration with the thalamocortical radiation.

Here, a number of experiments seem feasible although difficult. One is simply to search with a set of single-cell electrodes for corresponding responses in neurons of primary cortex and in neurons of a thalamic nucleus, using external signals as well as direct stimulation. The first task would be to look for corroboration of the hypothesis that clusters of individual neurons in the cortex will be in register with clusters of individual neurons in a particular thalamic nucleus. The second and more original task is to search for significant temporal relationships of the responses of those neurons found to be in register at the level of unit activity. According to the idea of reentry, a definite temporal correlation might be expected between the activity of thalamic cells and cells in the cortex, that is, between the activity of cells responsive to the thalamocortical radiation and the activity of thalamic cells upon which the corticothalamic radiation plays.

It would also be of distinct interest to test the arousal behavior and the responses to learning situations of primates in which bilateral total extirpation or lesioning of thalamic relay nuclei had been carried out. Such lesions might affect reentry properties in striking ways. Unfortunately for the corroborative aspects (but perhaps fortunately for us), there appear to be no well-documented cases of *isolated* bilateral lesions of the thalamic relay nuclei in human beings as the result of cerebral vascular accidents, for example.

One other possible test of the influence of sensory input upon reentrant signaling is via sensory-deprivation experiments in human beings. The prediction is that after a significant period of extensive sensory deprivation, the abstract routines of R-of-R neurons will need a considerable period to reestablish proper reentrant relationships with R neurons. That is, after such a period of deprivation, there would be well-defined disorders of perception that would not decay away unless sensory experience were again restored. Some evidence that this may be so has already been accumulated (Zubek, 1969). This paradigm might also be used in animals without verbal repertoires to test for variability in the subsequent responses of neurons in the parietal cortex, for example.

One of the most intriguing studies of timing in thalamocortical interaction has been that by Libet (1978) on neuronal versus subjective timing for conscious sensory experience. He finds that there is an almost immediate development of the awareness of sensory signals such as a skin pulse in short intervals after that pulse (latencies 25–50 msec). But direct stimulation of the SI cortex with a volley of signals required up to 500 msec. When the thalamus was stimulated by this volley, although a volley duration of at least 200 msec was required, the subject reported the time (subjectively) back to earlier times, and these times were of the same magnitude as those estimated after a skin pulse. According to Libet, this may represent a referral, for timing purposes, to early cortical responses evoked by the afferent signal of which the subject is not directly aware but which appear to serve as "time markers." The relation of this work to the hypothesis of reentrant signaling deserves closer exploration. Some of the delays occurring upon direct cortical stimulation may be related, for example, to the absence of a regular reentrant loop under these circumstances. The delay required for a response after stimulation of the thalamus may also be related to similar effects and may not be solely due to the time required to carry out some cortical "computation."

The Darwinian Computer

The analogy of many of the processes of brain function to computational processes has been pointed out repeatedly (see, e.g., Arbib, 1972; Marr and Poggio, 1979). This analogy has great heuristic value. Moreover, it is particularly persuasive if computer implementation of a particular

Gerald M. Edelman

Table I A qualitative comparison of features of the human brain and digital computers

Computer	Brain
1. Program and programmer	No external programmer, no internal homunculus
2. Strict symbol assignment in syntax and logic	Possibility of variable and ambiguous assignments, e.g., visual illusions
3. Computation fast relative to input–output	Input–output and computational speeds comparable
4. Few or no exploratory routines or action patterns	Exploration (behavior) and patterns of action
5. Sequential machine based on logic; slightly distributed	Largely parallel, less sequential, highly distributed
6. Number-addressable store	Content-addressable store
7. Storage of status registers or address tags on interrupts; context switching; "save the world" upon interrupts	No evidence for systematic storage of tags; possible reentry to features of sense object for continuity of representation
8. Operating systems and list hierarchies	Statistical resolution of conflicts or redundancies of potential command
9. Enqueuing of serially reusable resources	Redundancy of multiply used routines or "capture" by most active input
10. Designed for minimum complexity, minimum number of parts to carry out given function	Evolution toward greater complexity; least energy used to carry out function
11. Manufactured	Self-assembling during both development and learning

hypothesis about brain function can be successfully carried out. It is obvious, however, that there are enormous differences between the kinds of computation carried out by brains and computers. The most obvious difference lies in the parallel nature of many of the routines carried out by nervous systems. A successful phenomenological theory describing many of the features of such a parallel computation in the fly has been provided, for example, by Poggio and Reichardt (1973).

Clearly, we are very far from such a formulation for mammalian brains. But, at a more superficial and qualitative level, it may still be useful to point out a number of other features that distinguish such brains from digital computers (Table I). Some of these differences are superficial, some are profound; all of them are considerable.

From the point of view of the theory of group selection, the conclusion is that if the brain is a computer (as it must be at least in part), it must be a Darwinian computer. That is, the main problem posed in the evolution of primate brains is to assure that they can deal successfully with situations that were not foreseeable and that could not be preprogrammed in detail before actual encounters with such situations. The brain that is the outcome of such a requirement is built for action and exploration, works in a largely parallel fashion, and does multiple "quick and dirty" calculations subject to updating, although the depth of individual computations is likely to be much less than that employed in computers.

Under these circumstances, logic is but a small part of such a system which must not only "program" itself through action but must also develop means of access to a content-addressable store (Edelman, 1978; Cooper, this volume). To resolve the problem of access to such a memory, the group-selection theory proposes that the degeneracy of groups leads to an associative property (Edelman, 1978) which is continually exploited in multiple cyclic repetitions by the process of reentry. In the theory, this is also supposed to obviate the need for storage of multiple tags upon interruption of a task. The entire process is statistical and is subject to continual updating—in this view, there are no absolutely fixed operating systems in the brain, only *relatively* effective hierarchies that resolve the question of redundancy of potential command on a *statistical* basis.

While these various aspects of the group-selection theory clearly must be substantiated or excluded by experiment, it is useful to attempt to model some of its features in a computer. This is a formidable task, but some small beginnings have been made. As shown in the appendix, a selection algorithm can be made to operate upon bit strings having various representative forms. This may provide a basis for modeling some of the more sophisticated aspects of the theory; to some extent, it provides a specific example of how selection and repertoire alteration may change responses to inputs, and it also gives a deeper insight into the statistical behavior of systems of selective recognition.

Appendix: A Minimal Computer Model for a Selective Recognition System[1]

In order to explore how various selective recognition systems of the type described might operate in practice, we are developing a computer model which will ultimately incorporate the main features of the theory. We describe here an early portion of this model that simulates only the recognition process itself; later we briefly discuss methods for adding signaling among R groups and R-of-R groups, along with the amplification of the response of successful groups through modification of the efficiency of the various signaling pathways. The major aim of these efforts is to demonstrate the self-consistency of the group-selection theory; obviously, the successful functioning of a computer model does

1 Coauthored by G. N. Reeke, Jr., Rockefeller University.

not bear upon the correctness of the theory as a description of actual higher brain function.

At present, the model is already capable of displaying adaptive behavior with respect to recognition of "stimuli" (32-bit numbers) selected from a chosen domain of possible patterns. We are using it to explore the effects of various choices of matching functions and other parameters of the theory, such as repertoire size, thresholding, and the amount by which repertoire elements that succeed in recognizing a stimulus are amplified. The model has proved useful in stimulating further refinement of selective recognition theories and may have practical implications as well, serving as a prototype for a class of pattern-recognizing machines based on the selective-recognition principle.

While the model is not intended to correspond to any real nervous system, in what follows we will for convenience discuss its components in terms of certain nervous-system analogs. The repertoire elements and informational inputs manipulated by the program are implemented in the computer as bit strings. By the use of a suitable code, such strings in general can be made to represent any kind of information, including neuronal signals. In a real nervous system there are early processing centers that map the external stimuli by suitable transformations into combinations of signals appropriate for input to the higher-order recognition units. In the minimal model, these early processing centers are ignored. For this reason, the model has only to deal with already encoded bit strings, and the detailed nature of the code does not need to be specified exactly. We will often refer loosely to these encoded input strings as "stimuli." For the present purpose, working with arbitrary strings permits us to separate the encoding problem from the selective-recognition problem, although in an actual nervous system the two processes must to some extent overlap.

The essential features of the basic model are a repertoire generator, which produces a repertoire of random bit strings; a stimulus generator, which produces or reads from a file the inputs to be tested; a match seeker, which searches for correspondences between the inputs and individual elements of the repertoire; and an amplifier, which increases the probability of a response by those repertoire elements that have successfully been matched to input stimuli. These components interact as illustrated in Figure 2; each will be discussed in more detail later. Auxiliary routines record statistics on the selective performance of the model and permit the repertoire, as modified by the amplifier during a series of trials, to be saved for input to subsequent trials. Recognition of a "stimulus" at present results only in modification of the repertoire; we shall briefly discuss later some possible ways to incorporate associative recall and reentry of evoked responses into the model.

The model repertoire is generated as a set of random bit strings, arranged for convenience to be all of the same length. In the runs de-

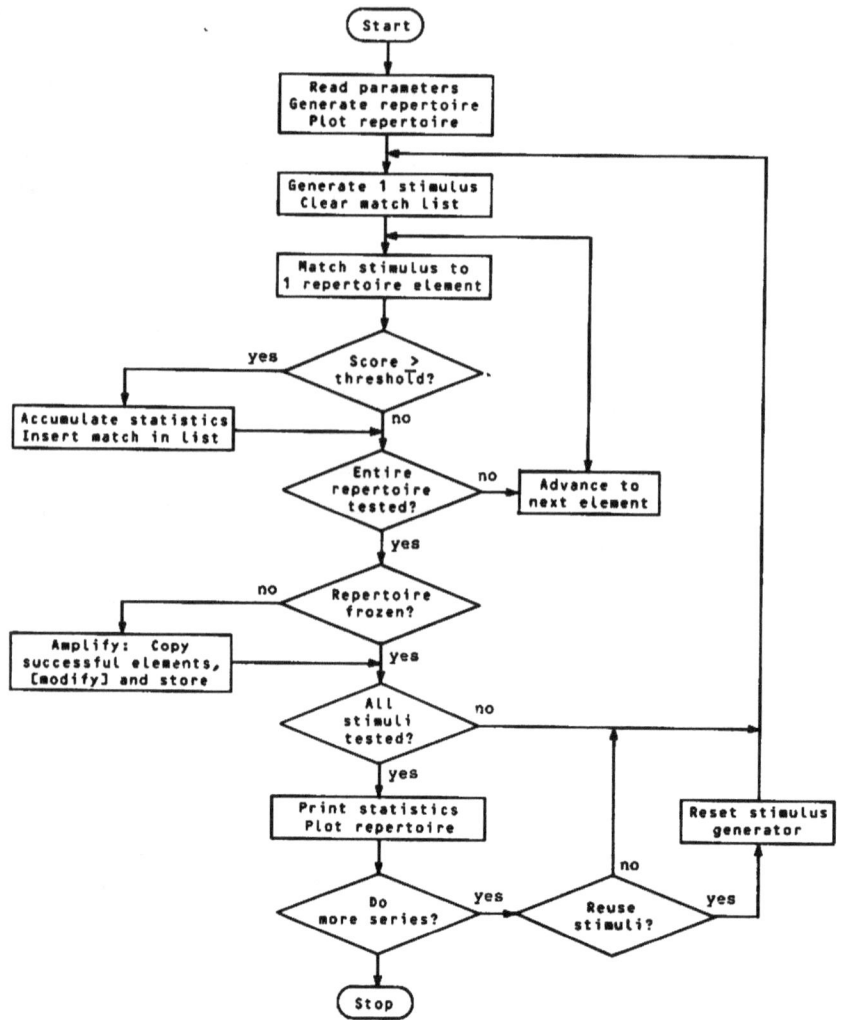

Figure 2 Scheme for a minimal model of a selective-recognition system. In each run the program performs one or more series of trials. In each series, a number of "stimuli" may be presented. These stimuli may be the same as or different from those used in previous series. Each stimulus is presented to all of the repertoire elements and a match score is evaluated for each presentation. After all possible matches have been tested, those elements meeting certain threshold criteria are amplified. Signaling between groups, present in our current models, is not shown.

552   Gerald M. Edelman

scribed here, each repertoire element contained 32 bits, permitting a total of $2^{32} = 4.3 \times 10^9$ possible patterns. Typically, 10^4 of these patterns were actually used. These collections of bit strings correspond to the predetermined, plurispecific repertoires of recognizer groups postulated in the theory. Individual bits or short substrings of bits represent particular features of the input signals to be matched. Various stimulus generators might be used according to the process being modeled, but we have worked mainly with stimuli chosen at random from one or a few subsets of the universe of all possible strings of the same length as that of the recognizers. In each such subset, half of the bits are fixed and the other half are allowed to vary randomly. These subsets could represent classes of objects that the system might be called upon to recognize. The necessary relationship between inputs or "stimuli" and the corresponding recognizers is determined entirely by an arbitrary "matching function," which is, in general, a real-valued function of two bit strings that returns a score indicating the degree of match between the two argument strings. In the implementation, the matching function is a replaceable subroutine that can be changed at will to investigate the effects of requiring various modes and degrees of fit for a successful match. For convenience, we have used matching functions in which the best possible fit is identity of the stimulus and recognizer bit strings, but we could equally well have required the strings to be complementary or related in any other way without changing the essential operation of the model. [For stimulus vector S, a coding function represented by matrix C, and two matching functions F and G, if $F^{-1}G$ exists, we have $GCS = (FF^{-1}) GCS = F (F^{-1} GC) S$. Thus, a change in matching function from F to G could be paired with a corresponding change in the external coding function from C to $F^{-1} GC$ to produce a run with identical matching statistics.] Typically, and for simplicity here, we have used a matching function that simply counts the number of bits that are identical in position and value in the two strings being compared. A threshold score is then set for accepting a match as a "recognition." This function gives equal weight to all bits in a stimulus; more complicated matching functions can easily be conceived that weight some bits ("recognition characteristics") more than others in arriving at a match score.

Given a matching function, a procedure is then necessary for presenting the stimuli to the repertoire in some order (the model being implemented in a sequential computer!) and taking appropriate action when a threshold match score is obtained. Because the repertoire elements are random, it is sufficiently general to scan through them in serial order searching for threshold matches. Statistics of such actual matches for various threshold scores M and numbers of repertoire elements N are shown in Figure 3. The results are entirely consistent with the theoretical distributions we have derived (Edelman, 1978). The

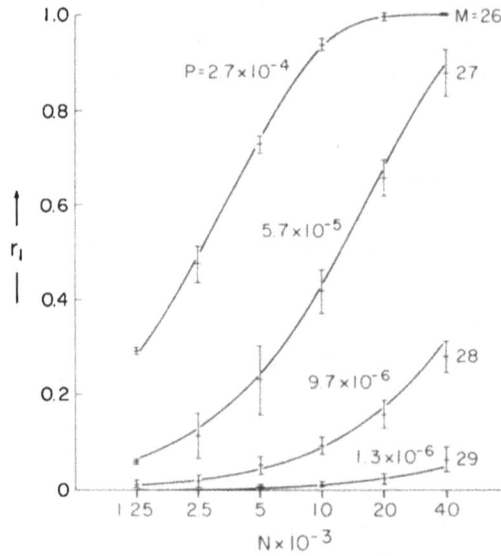

Figure 3 Comparison of theoretical and experimental recognition functions r_1 as a function of match threshold and repertoire size. r_1 = fraction of stimuli presented that are expected to be recognized. Solid curves were calculated according to $r_1 = 1 - (1 - P)^N$, where P = probability of recognizing any one stimulus, N = number of elements in repertoire. Experimental data are presented as dashes with vertical error bars, representing standard deviations of r_1 for four series of 100 trials each. Each curve is labeled with the match threshold M (number of bits out of 32 that must be identical in the stimulus and repertoire element for a "recognition" to occur) and the corresponding recognition probability P. As expected, the statistical distribution of matches obtained from the model closely approaches the theoretical values.

ranges of M and N tested cover the region of the sigmoidal transition between very poor and very efficient recognition.

A list of matches is made for each stimulus, and the responders giving the highest match scores are amplified. This amplification is of course at the heart of the adaptive behavior of the system. In the early model, amplification consists of making some predetermined number of copies of the successful recognizer and depositing these copies in random locations in the repertoire array. The number of copies made may depend on the match score. For implementation reasons, the size of the repertoire is kept constant and the amplified elements simply replace other elements at random. For a repertoire sufficiently large compared to the amplification factor, this procedure gives the same behavior as expansion of the repertoire during amplification. Alternatively, the repertoire list may be reordered so that successful elements are encountered earlier in subsequent scans.

In this early model, in which intergroup signaling is absent, these somewhat artificial amplification procedures at least make it possible to study a primitive form of adaptive behavior in the system. A more realistic amplification procedure based on changes analogous to a form of synaptic modification is being incorporated in current versions of the model. While the original procedure perhaps more closely resembles the behavior of the immune system than it does that of the nervous system, it basically serves to increase the response to later presentations of an already encountered stimulus, and this end result is the same in either system.

The model permits the state of the repertoire after a series of trials to be presented graphically. For this purpose, repertoire elements are considered to be vectors in an N-dimensional hyperspace, where N is the number of bits in each repertoire element. A projection of this hyperspace onto an ordinary 2-dimensional plane is made, and the number of elements falling in each unit square of the plane is recorded. The plane of projection can be selected in various ways to emphasize clustering of the repertoire that may occur as a result of the structure of the set of stimuli presented. Results of a typical series of trials are shown in Figure 4. In these series, 10,000 repertoire elements of 32 bits each were used. Stimuli always had the same pattern of ones in 16 of the 32 bits; the remaining bits were random, simulating the variation of sensory signals that might occur with presentation of a sequence of identical or similar stimuli. Successive panels of Figure 4 show how the repertoire responded to these stimuli by amplification of the ability to respond to any input similar in pattern to the actual inputs used. It is important to note that the particular pattern of similarity of these stimuli was in no way anticipated in the construction of the repertoire. Any other pattern could have been chosen as well and a similar adaptive response would have been seen.

The procedure employed in the model also incorporates degenerate recognition. Many repertoire elements can respond above threshold to any one stimulus, and in the computer an ordered list of these elements is made before amplification so that only the best responders can be selected for amplification. In addition, infidelity of amplification can be simulated by varying, with a predetermined probability, some bits in each copy of a "successful" repertoire element. This procedure permits the repertoire to acquire new properties in response to the overall structure of the set of inputs actually encountered, and is intended to model to some extent the unknown effects of the presumed plasticity of synaptic connections during early development.

In Table II are shown the statistical results obtained in typical runs with exact or inexact amplification. Amplification enhances the response to recognized stimuli roughly equally in the two cases, as measured by the mean number of matches above threshold, or "hits." However, amplification with copying errors (averaging one bit alteration per repertoire element copied during amplification in the runs shown) makes it possible for the repertoire to recognize nearly all (91%) of the related stimuli presented. The mean number of matches that must

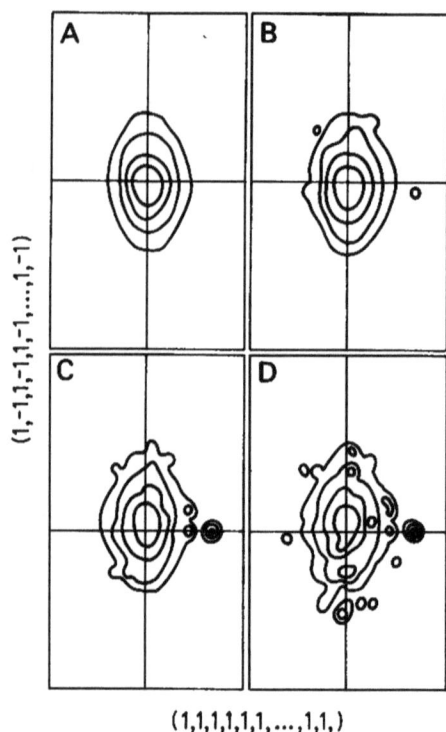

Figure 4 Alterations in the density distribution of repertoire elements after amplification. Repertoire elements are considered as points on a lattice in 32-space, each bit corresponding to one coordinate axis. Points are projected onto the plane defined by the vectors $(1,1,1,1,1,1,...,1,1)$ and $(1,-1,1,-1,1,-1,...,1,-1)$, and contours are drawn around equal densities of points at roughly equal intervals. In this run, the repertoire consisted of 10,000 elements of 32 bits each. Panels (A), (B), (C), (D) display the state of the repertoire after presentation of respectively 0, 100, 200, or 300 input patterns. The patterns were selected at random from one of four classes. Within each class, the patterns were identical in 16 of the 32 bit positions and random in the remaining 16 bits. For illustrative purposes, the identical bits within each class were chosen to place the classes at well-separated positions in the plane of projection. These positions are located approximately halfway from the center to the edge of the diagrams along the four axes drawn. The 16 random bits are different for all patterns, producing clustering around the center position of each class. The successive panels show the increase in the numbers of repertoire elements capable of matching the input patterns.

Table II Statistics of recognition in the minimal computer model[a]

	Before Amplification	After Amplification[b]	After Inexact Amplification[c]
Test Stimuli[d]			
% matched	44	38	91
Mean hits (all stimuli)	0.57	4.63	14.83
Mean hits (matched stimuli)	1.28	12.18	16.30
Mean trials to first match	4471	3289	1600
Control Stimuli[e]			
% matched	38	36	34
Mean hits (all stimuli)	0.48	0.46	0.53
Mean hits (matched stimuli)	1.28	1.28	1.54
Mean trials to first match	4801	4659	4476

a. Repertoire size was 10,000 × 32 bits.
b. Amplification: for each test stimulus, the best three matches above threshold were each replicated five times.
c. Inexact amplification: same, except individual bits were inverted at random with a probability such that, on the average, one bit was inverted in each copy of a replicated repertoire element.
d. Test stimuli: 400 stimuli were selected at random from one of four classes, each class having 16 bits fixed and 16 bits random. Test stimuli were amplified upon successful matching as described above.
e. Control stimuli: 200 stimuli with all bits random were used as controls. No amplification was performed when these stimuli were presented.

be tested for a match above threshold to be found is more than halved by this procedure. Under the conditions used, the response to unrelated control stimuli is virtually unaffected by amplification, showing that significant capacity remains for recognizing and responding to new stimuli of different classes that may be presented later. The only effects on control stimuli are a slight reduction in the percentage recognized as a result of the fixed repertoire size and an increase in the number of matches found for stimuli that are recognized as a result of cross-recognition of the test stimuli.

The possibilities for cross-recognition are illustrated in more detail in Table III. In this experiment, four different stimuli were used: S1 is the test stimulus that was used for amplification; S2 and S3 are "related" stimuli differing in 4 and 8 bit positions, respectively, from S1; and S4 is a "relatively unrelated" stimulus differing in 20 positions from S1. Before amplification, the four stimuli showed similar levels of response, averaging two hits each above a threshold match score of 27. One of these hits, element 3579, was common to two stimuli, S1 and S2. This element represents a preexisting, accidental cross-recognition. A more interesting kind of cross-recognition arises if the threshold for amplification is lowered during the presentation of S1. After all repertoire elements matching S1 in *24 or more positions* were replicated 10 times, an

Table III Cross-recognition of related stimuli[a]

	Stimulus	Bit Pattern	Bits Different from S1
1. Stimuli	S1	11110000111110011110001111110110	0
	S2 (X-R)[b]	01110000111111011110101101 10110	4
	S3 (X-R)	11111101111101001111001111111011	8
	S4 (NX-R)[c]	00011110010001101010101001011111	20

	Stimulus	Repertoire Position	Repertoire Element	Total Hits[d]
2. Response before	S1	3579	11110010111101101111000110110110	2
		6520	11110010011101101111000111110100	
Amplification	S2 (X-R)	3579	11110010111101101111000110110110	3
		3147	10100000011111111111010110110110	
		3575	01010100111111101101111110110110	
	S3 (X-R)	2336	11111101111100001011011111010011	2
		8289	11111001101111001111101111101011	
	S4 (NX-R)	1658	00011110001000101010101101010111	1

	Stimulus	Repertoire Position	Repertoire Element	Total Hits[d]
3. Response after Amplification[e]	S1	445	11110010111101101111000110110110	21
		2627	11110010111101101111000110110110	
		7751	11110010111101101111000110110110	
		9636	11110010011101101111000111110100	
			... 17 more ...	
	S2 (X-R)	2627	11110010111101101111000110110110	20
		3147	10100000011111111111010110110110	
		5090	10100000011111111111010110110110	
		8244	10100000011111111111010110110110	
			... 16 more ...	
	S3 (X-R)	2336	11111101111100001011011111010011	2
		8289	11111001101111001111101111101011	
	S4 (NX-R)	1658	00011110001000101010101101010111	1

a. Repertoire size in this run was 10,000 elements of 32 bits each.
b. X-R = related stimulus, possibly cross-recognized.
c. NX-R = relatively unrelated stimulus, not cross-recognized.
d. Number of matches with 27 or more bits identical in stimulus and repertoire strings.
e. Repertoire elements with match scores against S1 greater than 24 were each replicated 10 times.

increased response to S2 as well as to S1 was obtained at the original 27 *match-score level*. The elements giving rise to the matches above 27 for S2 were not all derived from element 3579, which matched originally; some were among the poorer (24–26 score) matches of S1 that were also amplified. Thus, elements that respond weakly to a particular stimulus (S1) can be amplified if the threshold is set low enough, strengthening the response to a related stimulus that has not yet been encountered (S2). These results show how cross-recognition arising from overlapping specificities in a degenerate repertoire can give the system an enhanced ability to recognize stimuli that are new but similar to some of those already encountered. This ability should be particularly advantageous in the early stages of adaptation, when relatively few stimuli have been encountered, but might later interfere with the highly selective processes needed for distinguishing among similar, familiar stimuli.

These considerations suggest the general need for some kind of gating system to vary the recognition thresholds at different times and in different subrepertoires of a selective system in order to adjust the degree of precision in matching so as to correspond with the degree of repertoire specificity already attained. Such a mechanism may be essential to the successful adaptation of the system to the overall structure of its inputs. It is well known that these thresholding systems are essential for assuring a highly specific immune *response* after a relatively broad cross-reactive *binding* to a large number of antigen-binding cells (Edelman, 1974). Of course, the cross-reactivity does not appear to be generally useful in the immune system, whereas cross-recognition can be highly important in an adaptive neural system. The requirement for alteration of thresholds in a selective system may help to explain some of the functions of the reticular activating system in "sensory" cortex and of the cerebellum in relation to "motor" cortex. In both cases, these systems may alter thresholds of recognition so as to refine the initial selection of repertoire elements and control the extent of cross-recognition.

These results represent a very preliminary development of the computer model. We are exploring further the properties of the model and are also adding additional features postulated to exist in selective neural networks. The basic recognizer groups are modeled as in the minimal model, but now we provide each repertoire element with an output channel on which it can transmit the results of recognition events to other units. Each such channel will carry at time $t + 1$ the match score resulting from input to the unit at time t. As before, the match score can be an arbitrary function of the signals on the input channels; we expect to use mostly, however, a linear summarizer (see, e.g., Kohonen, 1977), but with thresholding to provide some nonlinearity. Provision will also be made to allow strong signals to persist for a finite time, and to add fluctuating noise to the signal in each channel. Higher-level R-of-R groups will receive inputs from these primary recognizers, as well as reentrant inputs from other R-of-R groups. R-of-R groups will be designed on the same principles as R groups to recognize specific combinations of their inputs. Such R-of-R groups should display abstracting properties as a result of their ability to combine information from a variety of recognizers of simple characters. The channels between R-of-R groups will provide implicit reentrant signaling pathways that will permit associations to be formed between inputs that occur juxtaposed in time or space. Consistently occurring patterns of response will be reinforced by the amplification process, which will be carried out by modifying the *sensitivity* of each group to some of its inputs as a result of experience, rather than by changing the *number* or *arrangement* of the groups as described above. Amplification will be carried out by a scheme similar to that suggested in a different context by Hebb (1949) and since used in various forms by others (e.g., Brindley, 1969; Cooper, 1973; von der Malsburg, 1973; Perez, Glass, and Shlaer, 1975). The strength of each connection between two groups will be modified depending on the correlation between the input to the connection and the output of the unit according to

$$\delta c_{ij} = \phi(c_{ij})(s_i - \theta_{Mi})(s_j - \theta_{M'i}),$$

where

δc_{ij} = change in coefficient c_{ij} relating input j to output i,
$\phi(c_{ij})$ = saturation function, equal to 1 when $c_{ij} = 0$, 0 when $c_{ij} = c_{ij}(\max)$,
s_i = output signal from unit i,
θ_{Mi} = modification threshold for output level of unit i,
$\theta_{M'i}$ = modification threshold for input level to unit i.

The sensitivity thresholds (θ_{Mi} and $\theta_{M'i}$) for amplification will be varied according to the degree of selectivity already attained in order to optimize the responses. With all of these features, the model should emulate a selective, abstractive machine with significant resemblances to a primitive form of "Darwinian computer." While its information-handling capability will necessarily remain low because of limitations of the underlying sequential processor on which it is implemented, the model should prove useful in delineating some of the properties of systems based on the selective-recognition principle.

Acknowledgment

The author wishes to thank Vernon B. Mountcastle for his valuable comments.

Gerald M. Edelman

References

Arbib, M. A., 1972. *The Metaphorical Brain. An Introduction to Cybernetics as Artificial Intelligence and Brain Theory.* New York: Wiley-Interscience.

Barlow, H. P., 1972. Single units and sensation: A neuron doctrine for perceptual psychology? *Perception* 1:371–394.

Brackenbury, R., J.-P. Thiery, U. Rutishauser, and G. M. Edelman, 1977. Adhesion among neural cells of the chick embryo. I. An immunological assay for molecules involved in cell-cell binding. *J. Biol. Chem.* 252:6835–6840.

Brindley, G. S., 1969. Nerve net models of plausible size that perform many simple learning tasks. *Proc. Roy. Soc. B* 174:173–191.

Bullock, T. H., 1961. The problem of recognition in an analyzer mode of neurons. In *Sensory Communication.* W. A. Rosenblith, ed. Cambridge, MA: MIT Press, pp. 717–724.

Changeux, J.-P., and A. Danchin, 1976. Selective stabilization of developing synapses as a mechanism for the specification of neuronal networks. *Nature* 264:705–712.

Chung, S.-H., and J. Cooke, 1975. Polarity of structure and of ordered nerve connection in the developing amphibian brain. *Nature* 258:126–132.

Cooper, L. N., 1973. A possible organization of animal memory and learning. *Nobel Symp.* 24:252–264.

Cowan, W. M., 1978. Aspects of neural development. In *Int. Rev. Physiol. Neurobiology III, Vol. 17.* R. Porter, ed. Baltimore: University Park Press, pp. 150–191.

Cowan, W. M., 1979. Selection and control in neurogenesis. In *The Neurosciences: Fourth Study Program.* F. O. Schmitt and F. G. Worden, eds. Cambridge, MA: MIT Press, pp. 59–79.

Dostrovsky, J. O., J. Millar, and P. D. Wall, 1976. The immediate shift of afferent drive of dorsal column nucleus cells following deafferentiation: A comparison of acute and chronic deafferentiation in gracile nucleus and spinal cord. *Exp. Neurol.* 52:480–495.

Edelman, G. M., 1974. Origins and mechanisms of specificity in clonal selection. In *Cellular Selection and Regulation in the Immune Response.* G. M. Edelman, ed. New York: Raven Press, pp. 1–38.

Edelman, G. M., 1978. Group selection and phasic reentrant signalling: A theory of higher brain function. In *The Mindful Brain: Cortical Organization and the Group-Selective Theory of Higher Brain Function.* G. M. Edelman and V. B. Mountcastle. Cambridge, MA: MIT Press, pp. 51–100.

Glass, I., and Z. Wollberg, 1979. Lability in the responses of cells in the auditory cortex of squirrel monkeys to species-specific vocalizations. *Exp. Brain Res.* 34:489–498.

Hebb, D. O., 1949. *Organization of Behavior.* New York: John Wiley.

Hubel, D. H., and T. N. Wiesel, 1977. Functional architecture of macaque monkey visual cortex. *Proc. Roy. Soc. B* 198:1–59.

Kohonen, T., 1977. *Associative Memory: A System—Theoretical Approach.* Berlin: Springer-Verlag.

Lamport, L., 1978. Time, clocks, and the ordering of events in a distributed system. *Commun. ACM* 21:558–565.

Landmesser, L., and G. Pilar, 1976. Fate of ganglionic synapses and ganglion cell axons during normal and induced cell death. *J. Cell Biol.* 68:357–374.

Landmesser, L., and G. Pilar, 1978. Interaction between neurons and their targets during *in vivo* synaptogenesis. *Fed. Proc.* 37:2016–2022.

Libet, B., 1978. Neuronal vs. subjective timing for a conscious sensory experience. In *Cerebral Correlates of Conscious Experience. ISERM Symposium No. 6.* P. A. Buser and A. Rougeul-Buser, eds. Amsterdam: North Holland, pp. 69–82.

MacKay, D. M., 1970. Perception and brain function. In *The Neurosciences: Second Study Program.* F. O. Schmitt, ed. New York: Rockefeller University Press, pp. 303–316.

Marr, D., and T. Poggio, 1979. A computational theory of human stereo vision. MIT AI Lab Memo 451. (See also *Proc. Roy. Soc. B* 204:301–328, 1979.)

Millar, J., A. I. Busbaum, and P. D. Wall, 1976. Restructuring of the somatotopic map and appearance of abnormal neuronal activity in the gracile nucleus after partial deafferentiation. *Exp. Neurol.* 50:658–672.

Mountcastle, V. B., 1978. An organizing principle for cerebral function: The unit module and the distributed system. In *The Mindful Brain: Cortical Organization and the Group-Selective Theory of Higher Brain Function.* G. M. Edelman and V. B. Mountcastle. Cambridge, MA: MIT Press.

Mountcastle, V. B., 1980. *The Harvey Lectures.* New York: Academic Press.

Nass, M. M., and L. N. Cooper, 1975. A theory for the development of feature detecting cells in visual cortex. *Biol. Cybern.* 19:1–18.

O'Brien, R. A. D., A. J. C. Östberg, and G. Vrbová, 1978. Observations on the elimination of polyneuronal innervation in developing mammalian skeletal muscle. *J. Physiol.* 282:571–582.

Perez, R., L. Glass, and R. Shlaer, 1975. Development of specificity in the cat visual cortex. *J. Math. Biol.* 1:275–288.

Poggio, T., and W. Reichardt, 1973. A theory of the pattern-induced flight orientation of the fly *Musca domestica. Kybernetik* 12:185–203.

Rutishauser, U., W. E. Gall, and G. M. Edelman, 1978. Adhesion among neural cells of the chick embryo. IV. Role of the cell surface molecule CAM in the formation of neurite bundles in cultures of spinal ganglia. *J. Cell Biol.* 79:382–393.

Rutishauser, U., J.-P. Thiery, R. Brackenbury, and G. M. Edelman, 1978. Adhesion among neural cells of the chick embryo. III. Relationship of the surface molecule CAM to cell adhesion and the development of histotypic patterns. *J. Cell Biol.* 79:371–381.

Sahin, K., 1973. Response routing in Selcuk networks and Lashley's dilemma. *Int. J. Man-Machine Stud.* 5:567–573.

Scholes, J. H., 1979. Nerve fiber topography in the neural projection to the tectum. *Nature* 278:620–624.

Sohal, G. S., and T. A. Weidman, 1978. Development of the trochlear nucleus: Loss of axons during normal ontogeny. *Brain Res.* 142:455–465.

Thiery, J.-P., R. Brackenbury, U. Rutishauser, and G. M. Edelman, 1977. Adhesion among neural cells of the chick embryo. II. Purification and characterization of a cell adhesion molecule from neural retina. *J. Biol. Chem.* 252:6841–6845.

Uttal, W. R., 1978. *The Psychobiology of Mind.* Hillsdale, NJ: Lawrence Erlbaum Associates.

Von der Malsburg, C., 1973. Self-organization of orientation sensitive cells in the striate cortex. *Kybernetik* 14:85–100.

Wall, P. D., and D. Eggars, 1971. Neural connexions—functional reorganization after partial deafferentiation in the rat. *Nature* 232:542–544.

Wilson, H. R., and J. D. Cowan, 1973. A mathematical theory of the functional dynamics of cortical and thalamic nervous tissue. *Kybernetik* 13:55–80.

Zubek, J. P., ed., 1969. *Sensory Deprivation: Fifteen Years of Research.* New York: Appleton-Century-Crofts.

List of Authors

Giovanni Berlucchi   415
David M. Berson   285
Floyd E. Bloom   323, 359
M. Colonnier   125
Martha Constantine-Paton   47
Leon N Cooper   479
W. Maxwell Cowan   xi, 101
A. Cowey   395
Francis H. C. Crick   505
John E. Desmedt   441
Gerald M. Edelman   477, 535
P. C. Emson   325
Edward V. Evarts   263
Charles D. Gilbert   163
Patricia S. Goldman-Rakic   69
Ann M. Graybiel   195, 285
David H. Hubel   29
S. P. Hunt   325
Herbert H. Jasper   373, 375
E. G. Jones   199
J. H. Kaas   237
Simon LeVay   29
J. S. Lund   105
David C. Marr   505
M. M. Merzenich   237
R. J. Nelson   237
Tomaso Poggio   505
Pasko Rakic   3, 7
James M. Sprague   415
T. W. Stone   347
M. Sur   237
D. A. Taylor   347
Edward L. White   153
Torsten N. Wiesel   29, 163

Participants, Proceedings of a Neurosciences Research Program Colloquium on Cerebral Cortex, 1979

George Adelman
Neurosciences Research Program

Giovanni Berlucchi
Istituto di Fisiologia
Della Università di Pisa

Floyd E. Bloom
Arthur V. Davis Center
The Salk Institute

Marc Colonnier
Laboratory of Neurobiology
Hôpital de l'Enfant-Jésus

Martha Constantine-Paton
Department of Biology
155 Guyot Hall
Princeton University

Leon N Cooper
Department of Physics
Brown University

W. Maxwell Cowan
The Weingart Laboratory
for Developmental
Neurobiology
The Salk Institute

Alan Cowey
Department of Experimental
Psychology
University of Oxford
Lincoln College

Francis H. C. Crick
The Salk Institute

Stephen G. Dennis
Neurosciences Research Program

John E. Desmedt
Brain Research University
University of Brussels

Gerald M. Edelman
Department of Biochemistry
The Rockefeller University

Piers C. Emson
MRC Neurochemical Pharma-
cology Unit
Department of Pharmacology
Medical School
Cambridge

Edward V. Evarts
Laboratory of Neurophysiology
National Institute of Mental
Health

Charles Gilbert
Department of Neurobiology
Harvard Medical School

Patricia Goldman-Rakic
Laboratory of Neuropsychology
National Institute of Mental
Health

Ann M. Graybiel
Department of Psychology
Massachusetts Institute of
Technology

Herbert H. Jasper
Department of Physiology
University of Montreal

Edward G. Jones
Department of Physiology
Monash University

Jon H. Kaas
Department of Psychology
Vanderbilt University

Harvey J. Karten
Department of Psychiatry and
Behavioral Science
State University of New York
School of Medicine

L. Nicholas Leibovic
Neurosciences Research Program

Simon LeVay
Department of Neurobiology
Harvard Medical School

Jennifer S. Lund
Department of Ophthalmology
University of Washington School
of Medicine

Brenda A. Milner
Montreal Neurological Institute

Mortimer Mishkin
Laboratory of Psychology
National Institute of Mental
Health

Vernon B. Mountcastle
Department of Physiology
The Johns Hopkins University
School of Medicine

Walle J. H. Nauta
Department of Psychology
Massachusetts Institute of
Technology

Pasko Rakic
Yale University School of
Medicine

Francis O. Schmitt
Neurosciences Research Program

David A. Taylor
Merck Institute of Therapeutic
Research

Edward L. White
Department of Anatomy
Boston University School
of Medicine

Frederic G. Worden
Neurosciences Research Program

Name Index

Chapters in this volume are indicated by inclusive pages in boldface; discussions, by inclusive pages in italic.

Adams, J. C., 48, 167
Adelman, G., 567
Adrian, E. D., *376*
Aghajanian, G. K., 126, 348, 349, 363
Akert, K., 70, 461
Alexander, S. E., 464
Allman, J. M., 163, 286, 396, 397, 398, 408
Andén, N. E., 389
Andersen, P., 128, 137
Anderson, J. A., 480, 481, 487
Andres, P. F., 360
Angevine, J. B., Jr., 9
Antanitus, D. B., 13
Antonini, A., 431, 433, 434
Arbib, M. A., 109, *273–274*, 548
Arduini, A., 462
Armstrong-James, M., 126
Artyukhina, N. I., 136
Ary, M., 43
Asanuma, H., 219
Atencio, F. W., 418

Barbas, H., 418
Bard, P., *238–239*, 442
Barlow, H. B., 506, 515, 527, 537
Battig, K., 84
Baumann, T. P., 418, 419, 425, 426, 430
Beach, D. H., 50
Bear, M. F., 303
Beauchamp, M., 444
Beaudet, A., *130–131*, 348
Beck, J., 506
Begleiter, H., 442
Belcher, G., 365
Belford, G. R., 214

Ben-Ari, Y., 462
Bender, D. B., 403, 406
Benevento, L. A., 300, 301
Bennett, M. V. L., 141
Berger, B., 348
Berger, H., *375*, 376
Berkley, M. A., 426, 431
Berlucchi, G., **415–440**, 424, 426, 427, 428, 431, 433, 567
Berry, M., 9
Berson, D. M., **285–319**, 286, 288, 291, 299, 300, 301, 302, 303, 304, 306, 308–309, 311
Betz, V. A., *264*
Bianchi, L., 69
Bienenstock, E., 500
Bilge, M., 163
Birdsall, T. G., 444
Bishop, G., *375*
Bishop, P. O., 165, 166, 288, 426, 434
Bjorklund, A., 362
Blake, R., 434
Blakemore, C., 30, 42, 405, 435, 492, 500
Blinkov, S. M., 126, 127
Bliss, T. V. P., 50
Block, H. D., 480
Bloom, F. E., 126, 131, **323–324**, 326, 338, 348, 350, 351, 353, **359–370**, 360, 362, 363, 364, 459, 460, 567
Bodian, D., 78
Bodis-Wollner, I., *379*
Boothe, R. G., 43, 109, 112, 113, 115, 116, 139, 180, 206
Borghi, C., 365
Boulder Committee, 8n
Boycott, B. B., 167

Braak, H., 408

Brackenbury, R., 545

Brand, S., 86

Braun, J. J., 418, 426

Bremer, F., 461

Brindley, G. S., 418, 560

Broadbent, D. E., 455

Brodmann, K., 9, 10, 163

Brookhart, J. M., 462

Brooks, V. B., *280*

Brown, M., 365

Brown, R. M., 92

Brugge, J. F., 47, 90

Buchtel, H. A., 419, 426, 431

Bugbee, N., 77

Buisseret, P., 492, 493, 494

Bullier, J., 206, 220

Bullock, T. H., 539

Bunney, B. S., 349, 363

Burnstock, G., 352, 353

Burr, D. C., 517, 527, 528

Burton, H., 47, 203, 204, 205, 207, 210, 214, 216

Burton, M. J., 406

Busbaum, A. I., 546

Butcher, L. L., 85

Butler, A. B., 119, 171

Butters, N., 71

Camarda, R. M., 164

Caminiti, R., 25

Campbell, A., Jr., 424

Campbell, A. W., 163

Campbell, F. W., 409, 417, 531

Carey, R. G., 303

Carman, J. B., 84

Carpenter, M. B., 84

Catsman-Berrevoets, C. E., 201

Caviness, V. S., 21

Caviness, W. F., 78

Celesia, G. G., 390, 459

Chambers, B. E. I., 435

Champagnat, J., 365

Champlain, J. de, 390

Changeux, J.-P., 25, 545

Chapman, R. M., 459

Chavis, D. A., 461

Cheron, G., 444, 447, 455

Chiba, M., 177

Choi, B. H., 13

Chow, K. L., 70

Chung, S. H., 50, 545

Cicerone, C. M., 53, 60

Clanachan, A. S., 353

Clark, G., 407

Clarke, E., *264*

Clarke, P. G. H., 41

Cleland, B. G., 167

Clemente, C. D., 461

Cohen, L., 448

Colburn, T. R., 266

Cole, M., 406

Colman, D. R., 48

Colonnier, M., *102*, 106, 108, 109, **125–152,** 130, 131, 132, 133, 138, 139, 141, 142, 143, 404, 567

Constantine-Paton, M., **47–67,** 48, 50, 51, 53, 54, 55, 567

Cooke, J., 545

Cooper, L. N, *477–478,* **479–503,** 480, 483, 488, 489, 490, 491, 492, 495, 497, 498, 499, 500, 501, 537, *538– 539,* 550, 560, 567

Cornwell, P., 424

Correa, F. M. A., 365

Cotman, C. W., 89, 329

Coulter, J. D., 73, 90, 207, 208, 209, 211, 213, 214, 223, 246, *271, 272,* 447

Courchesne, E., 458

Cowan, J. D., 538

Cowan, W. M., **xi–xxi,** 50, 84, **101– 103,** 537, 538, 545, 567

Cowey, A., *374,* **395–413,** 396, 397, 400, 402, 404, 406, 407, 515, 541, 567

Coyle, J. T., 131, 363

Cracco, R. Q., 444

Cragg, B. G., 43, *126,* 127, 310

Crick, F. H. C., 477, **505–533,** 567

Csillik, B., 25

Cuello, A. C., 365

Cullen, A. M., 126

Cunningham, T. J., 25, 89

Currie, J., 50

Curtis, D. R., 361

Cynader, M., 165

Dahlström, A., 348

Daly, J. W., 352

D'Amato, C. J., 21, 89

Danchin, A., 25, 545

Daniel, P. M., 163, *396,* 401, 515

Danta, G., 406

Davidson, N., 328

Davies, J., 365

Davies-Jones, G. A. B., 406

Davis, T. L., 183

Dean, P., 406
Debecker, J., 442, 443, 445, 446, 447, 449, 450, 451, 452, 453, 455, 456, 457, 459, 461, 462, 463, 464
Deecke, L., 442, 443, 452
DeGroot, D., 126
DeLong, M. R., *280–281*
Dempsey, E. W., 379
Dennis, S. G., 567
Denny-Brown, D., 69, *265*
Descarries, L., *130–131*, 348
Desmedt, J., *374*, **441–473**, 442, 443, 444, 445, 446, 447, 448, 449, 450, 451, 452, 453, 454, 455, 456, 457, 458, 459, 460, 461, 462, 463, 464, 567
Detwiler, P. B., 528
DeVito, J. L., 84
Dews, P. B., 425
Diamond, I. T., 383, 418
Diamond, M. C., 127, 137
Diamond, T., 303
Dillier, N., 362, 363
Di Stefano, M., 427
Divac, I., 84, 328, 362, 459
Doane, B., 386
Dockray, G. J., 334
Dodd, J., 331, 334
Donaldson, H. H., 126
Donchin, E., 442, 443, 445, 447, 448, 449, 452, 459
Dostrovsky, J. O., 546
Doty, R. W., 116, 418, 419, 426
Dow, B. M., 116, 153
Dray, A., 365
Dreher, B., 166
Dreyer, D. A., 239
Droogleever-Fortuyn, J., 378
Dubin, M. W., 167
Durkovic, R. G., 166
Dye, P., 71
Dykes, R. W., 257, 258

Easter, S. S., Jr., 53, 56, 60
Ebner, F. F., 130, 131, 142, 143
Eccles, J. C., 128, 137, 205, 447
Edelman, G. M., 16, 409, **477–478**, **535–563**, 536, 537, 538, 539, 541, 543, 544, 545, 550, 553, 559, 567
Edwards, S. B., 164, 168
Eggars, D., 546
Egger, M. D., 256
Ellis, C. M., 396

Emson, P. C., 112, 229, *323*, **325–345**, 325, 326, 331, 337, 338, 360, 364, 365, 459, 567
Engberg, I., 389
Enroth-Cugell, C., 167, 168
Erlanger, B. F., *375*
Estevez, O., 443
Ettlinger, G., 405
Evarts, E. V., *196–197*, **263–283**, 265, 266, 267, 268, 276, 277, 279, *280*, 383, *387*, 388, *389*, 567

Faiers, A. A., 348
Fairén, A., 108, 111, 138, 139, 145, 154, 156, 157, 157, 326, 328
Falck, B., 325
Feldman, M., 142, 143, 154, 205
Feldman, M. L., 331, 333, 336
Felleman, D. J., 240, 251
Ferrier, D., 69, 264
Ferster, D., 113, 169, 177, 183, 184, 205, 217
Filimonov, I. N., 69
Finlay, B. L., 108, 116, 119, 165
Finley, J. C. W., 365
Fiore, L., 25, 138
Fischer, B., 116, 403
Fisken, R. A., 134, 141, 142, 404
Fite, K., 48
Fitzpatrick, D., 303
Flechsig, P., 11
Fleshman, J. W., Jr., 203
Fonnum, F., 328, 360
Foote, S. L., 362, 364
Ford, J. M., 448
Fraisse, P., 457
Frank, E., 167
Franz, S. I., 69
Frederickson, R. C. A., 350
Fredholm, B. B., 353
Freedman, R., 352, 362, 364
Freedman, S. L., 47
Freeman, D. C., 75
Freeman, R. D., 492
Frégnac, Y., 492, 493, 494, 497
Friedman, D. P., 217
Fritsch, G., 69, *263–264*
Fromm, C., 265, 268
Fujii, M., 293
Fukuda, Y., 167
Fulton, J. F., 69
Fuster, J. M., 461
Fuxe, K., 84, 348, 365

Galambos, R., 444, 452, 456
Gale, J. S., 365
Galkin, T. W., 22, 76, 79, 92
Gall, W. E., 545
Ganz, L., 425, 426
Garey, L. G., 30, 42, 132, 134, 138,
    141, 142, 143, 164, 299, 404
Gary-Bobo, E., 493, 494
Gasser, H. S., *375*
Gatter, K. C., 141, 363
Gauthier, L., 387, 389
Gautier-Smith, P. C., 418
Gaze, R. M., 50, 60
Gepts, W., 334
Giachetti, A., 331
Gibson, A., 177
Giese, S. C., 511, 531
Gilbert, C. D., *103*, 109, 119, 138, 142,
    143, **163–191**, 164, 165, 166, 167,
    168, 169, 171, 174, 177, 180, 184,
    201, 206, 220, 228, 299, 567
Giordano, D. L., 25
Giorguieff, M. F., 360
Glass, I., 546
Glass, L., 560
Glendenning, K. K., 286
Glezer, I. I., 126, 127
Gloor, P., 375
Glowinski, J., 360
Goldman-Rakic (Goldman), P. S., 22,
    25, 47, **69–97,** 71, 72, 73, 76, 77, 79,
    82, 84, 85, 86, 87, 88, 89, 90, 91, 92,
    174, 567
Goldring, S., 460
Golterman, N. R., 334
Goodin, D. S., 458
Goodman, H., *239*, 246, *252–253*, 270
Gordon, B., 427
Gould, H. J., 47
Grafstein, B., 22, 30
Grant, G., 47
Gray, E. G., 106, *127–128*, 137
Graybiel, A. M., 47, 85, **195–198,**
    197–198, **285–319,** 286, 288, 291,
    299, 300, 301, 302, 303, 304, 306,
    308, 311, 568
Greengard, P., 459
Greenough, W. T., 126
Gregory, R. L., 407
Grimson, E., 506
Groenewegen, H. J., 47
Gross, C. G., 403, 406, 428
Gruen, E., 363
Gudden, B., 153

Guillery, R. W., 167
Gummow, L., 427

Hall, W. C., 418
Halliday, A. M., 443
Hamberger, A., 329, 460
Hamlyn, L. H., 128
Hamori, J., 128
Hamsher, K. deS., 406
Hand, P. J., 77, 214
Hara, K., 424
Harlow, J. M., 69
Harris, J., 418
Harris, W. A., 167
Harvey, A. R., 119
Hassler, R., 167
Hayden, L. J., 336
Heath, C. J., 309
Hebb, D. O., 489, 560
Hecox, K., 444
Hedqvist, P., 353
Held, R., 435
Hendrickson, A. E., 47, 117, 119, 120,
    313
Hendry, S. H. C., 73, 90, 203, 246,
    271, 272, 447
Henn, F. A., 460
Henneman, E., 269
Henry, G. H., 119, 206, 220
Hersch, S. M., 154
Hewes, C. R., 350
Hickey, J. C., 47
Hicks, S. P., 21, 89
Hildreth, E., 511, 513, 514, 523, 530,
    531
Hillyard, S. A., 443, 448, 449, 452,
    453, 455, 456, 458, 464
Hilton, R. C., 406
Hiorns, R. W., 132, 138, 139
Hirsch, H., 326
Hirsch, H. V. B., 164, 326, 425, 426,
    434, 492
Hitzig, E., 69, *263–264*
Hodge, C. G., 85
Hodgkin, A. L., 528
Hoeltzell, P. B., 257, 258
Hoffman, K. P., 167, 183
Hökfelt, T., 336, 338, 358, 365
Hollander, H., 164
Hollyfield, J. G., 50, 59
Holmes, G., *396*, 406
Holmqvist, B., 137
Homskaya, E. D., 461
Hope, R. A., 60

Hore, J., *280*
Horne, M. K., 273
Hosli, E., 360
Hosli, L. P., 360
Hubel, D. H., 22, 24, **29–45**, 29, 30,
    31, 34, 41, 47, 48, 59, 60, 73, 75, 77,
    78, 81, 90, 113, 114, 115, 116, 117,
    119, 153, 163, 164, 165, 169, 171,
    174, 177, 183, 206, 211, 214, 220,
    226, 252, 286, 293, 361, 379, 403,
    405, 417, 419, 425, 426, 443, 492,
    531, 540
Hughes, H. C., 418, 419
Humphrey, A., 113
Hunt, R. K., 59
Hunt, S. P., 112, 229, *323*, **325–345**,
    364

Imbert, M., 492, 493, 494, 497
Imig, T. J., 47, 90
Ingham, C. A., 127
Ingle, D., 56
Innis, R. B., 365
Innocenti, G. M., 24–25, 138
Ito, M., 205
Itoh, H., 290
Iversen, L. L., 326, 329, 330
Iwama, K., 348
Iwamura, Y., 272

Jackson, H., *263*
Jacobsen, C. F., 69
Jacobson, M., 50, 53, 59, 60
Jacobson, S., 71, 329
Jane, J. A., 119, 171, 418
Jankowska, E., 166, 389
Jasper, H. H., **373–374**, **375–393**, 376,
    378, 380, 381, 382, 383, 384, 385,
    386, 390, 459, 568
Jewett, D. L., 444
Jhamandas, K. H., 353
Johns, A., 353
Johnson, F. R., 126
Johnson, R. E., 127
Johnson, T. N., 84
Johnston, G. A. R., 361
Jones, D. G., 126
Jones, E. G., 21, 47, 73, 90, 109, 132,
    134, 137, 138, *139*, 141, 142, *174*,
    195, **199–235**, 201, 203, 205, 206,
    207, 208, 209, 210, 211, 212, 213,
    214, 216, 217, 218, 219, 221, 222,
    223, 224, 225, 226, 227, 228, 229,

246, 270, 271, 272, 299, 309, 310,
    418, 447, 455, 461, 568
Jones, G., 364
Joosten, H. W. J., 338
Jordan, L. M., 348
Judge, S. J., 405
Jukes, M. G. M., 389

Kaas, J. H., 163, *195–196*, 219, **237–**
    261, 239, 240, 241, 242, 247, 251,
    252, 253, 256, 257, 258, 286, 396,
    397, 408, 447, 568
Kaiserman-Abramof, I. R., 132, 134,
    136
Kalaska, J., 256
Kalia, M., 287
Kalil, K., 84, 85
Kandel, E. R., 137, 481, 489
Karlsen, R. L., 360
Karten, H. J., 568
Kasamatsu, T., 43
Kato, H., 166
Kato, M., 276
Katz, A. M., 350
Kawamura, K., 177, 286, 303
Keating, M. J., 50
Kelly, J. P., 164, 166, 167, 169, 174,
    177, 180, 185, 201, *220*
Kelly, J. S., 331, 334
Kelovic, Z., 13
Kemel, M. L., 360
Kemp, J. A., 404
Kemp, J. M., 84
Kemper, T. L., 78
Kennedy, C., 77, 119, 221
Kennedy, M. B., 167
Kerkhof, G. A., 449
Kievit, J., 71
Killackey, H. P., 214, 418
Kimmel, J. R., 336
Kinston, W. J., 288
Kirchberger, M. A., 350
Kirkpatrick, J. R., 331, 365
Kitai, S. T., 166
Knapp, H., 48
Knight, B. W., Jr., 480
Knott, J. R., 442, 457
Kobayashi, R. M., 365
Kohonen, T., 481, 488, 559
Kollros, J. J., 50
Konno, T., 177
Kornhuber, H. H., 276, 442, 443, 452
Kostopoulas, G. K., 349, 352

Kostovic, I., 13, 79.
Knyihar, E., 25
Krettek, J. E., 311
Krishnamurti, A., 257
Krisst, D. A., 131
Kristeva, R., 276
Krmpotic-Nemanic, J., 13
Krnjević, K., 328, 348, 360, 361, 365, 459
Kuffler, S. W., 167, 373
Kuhar, M. J., 329, 348, 365
Künzle, H., 71, 84, 85
Kuo, J. F., 459
Kuroda, Y., 353
Kutas, M., 443, 445, 449, 452
Kuypers, H. G. J. M., 71, 78, 201, *264*, 270, 310, 403

LaGrutta, G., 460
Lake, N., 348
Lam, D. M. K., 22, 30, 47, 117
Lamont, P., 138
Lamport, L., 543
Landgren, S., 47
Landmesser, L., 545
Lapham, L. W., 13
Lapierre, Y., *130–131*
La Raia, P. J., 350
Larsson, L. I., 336
Lashley, K. S., 407, *480–481*
Law, M. I., 48, 50, 51, 53, 54, 55
Lázár, G., 48, 50
Lee, T. P., 459
Le Gros Clark, W. E., 515
Leibovic, L. N., 568
Lekić, D., 365
Lemon, R. N., 273
Lepore, F., 431
Lettvin, J. Y., 54
LeVay, S., 24, 25, **29–45**, 30, 31, 33, 34, 41, 42, 43, 47, 48, 59, 60, 73, 78, 81, 90, 106, 108, 109, 113, *132*, 134, 138, *139*, 142, 143, 164, 167, 168, 169, 177, 183, 184, 205, 206, 211, 217, 299, 515, 568
Leventhal, A. G., 164
Levey, N. H., 418
Levick, W. R., 167
Levine, R. L., 48, 53, 61
Levitt, P., 348, 363
Lewin, W., 418
Lewis, M. S., 338
Liberman, F., 495, 497, 498, 499, 500, 501

Libet, B., *445*, *449*, *548*
Lidov, H. G. W., 338, 363
Light, A. R., 166
Limacher, J. J., 352, 365
Lin, C.-S., 255
Lindsley, D. B., 442
Lindström, S. H., 47, 169
Lindvall, O., 325, 326, 337, 338, 348, 360, 362, 459
Livett, B. G., 365
Ljungdahl, A., 338
Llinas, R., 137
Logan, B. F., Jr., *529–531*
Lømo, T., 137
Loren, I., 336
Lorente de Nó, R., 73, 109, 163, 171, 180, 201, 220
Low, M. D., 458
Løyning, Y., 128
Lund, J. S., 89, *102*, **105–124**, 106, 108, 109, 111, 112, 113, 115, 116, 117, 118, 119, 138, 139, 141, 142, 163, 164, 171, 174, 180, 201, 205, 206, 229, 568
Lund, R. D., 21, 53, 54, 82, 89, 106, 108, 109, 115, 139, 142
Lundberg, A., *389–390*
Luria, A. R., 461
Lynch, G., 89

Maeda, T., 304
Maffei, L., 405, 417
Malmgren, L., 167
Manil, J., 442, 445, 447, 450, 456, 463
Manning, F., 406
Marin-Padilla, M., *139*, 225, 227
Marr, D. C., 409, 477, **505–533**, *505–506*, 510, 511, 513, 514, 530, 531, 536, 548
Marshall, W. H., *238–239*, 442
Marzi, C. A., 427
Mascetti, G. G., 426
Mason, R., 288
Mates, S., 108, 111, 112, 113
Matthews, B. H. C., *376*
Matthews, W. B., 444
Maturana, H. R., 54
McCallum, W. C., 442, 457, 462
McCarthy, G., 445, 449
McDonald, W. I., 443
McGeer, P. L., 328
McIlwain, H., 353, 363, 481
McKee, S. P., 506, 507, 527
McLaughlin, B. J., 108, 130

McLennan, H., 132
McNaughton, P. A., 528
Meadows, J. C., 406
Megelhaes-Castro, B., 177, 418
Megelhaes-Castro, H. H., 177
Mendelson, M. J., 92
Merzenich, M. M., **237–261,** *239*, 241,
    245, 246, 248, 249, 251, *252–253,*
    255, 256, 258, 270
Mesulam, M.-M., 167, 310, 459
Mettler, F. A., 70
Meyer, D. R., 419
Meyer, P. M., 419
Meyer, R., 53, 56, 60
Meyer-Lohmann, J., *280*
Michael, C. R., 116
Michel, F., 444
Millar, J., 546
Miller, B. F., 53, 54
Miller, J. W., 300, 301
Millhouse, O. E., 461
Milner, B., 407, 461, 568
Miner, M., 417
Miner, N., 428
Minsky, M., 480
Minzuno, N., 290
Miselis, R. R., 77
Mishkin, M., 84, 406, 428, 567
Mishra, R. K., 363
Mitchell, D. E., 492
Mitchell, E. D., 82
Mize, R. R., 418
Mogenson, G. J., 348
Møllgaard, K., 126
Mollon, J. D., 406
Molliver, M., 79
Molliver, M. E., 79, 131, 338, 363
Montero, V. M., 396
Moore, D. T., 418
Moore, R. Y., 348, 362, 363, 459, 460
Mora, F., 406
Morison, R. S., 379
Morkin, E., 350
Morrison, J. H., *131,* 363
Moruzzi, G., 461, 462
Moskovitz, N., 132, 134, 138, 139
Mountcastle, V. B., 16, 73, *101,* 211,
    213, 214, 220, 226, *239,* 252, 309,
    339, 373, 447, 538, 540, 546, 547, 568
Movshon, J. A., 435, 500
Moxley, G. F., 25
Muller, J. E., 334
Munro, P., 500
Murphy, E. H., 418

Murray, E. H., 223
Musgrave, F. S., 447
Mushkin, J., 443
Mutt, V., 329
Myers, R. E., 417, 427, 428

Nakamura, S., 348
Näsänen, R., 397
Nass, M. M., 488, 491, 539
Nathanson, J. A., 350
Nauta, W. J. H., 25, 47, 70, 71, 73, 77,
    84, 90, 119, 171, *198,* 461, 568
Neff, W. D., 383
Nelson, R. J., **237–261,** 240, 250, 251,
    253, 256, 257
Newman, J. D., 464
Nicholson, C., 137
Niimi, K., 303
Nikara, T., 165
Nilsson, G., 338
Nishihara, H. K., 505, 529, 530
Noël, P. 447
Nonneman, A. J., 424
Norris, F. H., 350
Nowakowski, R. S., 12
Nunes-Cardozo, J., 126

O'Boyle, D. J., 406
O'Brien, R. A. D., 545
Ogren, M. P., 47, 117, 313
Oja, E., 495, 497, 498, 499, 500, 501
O'Leary, J. L., 109, 163, 171, 180
Oliver, A. P., 364
Olson, L., 84
Olsson, Y., 167
O'Malley, C. D., *264*
Orban, G. A., 166
Oscarsson, O., 47, 258
Östberg, A. J. C., 545
Otsuka, R., 167
Otto, D. A., 442

Palay, S. L., 108, 136
Palmer, L. A., 119, 163, 164, 165, 166,
    168, 177, 205, 220, 286, 287, 293,
    304, 396, 418, 419, 420, 427
Pandya, D. N., 71, 246, 270, *271–272,*
    310, 363, 455, 461
Papert, S., 480
Parnavelas, J. G., 132, 138, 139
Pasek, P., 418, 419
Pasek, T., 418, 419
Patel, H. H., 361, 362, 404
Paton, D. M., 353

Paul, D. D., 449
Paul, R. L., *239*, 246, *252–253*, 270
Paxinos, G., 365
Pearlman, A. L., 396
Pearson, R. C. A., 246
Peck, C. K., 426
Penfield, W., 376
Perachio, A., 47
Perez, R., 560
Peronnet, F., 444
Pert, C. B., 331
Peters, A., 108, 111, 132, 134, *136*, 138, 139, 142, 143, 145, 154, 156, 157, 184, 205, 326, 328, 331, 333, 336
Petrusz, P., 336
Pettigrew, J. D., 43, 165, 405, 492
Phillips, C. G., 228, *264–265*, *269–270*
Phillis, J. W., 331, 348, *349*, 350, 352, 353, 365
Picton, T. W., 443, 449, 453, 455, 464
Pilar, G., 545
Pinget, M., 365
Poggio, G. F., 116, 214, 309, 403
Poggio, T., 409, 477, **505–533**, 505, 506, 510, 514, 530, 536, 548, 549
Poliakov, G. I., 8, 11
Pollack, H. G., 336
Pollack, J. G., 47
Pollen, D. A., 378, 385, 417
Pomeranz, B., 256
Porrino, K., 72
Porter, J., 406
Porter, R., 47, 207, 210, *264–265*
Potter, H. D., 48
Powell, T. P. S., 47, 84, 130, 132, 134, 136, *137*, 138, 139, 141, 142, 143, 164, 207, 211, 213, 226, *239*, 246, 270, *271*, 299, 310, 363, 404, 447, 455, 461, 515
Preobrazhenskaya, N. S., 11
Presson, J., 427
Pribram, K. H., 70
Price, J. L., 25, 311
Proskauer, C. C., *136*, 156
Pull, I., 353
Purpura, D. P., 447

Ragsdale, C. W., 85
Rakic, P., **3–5**, **7–28**, 8, 9, 10, 11, 12, 13, 14, 16, 19, 21, 22, 23, 24, 27, 28, *30*, 40, 59, 78, 79, 81, 86, 91, 568
Rall, T. W., 352
Rall, W., 126

Ramachandran, V. S., 41
Ramón y Cajal, S., 13, 25, 109, 128, 137, 138, 139, 141, 163, 171, 180, 205, 214, 218, 228, 229, *311*
Randolph, M., *248*
Ransom, B. R., 460
Rasmussen, P. D., 257, 258
Rasted, J., 166
Ratcliff, G., 406, 407
Reader, T. A., 352, 396
Rebert, C. S., 458
Rehfeld, J., 334, 336
Reichardt, W., 549
Reits, D., 443
Reivich, M., 77
Ribak, C. E., 108, 130, 131, 141, 225, 226, 228, 325, 326, 360
Ricci, G. F., 386
Rice, F. L., 338, 363
Ridley, R. M., 405
Riss, W., 48
Ritchie, D. G., 419
Ritter, W., 444, 448, 451, 463
Rizzolatti, G., 164, 428
Robertson, D., 443, 445, 446, 449, 450, 451, 452, 453, 454, 455, 456, 458, 463, 464
Robins, E. R., 326
Robson, J. G., 167, 168, 531
Rocha-Miranda, C. E., 403, 406
Rock, M. P., 157
Rockel, A. J., 47, 246, 515
Rodieck, R. W., 299
Rogers, A. W., 9
Røigaard-Petersen, H., 334
Rojas, A., 396
Rolls, E. T., 397, 402, 405, 406
Romano, N. N., 444
Ropollo, J. R., 220, 239
Rose, D., 166
Rose, J. E., 310
Rosen, I., 258
Rosenblatt, F., 480
Rosene, D. L., 310, 363
Rosenquist, A. C., 119, 163, 164, 165, 168, 177, 205, 220, 286, 287, 293, 304, 396, 418, 419, 420, 427
Roskoski, R., 360
Ross, J., 517
Rossignol, S., 142, *387*, 389
Rosvold, H. E., 84
Roth, R. H., 348
Rothstein, T. B., 406
Rovamo, J., 397

Rowe, M. H., 167, 168
Rowland, V., 459
Royce, J. G., 84
Ruchkin, D. S., 449, 459
Ruiz-Marcos, A., 112
Runnels, L. K., 421
Runnels, P., 421
Rutishauser, U., 545
Ryall, R. W., 365, 389

Sachs, J. G., 406
Sahin, K., 543
Said, S. I., 329, 331, 365
Saito, K., 108
Sakata, H., 272
Saldanha, J., 142, 154, 157, 205
Saletu, B., 445
Salhanda, J., 142
Sanghera, M. K., 405
Sanides, F., 257
Saraiva, P. E. S., 177
Sas, E., 404
Sattin, A., 352
Sawynok, J., 353
Scalia, F., 48
Schilder, P., 418, 419
Schiller, P. H., 108, 116, 119, 165
Schmechel, D. E., 13, 14
Schmidt, J. T., 53, 56, 60
Schmitt, F. O., 568
Schneider, 53, 54, 89
Scholes, J. H., 545
Schubert, P., 353
Schutta, H. S., 406
Schwartz, A., 364
Schwartz, B. E., 351
Schwartz, T., 506
Schwent, V. L., 452, 456
Schwob, J. E., 25
Scott, T. M., 50
Seacord, L., 428
Segraves, M. A., 303
Seiger, A., 84
Semmes, J., 70, *248*
Sétáló, G., 48
Shagass, C., 376
Shanks, M. F., 47, 246
Shannon, C., 523, 524, 526
Sharbrough, F. W., 444
Sharma, S. C., 56, 59, 60
Sharpless, S., 380, 381, 382, 383
Shatz, C. J., 22n, 24, 30, 33, 41, 47, 48,
    59, 82, 169, 202, 427
Shatz, C., 22n, 202, 427

Shepherd, G. M., 339, 348
Sherman, S. M., 167, 426
Shlaer, R., 560
Shofer, R. J., 447
Sholl, D. A., 201
Shumway, W., 48
Sidman, R. L., 8, 9, 21
Signeau, J. C., 334
Silfvenius, H., 47
Silinsky, E. M., 353
Sillito, A. M., 186, 361, 362, 404
Simoni, A., 427
Simons, D. J., 156
Simson, R., 448, 449, 451, 463
Singer, W., 165, 426
Skinner, J. E., 460, 461, 462, 464
Sloper, J. J., 130, 132, 134, 136, *137*,
    138, 139, 141, 142, 143
Small, D. G., 444
Smith, C. G., 127
Smith, D. E., 132, 134, 138, 139
Smith, L. M., 142, 143
Smith, O. A. S., 84
Snyder, M., 418
Snyder, S. H., 329, 365
So, K. F., 53, 54
Sohol, G. S., 545
Sokoloff, L., 77, 339
Somjen, G. G., 13, 460
Somogyi, P., 106, 108, 109, 111, 138,
    145, 229
Spatz, W. B., 118, 171
Spear, P. D., 418, 419, 425, 426, 430
Specht, S. C., 30
Spekereijse, H., 443
Spencer, W. A., 137
Sperry, R. W., 60, *417*, 428, 458
Spinelli, D. N., 492
Sprague, J. M., 303, **415–440**, 418,
    419, 420, 424, 426, 431, 433
Squires, K. C., 449, 457
Squires, N. A., 449
Stamm, J., 428
Stanfield, B., 89
Starr, A., 444, 457
Stefanis, C., *384*, 385
Stein, B. E., 418
Steinbusch, H. W. M., 338
Steriade, M., 386
Sterling, P., 132, 138, 143, 183, 418
Sterman, M. B., 461
Sternberger, L. A., 325
Stockard, J. J., 444
Stone, J., 167, 168, 183

Stone, L. S., 59
Stone, T. W., *323–324*, **347–357**, 329, 348, 349, 350, 351, 352, 353, 360, 362, 459
Storm-Mathisen, J., 328, 329, 330
Straus, E., 365
Straznicky, K., 50
Strick, P. L., 132, 138, 143, *280*
Sulakhe, P. V., 353
Sur, M., **237–261**, 240, 248, 251, 252, 253, 254, 256, 257
Sutherland, N. S., 404
Sutton, S., 442, 447, 448, 449, 459
Stryker, M. P., 24, 25, 30, 33, 41, 42, 43, 48, 59, 77, 119, 169, 226
Swets, J. A., 444
Swift, S. J., 459
Symmes, D., 464
Symonds, L., 299, 304
Székely, G., 48, 59
Szerb, J. C., 459
Szentágothai, J., 109, 115, 128, 139, 141, 171, 205, 221, 225, 228, 229, 447

Tada, M., 350
Talbot, W. H., 116
Tanaka, D., 71
Tanji, J., 276, 277, 279, *280*, *387*, 388, *389*
Tanner, W. P., 444
Tassin, J. P., 363
Taylor, A. C., 51
Taylor, D. A., *323–324*, **347–357**, 348, 349, 350, 351, 352, 353, 362, 459, 568
Taylor, D. P., 331
Taylor, J. H., 417
Tennyson, V. M., 84
Teuber, H.-L., 407
Thach, W. T., *280*
Thierry, A. M., 348, 363
Thiery, J.-P., 545
Thompson, R., 421, 430
Tieman, S. B., 426
Tigges, J., 47, 171
Tigges, M., 47, 171
Tomböl, T., 132, 138, 139
Torrealba, F., 396
Tovsky, N. J., 71
Towe, A. L., 456
Toyama, K., 164, 174
Tracey, D. J., 273
Treisman, A., 455
Tremblay, J. P., 132
Tretter, F., 165

Trojanowski, J. Q., 71
Tueting, P., 448
Tunkl, J. E., 432
Turlejski, K., 183
Tusa, R. J., 163, 286, 287, 293, 304, 396, 420, 427

Uchizono, K., 108, *128–129*
Udin, S., 60
Uhl, G., 365
Ullman, S., 505, 506, 513, 530
Ungerstedt, U., 348
Updyke, B. V., 288, 301, 307
Uttal, W. R., 539, 540

Vadas, M. A., 288
Vale, W., 365
Valverde, F., 106, 112, 163, 180, 205, 221, 222, 228, 229
van der Burg, J., 273
Vanderhaegen, J. J., 334
Van Essen, D. C., 112, 163, 166, 169, 177, 185, *220*, 286
Van Hoesen, G. W., 71, 84, 310, 459
Van Sluyters, R. C., 30, 42, 492, 500
van Winkle, T., 214
Varon, S. S., 13
Vaughan, H. G., 444, 448, 449, 451, 463
Vaughn, J. E., 108
Verhofstad, A. A. J., 338
Vignolo, L. A., 455
Virsu, V., 397
Vital-Durand, F., 30, 42
Vogt, B. A., 246, *271–272*, 363
Vogt, C., 163
Vogt, O., 163
Volman, S. F., 108, 116, 119, 165
von der Malsburg, C., 560
von Economo, C., 126
Von Grünau, M. W., 426, 434
Voogd, J., 47
Voorhoeve, P. E., 128, 137
Vrbová, G., 545
Vrensen, G., 126

Wagor, N. M., 396
Walker, A. E., 70, 310
Wall, P. D., 256, 546
Walshe, F. M. R., *264*
Walter, W. G., 442, 457
Ward, J. P., 418
Warren, J. M., 424
Warrington, E. K., 406

Wassle, H., 167
Watkins, K. C., *130–131*, 348
Webster, H. de F., 108
Webster, K. E., 84
Weidman, T. A., 545
Weiskrantz, C., 418
Weiskrantz, L., 406
Welker, C., 210, 257
Welker, W. I., 257
Weller, R. E., 240, 257
Werner, G., 220, *239*
West, R. W., 126
Westheimer, G., 506, 507, 527
Westman, J., 166
Westrum, L. E., 136
White, E. L., *102*, 106, 138, 145, **153–161,** 154, 156, 205, 339, 568
Whitsel, B. L., 220, *239*
Whittaker, V., 523
Whitteridge, D., 41, 163, 287, **396,** 401, 515
Wickelgren, B. G., 418
Wiesel, T. N., 22, 24, **29–45,** 29, 30, 31, 34, 41, 47, 48, 59, 60, 73, 75, 77, 78, 81, 90, *103*, 109, 113, 114, 115, 116, 117, 119, 138, 153, **163–191,** 163, 164, 165, 166, 169, 171, 174, 177, 183, 206, 211, 214, 220, 226, 228, 252, 288, 293, 361, 379, 403, 405, 417, 419, 425, 426, 443, 492, 531, 540
Wikmark, G., 79
Williston, J. S., 444
Wilson, H. R., 511, 531, 538
Wilson, J. R., 47, 117, 119, 120
Wilson, P. D., 167, 168
Winans, S. S., 419
Winfield, D. A., 142
Wise, S. P., 21, 47, 201, 203, 204, 207, 208, 209, 210, 211, 212, 213, 214, 218, 223, 224, 246
Wofsey, A. R., 329
Wolfe, J. M., 435
Wollberg, Z., 546
Wood, C. C., 426
Woodward, D. J., 460
Woodworth, R. S., *274*
Woody, C. D., 351, 363
Woolsey, C. N., *238–239*, 240, 310, 442
Woolsey, T. A., 156
Worden, F. G., 568
Wurtz, R. H., 459

Yakovlev, P. I., 78
Yalow, R. S., 334, 365
Yamamura, H. I., 459
Yasargyl, G. M., 137
Yeterian, E. H., 84
Yingling, C. D., 461, 462, 464
Yoon, M. G., 60
Yoshii, N., 293

Zeki, S. M., 112, 163, 211, 286, 399, 403, 405, *406*, 517
Zieglgansberger, W., 365
Zubeck, J. P., 548
Zubin, J., 448

Subject Index

Ablation. *See also* Lesion studies;
  specific cones
  auditory cortex, 381–383
  receptive fields and, 418–419
  tectum, 51–59
  visual areas, 406
Abstraction, 487, 540–541
Acetylcholine (ACh), 351
Acetylcholinesterase (AChe), 290,
  338
Achromalopsia, 406
Acuity, 506–507
Adaptation, and development of
  logic, 487
Adenine nucleotides, 352, 353
Adenosine, 349
  interaction with norepinephrine,
  351, 352–353
Adenosine triphosphate. *See* ATP
β-Adrenergic blocking agents, 349
Afferent input
  to motor cortex, 270–273
  to neocortex, 337–338
  types of cortical, 167–169
Alerting response, 377
Alpha motoneuron loop, 270
Amino acid neurotransmission, 360–
  362
Amino acids, excitatory, 328–329
Amphibian retinotectal specificity,
  60–61
Amplification, 551, 554–557
Anatomical chemistry, cerebral cor-
  tex, 325–345
Anatomy
  cerebral cortex, 199–235
  cortical variation, 407–408
Animal logic, 487
Anterior commissure, 428
Anterograde degeneration, 142

"Antireflex" preprogrammed movements, 276–277
Apical dendrites, 113, 115, 447
Aplysia, 489
Area dentata, autoradiograph, 330
Area 17
  ablation studies, 419–435
  corticothalamic projections, 297
  neuron morphology, 105–109
  noncortical connections, 303–304
  primate visual cortex, 105–124
  zero-crossing segments and, 513
Area 19, crossover links, 306–308
Areal organization, of neocortex, developmental events leading to,
  7–28
Areal positions, acquisition of neocortical, 16–21
Areas 3a and 2, multiple representations in, 244–248
Areas 3b and 1,
  convergence in, 255–256
  double representation in, 241–244
  modular and microorganization of,
  252–255
Arousal reflex, 461
Arousal response, 377, 380–383, 543
Aspartate, 328–329, 360
Aspecific cells, 493–494
Association, in distributed memories,
  485–487
Association cortex
  development and plasticity of, 69–97
  monoamine distribution, 362–363
  new methods of studying, 70
  prenatal development, 81
  proximal and distal, 305–306
  and sensory, differences in columnar
  organization of, 73
  terminal fibers, 141–145

Associative memory, 489
Associative storage and recall, 539
Asymmetrical membrane differentiation, 130–141
Athalamic cortex, 310
ATP (adenosine triphosphate), 352
Atropine, 351, 352
Auditory cortex
  callosal columns in, 209
  habituation and, 381–383
Auditory evoked potentials (AEP), 444
Auditory signals, model of optical connections, 488
Averaging, ERPs, 443
Avian pancreatic polypeptide (APP), 336
Axon
  initial segment, 136
  LGN projections, 515
  pyramidal cell collaterals, 226–227
Axonal bundling, 212–219, 221
Axonal connections, neocortical, 285–286
Axonal regeneration, tectal, 51–54
Axonal resprouting, with monocular deprivation, 42

Ballistic movements, 274–275
Banding. See also Ocular-dominance columns
  determinants of, 59–61
  genesis of, 50–54
  in three-eyed frogs, 48–50
  width, 50–51
Band-pass channels, 511
Basal dendrites, 185
Basal ganglia, 280–281
Basket cell circuitry, 223–225
Betz cells, 264
Bicuculline, 361–362
Binocular interactions, 427–428, 431–435
Bradykinin, 365
Brain, compared to computers, 549
Brain damage, visual, 406–407
Brain function, higher
  group selection as basis for, 535–563
  role of cerebral cortex in, 371–473
Brain stem, focal pathology, 444
Branching, pyramidal cell, 226–228
Brightness discrimination, 423

Calcium flux, 350, 351

Callosal connections
  columnar organization, 207–212
  development and plasticity, 78–82
  laminar distribution, 207
  prefrontal, 75
  relationship to ipsilateral connections, 212
  relationship to thalamic connections, 210–211, 213
Callostomy, 209
Ca^{++}-Mg^{++} ATPase, 350
Cat
  auditory cortex, callosal columns in, 209
  cortical connections in, 144, 301–302
  extrastriate cortex, 292
  habituation of arousal response in, 380–383
  interhemispheric transfer in, 415–440
  LP-pulvinar complex, 288–290, 291, 295
  ocular-dominance columns, 33, 41
  reactive states, 389
  thalamic pathways, 297, 299, 304, 305
  visual cortex, 396
    ablation studies, 419–435
    laminar specialization, 163–191
    pyramidal cells, 133
    role of GABA in, 361
    stellate cells, 140
    synaptic contacts, 126, 128
    thalamic terminations, 205
Caudate nucleus, 84, 86–89
Cebus monkeys, 251
Cell. See also specific types
  death, 537
  differentiation, and neuronal origin, 11
  discharge, and surface rhythms, 383–386
  groups, tuning, 538
  modifiability, and visual experience, 494
  processes, in selection for circuitry, 537
  properties of in visual areas, 403–405
  specificity, and cognitive functions, 375–393
  specificity, retinotectal, 60–61
Central nervous system, distributed memory in, 479–503

Central programs, servo control and, 278–280
Centroparietal region, and P300s, 451
Cerebellar cortex, 201, 205, 280–281
Cerebello-thalamocortical pathway, 280
Cerebral cortex
  anatomical chemistry, 325–345
  chemical signaling and circuitry, 321–370
  electron microscopy, 125–152
  ERPs, and cognitive processing, 441–473
  functional microorganization, 99–192
  lesion studies, 416–417
  neurotransmission
    amino acid, 360–362
    monoaminergic, 348–349, 362–364
    peptidergic, 364–365
  neurotransmodulatory control, 347–357
  role in higher brain function, 371–473
  synaptic contacts in, 125–127
  in visual learning, memory, and interhemispheric transfer, 415–440
Chandelier cell, 109, 111, 228–229
Chemical signaling, and cortical circuitry, 359–370
Cholecystokinin (CCK), 334–336, 339–341, 365
Choline acetyltransferase (ChAT), 338
Circuitry
  basket cell, 223–225
  cerebral cortex, 229–230, 321–370
  cerebellar cortex, 205
  intrinsic, 199–235
  selection and, 537
  thalamocortical, 310–314
Class formation, in distributed systems, 488
Claustrum, 303
Cl conductance, 361
Closed-loop negative feedback, 273, 278–280
CLO theory, 495–501
Clustering, corticostriatal, 84
Cognition, sleep and, 379
Cognitive functions, and cellular or modular specificity, 375–393
Cognitive processing, and ERPs, 441–473
Colchicine, 334

Collateral branching, 226–228
Color, columnar arrangement for, 405
Columnar organization. See also
    Hypercolumns; Minicolumn;
    Modular organization; Ocular-dominance columns; Orientation columns; Vertical interactions
  within the cortex, 219–221
  corticocortical connections and, 73
  effect of lid suture on, 33–40
  input-output, in cerebral cortex, 199–235
  monkey visual field, 29–30
  normal development, 31–33
Columns
  callosal, 207–210
  input, as output columns, 221–223
  receptive field studies of, 252–253
  role of putative neurotransmitters and, 339–341
  and selection, 537
  synaptic modification and, 399–400
  as translators, 540
  V1, 404–405
Commissural connections, 141–145
Communication, internal neuronal, 489–490
Complex cells
  and directional specificity, 361–362
  intracortical pathways of, 183–184
  laminar distribution of, 165–166
Computer memories, 480
Computer model
  for selective recognition system, 550–560
  of visual system, 508–513
Computers, compared to human brain, 549
Conditional responses, 386–390
Congruent borders, 249–251
Connectivity, selective forces, 537–539
Consciousness, states of impaired, 379
Content-addressable memory, 544
Contingent negative variation (CNV), 458–459, 460, 461–462
Continuous distribution, computer model of, 508–513
Contrast sensitivity, 397
Convergence, cytoarchitectonic, 255–256
Convolution, 517–518
Corpus callosum, 24–25, 428–431

Corpus striatum, 331

Correlation, in group selection theory, 544

Cortex. *See* Cerebral cortex; Neocortex

Cortical
activity, during habituation, 380–383
cells, classification by visual stimuli, 493
circuitry, 229–230, 320–370
damage, 480
excitatory state, 375–379
function, impact of theoretical constructs and modeling of, 475–563
input-output columns, 221–223
lamination, 201–203
lesions, effect on pattern discrimination, 419–435
magnification, relation to receptive-field size, 251–252
maps, 256–257
organization, and anatomical chemistry, 339–341
organization, of monoamine afferents, 362–363
plate, 16–21
processing, 251–252, 310–314
surface rhythms, 383–386
synapses, 126–127
variation, 407–408
wiring diagram, 182

Corticocortical connections
adult organization, 73–77
and corticothalamic projections, 309
laminar terminations, 207
mode of development, 78–81
plasticity of, 81–82
of somatosensory cortex, 270

Corticofugal connections, classes of, 301–302

Corticospinal projections, 265

Corticostriatal connections, 82–89

Corticotectal terminations, 205

Corticothalamic projection, 290, 309, 547–548

Cortico-thalamo-cortical circuits, 296, 310–314

Critical period, for visual experience, 492–494

Cross-recognition, 557–559

Cyclic AMP
and ERPs, 459–460

interaction with norepinephrine, 350, 352
length of inhibition by, 349

Cyclic GMP, 350–352, 459–460

Cytoarchitectonic areas
electrophysiological properties, 246–248
as functionally distinct, 248
multiple representations hypothesis, 241–248
organization, 9–12, 125–124
receptor modalities, 271–272

Darwinian computer, 548–550, 560

Decision, and P300s, 447–452

Degeneracy, 540, 545–547

Degenerate recognition, 555

Degenerate systems, 536–538, 542–543

Degenerating terminals, 141–145

Dendrite
apical, 113, 115, 447
basal, 185
morphology, 106–109, 184–186
smooth and sparsely spined, 109–112

Dendritic field, intermediate interneuron, 221

Dendritic shaft, 134, 143–145

Dendritic spine
functional significance, 137
synaptic contacts on, 134, 135, 160
thalamocortical projections, 143

2-Deoxyglucose method, 77

Development
and circuitry, 537
cortical connections, 78–81, 85
neocortex, 7–28
and plasticity, evolution of neocortex and, 1–98
and plasticity, primate frontal association cortex, 69–97
selective aspects of, 545–546

Directional specificity, 361–362, 403, 405

Distance, columnar arrangement for, 405

Distributed mapping, 481–489

Distributed memory, 479–503

Distributed systems, 535–539, 542–543

L-Dopa, 390

Dopamine, 348–349, 362–363

Dorsal thalamus, 70–71. *See also* Lateral geniculate nucleus

Efferent connections, striate cortex, 301–302
Electrical activity, variations in, 491, 492
Electrical signals, and synaptic modification, 489
Electrical signs
  of cortical excitatory state, 375–379
  of reactive state, 387–390
Electroencephalogram (EEG), 376–377, 379, 380–383
Electromyogram (EMG), 275–276, 389
Electron microscopy, of cerebral cortex, 125–152
End inhibition, 166
  neural basis, 458–462
  study methodology, 449
  time features, 456
Enkephalin, 365
Epilepsy, 377–379
Event-related potentials (ERPs), in man,
  and cognitive processing, 441–473
  components, 443–458
  eliciting, and primary components, 443–444
  to faint skin stimuli, and liminal sensation, 444–447
Evolution
  neocortex, 1–98
  synaptic modification, 490
Excitation, 108, 130
  amino acid, 328–329, 360
  electrical signs of, 375–379
Extrageniculate thalamus, 288–293
Extrastriate cortex
  connections, 286–288
  families of, 304–308
  pattern recognition and, 418–419
  thalamocortical projections to, 293–296
Eye preference, cortical columns and, 163
Eye-specific termination bands, 51–53

Family clusters, 296–310
Far-field potentials, 444
Feedback, closed and open loop, 273–280
Fetal neurosurgery, 22

Firing rate, neuronal communication of, 489–490
5-HT. *See* Serotonin
Focal input, 212–219
Forebrain circuits, 312
Four-fingers paradigm, 447–458
Fovea eccentricity, 396–397
Frogs, banding in, 48–61
Frontal association cortex. *See also* Association Cortex; Prefrontal association cortex
  monoaminergic distribution in, 362–363
  new methods of studying, 70
  primate, development and plasticity of, 69–97
Frontoparietal cortex, lesion studies, 329
Functional organization, lesion studies and, 416–417
Functional studies, of motor cortex, 263–283

GABA (gamma-aminobutyric acid)
  as inhibitory neurotransmitter, 326, 360–361
  interaction with norepinephrine, 352
  membrane differentiation and, 130
  thalamic stimulation and, 339–341
GAD. *See* Glutamic acid decarboxylase
Ganglion cell, axonal specificity, 60–61
Gap junctions, 139
Gating system, 559
Geniculate family, 296–304
Geniculocortical pathway, 299
  development, 22–24, 31–33
  distribution of callosal fibers and, 82
  monkey, 29–30
  monocular deprivation and, 30–31
  parallels to eye-specific banding, 59–60
Geniculorecipient cortex, 296
Glial cells, 13–21, 460
Glutamate, 328–329, 360
Glutamic acid decarboxylase (GAD), 326, 360
  localization of, 130, 141
Goldfish, 53, 60–61
Gold-treated neurons, 154
Golgi-electron-microscope technique, 154

Golgi preparations, primate visual cortex, 105–124
Golgi type II cell, 228. *See also* Interneuron
Granule cell, 203, 271
Group selection, 535–563
Growth hormone-release-inhibiting factor, 336

Habituation, 380–383
Hemispheric transfer, pattern recognition and, 426–435
Hierarchical organization
  nested, 300–301
  neuronal, 153, 156–157
  somatosensory cortex, 272
Higher brain function
  group selection as basis for, 535–563
  role of cerebral cortex in, 371–473
  and surface slow waves, 385–386
Homotypical cortex, 541
Homunculus, 238–239
Horizontal interactions, 223–228
Horseradish-peroxidase labeling, 166–167
5-HT. *See* Serotonin
Human brain, compared to digital computers, 549
Hyperacuity, 506–507, 515, 516–517
Hypercolumn, 252, 404–405. *See also* Columnar organization
Hypercomplex cell, 166, 362
Hyperpolarization, 377–378, 385

Immature cells, 493–494
Immunoreactivity
  colchicine, 334
  GAD, 326–327
  VIP, 331
Inferotemporal cortex, 403, 406, 428
Information processing, 180, 399–403, 409
Information-processing approach, to visual cortex, 505–533
Information storage and retrieval systems, 480
Infragranular layers, 202
Inhibition, 108, 130, 141
Inhibitory amino acids, 360–362
Inhibitory interneurons, 225–226, 228–230
Input columns, 221–223
Interhemispheric transfer, 415–440

Interneuron
  classes, 228–230
  GABAergic, 360–361
  horizontal, 223–228
  inhibitory, 225–226, 228–230
  intermediate, 221
  receptive-field tuning, 404
  thalamic pathways, 205, 219
  vertical, 219–221
Interocular recognition, 426–435
Intracellular recording and marking techniques, 166
Intracortical connections, in cat visual cortex, 163–191
Intrinsic circuitry, 199–235
Invertebrates, 481
Ipsilateral fibers, 212
Isofunctional nonisomorphic groups, 545

Kitten, normal and dark-reared, 493

Laminar distribution
  CCK, 336
  corticocortical fibers, 207
  monoamines, 363
  pyramidal neuron, 112–113, 115
  receptive-field classes and, 164, 165–166
  stellate neuron, 112–113
  thalamic fibers, 203–207
  VIP neurons, 331
Laminar interactions, 223–228
Laminar organization, developmental events leading to, 7–28
Laminar positions, 8–16
Laminar specialization, 163–191
Lamination, cortical, 201–203
Lateral constraints, 16
Lateral geniculate nucleus (LGN)
  axonal relays, 112, 117–118
  cat, 420
  laminar distribution in, 164, 183, 184
  mapping, 168–169
  model, 515–516
  and pattern recognition, 417–418
  and synaptic modification, 495
Layers I–VI
  development, 22–25
  geniculocortical pathway, 299
Layers II and III
  intracortical pathways, 180, 183
  receptive fields, 171–174

Layer III, thalamic terminals, 203–205
Layer IV
 computer model, 513–515
 in intracortical pathway, 180, 183–184
 monocular deprivation effects on, 36–40
 normal development, 31–36
 ocular-dominance columns and, 29–30, 31
 plasticity, 43
 receptive fields, 169–171
 stellate cells, 154, 157–160
 thalamic terminals, 154, 203–205
Layer V, 174–177, 180, 183–184, 329
Layer VI, 177–181
Learning
 active and passive, 489–492
 tuning and, 496–497
Lemniscal fibers, 214
Lesion studies, 416–419, 423. *See also* Ablation
 cat visual cortex, 419–435
 and reentry, 548
Lid suture, 33–40
Limbic cortex, 73
Liminal sensation, and ERPs, 444–447
Linearity, and distributed systems, 488
LM-Sg complex, 308–309
Local circuit neuron. *See* Interneuron
Localization, assumptions, 535
Local storage, 481
Locus coeruleus, 348, 353, 364, 459–460
Logan's theorem, 509–510, 529–531
Logic, 483, 486–488
Low-pass filter, 508
LP-pulvinar complex, 288–293

Macaca nemestrina, 107
Macaque monkey
 intrinsic organization of visual cortex of, 105–124
 laminar distribution in, 116–117
 lateral dendritic spread in, 114
 postnatal development and plasticity of ocular-dominance columns in, 29–45
 somatosensory representation in, 239
Magnification factor (MF), 396–397, 399, 403, 515

Magnocellular axonal relays, 117–118
Magnocellular geniculate afferents, 39–40, 42–43
Mammals, single-tectum ablations, 53–54
Man
 computer and brain compared, 549
 ERPs in, and cognitive processing, 441–473
 synaptic contacts in, 126–127
 visual areas in, 397–399, 406–407
Manipulation, role of motor cortex in, 264
Mapping
 cortical, 256–257
 group selection and, 539–541
 and multiple representation, 241–248
 topological, 395
Match seeker, 551, 553–554
Mathematical tools and definitions, 517–518
Medial interlaminar nucleus, 299
Medial thalamus, 378–379
Median nerve, effect of cutting on cortical map, 256–257
Mediodorsal nucleus (MD), 70–71
Membrane differentiation, 130–141
Memory
 distributed vs. local, 480–481
 and group selection theory, 550
 machine vs. animal, 483
Mesencephalic reticular formation (MRF), 459, 460–462
Microelectrode multiunit mapping, 240–246
Microorganization, areas 3b and 1, 252–255
Minicolumn, cortical plate, 16. *See also* Columnar organization
Modeling, cortical function, 475–563
Modular organization, areas 3b and 1, 252–255. *See also* Columnar organization
Modular specificity, and cognitive function, 375–393
Modulation, 265–270, 276–278, 365. *See also* Neuromodulation
Modules, assumptions, 535. *See also* Columns
Monkey. *See also* specific species
 callosal columns, 207–209, 210
 callosal fibers, 80

Monkey (cont.)
  caudate nucleus, 88
  cortical degenerating terminals, 144
  corticofugal connections, 301–302
  inferotemporal cortex, 287
  interhemispheric transfer, 428
  motor cortex, 274–278
  ocular-dominance columns, post-
    natal development and plasticity
    of, 29–45
  PTNs, 265–270
  reactive states, 387–390
  sensory-motor cortex, 227
  somatosensory cortex, 214
  somatosensory representation, 239
  visual areas, 396–399
Monoamine, 130–131. *See also* specific types
  cortical afferents, 362–363
  neurotransmitters, 348–349, 362–364
  neurotransmodulators, 347–357
  receptor mechanisms, 363–364
Monocular deprivation, 30–45, 425
Motoneuron loop, alpha, 270
Motor control, 265
Motor cortex
  afferent feedback pathways, 270–273
  correlation and, 544
  degenerating terminals, 144
  functional studies, 263–283
  modulation, 265–270, 276–278
  reactive states, 387
  role of cerebellum in discharge of,
    280–281
  role in speech and manipulation, 264
Motor ERPs, 443
Motor programs, 278–281
Motor set, 276–278, 387
Mouse
  primary somatosensory cortex, 156,
    158
  sensorimotor cortex, 339
  visual areas, 396
Movement
  brain cell activity during, 265–281
  columnar arrangement for, 405
Moving patterns, sampling theorem,
  525–527
Multiple representation, 270–271,
  406–407, 409
  areas 3b and 1, 241–244. *See also*
    Representation
  in distributed degenerate systems,
    543

in extrageniculate thalamus, 288–293
  hypothesis, 238–248
  mapping evidence for, 241–248
  parallel and congruent, 249–251
  as somatotopic composites, 248–249
  in visual association cortex, 286–288
Muscarinic effects, and ERPs, 459–460

Na⁺-K⁺ ATPase, 350, 351
Neocortex
  afferent inputs, 337–338
  axonal connections, 285–286
  developmental events leading to
    laminar and areal organization of,
    7–28
  development, plasticity, and evolu-
    tion, of, 1–98
  evolutionary modifications of, 339–
    341
  patterns of access to, 312
  subdivisions, 71
  synaptogenesis in, 21–25
Neostriatum, 82–86
Nerve regeneration, and column size,
  253–256
Network modification, 489
Neural basis, of ERP components,
  458–462
Neural coding, assumptions, 535–536
Neurogenesis, 9–11
Neurological disorders, SEP approach
  to, 444
Neuromodulation. *See also* Neurotransmodulation
  in association cortex, 456
  ERPs and, 460
  glial cells and, 460
  MRF and, 460–462
Neuron. *See also* types of neurons
  internal communication, 489–490
  morphology, area 17, 105–109
  smooth and spiny, 109–116
Neuronal
  activity, neurotransmodulatory con-
    trol, 347–357
  and group selection, 537
  migration, 11–21
  modification, 494–496
  organization, electron-microscopic
    analysis, 125–152
  pathways, tracing, 22
Neurospecificity, and synaptogenesis, 61
Neurosurgery, fetal, 22

Neurotransmission
  candidates, 325–345
  and cortical circuitry, integration,
    359–370
  and peptide modulation, 364–366
Neurotransmodulation, 347–357
Noiseless patterns, 498
N140, 452, 453–458
Nonretinotopic representations,
  405–406
Noradrenergic pathways, 459–460
Norepinephrine
  adenosine and GABA and, 352–353
  circuitry constraints, 362–363
  distribution, 338
  inhibition by, 340–350
  modulation by cyclic AMP, 351, 352
  as neurotransmodulator, 353
  receptor mechanisms, 363–364
  role in cortical plasticity, 43
  role in reactive states, 389–390
Nucleus interlaminaris medialis
    (NIM), 420
Nucleus lateralis posterior pulvinar
    complex. See LP-pulvinar complex

Occipital cortex, 387
Ocular-dominance columns, 73. See
    also Banding; Visual cortex
  development of, 22–24
  induced, 47–67
  monkey, 29–45
  overlap, 215–219
  prenatal development and plasticity
    of, 22–24
  postnatal development and plasticity
    of, 29–45
  width, 114
  Y afferents, 168–169
Ontogenetic columns, 16–21
Opacity, postsynaptic, 129, 130
Open-loop control, 273–276, 278–280
Opponent color coding, 403
Optical-auditory system model, 488
Optical signals, 488
Optimal filter, 510–513
Organization
  cerebral cortex, 535
  cytoarchitectonic, 9–12, 105–124
  hierarchical, 153, 156–157, 272,
    300–301
  neocortex, 7–28
  somatosensory cortex, 237–261

Orientation columns, 404–405, 499–
    500. See also Columnar organiza-
    tion
Orientation specificity, 163, 403, 493
Orienting reflex, 377, 461
Output columns, as input columns,
    221–223
Owl monkey, 241–248, 396, 398
2-Oxyglucose method, 77

Parallel representations, 249–251
Parietal cortex, 406, 540
  and ERP components, 455
  organization, 248–255
  unit responses, 386–387
Parvocellular afferents, 39–40, 42–43,
    117
Passive modification, 490–492, 495
Patterned information, 494
Pattern recognition, 417–435
Peptide modulation, 364–366
Peptides. See types of peptides
Perception, 539
Perceptual models, 409
Perforant pathway, 329, 330
Petit mal EEG, 377–378
Phosphodiesterase, 350
Plasticity
  of callosal connections, 81–82
  and evolution of neocortex, 1–98
  of ocular-dominance columns, 29–45
  primate frontal association cortex,
    69–97
  prefrontocaudate projection, 86–89
  and segregation, 43
  and visual experience, 492
Positional accuracy, 506–507
Postnatal development, and plasticity
    of ocular-dominance columns,
    29–45
Postsynaptic opacity, 129, 130
Precentral gyrus, 265
Prefrontal cortex, 70–72, 461. See also
    Frontal cortex
Prefrontal resection, 86–89
Prefrontocaudate projection, 86–89
Prenatal development, and plasticity
    of ocular-dominance columns,
    22–24
Preparatory set, 276–278
Preprogrammed movement, 276–281
Prestriate cortex, 406, 408
Presylvian crown, 305–306

Pretectorecipient zone, 288–290, 293, 304–306
Primary reportoires, 537, 538
Primary somatosensory cortex (SI), 156, 257–258, 270–272, 540. *See also* Somatosensory cortex
Primary visual cortex, 164–166, 418–419. *See also* Visual cortex
Primate
  cortical processing, 207, 313
  development and plasticity in frontal association cortex of, 69–97
  intermediate interneuron in cortex of, 221
  laminar organization in, 203
  neocortex, 7–28
  somatosensory cortex, 237–261
  synaptic contacts in, 126
  visual cortex, 105–124, 211, 396–399
Principal sulcus, 75–77
Processing units, cortical, 251–252
Proliferative zones, 8, 16–21
Psychophysical experiments, 527–531
P300, 447–452, 453, 456, 458–459
  and neuromodulation, 461–462
PTN. *See* Pyramidal tract neuron
PTW loop, 270
Putamen, 85
Pyramidal neuron
  apical dendrites, 113, 115, 447
  axon collaterals, 226–228
  ERP components, 447
  as efferent cell, 201–202
  as excitatory, 138
  laminar distribution, 113–114, 155, 173, 176, 179, 329
  Macaca nemestrina, 107
  receptive fields and, 173, 185
  synaptic contacts, 132, 134–137
  terminations, 145, 205–207
  types, 109–112
Pyramidal tract neuron (PTN)
  adenine nucleotides and, 353
  during movement, 274–278
  norepinephrine and, 348
  sensory feedback and, 266–270
  servo control and, 278–280
Pyriform cortex, 25

Rabbit, 126
Rana pipiens, 48–61
Rapidly adapting inputs, 254
Rat cortex
  CCK in, 334

GAD in, 327
  laminar organization of, 203
  nonspiny bipolars in, 333
  peptides of, 336
  synaptic contacts, 126, 127, 136
  terminations, 210, 212
  VIP in, 331–334, 335
  visual, 131, 226, 396
Reactive states, 386–390, 449–451
Readiness, 276–278
Recall, in distributed memory model, 484–485
Receptive fields
  and ablation, 418–419
  characterization of, 165–167
  construction of, 180–186
  cortical columns and, 252–253
  cytoarchitectonic, 246–248
  hierarchical sequence, 153, 156–157
  laminar distribution, 164, 165–166
  multiple representation and, 243–244
  pattern discrimination and, 426
  size, 251–252, 540
  of superior colliculus, 434
  visual areas, 403–405
Receptor mechanisms, 363–364
  α-Receptors, 350
  β-Receptors, 350
Recognition, in distributed memory model, 484–485, 487
Recognizer (R) groups, 540, 541
Recognizer-of-recognizer groups. *See* R-of-r groups
Reentry, 543–545, 547–548
Relay nucleus, 312
Reportoire generator, 551–559
Representation, 492. *See also* Multiple representation
  group selection and, 539–541
Retina, 395–397, 403, 404
  model, 508–510
Retinotectal system, 48–54, 60–61
Retrograde axonal transport, 201–202
Retrosplenial cortex, 74
Reverse lid suture, 36–40
R groups, 540, 541
Rhesus monkey
  neocortex, 7–28
  prefrontal cortex, 83–87
  retrosplenial cortex, 74
  visual areas, 396
Rodents, 205
R-of-r groups, 541–544, 547, 560

Sampling theorem, 508–509, 518–525
Scalp-recorder ERPs, 441–473
Secondary reportoire, 538
Segregation, 25, 86
  in frog tectal cortex, 47–61
  visual, 31–43
Selective attention, 447–452, 456
Selective recognition model, 550–560
Sensory cortex, 73, 207–210, 265–266, 452–458
Sensory deprivation, and reentry, 548
Serial reconstruction, 157–160
Serotonin, 338, 348–349, 389–390
Servo control, 265–266, 269, 278–280
SI. *See* Primary somatosensory cortex
Siamese cats, 427
Simple cells, 165, 183–184, 361, 531
Simple memory model, 489
Single-unit studies, 240, 254, 266–270
  pattern recognition, 417–418
  reactive states and, 386–390
Sleep, 383
Slowly adapting inputs, 254
Slow potential shifts (SPS), 459–460
Somatosensory cortex, 144, 211–212.
    See also Primary somatosensory
    cortex
Somatosensory evoked potentials
    (SEPs), 444, 445–447
Somatostatin, 336, 365
Spatial-frequency-tuned channels, 531
Spatial periodicity, 405
Special complex cells, 165, 174–177
Specificity loss, 497–501
Speech, 264
Spider web cell, 228
Split-chiasm cats, 428–431
Squirrel monkey, 546
Standard complex cells, 165, 174–177
State-dependent reactions, 375–393
Stellate neurons, 154, 185
  nonspiny bipolars, 326, 328, 331, 336
  smooth, 109–112, 138–139, 141–145, 172
  spiny, 112–120, 132–138, 157–160, 170, 172
Stereoblindness, 434–435
Stereopsis, 507
Stereoscopic depth perception, 406
Stimulus generator, 551
Striate cortex
  connections, 301–304

lesions, and visual field defects, 396–397
  laminar distribution, 396, 513–515
  number of cells in, 515
Striate recipient cortex, 290, 293, 296–304
Structure-function studies, 70
Subcortical pathways, 280–281, 311
Subjective sensation, 444–447
Substance P, 338, 365
Substantia nigra, 348
Superior colliculus
  binocularity and, 427
  cortical pathways, 178, 303
  distributed mappings, 481
  and pattern discrimination, 431, 433, 434
Superior temporal sulcus (STS), 112
Supragranular layers, 202
Suprasylvian lesions, 423
Surface slow waves, 377–378, 385–386
Surface-unit mapping, 240–241
Symmetrical membrane differentia-
    tion, 130–141
Synapses, temporary, 25
Synaptic contact, 106–108, 136, 172
  formation, 21–25
  ideal, 483
  number in cortex, 125–127
Synaptic control, 456
Synaptic density, 126
Synaptic elimination, 537
Synaptic membrane differentiation, 130–141
Synaptic modification, 536, 545
  in distributed systems, 481, 494–496
  evidence for, 547
  passive, 490–492
  two-point, 489, 490
  synaptic potential, 447
Synaptic relations, thalamocortical, 153–161
Synaptic types, 127–141
Synaptogenesis, 21–25, 61

Task-related ERPs, 449
Taurine, 361
Tectal cortex, induced ocular-
    dominance columns in, 47–67
Tectorecipient zone, 288–290, 293, 304–306
Temporal lobe, 405–407
Terminal fields, diffused and pat-
    terned, 91

Thalamic fibers, 156–157, 160, 210–219, 221
  callosal, 210–211, 213
  laminar terminations, 203–207
  stimulation, 339–341
Thalamic bypass, 311, 314
Thalamocortical fibers, 21–25, 82, 142–143
  circuitry, 310–314
  to extrastriate cortex, 293–296
  to motor cortex, 273, 280–281
  to prefrontal cortex, 72
  to somatosensory cortex, 270–272
  synaptic relations, 153–161
  terminal sites, 141–145
Thalamus, 280–281, 378–379. *See also* Geniculate family; Lateral geniculate nucleus; LP-pulvinar system
Theophylline, 352
Thin-section reconstruction, 157–160
Three-eyed frog, 48–61
Threshold passive modification, 495
Tight coupling, 206
Topological maps, 395
Transcortical pathways, 269, 285–319
Transthalamic pathways, 285–319
Tuning, 496–501
Turtle cortex, 131, 142
Two-dimensional distribution, 509–510, 530–531
Type 1 and 2 synapses, 106–108, 112, 127, 128

Vasoactive intestinal peptide. *See* VIP
Ventrobasal complex, 271
Vertical interactions, 219–221, 417, 447. *See also* Columnar organization
VIP, 329–335, 339–341, 364–365
Visual association cortex, 285–319
Visual cortex, 9–11, 144, 166–167, 492–496. *See also* Ocular-dominance columns
  areas, 395–413
  cat, 163–191
  connections, 22–25
  distributed memory and, 479–503
  information-processing approach, 505–533
  lesion studies, 418–419
  organization, 105–124, 296–304
  and pattern recognition, 417–435

Visual deprivation. *See* Monocular deprivation
Visual evoked potentials (VEPs), 443
Visual experience, 493–494
Visual learning, 405–406, 415–440
Visual pursuit tracking paradigm, 266–270
Visual system, theoretical model, 508–513
Voluntary movements, 265–270
V1, 396–401, 406
V2, 397–403, 406

Waiting compartment, 22, 24–25, 90
Warning, and selective attention, 450, 458–459
Wiring diagram, cortex, 182

X cells, 167–169, 180, 183, 513

Y cells, 167–169, 180, 183, 513

Zero-crossing theorem, 509–510, 512–513